EPIDEMIOLOGY OF ARTERIAL BLOOD PRESSURE

DEVELOPMENTS IN CARDIOVASCULAR MEDICINE

VOLUME 8

1. C.T. Lancée, *Echocardiology,* 1979. ISBN 90-247-2209-8.
2. J. Baan, A.C. Arntzenius, E.L. Yellin, *Cardiac Dynamics.* 1980. ISBN 90-247-2212-8.
3. H.J.Th. Thalen, C.C. Meere, *Fundamentals of Cardiac Pacing.* 1979. ISBN 90-247-2245-4.
4. H.E. Kulbertus, H.J.J. Wellens, *Sudden Death.* 1980. ISBN 90-247-2290-X.
5. L.S. Dreifus, A.N. Brest, *Clinical Applications of Cardiovascular Drugs.* 1980. ISBN 90-247-2295-0 (hardcover); ISBN 90-247-2369-8 (paperback).
6. M.P. Spencer, J.M. Reid, *Cerebrovascular Evaluation with Doppler Ultrasound.* 1980. ISBN 90-247-2384-1.
7. D.P. Zipes, J.C. Bailey, V. Elharrar, *The Slow Inward Current and Cardiac Arrhythmias.* 1980. ISBN 90-247-2380-9.
9. F.J.Th. Wackers, *Thallium-201 and Technetium-99m-Phyrophosphate Myocardial Imaging in the Coronary Care Unit.* 1980. ISBN 90-247-2396-5.

series ISBN 90-247-2336-1

EPIDEMIOLOGY OF ARTERIAL BLOOD PRESSURE

edited by

H. KESTELOOT

Department of Cardiology
St.-Rafaël University Hospital
Leuven, Belgium

and

J.V. JOOSSENS

Department of Epidemiology
St.-Rafaël University Hospital
Leuven, Belgium

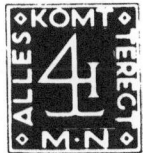

1980

MARTINUS NIJHOFF PUBLISHERS
THE HAGUE / BOSTON / LONDON

Distributors:

for the United States and Canada

Kluwer Boston, Inc.
190 Old Derby Street
Hingham, MA 02043
USA

for all other countries

Kluwer Academic Publishers Group
Distribution Center
P.O. Box 322
3300 AH Dordrecht
The Netherlands

Library of Congress Cataloging in Publication Data   CIP

Main entry under title:

Epidemiology of arterial blood pressure

    (Developments in cardiovascular medicine; v. 8)
    1. Hypertension. 2. Hypertension – Statistics.
    3. Blood pressure – Statistics. 4. Epidemiology.
    I. Kesteloot, H. II. Joossens, J. V. III. Series.
    [DNLM: 1. Blood pressure determination.
    2. Epidemiologic methods. WI DE997VME v. 8 / WG106 E64]
    RC685.H8E59   616.1'32   80–36870

ISBN-13: 978-94-009-8895-8   e-ISBN-13: 978-94-009-8893-4
DOI: 10.1007/978-94-009-8893-4

PREFACE

Hypertension is a major health problem and contrary to ischemic heart disease, which occurs only in Western countries, its distribution is almost universal. It is this universality that has prompted us to gather, in this book, data on arterial blood pressure obtained in different parts of the world. Moreover, cerebrovascular mortality, which is the commonest cause of death from hypertension, is decreasing in most Western countries and in Japan, and the reasons for this are still far from clear.

A major problem in comparing blood pressure values from different centers is the standardization of the measurement. Complete standardization will never be achieved if one takes into account the numerous factors that may influence blood pressure in epidemiological studies. Whether blood pressures are measured by doctors or by technicians, are recorded at home, in the working place or in a hospital, in sitting, standing or supine position, and whether a blood sample is taken during the same examination—all of these factors can influence blood pressure measurement. But meals, time of day (blood pressure being higher in the evening), heart rate, cuff size, stethoscope used, digit preference, month of year, temperature, etc., can equally influence the measurement.

Home reading of arterial blood pressure at standardized times is probably the best answer to all of these problems and has been used with gratifying results in a comparative study between Belgium and Korea.

The ratio of systolic to diastolic pressure appears to be an indicator of whether or not blood pressure has been recorded in basal conditions. The ratio is less than 1.55 when home reading of blood pressure is used, and it is substantially higher when casual readings of blood pressure are recorded. Higher values are obtained in subjects below age 20 and above age 60, and this can be due to sympathic influences in younger subjects and to hardening of the arteries in older subjects.

In our opinion, it is dissatisfactory to draw conclusions from blood pressure data obtained in different population groups when the age-specific systolic to diastolic ratio is markedly different. Optimally this ratio should be below 1.6.

Although theoretically most of the problems mentioned above can be standardized, the problem remains that anthropometric differences between populations may also influence the measurement of blood pressure. When comparing Koreans with Belgians, and with Japanese living in Japan and in California, differences in height and weight should be taken into account. The only way out of this problem appears to be to calculate the blood pressure of a subject, e.g., age 40, height 170 cm, weight 67 kg, by using the multiple regression equation obtained between blood pressure and age, height, and weight in each population separately. Height and weight must be chosen in such a way that a minimum of extrapolation is necessary.

An even more exact way is to use covariance analysis, introducing a group dummy variable, and the interaction variables obtained from combining the group factor with the other independent variables.

The problem of the importance of salt intake as a determinant of the blood pressure in a population remains an intricate one. A large amount of circumstantial evidence points to sodium as the major factor positively influencing blood pressure in a population. Recently, evidence has been gathered pointing to a decreasing effect of potassium on blood pressure levels. Whether potassium acts as an independent factor, or through the sodium to potassium ratio, remains to be established. Measuring sodium and potassium intake, however, remains a tedious task. The recall method for estimating salt intake is not very accurate, and taking samples of all food consumed is a time-consuming and expensive procedure.

In countries with a temperate climate, collection of 24-h urine is theoretically the easiest way to measure 24-h sodium and potassium intake. Moreover, all excreted electrolytes have to pass through the kidney, and this quantity could be more important than the total intake. However, the accurate collection of 24-h urine has its own problems. Collection seems to be more accurate in population groups above age 30, probably due to better motivation. Collection is more difficult in women than in men; this problem could be overcome by using plastic bags that can easily be closed after the removal of air. For certain purposes, the urine should be slightly acidified, and thymol can be used to avoid unpleasant odors. For volunteers, all of these problems of accurately collecting the 24-h urine can be solved, but they are prohibitive if one wants to obtain a random sample of the population.

Measuring the 24-h creatinine excretion is probably the best way to estimate the correction of the 24-h urine collection. Due to variations in creatinine excretion, the method is probably more valuable for comparing population groups than as an estimate of the correctness of the collection in the individual. At least for Western countries, the correction of urinary excretion values to a urinary creatinine excretion value of 1.77 g seems recommendable, if one wants to compare the values obtained in different studies. This has as a prerequisite that the method for the measurement of creatinine should be standardized. The value of 1.77 g is an arbitrary one, but was obtained in a rather large Belgian study performed in 1968–1969. Whether this method could also be employed to correct for body mass or muscular weight differences between Western and Oriental populations remains to be established.

Cross-sectional studies of the relationship between sodium intake and blood pressure have resulted in conflicting findings, particularly in Western countries where actually a negative relationship between sodium intake and blood pressure has been obtained in several studies.

Since more and more hypertensive people believe that they should reduce salt intake, consciously or unconsciously, it could be impossible in Western populations to obtain an unbiased sample in order to study the problem. Moreover, very little data is available on the longitudinal evolution of sodium intake by the population. Evidence from Japan and from Belgium points to a reduction in salt intake that could be due more to the introduction of refrigerators than to medical education. The acceleration of the decrease in cerebrovascular mortality occurring during the last 6–8 years is probably due to an effective treatment of the disease by antihypertensive drugs. The lack of data on the longitudinal evolution of salt intake in the population is only matched by a similar lack of data on the longitudinal evolution of blood pressure in the population. The increasing interest in the study of blood pressures in children is heartily welcome because influences acting at a young age may well play an important role in the occurrence of high blood pressure at a later age. Migrant studies are also of high value since they enable the differentiation between genetic factors and environmental determinants of blood pressure. Nobody will deny the importance of genetic factors, but their influence is probably only minor in population groups characterized by a low salt intake.

Every researcher working in the field of epidemiology knows the important difficulties that have to be surmounted in order to organize a successful study. Moreover, such studies can be frustrating since sometimes the final results become available only after many years of hard work, and because the results are not readily accepted by the medical community. Statistical support and background are also of the highest importance.

For all these reasons, we wish to thank the many epidemiologists who have contributed to the realization of this book. Although many problems remain to be solved and many contradictions are to be clarified, we hope that this book will be a source of scholastic thought both for researchers and clinicians.

viii

Acknowledgment. The editors wish to thank Miss Roos Struyven for her invaluable organizational and secretarial help, which has greatly facilitated the editing of this book.

H. KESTELOOT, M.D.
J.V. JOOSSENS, M.D.

CONTRIBUTORS

Arntzenius, Alexander C., M.D., Department of Cardiology, Leiden University, Rijnsburgerweg 10, 2333 AA Leiden, The Netherlands

Berenson, Gerald S., M.D., Professor of Medicine, Head for Section of Cardiology, Department of Medicine, Director Specialized Center of Research – Arteriosclerosis, Louisiana State University Medical Center, 1542 Tulane Avenue, New Orleans, LA 70112, USA

Berglund, Göran L., M.D., Assistant Professor, University of Göteborg, Department of Medicine I, Sahlgren's Hospital, S-413 45 Göteborg, Sweden

Bloch, Chantal M.A., Technicienne, Equipe de Recherche Cardiologie, INSERM (Institut National de la Santé et de la Recherche Médicale), 15 Rue de l'Ecole de Médecine, F-75006 Paris, France

Bonjer, Frederik H., M.D., Department of Cardiology, Leiden University, Rijnsburgerweg 10, 2333 AA Leiden, The Netherlands

Böthig, Ingrid, M.D., Working Group of Epidemiology, Central Institute of Cardiovascular Regulation Research, Academy of Sciences of the GDR, Wiltbergstr. 50, DDR-1115 Berlin, German Democratic Republic

Böthig, Siegfried, Docent Dr.sc.med., First Medical Clinic, County Hospital 'Heinrich Braun', Karl-Keil-Str. 35, DDR-9500 Zwickau, German Democratic Republic

Brems-Heyns, Els, Lic. Math., previously working in the Division of Epidemiology, School of Public Health, Catholic University of Leuven, Capucijnenvoer 35, B-3000 Leuven, Belgium; present address: Middelweg 166, 3030 Heverlee, Belgium

Claes, Jozef H., Pharm., Central Clinical Laboratory, St.-Rafaël University Hospital, Capucijnenvoer 35, B-3000 Leuven, Belgium

Claessens, Jan, M.D., previously working in the Division of Cardiology, Department of Internal Medicine, Catholic University of Leuven, Capucijnenvoer 35, B-3000 Leuven, Belgium; present address: Bellevuedreef 42, B-2230 Schilde, Belgium

Costenoble, André, Pharm., Head of the Clinical Laboratory, Military Hospital, Kroonlaan 145, B-1050 Brussels, Belgium

Coussaert, Eddy J.A.P., Lic. Sc. Phys., University of Brussels, Faculty of Medicine and Pharmacy, Department of Scientific Data Processing, Rue Heger Bordet 7, B-1000 Brussels, Belgium

Demanet, Jean-Claude F.R., M.D., Ph.D., Professor of Medicine, University of Brussels, Department of Internal Medicine, Saint-Pierre Hospital, 322 Rue Haute, B-1000 Brussels, Belgium

de Pádua, Fernando, M.D., Ph.D., Chairman of Internal Medicine, Faculty of Medicine of the University of Lisbon, Centro de Estudos de Cardiologia Preventiva, Serviço de Medicina IV, Hospital Universitário de Santa Maria, Cadeiras de Terapêutica Médica e Higiene e Medicina Social, Instituto Nacional de Saúde, Lisboa; Hospital Universitario de Santa Maria, Faculdade de Medicina, Universidade de Lisboa, Hospital de Santa Maria, Av. Egas Moniz, 1699 Lisboa-Codex, Portugal

Elo, Jyrki, M.D., Research Investigator, Research Institute for Community Health of the University of Kuopio, Box 40, 70101 Kuopio 10, Finland

Fodor, J. George, M.D., Ph.D., Division of Community Medicine, Memorial University of Newfoundland, Health Sciences Centre, St. John's, Newfoundland A1B 3V6, Canada

Geboers, Jozef, Lic. Math., Division of Epidemiology, School of Public Health, Catholic University of Leuven, Capucijnenvoer 35, B-3000 Leuven, Belgium

Geizerová, Helena, M.D., Department of Medicine II, Institute for Clinical and Experimental Medicine, Vídeňská 800, 146 22 Praha 4, Czechoslovakia

Guillaneuf, Marie-Thérèse, M.D., Technicienne, Equipe de Recherche Cardiologie, INSERM (Institut National de la Santé et de la Recherche Médicale), 15 Rue de l'Ecole de Médecine, F-75006 Paris, France

Hatano, Shuichi, M.D., Department of Epidemiology, Tokyo Metropolitan Institute of Gerontology, 35-2 Sakaecho, Itabashi-ku, Tokyo 173, Japan

Hejl, Zdeněk, M.D., Department of Medicine II, Institute for Clinical and Experimental Medicine, Vídeňská 800, 146 22 Praha 4, Czechoslovakia

Hofman, Bert, M.D., Department of Epidemiology, Erasmus University, P.O. Box 1738, 3000 DR Rotterdam, The Netherlands

Huige, Marinus C., M.D., Department of Cardiology, St.-Joseph Hospital, 259 Aalsterweg, 5644 RC Eindhoven, The Netherlands

Hurych, Jiří, M.D., Department of Medicine II, Institute for Clinical and Experimental Medicine, Vídeňská 800, 146 22 Praha 4, Czechoslovakia

Joossens, Jozef V., M.D., Department of Epidemiology, School of Public Health, Catholic University of Leuven, Capucijnenvoer 35, B-3000 Leuven, Belgium

Kagan, Abraham, M.D., Honolulu Heart Study, National Heart, Lung and Blood Institute, 347 North Kuakini Street, Honolulu, HI 96817, USA

Kannel, William B., M.D., M.P.H., FACP, FACC, Department of Medicine, Chief of Section of Preventive Medicine and Epidemiology, Evans Research Foundation, Boston University School of Medicine, Room E-124, 80 East Concord Street, Boston, MA 02118, USA

Kato, Hiroo, M.D., Department of Epidemiology and Statistics, Radiation Effects Research Foundation, 5-2 Hijiyama Park, Hiroshima 730, Japan

Kesteloot, Hugo, M.D., Department of Cardiology, St.-Rafaël University Hospital, Capucijnenvoer 35, B-3000 Leuven, Belgium

Komachi, Yoshio, M.D., Department of Community Medicine, Institute of Community Medicine, Tsukuba University, 1-1-1 Tennodai Sakura-mura, Niihari-gun, Ibaragi-ken, 305 Japan

Kottke, Thomas E., M.D., M.P.H., Research Fellow, Laboratory of Physiology and Hygiene, University of Minnesota, 611 Beacon Street SE, Minneapolis, MN 55455, USA

Kozarević, Djordje, M.D., Ph.D., M.P.H., Institute of Chronic Diseases and Gerontology, Center for Hypertension, Slobodana Penezića, 11000 Beograd, Yugoslavia

Laaser, Ulrich, M.D., Medizinische Universitäts-Poliklinik, Köln, Josef-Stelzmann-Str. 9, D-5000 Köln 41, Federal Republic of Germany

Lee, Chan Sae, M.D., Department of Internal Medicine, Kyung Hee University, Hoikidong 1 Dongdae Mun-ku, 131 Seoul, Korea

Lellouch, Joseph, Directeur de Recherche, Unité de Recherche sur les Méthodes Statistiques et Epidemiologiques et leurs applications à l'Etude des Maladies, INSERM (Institut National de la Santé et de la Recherche Médicale), 16 bis, Avenue Paul Vaillant Couturier, F-94800 Villejuif, France

Lubin, Nancy K., B.A., Data Processor, Newton-Wellesley Hospital, 17 Ascenta Terrace, West Newton, MA 02165, USA

Marmot, Michael G., MB, BS, MPH, PhD, Department of Medical Statistics and Epidemiology, London School of Hygiene and Tropical Medicine, Keppel Street, London WC1E 7HT, England

Maus, Yvon J.M., M.D., Université de Liège, Institute of Medicine, Hôpital de Bavière, Boulevard de la Constitution 66, B-4020 Liège, Belgium

McGee, Daniel L., Ph.D., National Institutes of Health, Honolulu Heart Study, National Heart, Lung, and Blood Institute, 347 North Kuakini Street, Honolulu, HI 96817, USA

Nader, Karim, M.D., Director of Auxiliary Health Programs, Fars Province, Ministry of Health, Shiraz, Iran

Nissinen, Aulikki, M.D., N.T., Senior Investigator, Research Institute for Community Health of the University of Kuopio, Box 40, 70101 Kuopio 10, Finland

Oliver, William J., M.D., Department of Pediatrics, University of Michigan Medical Center, Box 66, F7814 Mott Children's Hospital, Ann Arbor, MI 48109, USA

Page, Jesse R., Research Assistant, Newton-Wellesley Hospital, Conant Road, Lincoln, MA 01773, USA

Page, Lot B., M.D., Professor of Medicine, Tufts University School of Medicine, Chief of Medicine, Newton-Wellesley Hospital, 2000 Washington Street, Newton Lower Falls, MA 02162, USA

Park, Byoung Chae, M.D., Ph.D., Department of Internal Medicine, Kyung Hee University Medical Center, Hoikidong 1 Dongdae Mun-ku, 131 Seoul, Korea

Pereira Miguel, José M., M.D., Centro de Estudos de Cardiologia Preventiva, Serviço de Medicina IV, Hospital Universitário de Santa Maria, Cadeiras de Terapêutica Médica e Higiene e Medicina Social, Instituto Nacional de Saúde, Lisboa; Hospital Universitário de Santa Maria, Faculdade de Medicina, Universidade de Lisboa, Hospital de Santa Maria, Av. Egas Moniz, 1699 Lisboa-Codex, Portugal

Pietinen, Pirjo I., Lic. Sc. (Nutrition), Department of Nutrition, University of Helsinki, SF-00710 Helsinki 71, Finland

Píša, Zbyněk, M.D., Prof., Chief, Cardiovascular Diseases, W.H.O., 1211 Geneva 27, Switzerland

Pistulková, Helena, M.D., Department of Medicine II, Institute for Clinical and Experimental Medicine, Vídeňská 800, 146 22 Praha 4, Czechoslovakia

Prior, Ian A.M., M.D. (NZ), FRCP, FRACP, Epidemiology Unit, Wellington Hospital, Private Bag, Wellington, New Zealand

Puska, Pekka, M.D., M.pol.Sc., Director, Epidemiological Research Unit of the National Public Health Laboratory, Mannerheimintie 166, 00280 Helsinki 28, Finland

Richard, Jacques L., M.D., Maître de Recherche, Equipe de Recherche Cardiologie, INSERM (Institut National de la Santé et de la Recherche Médicale), 15 Rue de l'Ecole de Médecine, F-75006 Paris, France

Rorive, Georges L.S.J., M.D., Ph.D., Université de Liège, Institute of Medicine, Hôpital de Bavière, Boulevard de la Constitution 66, B-4020 Liège, Belgium

Rusted, Ian E.L.H., M.D., F.R.C.P. (C), Faculty of Medicine, Memorial University of Newfoundland, Health Sciences Centre, St. John's, Newfoundland A1B 3V6, Canada

Samii, Kambise, M.D., University of Brussels, Department of Medicine, Saint-Pierre Hospital, 322 Rue Haute, B-1000 Brussels, Belgium

Sasaki, Naosuke, M.D., D.med.sc., Professor, Department of Hygiene, Hirosaki University School of Medicine, 5 Zaifu-cho, Hirosaki 036, Aomori Prefecture, Japan

Schütt, Alexander, Dipl.-Math., Institut für medizinische Dokumentation und Statistik der Universität Köln, Josef-Stelzmann-Str. 9, D-5000 Köln 41, Federal Republic of Germany

Shimamoto, Takashi, M.D., Department of Epidemiology and Mass Examination for Cardiovascular Diseases, The Center for Adult Diseases, 1-3-3 Nakamichi, Higashinari-ku, Osaka 537, Japan

Smets, Philippe, M.D., Ph.D., Chargé de Cours, Director of the Department of Scientific Data Processing, University of Brussels, Faculty of Medicine and Pharmacy, Rue Heger Bordet 7, B-1000 Brussels, Belgium

Stanhope, John M., M.B., B.S., D.T.M.&H., Epidemiology Unit, Wellington Hospital, Private Bag, Wellington, New Zealand

Svärdsudd, Kurt S., M.D., Assistant Professor, University of Göteborg, Department of Medicine, Östra Hospital, S-416 85 Göteborg, Sweden

Tuomilehto, Jaakko, M.D., M.pol.Sc., Principal Investigator, Epidemiological Research Unit of the National Public Health Laboratory, University of Kuopio, Box 40, 70101 Kuopio 10, Finland

Valkenburg, Hans A., M.D., Ph.D., Department of Epidemiology, Erasmus University, P.O. Box 1738, 3000 DR Rotterdam, The Netherlands

Vandevert, David, B.A., M.A., Research and Administrative Assistant, Department of Community Medicine, Shiraz University School of Medicine, Shiraz, Iran; present address: 1798 Lake Street, Salt Lake City, UT 84105, USA

Van Vollenhoven, Erik, M.Sc., Department of Cardiology, Leiden University, 10 Rijnsburgerweg, 2333 AA Leiden, The Netherlands

Voors, Antonie W., M.D., Dr.P.H., Professor of Public Health and Preventive Medicine, Department of P.H. and Preventive Medicine, Louisiana State University Medical Center, 1542 Tulane Avenue, New Orleans, LA 70112, USA

Vuylsteke-Wauters, Magda, M.Sc., Computer Center, Catholic University of Leuven, de Croylaan, B-3030 Heverlee, Belgium

Walker, W. Gordon, M.D., Professor of Medicine, Director, Renal Division, Department of Medicine, Johns Hopkins University School of Medicine; Director, Clinical Research Center, Johns Hopkins University School of Medicine and Johns Hopkins Hospital; Physician, Johns Hopkins Hospital; Physician, Good Samaritan Hospital; Director, Renal Division, Good Samaritan Hospital, Baltimore, MD 21205, USA

Webber, Larry S., Ph.D., Associate Professor of Biometry and Medicine, Departments of Biometry and Medicine, Louisiana State University Medical Center, 1542 Tulane Avenue, New Orleans, LA 70112, USA

Widimský, Jiří, M.D., Professor, Head of the Department of Medicine II, Institute for Clinical and Experimental Medicine, Vídeňská 800, 146 22 Praha 4, Czechoslovakia

Wilhelmsen, Lars W., M.D., Associate Professor, University of Göteborg; Head, Department of Medicine, Östra Hospital, S-416 85 Göteborg, Sweden

CONTENTS

PART ONE

METHODOLOGICAL STUDIES

1. MEASUREMENT OF BLOOD PRESSURE

A.C. ARNTZENIUS, F.H. BONJER, M.C. HUIGE, and E. VAN VOLLENHOVEN

1. HISTORICAL DEVELOPMENT

The historical development of blood pressure measurement has been reviewed extensively by various authors, but in this presentation we will mention the most important steps only [1–4].

1.1. Oscillometric method

The first attempts to measure man's blood pressure noninvasively were initiated in the last decades of the 19th century. In this period, values of blood pressure determined with the indirect method could not be compared sufficiently, accurately, or reliably with those obtained when using invasive techniques. This became feasible only when intraarterial blood pressure could be determined with sufficient accuracy.

The oscillometric method, as developed by Marey, was available for noninvasive measurement. By this technique, pressure in the cuff—which partly encircles the arm—is measured with a mercury manometer, and the oscillations are recorded while pressure in the cuff is gradually reduced. At the moment when the first oscillations appear, systolic pressure is determined from a scale. Diastolic pressure is thought to occur when oscillations show their largest amplitude. Since the maximum is reached only very gradually, diastolic pressure cannot be measured accurately by the oscillometric method.

1.2. Palpatory method

Riva-Rocci in Italy in 1896 introduced the palpatory method for indirect measurement of blood pressure [5]. He used a mercury manometer and a small air-filled rubber tube which was to be applied around the upper arm. The simple instrument really signified a considerable improvement on all indirect blood pressure measuring devices so far developed. Systolic pressure could now be measured easily and rapidly by palpation of the radial artery;

the oscillometric methods in comparison were rather clumsy and complicated.

1.3. Auscultatory method

Korotkoff in 1905 invented the auscultatory method. In his original publication in Russian he gave a detailed description of all auscultatory findings. His article, translated into English, was entitled: 'On the subject of methods of determining blood pressure' [6]. The sounds which can be observed with the use of a stethoscope when the pressure in the cuff is lowered are quite rightly named after him. Korotkoff utilized the original (rather small) Riva-Rocci cuff. In a relatively short period, three separate techniques for determination of blood pressure were thus developed: the oscillometric, the palpatory, and the auscultatory methods. Von Recklinghausen in 1901 did some experiments which contributed considerably to the further development of noninvasive measurement of blood pressure [7]. He emphasized the importance of the choice of a proper cuff and considered the cuff to be the most essential part of measuring equipment. A double-layered cuff 13 cm wide was his choice and he was able to show that the original cuff used by Riva-Rocci undoubtedly was too narrow. As a result of Von Recklinghausen's work, the cuff width of 13 cm was introduced and has since been used universally in measuring blood pressure.

In spite of the great progress in medical technology in the last decades, no essential changes have been made with respect to the instrumentation of noninvasive measurement of blood pressure. The stethoscope, the mercury manometer, and the cuff are used nearly everywhere, though occasionally a microphone or an ultrasonic transducer are used to detect systolic and diastolic end points [8]. No other clinical method has been used as long and as frequently as the 'classic' noninvasive method for measurement of blood pressure. The method itself has been the subject of study for a long period and, for instance, the auscultatory method has been compared with the oscillometric technique and with the palpatory method of blood pressure measurement. Many studies in which results of the noninvasive method have been compared with invasive determination of blood pressure have been published [9–11]. In one of them, Ragan and Bordley made an extensive investigation comparing both methods in 50 adult subjects [11]. It left no doubt that values of blood pressure obtained with noninvasive measurement could show large errors when compared with invasive determination, and this proved to be particularly the case when the occlusive cuff was applied to obese upper arms. The authors concluded that with the standard cuff, no reliable noninvasive measurement of blood pressure could be obtained for obese adults. They recommended further research in order to find the optimum ratio of cuff width and limb circumference. Thereafter, many experiments were performed in which the auscultatory method each time was compared with intraarterial determination using cuffs of different sizes; with moderate success only, as we shall see.

2. METHODOLOGY OF BLOOD PRESSURE MEASUREMENT

2.1. Direct versus indirect measurement

A distinction is to be made between direct and indirect blood pressure measurement. For the *direct* measurement, a cannula attached to a manometer (pressure gauge) is inserted into an artery. This method enables great freedom in choosing the artery in which the measurement is to be carried out and offers the possibility of continuous recording, but since the insertion of a needle or catheter is a prerequisite, the direct measurements can be carried out only on special indications, and only by physicians trained in arterial puncture.

Indirect measurement can be applied to extremities only, and the result will often deviate considerably from the actual pressure which exists in the arteries. In fact, what is determined by this technique is the external pressure in the cuff around the arm at which the arterial blood just commences to flow (systolic blood pressure) or is completely restored (diastolic blood pressure). For indirectly measured values to be mutually comparable and so as to enhance reproducibility, certain specific standardized procedures are recommended.

2.2. Physical principles of auscultatory phenomena of blood pressure

To study this, Freis and Sappington [12] used blood pressure cuffs with an inflatable bladder which measured 23×12.5 cm, and a nylon covering of 58×14 cm. A catheter was inserted in the brachial artery, which could be occluded by means of a cuff, thus enabling comparison of cuff pressure with intraarterial pressure. At the same time, Korotkoff sounds were recorded by using a microphone during the blood pressure measurement. Freis and Sappington concluded from their experiments that the cuff pressure was incompletely transmitted to the compressed arterial segment, resulting in a slightly higher cuff pressure at 'muffling' than in the artery. The experiment showed that systolically there is good agreement between cuff pressure at appearance of the first Korotkoff sound and systolic pressure as measured with the cuff. Possibly this is due to a delay in penetration of pressure waves in the distal segment of the artery, which compensates for the loss of pressure due to incomplete transmission of the cuff to the artery. McCutcheon and Rushmer [13] concluded from angiographic experiments that when the cuff pressure is lowered to arterial pressure, the pulsating fluid column under the cuff approaches the center of the cuff with each beat. Just below systolic pressure, a brief, tiny jet could be seen distal to the constricted region under the center of the cuff. These experiments therefore agree with those of Freis and Sappington [12]. In yet a third series of experiments, with an ultrasonic transcutaneous transducer, results showed that the first appearance of Korotkoff sounds coincided with the ultrasonic signal, which indicates movement of the arterial wall due to the sudden opening of the occluded segment of the artery [8, 13–15]. At that instant, cuff pressure closely approximates systolic blood pressure. It is important to note that Alexander et al. [14] showed that the accuracy of the measurement of systolic blood pressure is influenced by the choice of the width of the blood pressure cuff. They advocated the use of a cuff which is larger than 1.2 times the diameter of the arm, and a bladder that completely encircles the arm.

Noninvasive blood pressure to be measured in subjects with obese upper arms creates a problem in itself. There appears to be great difference in fat upper arms when cuff measurements are compared with intravasal blood pressure determination [16]. Blood pressures of subjects with muscular arms do not show such large differences. The explanation of this phenomenon is thought to lie in the compressible properties of fat arms, causing incomplete transmission of cuff pressure to the occluded arterial segment. In conclusion, we can state that the first Korotkoff sound is caused by the sudden distension of the arterial wall [13, 14]. The Korotkoff sounds can be heard when the pressure is decreasing, and are probably of mixed origin (vibration of the wall and sound caused by moving vortices). The Korotkoff sounds get muffled when the intensity of their high-frequency components is diminished [13, 17, 18].

2.3. Instrumentation

2.3.1. The cuff. Note: perhaps it would be better to speak of the bag or bladder, since the word cuff would include the nylon covering, to which the sizes mentioned here have no bearing.

Three standardization committees of the American Heart Association (AHA) in 1939, 1951, and 1967 successively have given recommendations on auscultatory measurement of blood pressure, including specifications for the width and length of the cuff [19–21]. In *1939* the cuff size to be used was specified as 13×12 cm, but in *1951* the committee recommended that the width of the bag be adapted to the diameter of the upper arm, and postulated that the width of the bag should be 20% larger than the diameter of the upper arm. This is not very practical advice since it is not easy to measure the diameter of the upper arm. In 1967 the recommendation reads as follows:

The inflatable bag must be the correct width for the diameter of the patient's arm; for if it is too narrow, the blood pressure reading will be erroneously high, if it is too wide, the reading may be erroneously low. The inflatable bag should be 20% wider than the diameter of the limb on which it is to be used. For the average adult, a bag of 12 to 14 cm wide has been found to be satisfactory. Smaller cuffs are available for patients with small arms, as are larger (18 to 20 cm) ones for measurement for obese persons or in the thigh. The diameter of the arm is the factor which determines whether 'children cuff' or 'adult cuff' is used, not the age of the patient.

In *1967* the committee for standardization recommended that the width of the air chamber be 1.2 times the diameter of the arm, which is assuming the arm is of cylindrical shape, which can also be formulated as follows: width of the bag to be 40% of the circumference of the arm. According to this rule, an adult with an arm circumference of 30 cm would need a bag of 12 cm width, for which the standard-sized bag is just acceptable. The phrase 'as are larger (18 to 20 cm) ones for measurement in obese persons or in the thigh' seems to be incorrect. A bag of 20 cm width has been used in one study only, i.e., by Ragan and Bordley [11], and it certainly did not prove to be a good solution. Such a very wide bag can possibly be used for the upper leg, but is not appropriate for the shape of the upper arm. The type of cuff to be used for obese upper arms has not been sufficiently discussed in the AHA reports.

The chairman of the committee of standardization (Bordley) concluded in *1951:* 'A length of bag sufficient to half-encircle a limb is adequate, provided care is taken by the operator to place it on the side of the compressed artery. However, some authorities believe that any rule of misapplication should be obviated by use of a bag that nearly or completely encircles the limb.' In *1967* the committee of standardization made a recommendation with respect to the length of the bag: 'The inflatable bag should be long enough to go halfway around the limb if care is taken to put it directly over the compressible artery. A bag 30 cm in length which nearly (or completely) encircles the limb obviates any risk of misapplication'. The committee thus prefers a bag which completely or nearly completely encircles the arm.

Most physicians, since the recommendation of the AHA committee for standardization in 1951, have used bags with dimensions of 23×12 cm. The World Health Organization (WHO) recommendations on the size of the bag differed clearly from those of the AHA: WHO recommended a bag of 14 cm width and with various lengths to be used so that the upper arm could be completely encircled [22]. It should be noted that space does not allow us to present here the particular problem which blood pressure measurement in children poses. We can therefore only refer to the many publications on this subject [23–27].

2.3.2. Systems for detecting systolic and diastolic end points. The matter of detection systems to be used to measure blood pressure noninvasively has been well documented by Geddes [2] and Greatorex [3, 4]. A stethoscope is commonly used to detect Korotkoff sounds. Instead of a stethoscope, Geddes and Moore [2] mounted a small piezoelectric crystal inside the bladder just beyond its center. When the transducer is positioned in this way, the Korotkoff sounds are louder than when placed at the antecubital fossa, where Korotkoff sounds are generally observed, and moreover it is better shielded from environmental noise. De Dobbeleer [28] used three cuffs; in one of these, an extra cuff in which a thermistor was mounted. The commercial version of his apparatus is the Godart Haemotonograph. Recently also other methods of detection have been used: impedance plethysmography [29] and ultrasonics [8, 14, 15, 29–32, 36]. The choice of good detection systems is very important for devices aimed at the automatic recording of blood pressure, a matter which is dealt with in various publications [3, 4, 33–37]. Six different types of sphygmomanometers and their characteristics are listed in Table 1.

2.3.3. The manometer. The mercury manometer is easily calibrated. The graduations on the glass tube should be checked before delivery. It is essential, in view of the great importance of blood pressure measurement to public health, that the instrument bear a national hallmark. With the cuff empty, the mercury level should stand at 0 mm. If it is higher, the reservoir contains too much mercury; and if it is lower, the reservoir contains too little mercury. When stopped after the mercury level has been rapidly inflated to 200 mmHg (with the cuff round a one-liter bottle), the mercury should not climb any further. If it does, the filter at the top of the tube is not sufficiently permeable. If the mercury column falls after the valve has been closed, there is a leak in the instrument. Too slow a fall with the valve open indicates a clogged dust filter in the valve. The mercury manometer is preferable to the membrane manometer, the use of which in general cannot be recommended because its reliability and durability have not received enough objective study. But as the use of the membrane manometer can now hardly be suppressed, there is a need for research into its reliability and durability. In view of the urgent need to eliminate shortcomings in measurement equipment, we believe that a system of periodic calibration should be introduced. The frequency of the calibration should depend on the nature of the instrument used, a limited reliability calling for more frequent calibration [43, 44].

2.4. Procedure and standardization of measurement [38–40]

1) Fasten the cuff snugly around the upper arm with its lower edge 2–3 cm above the flexure on the upper arm. Use self-adhesive type of wrapping. There should be no tight clothing on the upper arm.
2) The blood pressure values should be recorded to the nearest 2 mmHg.

Table 1. Six types of sphygmomanometers and their characteristics.

	Pressure in bag			Detection of systolic and diastolic end points		Measurement (of pressure)
	Inflation	Deflation	Measurement	Korotkoff sounds	Arterial wall flutter	
Conventional	Bulb assembly + valve	Needle valve (bleed)	Open column of mercury	Stethoscope	—	On moving column of mercury with visible scale.
London School of Hygiene Sphygmomanometer (LSHS)[41]	Compressed gas	Fixed rate of descending	Open column of mercury	Stethoscope	—	Column of mercury is halted when systolic or diastolic end points are reached. Scale is not visible during observation.
Random zero (Hawksley) Sphygmomanometer [42]	Bulb assembly + valve	Needle valve (bleed)	Open column of mercury	Sthethoscope	—	Column of mercury is moving during measurement.
Physiometrics	Pump driven by electricity	Fixed rate of descending	Aneroid manometer	Microphone	—	Recording of Korotkoff sounds on a disk. The disk revolves as a function of pressure.
Bosch Tonomat	Bulb assembly + valve	Fixed rate of descending	Aneroid manometer	Microphone	—	Indication of pointer.
Arteriosonde	Automatic by means of pump driven by electricity	Rate of descending is variable	Column of mercury	—	Ultrasonic	Column of mercury is halted when systolic or diastolic pressure is read.

3) The time of the day when the blood pressure measurement is made should be recorded (in view of the large differences that can occur between morning and evening values).

4) Record whether the blood pressure was obtained with the subject in the sitting, recumbent, or standing position.

5) Record whether as part of the examination a venous puncture is performed. The blood pressure measurement should be made before the venous puncture. The examination procedure, of which the blood pressure measurement is part, should be specified.

6) Describe the type of device used for measuring blood pressure. Aneroid manometers should be calibrated regularly.

7) The blood pressure measurement should be made during the continuous deflation, and be measured twice. The number of measurements made should be specified, and the time interval between measurements should be recorded.

8) Phases 4 and 5 of diastolic blood pressure should be recorded.

9) The qualifications of the person recording blood pressure should be given (e.g., physician, nurse, technician). The blood pressure should preferably be recorded by a trained nurse or technician. The recording observer should be given a code number, in order to be able to check the results obtained by each observer.

10) Information should be given about the training program for observers. Theoretical information should be given to the observers making the blood pressure measurements in order to make them understand the procedure. The observers should learn to locate the cubital artery.

3. RELIABILITY OF BLOOD PRESSURE MEASUREMENT

3.1. Accuracy of indirect auscultatory measurement

In the various studies in which invasive pressure measurements have been compared with noninvasive blood pressure measurements, there has been no agreement on the procedures which should be applied or on the instrumentation used. For instance, the first publications on this subject did not specify cuff dimensions and it appears that the two blood pressure measurements, as determined by the noninvasive method, were not taken simultaneously. The latter is very unfortunate since it is known that blood pressure can show variations even over a short period of time. Also, generally only a small number of measurements were carried out.

After 1960, most of the research was directed toward developing a cuff of optimum design. Karvonen et al. [45, 46], Simpson et al. [47], and King [48] all

Table 2. Differences between intraarterial and cuff blood pressure.

Intraarterial pressure cuff pressure (mmHg)	Systolic	Diastolic 1 (phase 4)	Diastolic 2 (phase 5)
+43 – +47	4		
+38 – +42	4		1
+33 – +37	3	1	2
+28 – +32	6	2	1
+23 – +27	7	2	3
+18 – +22	6	3	5
+13 – +17	9	3	9
+8 – +12	5	7	10
+3 – +7	1	7	11
+2 – 2	1	11	5
−3 – −7	1	5	
−8 – −12		4	
−13 – −17			
−18 – −22		1	
−23 – −27			
−28 – −32		1	
Total	47	47	47 n
Mean difference	+24.6	+ 5.3	+13.1 mmHg
Standard deviation	14.0	13.9	9.5 mmHg

From Holland et al., *Br. Med. J.* 2:1241, 1964 [49].

stated that the length of the bag is an important factor, and each of them found that when the bag completely encircles the upper arm the reliability of the measurement is considerably improved. Alexander et al. [14, 15] deduced from their theoretical model, and after experimental research with it, not only that the bag should completely encircle the arm but that the width of the cuff should be at least 1.2 times the diameter of the upper arm. Holland and Humerfelt [49] performed thorough research with respect to the reliability of the auscultatory measurement of blood pressure for adults whose upper arms were not obese. Table 2 is taken from their publication and shows the differences as found between the intraarterial pressure determination and the blood pressure as measured with the auscultatory method.

Systolically the mean pressure difference amounted to 24.6 mmHg, diastolically it was 5.3 mmHg, and for the diastolic phase 5 it was 13.1 mmHg. The correlation between the difference between systolic intraarterial versus cuff pressures and arm circumference was barely significant at the 5% level. Neither for phase 4 nor for phase 5 were the correlation coefficients statistically significant. Geddes and Whistler [50, 51] concluded from analysis of results of different research workers that a too narrow cuff will show too high values of blood pressure whereas a too wide cuff will show too low values.

3.1.1. Fat upper arms. Very large errors are introduced when blood pressure is indirectly measured in individuals with obese upper arms. Ragan and

Bordley in 1941 pointed out these errors for the first time: in 11 subjects with adipositas, they found the error with a cuff of 13 cm width to vary from -7 to $+47$ mmHg systolically, and for diastolic pressure it varied from -1 to $+39$ mmHG [11]. Trout et al. [16] examined another 11 individuals with large-sized upper arms, and their results were even worse: errors varying between $+32$ and $+102$ mmHg were found for systolic pressures. The values for diastolic pressure varied from $+18$ to $+66$ mmHg. Berliner et al. [52] and Kvols et al. [53] also found large errors in carefully executed comparisons. These authors believe the error of the measurement to lie in the loss of pressure transmission which occurs across compressible substances, resulting in falsely high readings (cf. p. 6).

3.1.2. Can the measurement be improved? To find more accurate values when measuring blood pressure, various suggestions have been proposed. Geddes and Whistler [51] and Pickering et al. [54] reviewed the original measurements of Ragan and Bordley [11] and suggested the introduction of corrections to be used in fat upper arms, which were derived from tables by them. Some investigators applied these tables, but later it was concluded that the error in measurement did not clearly correlate with the circumference of the arm, and their use was therefore discontinued. Several researchers advocated measuring blood pressure with the auscultatory technique on the lower arm, putting the stethoscope above the radial artery [16, 49, 52, 53, 55], but Kvols et al. [53] found this method to be very unsatisfactory. These authors instead used three rectangular cuffs of various sizes in 16 subjects with obese upper arms, but with none of the three cuffs was satisfactory agreement between invasive and noninvasive measurement of blood pressure obtained. It is clear from all these observations that the auscultatory measurement of blood pressure for obese upper arms by using cuffs with standard shape and size has very limited value, and when there exists serious doubt on the reliability of the measurement, intraarterial pressure determination is preferred. In general, it can be stated that we should always be very careful when measuring blood pressure with a cuff and stethoscope, and that we should be on our guard not to mistake cuff hypertension for real hypertension.

3.1.3. The conically shaped cuff. In Leiden recently, we evaluated the accuracy of auscultatory blood pressure measurement of subjects with obese upper arms [56–58]. All measurements were done selectively. Blood pressure was measured in 70 subjects who had obese upper arms. In the first part of the experiments, the standard 23×12 cm bladder was compared with a larger rectangular type: 28×15 cm in a subgroup of 20 obese subjects. Each time, the cuff was applied to the left arm and the intrabrachial artery blood pressure, which was recorded continuously, was determined simultaneously on the right arm. In a second subgroup of 50 subjects, the results obtained by using a cuff sized 28×12 cm were compared with those obtained by using three conically shaped cuffs (large, medium, and rather small) specially designed for the purpose.

3.1.4. Methods. The subject, who was in the recumbent position, had both arms positioned to the level of the right atrium, to avoid any correction necessary for hydrostatic pressure difference. We first checked each individual to ensure that systolic and diastolic pressure on left and right arm did not differ by more than 5 mmHg. For the intrabrachial method, a Cournand needle no. 18 was inserted into the right brachial artery, the needle being connected by means of a three-way stopcock and a protected Teflon tube of 30 cm length to a Statham P23 Db pressure transducer. Use was made of an amplifier type Elema EMT31 and a six-channel recorder type Elema EMT81. For calibration, a stepwise total pressure change of 100 mmHg produced a 5-cm step on the recording paper, marked by position 100 on the Elema recorder. Changes in the recorded pressure were proportional to the pressure applied to the input of the strain-gauge manometer. The pressure was calibrated by using a mercury manometer. The frequency response of the needle connected with a fluid-filled Teflon tube to the manometer was determined with a method developed by Stegall [8]. The frequency response of the fluid-

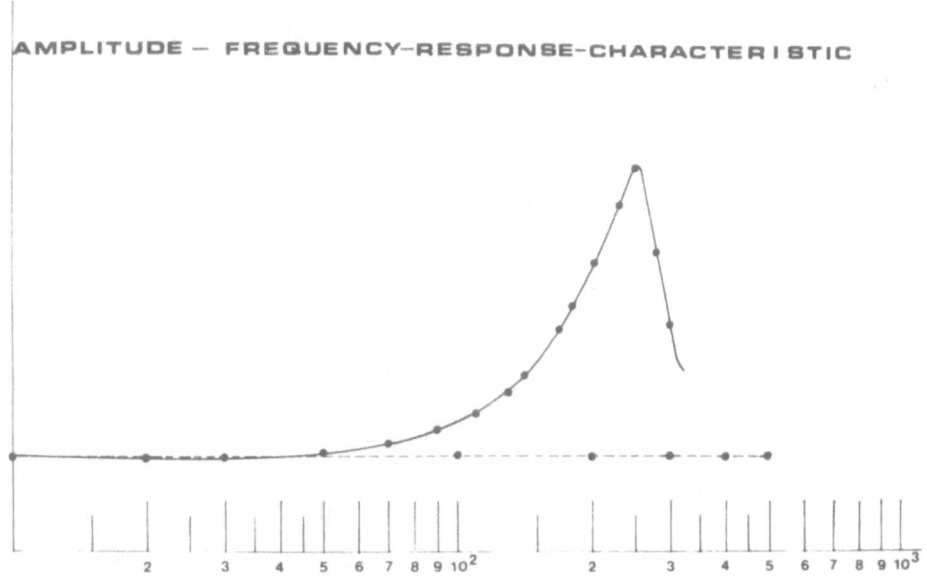

Figure 1. Frequency response of the fluid-filled system (Cournand needle, plastic tube, and Statham pressure gauge). Amplitude: linear scale, frequency in Hz.

filled system was determined while the Cournand needle dwelled in the brachial artery by a stepwise pressure change in the fluid-filled system. From these experiments, the resonance frequency and coefficient of damping were measured. With no air bubbles (which can be accomplished after careful flushing), a resonance frequency of 25 Hz and a coefficient of damping of 0.13 in the frequency response were obtained (Fig. 1). Pressure recordings with such an underdamped fluid-filled system will show an overshoot, as high-frequency components will be recorded with amplitudes which are relatively too large. Fortunately, however, the magnitude of this effect is not very great, since amplitudes of high-frequency components rapidly decrease with increasing frequency, as was demonstrated by Patel et al. [59]. The overshoot of the pressure curve was measured experimentally and theoretically [58–60]: Figure 2 shows the results. The pressure overestimation is more pronounced with a steep rise in the pressure curve, which of course is the case in systole and hardly at all in diastole. In the experiment shown, overshoot amounts to 13 mmHg with the systolic pressure at 114 mmHg. Clearly, values of systolic pressure measured with an underdamped fluid-filled system should be corrected for the overshoot.

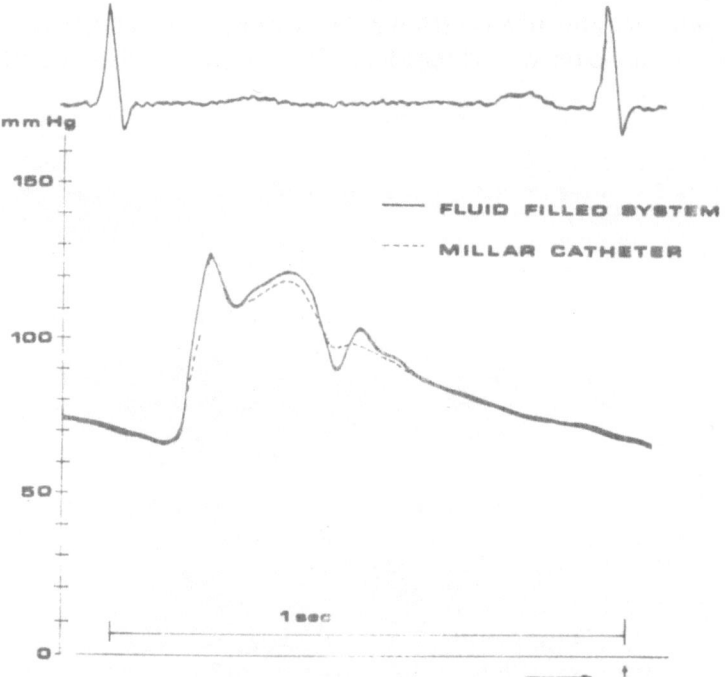

Figure 2. Two superimposed intrabrachial blood pressure tracings. One obtained by our fluid-filled system, the other by catheter tip manometer (Millar). In our fluid-filled system in the case shown, the overshoot amounts to 13 mmHg with a systolic pressure of 114 mmHg. From Huige [58].

An event marker was used to compare data of the direct with those of the indirect measurement of blood pressure. In this way, instants of systolic and diastolic end points determined by the Riva-Rocci method were marked on the continuous intraarterial blood pressure recording. Systolic and diastolic end points were determined by using the instrument of the London School of Hygiene [41]. All measurements were performed by two observers and each observer did two measurements with each cuff. The bell of the Rappaport stethoscope manufactured by Hewlett and Packard was placed on the distal end of the brachial artery. The Korotkoff sounds, which often have a low frequency, can be heard adequately with this type of stethoscope for this category of patients. For the diastolic pressure, phase 5 was taken. The investigation was aimed at determining the influence of the shape and size of cuffs on the accuracy of blood pressure (BP) measurements, especially in subjects with obese upper arms. Experiments have shown that, in these subjects, often great differences exist between pressures measured invasively and noninvasively.

3.1.5. Comparison of two rectangular cuffs. Table 3 shows the number of subjects in groups according to the circumference of the upper arm, a classification which can be interpreted as normal, moderate, and extremely fat upper arms.

Table 3.

Circumference upper arms	n
27 – 30 cm	9
31 – 34 cm	7
≥ 35 cm	4
Total	20

Figures 3a–d show the results of measurements in the first 20 individuals. It is clear that the accuracy of blood pressure measurement with the wider rectangular cuff is only slightly better than that with the smaller cuff. For the systolic pressure, considerable scattering around the line of identity exists. The diastolic pressure measured indirectly with both cuffs proved to be systematically too high.

3.1.6. Comparison of conical cuffs with rectangular cuffs: obese upper arm and cuff shape. Obese upper arms are often not cylindrical, but instead have a conical geometric form: the circumference of the upper arm at the shoulder is much larger than at the elbow site and there are even quite considerable differences between the circumference of the arm at the upper end of the cuff when compared with the lower border. A relatively narrow cuff will fit around

16

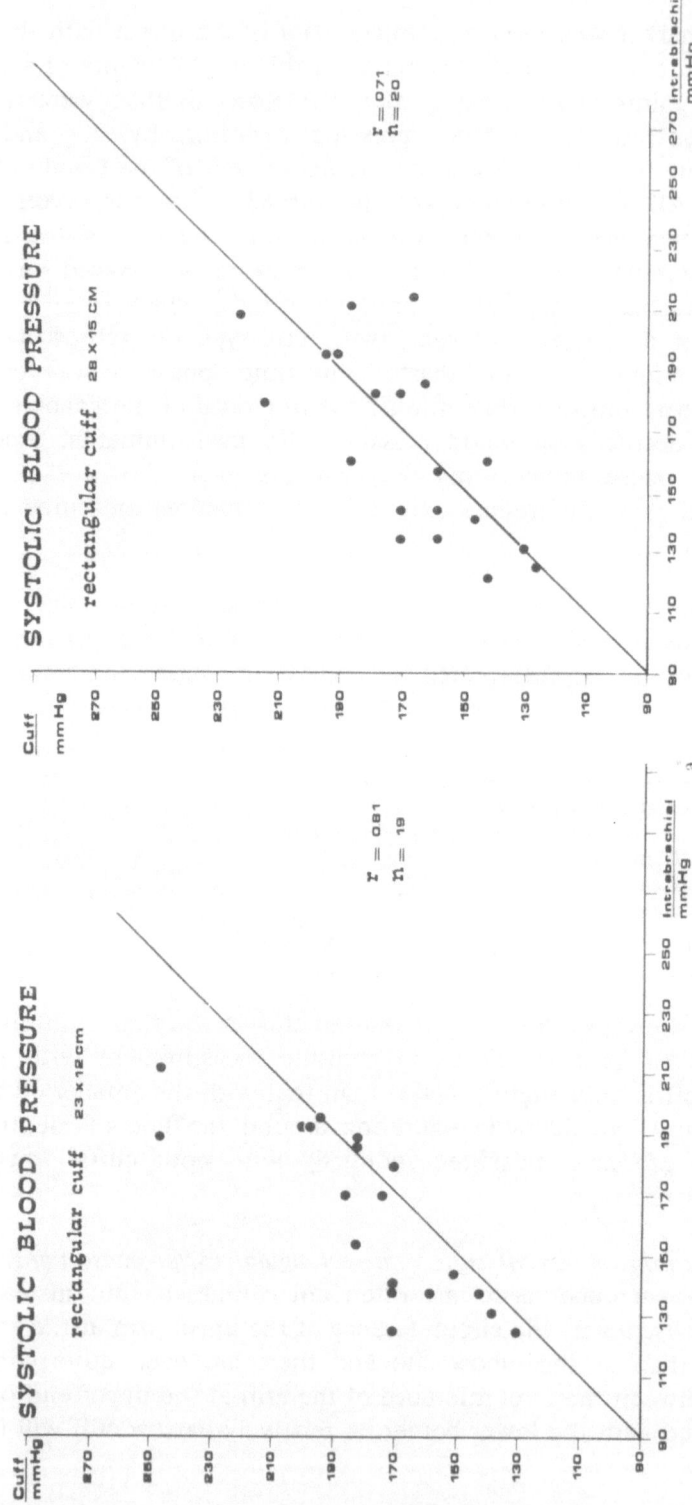

Figures 3a and b. Two diagrams for observer A. Systolic cuff pressure (small and large rectangular cuffs) versus intrabrachial blood pressure determination.

17

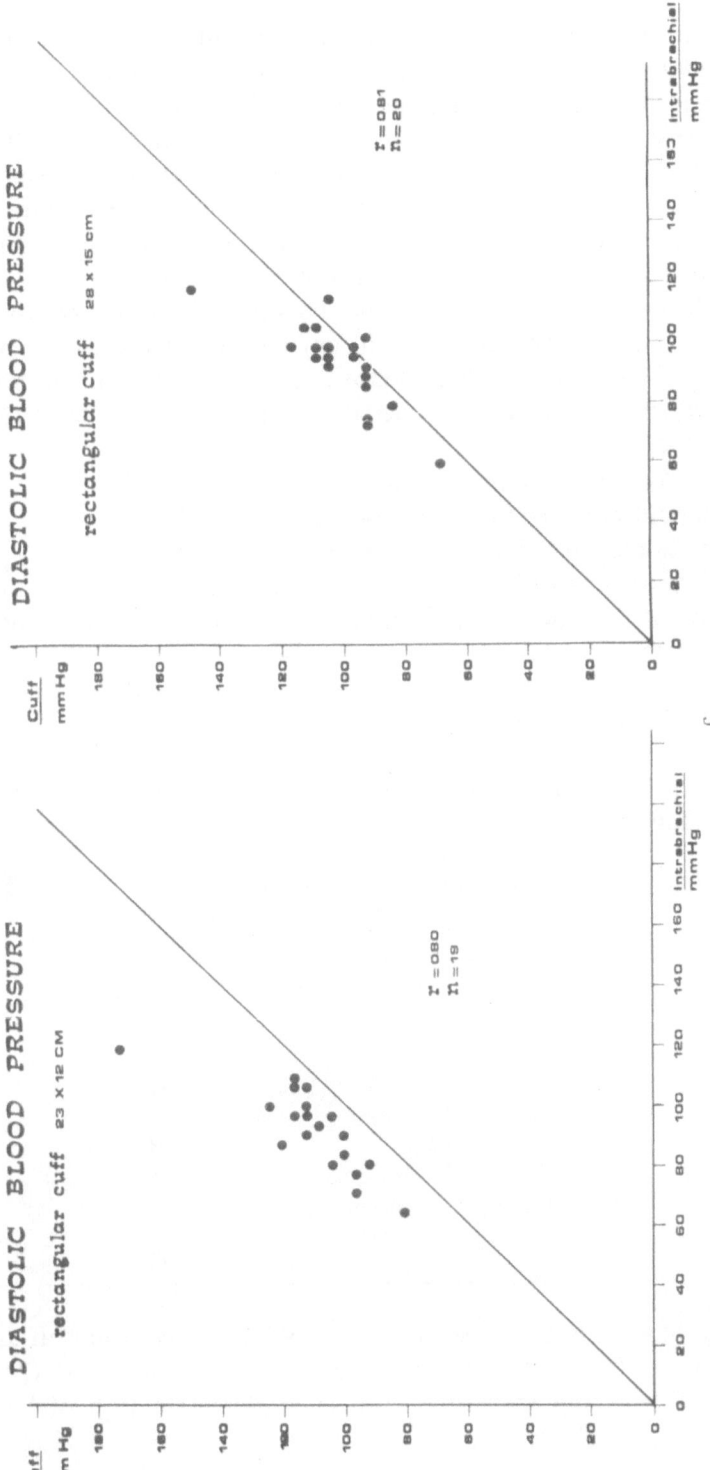

Figures 3c and d. Two diagrams for observer A. Diastolic cuff pressure (small and large rectangular cuffs) versus intrabrachial blood pressure determination.

the arm, but it does not solve the problem as it will not occlude the brachial artery. A wider cuff when put around a fat upper arm will function as a narrow cuff since it cannot be applied snugly at the lower part of the upper arm, leaving free space there. Some physicians try to make the cuff fit better by crossing the ends of the cuff over the arm. Such a procedure has its disadvantages: it requires extra space and leaves too little space to apply the bell of the stethoscope in the elbow region. The most important disadvantage, however, is that the ends of the bag will not meet at the upper side, and the two flaps will overlap at the lower side. Therefore, uniform compression of the tissue of the arm under the cuff will not be obtained. It is our belief that the nonfitting of large rectangularly shaped cuffs around fat upper arms is the main cause of errors. We therefore decided to adapt the shape of the cuff to the shape of the arm.

Our criteria for an optimum cuff are:
1) The bag should encircle the upper arm completely.
2) The width should be 1.5 times the diameter of the upper arm.
3) The shape must at all places fit snugly around the arm.
4) The interior of the bag should consist of silicone rubber and the exterior part of nonelastic rubber, 0.5 mm thick.
5) The cuff should be attached with adhesive cellotape and the length and the slip be sufficiently long so that it is well attached.

The most important data of the conically shaped cuff and patient material are presented in Tables 4 and 5.

Table 4. Conical cuff measurement data ($n = 50$). From Huige [58].

	Years of age	n
In age groups:	<20	1
	20 – 29	7
	30 – 39	12
	40 – 49	12
	50 – 59	11
	≥60	7
According to sex:	Men	24
	Women	26
According to arm circumference:	≤30 cm	14
	31 – 34 cm	25
	≥35 cm	11

In this setup, blood pressure measurements with the conical cuff as well as those obtained with a commercially available rectangular cuff (28×12 cm) were compared with the intraarterial pressure determination of blood pressure.

Table 5. Results of comparison between rectangular and conically shaped cuff measurements to intrabrachial blood pressure determinations for observers A and B. From Huige [58].

Systolic blood pressure (mmHg) Rectangular cuff					$n = 50$ Conical cuff				
Obs	n	Δp	SD	r	Obs	n	Δp	SD	r
A	45	−0.3	11.0	0.94	A	44	−7.7	8.7	0.97
B	45	+3.0	14.7	0.87	B	46	−5.4	7.6	0.97
Diastolic blood pressure (mmHg) Rectangular cuff					$n = 50$ Conical cuff				
Obs	n	Δp	SD	r	Obs	n	Δp	SD	r
A	41	+6.4	10.4	0.79	A	44	−2.3	7.9	0.87
B	44	+8.7	11.6	0.71	B	46	+0.9	9.6	0.83

In Table 5, the measurements for two observers A and B are given as indicated by A and B in the columns marked Obs; Δp is the mean of the differences of noninvasive and invasive blood pressure measurement and SD is the standard deviation of these differences; and r is correlation coefficient of both methods of measurement.

In Figures 4a–d, four scatter diagrams for observer B are displayed for the systolic and diastolic pressure and for results with rectangular as well as for those obtained with the conical cuff. Along the vertical axis are the data for the noninvasive (cuff) measurement and along the horizontal axis the values of the intraarterial pressure.

3.1.7. Discussion. Large errors clearly are often introduced when blood pressure is measured with cuff and auscultation on obese upper arms, especially if relatively narrow cuffs are used [11, 49, 52, 53].

The thus measured systolic values will often be too high and occasionally be too low. Diastolic pressure determined by cuff and auscultation will systematically produce readings that are too high. As a result, diagnosis of hypertension will erroneously be made while blood pressure as determined intraarterially proves to be normal. Various proposals have been made to improve on the accuracy of the measurement: correction tables, cuffs with long rectangular bags, and different sizes of cuffs: wide and narrow [51–54]. In none of these proposals, however, was a satisfactory agreement between auscultatory and direct intraarterial blood pressure measurement observed. The conclusion must be that, in case of serious doubt of measurement data, intraarterial measurement should be carried out. In a comparative study, results of which are presented here, on 50 subjects with predominant fat upper arms, a conically shaped cuff proved to do better: agreement between its blood pressure readings and intraarterial determinations is good. The fluid-filled manometer system used for the direct blood pressure measure-

20

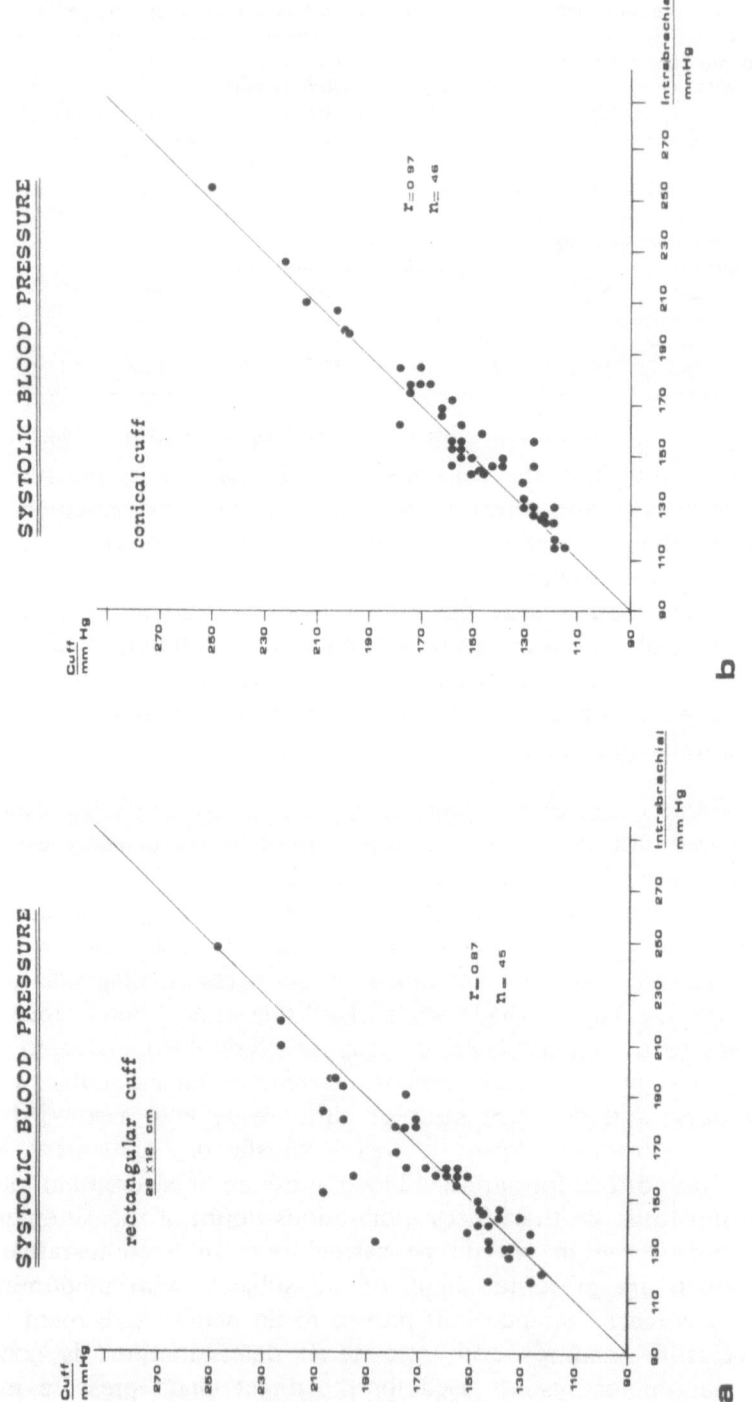

Figures 4a and b. Two scatter diagrams for observer B. Systolic cuff pressure (rectangular and conical) is shown versus intrabrachial determination.

21

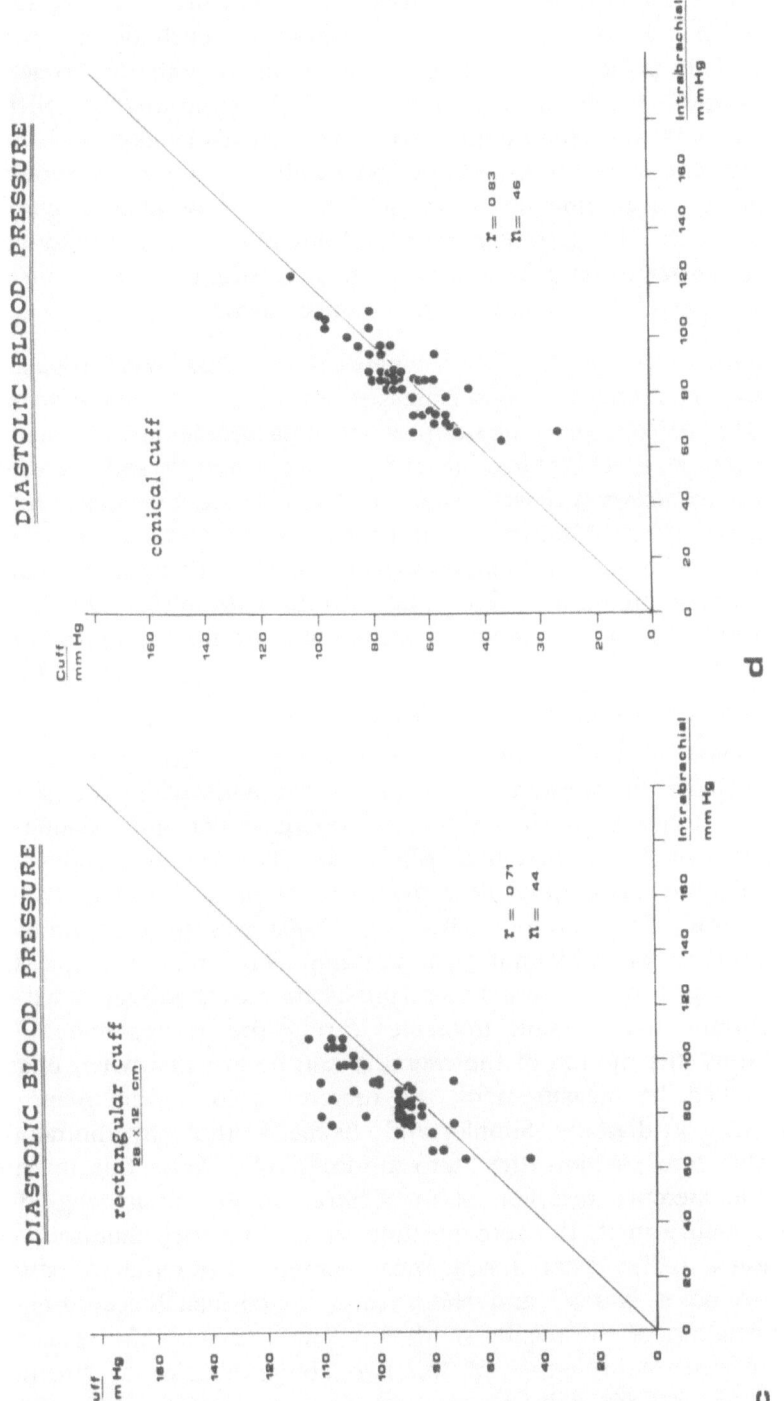

Figures 4c and d. Two scatter diagrams for observer B. Diastolic cuff pressure (rectangular and conical) is shown versus intrabrachial determination.

ment showed a resonance peak for systolic blood pressure. This explains why results of systolic blood pressure measurements for each of the measured intraarterially had higher values than those obtained with the conical cuff. The error of measurement did not correlate with the circumference of the arm and correlated only to a small degree with the height of blood pressure. The number of measurements was perhaps too small to show such correlations, but Holland and Humerfelt [49] were not able to show such a correlation either. In this study, the presented results obtained with a fairly large cuff of conical shape appear to be a promising kind of technique to measure noninvasively blood pressure in people with fat upper arms.

3.1.8. Summary of the results of investigation into an 'ideal' cuff. Invasive and noninvasive measurements of blood pressure on obese arms have been compared using 70 subjects. In a subgroup of 20, measurements were made with a standard and a wide rectangular cuff, which showed serious errors of measurements whatever cuff was used. The systolic pressure measured often too high and occasionally too low a value; the diastolic values (phase 5) were systematically too high. In a second subgroup of 50 patients, the accuracy of noninvasive blood pressure measurement could substantially be improved upon by using a conical cuff which fitted snugly around fat upper arms.

3.2. Elimination of bias and terminal digit preference

There are several ways to eliminate bias and terminal digit preference. The simplest is to have the measurement done by someone with no expectations of the results. It has been shown that paramedical personnel usually work more accurately in this respect than physicians. The use of an apparatus by which readings are taken only after the measurement considerably reduces the risk of error. The London School of Hygiene sphygmomanometer is extremely suitable for epidemiological research. This not only releases the pressure in the cuff at the correct rate, but is moreover provided with three mercury columns that remain invisible during the measurement [41]. By pressing buttons, the motion of the mercury can be arrested when phase 4 or 5 is heard. After the measurement, the mercury columns are made visible and can be read off digitally. Simpler and cheaper is the sphygmomanometer with a variable zero position (the 'zero-muddler') [42]. With this instrument, by setting the mercury reservoir at an arbitrary angle, or by changing the volume of mercury in it, the zero position of the mercury meniscus can be made unknown to the tester during measurement. After the measurement, the true zero point is read and the reading is corrected accordingly. For critical appreciation of the results of therapy and for scientific research into the effects of treatment, either of the two above-described instruments is recommendable. But for daily medical practice, at least for individuals not having obese upper arms, a conventional mercury manometer with a cuff of at least 13×30 cm is usually adequate.

3.3. Hydrodynamical phantom arm

The reproducibility of blood pressure measurement by one observer or between observers is difficult to determine on living subjects, as the measurement itself will cause a change in blood pressure. Unfortunately, there is as a result of this no reliable way to test the accuracy by which a person measures blood pressure on a living subject. Moreover, since consecutive measurements are not identical, it is difficult to compare properties of the various blood pressure devices (e.g., sphygmomanometers) with one another. The above problems can be bypassed with the development and application of a model of the upper part of the human arm, which naturally must have the same physical properties as regards shape, dimensions, compressibility of the soft parts, the viscoelastic properties of the artery, and the occurrence of vascular Korotkoff sounds. Previous studies on the development of a model for the sake of blood pressure measurement have been carried out and have been published [12–14, 17, 18, 62–66].

We want to report here briefly on a model in which artificial blood flow is generated with a pattern of pressure changes comparable to that in the brachial artery, an apparatus developed at the Institute of Medical Physics

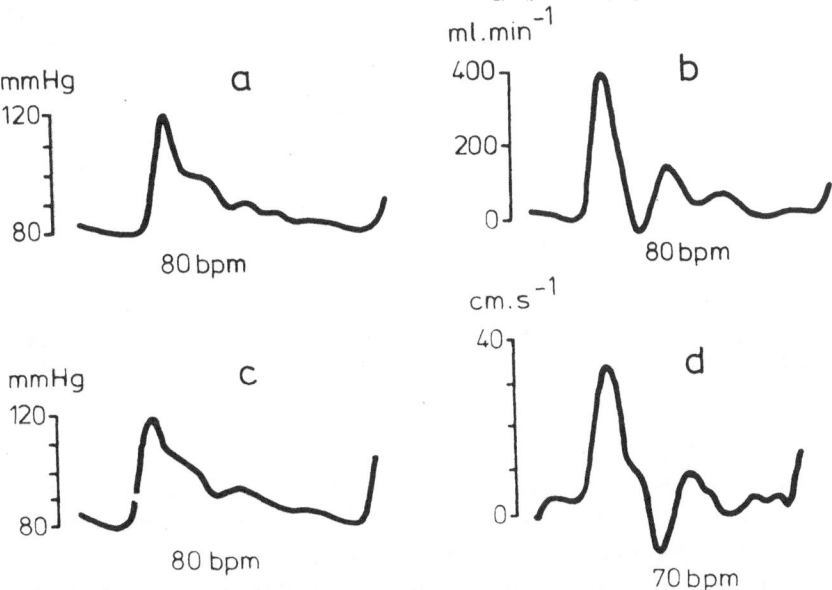

Figure 5. Model generated blood pressure (a) and flow (b) curves and 'real' intrabrachial blood pressure (c) and flow velocity (d) curves of the brachial artery, measured on a human arm by using Doppler techniques. From Hekkenberg, MFI Inf. 2, *Inst. Med. Phys. TNO,* 1978 [67].

24

TNO, Department of Medical Technology [67]. Some characteristics of the model are depicted in Figures 5 and 6. In Figure 5, the pressure and flow curves generated by the model are seen as a and b. The lower part of Figure 5 shows a blood pressure and a blood flow velocity curve of the brachial artery measured on a human arm by using Doppler techniques (c and d). The shape of the blood flow velocity curve of the arteria brachialis can be compared with the shape of the flow curve of the model arm, if we assume that the changes in diameter of both vessels do not differ considerably. The sounds generated by the model (shown in the upper part of Fig. 6) contain clear tapping sounds which change in nature during the measurement of blood pressure. This is similar to what happens during measurement of real blood pressure (the lower part of Fig. 6). Clearly, there is good qualitative agreement between a number of phenomena which occur in reality and which have been observed with the model arm. To reach also good quantitative agreement, the components in the model should be improved upon. More thorough investigation toward this aim is now being set up.

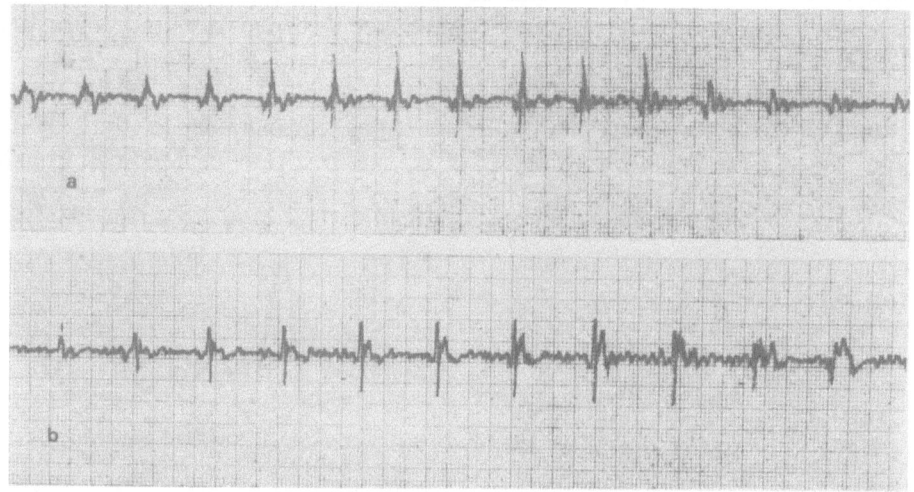

Figure 6. Korotkoff sounds generated by the model (a) and Korotkoff sounds in the human arm during measurement of blood pressure. From Hekkenberg, MFI Inf. 2, *Inst. Med. Phys. TNO*, 1978 [67].

3.4. Interpretation

Interpretation of results of measurement of blood pressure is more difficult than appears at first sight. The large variations of blood pressure over time and the fact that the observer obtains a momentary value only, are the main causes for problems with interpretation. Continuous measurement no doubt would be preferable, but is hardly feasible at present. Averaging a number of measurements would be 'next best' but even this is difficult to accomplish. Large errors can be introduced when values of blood pressure measurements are compared with previous ones, and this is all the more important since we often try to evaluate therapeutic effects that way. We will illustrate this with an example showing how unjustifiable a conclusion can be when it is based on what, at first sight, would seem to be good therapeutic intervention. A group of more than 4000 apparently healthy men is examined. Among them, 61 persons prove to have a systolic blood pressure of between 180 and 189 mmHg. After three years, in which some intervention took place, blood pressure is measured again in the 61 individuals. It now appears that only 8 persons out of 61 still have a blood pressure of between 180 and 189, while 8 others have values of 190 mmHg and higher, whereas in the remaining 45, blood pressure values have dropped to values below 180 mmHg. This would appear to be an encouraging result of the intervention. However, when we examine the results more closely, it shows that the mean lowering of blood pressure of the group of 61 amounted to approximately 20 mmHg. A large proportion of this, namely 17 mmHg can be 'explained' on the basis of statistics (so-called regression to the mean) and pressor effect and only 3 mmHg should actually be attributed to the therapeutic intervention. Undoubtedly results of therapeutic intervention should be interpreted with the greatest of care when the selection is based on elevated blood pressure as found with screening and particularly if only one casual measurement is made. Repeated measurements, preferably on two separate days, reduce chances of overinterpretation.

Acknowledgments. Technical assistance of Mr. J. Koops is gratefully acknowledged. The experimental part of this work has been carried out at the department of Exercise Physiology, head Dr. H.W.H. Weeda. He performed also the intraarterial blood pressure determinations and was observer A of the indirect (cuff) blood pressure measurements. The contribution to editing and typing of Patricia Steen is also gratefully acknowledged.

REFERENCES

1. Von Bonsdorf B: Zur Methodik der Blutdruckmessung mit besonderer Berücksichtigung der Registrierung absoluter Sphygmogramme beim Menschen. Acta Med Scand Suppl 51, 1932.
2. Geddes LA: The direct and indirect measurement of blood pressure. Chicago: Year Book Medical, 1970.
3. Greatorex GA: Indirect methods of blood pressure measurements. Watson (ed) IEE Monographs on Medical Electronics 1-6. Perigrinus Hers England, 1971.
4. Greatorex GA: Non invasive blood pressure measurement. In: Rolfe P (ed) Non invasive physiological measurements. London: Academic Press, 1979, pp 193-217.
5. Riva-Rocci S: Un nuovo sfigmanometro. Gaz Med Ital (Torino) 47:981-996, 1896.

26

6. Korotkoff NS: On the subject of methods of measuring blood pressure. Bull Imp Mil Med Acad St Petersburg 11:365-367, 1905. Translation: Geddes LA, Hoff HE, Badger AS: Introduction of the auscultatory method of measuring blood pressure. Cardiovasc Res Cent Bull (Houston) 5:57-74, 1967.

7. Von Recklinghausen H: Ueber Blutdruckmessung beim Menschen. Arch Exp Pathol Pharmakol 46:78-132, 1901.

8. Stegall HF: A simple inexpensive sinusoidal pressure generator. J Appl Physiol 22:591-592, 1967.

9. Wolf HJ, Von Bonsdorf B: Blutige Messung der absoluten Sphygmogramme beim Menschen. Z Gesamte Exp Med 79:569-577, 1931.

10. Hamilton WF, Brewer G, Brotman I: Pressure pulse contours in the intact animal. Analytical description of a new high-frequency hypodermic manometer with illustratic curves of simultaneous arterial and intercardiac pressures. Am J Physiol 107:427, 1934.

11. Ragan C, Bordley J: The accuracy of clinical measurements of arterial blood pressure. Bull Johns Hopkins Hosp 69:504-528, 1941.

12. Freis ED, Sappington RF: Dynamic reactions produced by deflating a blood pressure cuff. Circulation 38:1085-1096, 1968.

13. McCutcheon EP, Rushmer RF: Korotkoff sounds. An experimental critique. Circulation Res 20:149-161, 1967.

14. Alexander H, Cohen NL, Steinfeld L: The criteria in the choice of an occluded cuff for the indirect measurement of blood pressure. Med Biol Eng 15:2-10, 1977.

15. Steinfeld L, Alexander H, Cohen NL: Updating sphygmomanometry (Editorial). Am J Cardiol 33:107-110, 1974.

16. Trout KW, Bertrand CA, Williams MH: Measurement of blood pressure in obese persons. JAMA 162:970-972, 1956.

17. Maurer AH, Noordergraaf A: Korotkoff sound filtering for automated threephase measurement of blood pressure. Am Heart J 91:584-591, 1976.

18. McCutcheon EP, Baker BW, Wiederhelm CA: Frequency spectrum changes of Korotkoff sounds with muffling. Med Res Eng 8:30-33, 1969.

19. American Heart Association. Special article: Standardization of blood pressure readings. Am Heart J 18:95-101, 1939.

20. American Heart Association. Bordley J, Connor CAR, Hamilton WF, Kerr WJ, Wiggers CJ: Recommendations for human blood pressure determinations by sphygmomanometers. Circulation 4:503-509, 1951.

21. American Heart Association. Kirkendall WM, Burton AC, Epstein FH, Freis ED: Recommendations for human blood pressure determinations by sphygmomanometers. Circulation 36:980-988, 1967.

22. World Health Organization. Community control of hypertension. CVD/74, 4 (II). Appendix I. Geneva, 1973.

23. Woodbury RA, Robinow M, Hamilton WF: Blood pressure studies on infants. Am J Physiol 122:472-479, 1938.

24. Robinow M, Hamilton WF, Woodbury RA, Volpitto PP: Accuracy of clinical determination of blood pressure in children. Am J Dis Child 58:102-108, 1939.

25. Moss AJ, Adams FH: Auscultatory and intra-arterial pressure. A comparison in children with special reference to cuff width. J Pediatr 66:1094-1097, 1967.

26. Park MK, Guntheroth WG: Direct blood pressure measurements in brachial and femoral arteries in children. Circulation 41:231-237, 1970.

27. Park MK, Kawabori I, Guntheroth WG: Need for an improved standard for blood

pressure cuff size. The size should be related to the diameter of the arm. Clin Pediatr (Phila) 15:784-787, 1976.

28. De Dobbeleer GDP: Measurement of systolic and diastolic blood pressure by means of phase shift. World Med Electron Instrum 3:122-126, 1965.
29. Janssen FJ: The rheographic determination of systolic and diastolic blood pressure. Digest 7th Int Conf Med Biol Eng Stockholm, p 221, 1967.
30. Kirby RR, Kemmerer WT, Morgan JL: Transcutaneous Doppler measurement of blood pressure. Anaesthesiology 31:86-89, 1969.
31. Zahed B, Sadove MS, Hatano S, Wu HH: Comparison of automated Doppler ultrasound and Korotkoff measurements of blood pressure of children. Anesth Anal 50:699-704, 1971.
32. Buggs H, Johnson PE, Gordon LS, Balguma FB, Wettach GE: Comparison of systolic arterial blood pressure by transcutaneous Doppler probe and conventional methods in hypotensive patients. Anesth Anal 42:443-452, 1973.
33. Labarthe DR, Hawkins CM, Remington RD: Evaluation of performance of selected devices for measuring blood pressure. Am J Cardiol 32:546-553, 1973.
34. Labarthe DR, Hawkins CM, Remington RD: An evaluation of measurement performance of selected blood pressure devices. Hypertension manual. In: Laragh JH (ed) Mechanisms methods management. New York: York Medical Books Dun Donnelley, 1976, pp 585-603.
35. Labarthe DL: Comparative assessment of non-invasive techniques for blood pressure measurement. Acta Cardiol 33:87-88, 1978.
36. Hunyor SN, Flynn JM, Cochineas C: Comparison of performance of various sphygmomanometers with intra-arterial blood pressure readings. Br Med J 2:159-162, 1978.
37. Ramsey M: Non invasive automatic determination of mean arterial pressure. Med Biol Eng Comput 17:11-18, 1979.
38. Rose GA, Blackburn H: Cardiovascular survey methods. Geneva: WHO, 1968.
39. Kesteloot H: Problems related to the standardization of blood pressure measurement. Methodology and standardization of non-invasive blood pressure measurement in epidemiological studies. Proceedings Workshop Leuven, 6-7 December 1974. Commission of European Communities, EUR 5544 e, 1976.
40. Kesteloot H, Joossens JV: Methodology of blood pressure measurement and epidemiology of hypertension. Acta Cardiol 33:67-70, 1978.
41. Rose GA, Holland WW, Crowley EA: A sphygmomanometer for epidemiologists. Lancet 1:296-300, 1964.
42. Garrow JS: Zero muddler for unprejudiced sphygmomanometry. Lancet 2:1205, 1963.
43. Report. Evaluation of sphygmomanometers. Health devices. August:99-118, 1971.
44. Report. Evaluation of sphygmomanometers. Health devices. August:227-242, 1975.
45. Karvonen MJ: Effect of sphygmomanometer cuff size in blood pressure measurement. Bull WHO 27:805-808, 1962.
46. Karvonen MJ, Telivho LJ, Jarvinen EJK: Sphygmomanometer cuff size and the accuracy of indirect measurement of blood pressure. Am J Cardiol 13:688-693, 1964.
47. Simpson JA, Jamieson G, Dickhaus DW, Grover RF: Effect of cuff bladder on accuracy of measurement of indirect blood pressure. Am Heart J 70:208-215, 1965.

48. King GE: Errors in clinical measurement of blood pressure in obesity. Clin Sci 32:223-237, 1967.
49. Holland WW, Humerfelt S: Measurement of blood pressure: comparison of intra-arterial and cuff values. Br Med J 2:1241-1243, 1964.
50. Geddes LA, Tivey R: The importance of cuff width in measurement of blood pressure indirectly. Cardiovasc Res Cent Bull 14:69-79, 1976.
51. Geddes LA, Whistler SJ: The error in indirect blood pressure measurement with the incorrect size of cuff. Am Heart J 96:4-8, 1978.
52. Berliner K, Fujiy H, Lee DH, Yildiz M, Garnier B: Blood pressure measurements in obese persons. Comparison of intraarterial and auscultatory measurements. Am J Cardiol 8:10-17, 1961.
53. Kvols LK, Rohlfing BM, Alexander JK: A comparison of intraarterial and cuff blood pressure measurements in very obese subjects. Cardiovasc Res Cent Bull 7:118-123, 1969.
54. Pickering GW, Roberts JAF, Sowry GSC: The aetiology of essential hypertension. The effect of correcting for arm circumference on the growth rate of arterial pressure with age. Clin Sci 13:267-271, 1954.
55. Devetski RL: A modified technique for the determination of systemic arterial pressure in patients with extremely obese upper arms. N Engl J Med 269:1137-1138, 1963.
56. Huige MC, Van Vollenhoven E, Weeda HWH, Arntzenius AC: Influence of cuff size and design on indirect blood pressure measurement. Acta Cardiol 33:88-90, 1978.
57. Huige MC, Weeda HWH, Arntzenius AC, Van Vollenhoven E: Cuff size and shapes in blood pressure measurements on the fat upper arms. 8th World congress of cardiology, Tokyo, Sept 1978 (Abstr I), no. 0998, p. 340.
58. Huige MC: Thesis, University of Leiden, 1980.
59. Patel D, Mason DT, Ross J, Braunwald E: Harmonic analysis of pressure pulses obtained from the heart and the vessels of man. Am Heart J 69:785-794, 1965.
60. Krovetz LJ, Jennings RB, Goldbloom SD: Limitation of correction of frequency dependent artefact in pressure recordings using harmonic analysis. Circulation 50:992-997, 1974.
61. Holland WW: The reduction of observer variability in the measurement of blood pressure. In: Pemberton J (ed) Epidemiology. Reports on research and teaching, 1962. London: Oxford Medical, 1963, pp 271-281.
62. Gupta R, Miller JW, Yoganathan AP, Udwadia FE, Corcoran WH, Kim BM: Spectral analysis of arterial sounds: a noninvasive method of studying arterial disease. Med Biol Eng 13:700-705, 1975.
63. Anliker M, Raman K: Korotkoff sounds at diastole — a phenomenon of dynamic instability of fluid filled shells. Int J Solid Struct 2:467-491, 1966.
64. Cohen ML: Korotkoff sounds. Thesis, Technion Israel Institute of Technology, Haifa, Israel, 1970.
65. Conrad W: Pressure flow relations in collapsible tubes. IEEE Trans Biomed Eng BME 16:284-295, 1969.
66. Smolders DJ: Modelonderzoek naar het gedrag van een arterie onder een manchet tijdens indirecte bloeddrukmeting. Rep Univ Nijmegen Lab Med Phys, Feb 1972.
67. Hekkenberg R: De ontwikkeling van een bovenarmfantoom voor bloeddrukme-tingen. MFI Inf 2, Sept 1978. Inst Med Phys TNO.

2. ESTIMATING SODIUM INTAKE IN EPIDEMIOLOGICAL STUDIES
Review and results of a methodological pilot study in Finland

P. Piétinen and J. Tuomilehto

Sodium is probably important in the etiology of hypertension, but its role needs further clarification. The results of previous studies have been controversial and the nature of the relationship between salt and blood pressure is still unknown. Among the many factors that cause this controversy is the difficulty of measuring sodium intake.

There is no reliable and, at the same time, practical way of measuring an individual's true sodium intake. Even the standard method, the 24-h urinary sodium excretion, is an indirect estimation and subject to interpretation error. In addition to intra- and interindividual differences in the rate of urinary sodium excretion, day-to-day fluctuations in sodium intake itself confound the analysis[1].

Problems of measuring individual sodium intake levels arise in epidemiological studies testing for a correlation between sodium intake and blood pressure within a population. According to Liu et al.[2] nine 24-h urine collections are needed to characterize an individual's sodium intake. Most published studies correlating sodium output and blood pressure are unsatisfactory because they included only one 24-h urine.

Compliance problems limit the usefulness of 24-h urine samples. In studies where group comparisons are made, easier methods have been used successfully. For example, in a large intervention study, Farquhar et al.[3] used spot urine specimens collected after a 12-h fast to compare sodium/potassium ratio changes. The advantage of collecting urine samples while measuring blood pressure at the study site is enormous and makes it possible to study large population groups.

The methodological needs of clinical studies differ in many respects from those in epidemiological studies. Often, not only quantitative but also qualitative information about salt consumption is needed. Sodium excretion in even 24-h urine collections does not indicate the sources of dietary salt. Source is an important question in intervention studies where efforts are concentrated on decreasing the dietary intake of salt. Because of methodological problems, efforts to find a simple dietary method to estimate sodium intake have not been successful and, therefore, nutritional aspects of salt analysis have been neglected.

H. Kesteloot, J.V. Joossens (eds.), Epidemiology of Arterial Blood Pressure, 29–44.

1. DIETARY MEANS OF MEASURING SODIUM INTAKE

Nutrition surveys have rarely included estimated sodium intake. Measuring sodium intake by food consumption data requires accurate food composition tables for both sodium content of basic food ingredients and average salt content of typical local dishes. Because this requires a large effort with possible sources of error, the task is usually avoided by investigators.

Most of the studies reporting data on estimated salt intake have been done in areas where the diet contains relatively few food items. The largest epidemiological study using food consumption data in salt consumption estimations comes from Japan [4]. In a nutrition survey of farmers, regional salt intake was estimated based on Japanese food composition tables. The main sources of salt in the diet were soy sauce, table salt, miso (salty fermented soybean), and pickles. The salt intake figures agreed well with the regional 24-h urinary sodium analyses. (A significant correlation between mortality from apoplexy and the total salt consumption and the salt content of the local miso was present in different regions.)

In addition to one 24-h urine collection, precise weighing of food for three days has been used in age group comparisons in Korea [5]. Sodium intake estimates based on food composition tables correlated well with the average group sodium output. The sodium output averaged 87% of the intake. Since weighing food is time-consuming and can alter dietary intake, it has not been used very often. Komachi et al. [6] used this method in Japan and weighed the food in groups of 5–13 men for three days. They considered that this method gave a good estimate of salt consumption, but validity was not documented.

Tillotson and co-workers [6a] following up on a study of cardiovascular diseases among Japanese men living in Japan, Hawaii, and California, used both 24-h interviews and seven-day food records in estimating sodium intakes. The results were not verified by urinary analyses, but the mean sodium intakes were found to be similar to those previously measured in the same area by using urinary analyses. This, again, shows the value of carefully compiled local food composition tables in group level estimations of sodium intakes.

Prior et al. [7] also used the one-day recall method when studying two Polynesian populations. Salt used in cooking and at the table was also estimated. The group mean sodium intake values agreed well with the 24-h urinary outputs of sodium on the two islands.

There have been few efforts in epidemiological studies to correlate individual sodium intake levels based on food consumption data with reliable urine samples. Adlin et al. [8] found an insignificant correlation between one 24-h urine sodium excretion and sodium intake based on 'a typical day's food intake.' The result might be expected since neither of the methods allowed for large day-to-day variations in salt consumption.

Measuring sodium intake with the 'duplicate portion technique' would be the only direct way of determining sodium intake. In this method, a duplicate portion of all foods and beverages consumed during a designated period is taken for chemical analysis. This method has been applied only in small population groups of high school and college students or elderly people [9, 10]. Besides being difficult and costly, the intake of energy and nutrients with the duplicate portion technique tends to be low due to the difficulties the subjects experience in maintaining their ordinary food habits in the experimental setting. This method is not feasible in epidemiological studies.

Hankin and co-workers [11–13] have searched for a short dietary method of estimating individual sodium intakes in epidemiological studies. In a group of Japanese-American men, they developed a method based on selected food items. The calculation of the total sodium intake for the week was based on food consumption data and personal salting habits. A regression equation explained 69% of the total variance in sodium intake during a week, but most of the food items that predicted sodium intake were Japanese. The value of this equation is obviously limited to this population group. No urine analyses were done concurrently. This methodology needs further research in different populations and should include simultaneous collection of urine samples.

Dahl and Love [14] proposed a simple questionnaire for classifying people into low, moderate, or high salt users. Persons who never added salt to their food were 'low' salt users, those who added salt after tasting were 'moderate' salt users, and persons always salting their food before tasting were 'high' salt users. In a population of over 1000 adults, these authors found significant differences in the prevalence of hypertension in these three groups. These 'salt shaker' questions have been used also in other studies [15, 16], but no statistically significant differences in the prevalence of hypertension in the different groups have been found. The ability of these questions to classify a person's sodium intake was tested in the Framingham study and a poor correlation between 24-h sodium excretion and the use of table salt was found [17].

2. ASSESSMENT OF SODIUM INTAKE BY SODIUM OUTPUT

2.1. Sodium loss

The best measure of total sodium intake is the 24-h urinary excretion. Normal stool excretion of sodium is less than 5 mmol/day so that stool loss can be disregarded [18–20]. The chief source of unaccounted sodium loss is through sweat. Sweat usually contains 20–50 mmol sodium/l, so sweating associated with exercise, heat, or fever can lead to sodium losses of as much as 350 mmol/day [21]. On the other hand, when sweat excretion is low, most of the sodium and chloride ions are reabsorbed from the precursor secretion so that their concentrations in sweat are sometimes as low as 5 mmol/l [22]. In cases such as these, the total sodium loss in metabolic studies with free-sodium intake has been no more than 10 mmol/day [23].

It is usually assumed that about 90% – 95% of the ingested sodium appears in the urine [24]. This estimation has been confirmed in and out of the laboratory setting in conditions of minimal sweating. Mickelsen et al. [25] carried out a carefully designed study with healthy volunteers and analyzed the sodium in both food and urine for 28 days. On the average, 96% of the sodium ingested during this period was excreted in the urine, and individual average outputs varied between 89% and 106% of intake. Urine analyses appear to give a reliable estimate of individual sodium intake when the observation period is long enough.

Studies with fixed sodium intake levels have demonstrated a marked day-to-day and individual variation in sodium excretion [19, 20, 26]. The error variance of excretion seems to be a linear function of the sodium load given to the patient. The mean sodium excretion was 95% of the intake in patients at bed rest [20] and 70% – 80% among healthy volunteers [19]. Presumably the differences in the rate of perspiration explain the differences.

Because of these fluctuations in sodium excretion, clinical and physiological interpretations of single 24-h urinary sodium excretion data must be made with caution, and sweating should be minimized during the urine collection period. There does not seem to be any reliable correction factor for estimating intake on the basis of output, since sodium loss in sweat cannot be measured.

2.2. Estimating individual sodium outputs

Dahl [18] noticed a wide intraindividual variation in urinary sodium and concluded that one 24-h collection can be misleading. Langford and Watson [27] suggested at least three 24-h collections based on a good correlation with a six-day collection. This is comparable to the measurement of other nutrients in nutrition surveys where one week's food record is often used but a three- to four-day record is also considered sufficient, providing it includes one weekend day [28]. Kesteloot and co-workers [29] studied the relationship between blood pressure and sodium excretion among over 300 people in both Belgium and Korea using 24-h urine collections over at least three consecutive days. Blood pressures were measured while the people were lying and standing, in the morning and at bedtime, by using home readings. A significant positive correlation between blood pressure and sodium output was found among both populations.

Liu and co-workers [1] studied the methodological problems in measuring individual habitual salt intake which, by definition, should include a longer time period. They collected four 24-h urine samples from 167 business and administrative personnel at two work sites. The urines were collected in two sets each, for one weekday and for one weekend day; the interval between collection of the two sets was on the average three months. The ratio of intra- to interindividual variances in the sodium output was so great (over 3) that for ranking into three groups (tertiles), ten specimens would have been necessary to distinguish the highest and lowest with a ≤ 0.01 probability of misclassification; 14 collections of 24-h urine would have been necessary to limit the weakening of the correlation between salt intake and blood pressure to less than 10% and even with four measurements of urinary sodium, potential correlations could still be underestimated by 25%. With a single 24-h collection as the estimate of sodium intake, the correlation coefficient between sodium and another variable could be diminished by 52%.

Collecting several 24-h urines in large populations causes great compliance problems and so far no epidemiological studies based on this type of method have been reported. There is no reliable way of testing whether urine collection has been complete. Individual variations in creatinine excretion limit its use as an index of sample completeness [30–33]. Another problem which is seldom discussed is the overcollection. Collections usually do not cover exactly a 24-h period.

Despite the weaknesses of this method, 24-h urine collection still has to be considered the best method of measuring sodium intake. One 24-h urine collection is sufficient to estimate mean group intake levels, but is inadequate when individual sodium intake levels are being estimated. This is not only because of day-to-day variation in the sodium excreted in the urine, but also because of the great daily variation in dietary sodium intake.

2.3. Methods for group level estimations

In epidemiological studies where only group level comparisons are needed, easier methods than the 24-h urine collection have been developed and successfully used. Spot urine sodium concentrations have been used by Prior et al. [7] in comparing two different populations. The results obtained by this method were similar to those found on the basis of 24-h collections, indicating the usefulness of casual urine samples in rough group comparisons.

Sodium/creatinine ratios have been used in some studies. This ratio is considered useful because the diurnal pattern of creatinine excretion is similar to those of sodium and other minerals. It is lowest during the night and highest during the working hours [34–37]. Because of irregular daytime peaks in both patterns, the time period between early morning and noon is the best for collection.

Widdowson and McCance [38] used random specimens obtained during the forenoon for comparing groups of African and British children. Estimates of total sodium and other mineral intakes were based on assumed creatinine excretion in children. According to Dauncey and Widdowson [39], the analyses of single specimens of urine collected between 8 a.m. and 10 a.m. can give a valid estimate of the 24-h excretion of sodium, potassium, magnesium, and calcium for a group of men. Moore et al. [40] concluded the same for young adults, but not for older people. Fukase [41] also found good correlations between sodium/creatinine ratios of time-deposit urine samples and 24-h sodium excretion for groups of people.

The use of creatinine in estimating the 24-h sodium excretion has been criticized [30, 42, 43]. Creatinine excretion depends on age and the amount of lean body mass. This makes its use unreliable in aged overweight populations.

Langford and Watson have systematically studied the usefulness of overnight urine samples [27, 44–46]. The overnight sodium hourly output correlates well with the 24-h output and can be used for groups. Equally good correlations were found by Pietinen et al. [47, 48].

Although 24-h urinary sodium output can be misleading in estimating individual salt intake levels, even shorter methods have been used in correlation analyses within a population. Froment et al. [49] found a weak positive correlation between the overnight sodium/potassium ratio and diastolic blood pressure in school boys. Lucas et al. [50] found a correlation between sodium/creatinine ratio taken between 7 a.m. and 12 noon after a fast and blood pressure in a group of normotensive adults. Pietinen et al. [48] found a good correlation between the mean of three overnight hourly sodium excretions and blood pressure in a group of young normotensive adults with family histories of hypertension.

The above discussion has reviewed the variety of methods used in studies on salt and blood pressure. Large epidemiological studies using random samples of people and repeated reliable methods are still missing.

3. BACKGROUND OF THE METHODOLOGICAL STUDY IN NORTH KARELIA

An intervention study to reduce salt consumption in the population was started in North Karelia in 1979. This study is a part of a comprehensive community-based cardiovascular disease control program [51]. Primary prevention data on hypertension control are not available and, therefore, the main purpose of this study is to clarify the effects of a health education program designed to lower blood pressure levels in a population. A small pilot study was designed to find suitable sodium intake estimation methods and to determine the main sources of dietary salt. Another purpose was to find methods of following the changes in salt intake related food habits.

4. MATERIAL AND METHODS USED IN NORTH KARELIA

In 1977 a 6.6% random sample of men and women aged 24–64 living in a small industrial town, Outukumpu, in North Karelia were asked to participate in a cardiovascular survey [51]. One year later a random sample of 256 men and women taken from those 308 responders to the 1977 survey were invited to participate in a further study. The participation rate was 68% (177 of 256).

The study participants were asked to collect three consecutive 24-h urines, keeping the overnight urine samples separate, and to start a four-day food record the day before the first urine collections. A nutritionist made a 24-h food recall interview and instructed the subjects on keeping the food diary. A public health nurse who measured the blood pressure gave instructions for the urine collections and asked the subjects to give a spot urine sample both at the beginning of the study and when the completed food records and urine collections were returned. At the end of the study she also administered a short dietary questionnaire on the frequency of use of salty food items (Fig. 1).

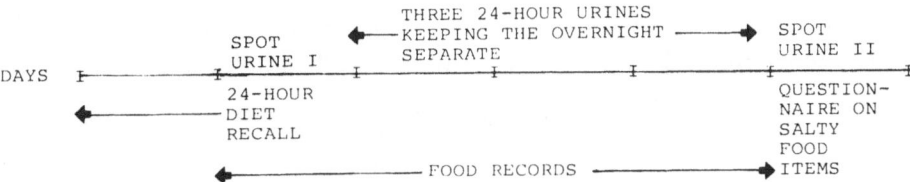

Figure 1. Description of the study design.

Of the subjects, 164 collected at least one 24-h urine which was complete according to the person's own report, gave both spot urine samples, and filled the dietary questionnaire; 102 men and women provided full information which included all the urine samples and a completed food record. The following results are for the subjects who provided full data.

The urines were analyzed for sodium and potassium by flame photometry, and for creatinine by the Technicon method. Food consumption data were calculated by automatic data processing. The calculation of daily sodium intakes was based on the average sodium content of basic food ingredients and on the average salt content of Finnish foods. Information on the sodium contents was collected from Finnish food manufacturers, research laboratories, cookbooks, and foreign food composition tables.

Table 1. Means and standard deviations (SD) of sodium and potassium excretion values in different urine collections ($n = 102$).

	Day 1		Day 2		Day 3	
	Mean	SD	Mean	SD	Mean	SD
24-h Na mmol/h	6.5	2.6	6.7	2.6	6.7	2.7
Overnight Na mmol/h	6.0	3.5	6.1	3.3	·6.2	3.9
Overnight Na mmol/l	127.6	56.6	129.1	52.5	127.1	60.0
Overnight Na/creatinine	1.4	0.4	1.4	0.5	1.4	0.4
24-h K mmol/h	3.6	1.0	3.7	1.3	3.7	1.2
Overnight K mmol/h	2.4	1.3	2.4	1.1	2.4	1.3
Overnight K mmol/l	53.9	21.7	52.2	21.9	51.8	22.9
Overnight K/creatinine	0.5	0.2	0.5	0.2	0.5	0.2
24-h Na/K	1.8	0.6	1.9	0.6	1.8	0.6
Overnight Na/K	2.6	1.2	2.7	1.2	2.7	1.3

5. RESULTS

Electrolyte excretion rates in both 24-h and overnight urine collections were consistent at the group level over three consecutive weekdays (Table 1). This consistency exists also between the two spot urine samples which were collected four days apart (Table 2). The slightly higher sodium concentration in the first spot urine sample is probably explained by the study design. The subjects gave the first spot urine samples when coming to the dietary interview between 8 a.m. and 5 p.m. but gave the second samples on returning the

Table 2. Means and standard deviations of sodium and potassium excretion values in spot urine samples ($n = 102$).

	Sample 1		Sample 2	
	Mean	SD	Mean	SD
Na mol/l	133.2	53.5	123.4	51.4
Na/creatinine	1.5	0.8	1.4	0.7
K mmol/l	79.5	25.6	79.3	25.0
K/creatinine	0.9	0.3	0.9	0.3
Na/K	1.8	1.0	1.7	1.0

three-day urine collections before noon at the end of the study. Since the peaks in the electrolyte excretion usually appear around noon and in the afternoon, the first spot samples probably include more of these peaks than do the second ones.

The correlation coefficients between the overnight hourly sodium outputs and the respective 24-h excretion values were 0.71–0.78 for the three consecutive days (Table 3). The respective correlations for potassium were 0.51–0.65 and 0.62–0.71 from the sodium/potassium ratio (all significant at $P<0.001$). The concentrations of overnight samples gave somewhat lower correlations, and those of potassium were not statistically significant.

Table 3. Correlation coefficients between overnight (ON) and respective 24-h electrolyte outputs for three consecutive days ($n = 102$).[a]

		Day 1	Day 2	Day 3
ON Na/h	vs 24-h Na	0.76	0.71	0.78
ON Na/l	vs 24-h Na	0.61	0.55	0.58
ON Na/creatinine	vs 24-h Na	0.57	0.51	0.64
ON Na/creatinine	vs 24-h Na/creatinine	0.59	0.52	0.51
ON K/h	vs 24-h K	0.51	0.60	0.65
ON K/l	vs 24-h K	0.14	0.17	0.20
ON K/creatinine	vs 24-h K	0.18	0.27	0.43
ON K/creatinine	vs 24-h K/creatinine	0.34	0.48	0.59
ON Na/K	vs 24-h Na/K	0.71	0.62	0.69

[a] Levels of significance:

P	r
5.0%	0.19
1.0%	0.25
0.1%	0.32

Creatinine as a reference standard was not as effective as the absolute overnight output rate (Table 3). The potassium/creatinine ratio in the overnight urine correlated poorly with the total 24-h potassium output ($r = 0.18$–0.43). The correlations between this overnight ratio and the same

Table 4. Correlation coefficients between the electrolyte output in different urine collections and the three-day mean of the same values ($n = 102$).[a]

Urine collections	Mean values of three consecutive 24-h periods				
	Na	K	Na/K	Na/creat	K/creat
1) 24-h output	0.91	0.85	0.88	0.86	0.85
2) 24-h output	0.86	0.91	0.86	0.83	0.91
3) 24-h output	0.83	0.86	0.84	0.73	0.90
1) Overnight output/h	0.69	0.33	0.58	0.59	0.34
2) Overnight output/h	0.65	0.57	0.53	9.52	0.48
3) Overnight output	0.62	0.58	0.53	0.51	0.59
1) Spot urine concentration	0.47	0.19	0.25	0.22	0.35
2) Spot urine concentration	0.43	0.16	0.20	0.27	0.40

[a] Levels of significance as in Table 3.

ratio in the 24-h urine were 0.34–0.59, indicating that the excretion patterns of these two were not similar.

Table 4 summarizes the correlations of sodium and potassium in the different urine collections with the three-day mean 24-h urine collection. Each separate 24-h sodium output correlated well ($r = 0.83$–0.91) with the three-day mean. The overnight outputs had lower correlation coefficients (0.62–0.69) and the spot urines the lowest (0.43–0.47) (all significant at $P < 0.001$ level).

The same order was also found in the correlation coefficients of potassium and sodium/potassium values. The correlations of the potassium concentrations in spot urines with the mean potassium output of three 24-h urine collections were not statistically significant.

The question of how many 24-h urine sodium measurements are needed to characterize individuals for assessing the relationship between salt intake and blood pressure within this population was studied. In our population, sixteen 24-h urine collections would be necessary to distinguish the sodium output in the upper and lower tertiles with $P < 0.05$. This large number was not the result of intraindividual variation ($F_{2;198} = 0.63$, which is nonsignificant), but the result of the relatively small range in the output values. The ratio of intra- to interindividual variance was 9.2, which makes the assessment of a correlation between sodium output and, for example, blood pressure, worthless in this population.

The three-day sodium output averaged 93% of the calculated sodium intake based on the four-day food record. The correlation between the intake and output was 0.61 for the whole time period and 0.55, 0.47, and 0.62 for the three separate days. The detailed data on the sodium intake as well as the value of a short series of questions about the use of certain salty food items are under further analyses.

6. COMMENTS

Compliance is the main problem in a study where the subjects are asked to collect many urine samples and record their food intake. Only 102 (58%) of 177 men and women who entered the study were able to provide complete data. Keeping the food record was not very difficult (87% completed records), but collecting the urines was (61% gave presumably reliable complete collections). In studies correlating individual levels of sodium intake and blood pressure, the problem of compliance is even greater since several urine collections over a long period of time seem to be needed. Even the value of the information on the present intake level is questionable since present blood pressure is probably affected by sodium intake over previous years or decades.

Against this background, cross-sectional observations of the relationship between sodium intake and blood pressure may be inappropriate. More efforts should probably be concentrated on studying sodium intake levels and blood pressures among different population groups.

In group comparisons, a variety of sodium intake estimation methods are available. One 24-h urine collection is best, but the overnight urine collection appears to be adequate. Compliance is better for the latter because of easier collection. The overnight sodium excretion rate is about 90% of the mean 24-h output rate and the rate of potassium is about 65%. Because the rate of potassium excretion is especially low during the night, the overnight Na/K is almost 150% of the 24-h ratio. These under- and overestimations have to be considered if the overnight values are used in the estimations of total outputs rather than between group comparisons.

The use of timed urine samples between early morning and noon is also a possibility in schools or in settings where the subjects can spend many hours at the study site. In other study situations, it may be easier for the subjects to collect overnight urines than to stay at the study site for a long time.

From our data, the value of creatinine as a reference standard and the values of spot urines collected at various times during the day seem to be questionable. If, however, the time range of spot urine collections is narrow enough, the data obtained may be used in group comparisons, but not in estimations of total outputs. Furthermore, the possibilities for methodological standardization are relatively good and, therefore, this simple method could be valuable under certain conditions.

Calculating sodium intakes by food consumption data seems to be worth trying. Although the intake estimates were based on the mean salt content of Finnish food, the correlation between individual intake and output was high and significant. The main use of this estimation is not, however, for measuring individuals, but is for determining dietary salt sources of different population groups. This is important in intervention studies aimed at changing salt consumption.

7. CONCLUSIONS

The problem areas comparing sodium intake and blood pressure are the same as in any dietary epidemiology: first, the choice of cross-sectional studies correlating dietary and biochemical-physiological variables within a population versus studies on the effects of changes in the dietary variable. Secondly, appropriate methods must be developed in both types of studies. So far, the unclear relationship between salt intake and blood pressure has aroused discussions on methodology and study designs which are similar to the discussion in the diet-cholesterol question [52, 53].

Liu and co-workers list several requirements that must be met in surveys assessing the relationship between dietary and biochemical-physiological factors. Among others, the requirements include the following:

1) The sample must be randomly selected and of sufficient size.
2) The problem of intraindividual variation must be overcome by following the sample over an adequate time period.
3) The sample must exclude individuals who have modified their dietary intake.
4) The methods used to estimate dietary intake must be appropriate for classifying individuals.
5) The measurements must be scheduled in such a way as to estimate individual means and intraindividual variations about those means without changing eating patterns.

So far none of the studies searching for a correlation between sodium intake and blood pressure have met these requirements.

Even if the methodological problems can be overcome in diet-cholesterol studies, the problem of a zero correlation may remain even if there is cause and effect [53]. This is caused by the great variances in the factors involved. This seems also to be the case in sodium intake–blood pressure studies. Therefore, cross-sectional study designs may not be suitable for studying this relationship. The emphasis should lie more and more on longitudinal studies that measure changes in sodium intake.

Besides these methodological difficulties, there are also other important reasons why studies attempting to seek evidence for a within-population correlation between salt intake and blood pressure have generally failed. The range of salt intake in a given population is not likely to be large enough to bring out a clear correlation. In most modern societies, the salt intake level greatly exceeds its physiological requirement and thus the effect of salt on blood pressure can be called the saturation effect. That means that almost all persons susceptible to its harmful effects have already been affected by it as much as they likely can [54].

The development of valid methods and study designs is of great importance in clarifying sodium's relation to high blood pressure. General recommendations are needed in order to provide a better basis for comparing studies. There are standard procedures for blood pressure measurement, but very little attention has been paid to standardizing the techniques of measuring those variables that we are trying to associate with blood pressure [1]. Maybe because sodium intake has so long been measured by urinary output, it has been forgotten that it is actually a highly variable dietary factor and not a relatively stable biochemical parameter. Its methodology needs further research so that appropriate and accepted guidelines are available for epidemiological studies.

Acknowledgments. This study was supported by the National Research Council for Agriculture and Forestry in Finland. We gratefully acknowledge the cooperation of Dr. Thomas E. Kottke in editorial assistance.

REFERENCES

1. Liu K, Cooper R, McKeever J, McKeever P, Byington R, Soltero I, Stamler R, Gosch F, Stevens E, Stamler J: Assessment of the association between habitual salt intake and high blood pressure: methodological problems. Am J Epidemiol 110:219-226, 1979.
2. Liu K, Cooper R, McKeever J, McKeever P, Byington R, Stamler R, Stamler J: How many measurements of 24-hour urine Na are needed to characterize an individual for assessment of the relationship between salt intake and blood pressure within a population? (Abstr). In: 8th World Congress of Cardiology, Matsue, Japan, 1978.
3. Farquhar JW, Wood PD, Haskell WL, Williams P, Fortmann SP: Relationship of urinary sodium/potassium ratio to systolic blood pressure: The Stanford three community study (Abstr). In: 18th Conference of Cardiovascular Disease Epidemiology. Orlando, FL: Am Heart Assoc, 1978.
4. Sasaki N: The relationship of salt intake to hypertension in the Japanese. Geriatrics 19:735-744, 1964.
5. Lee KY: A study on sodium chloride of Korean diet. In: Scheniazono N (ed) Influence of environmental and host factors on nutritional requirements. Proceedings of the Symposium sponsored by the Malnutrition Panels of the US-Japan Cooperative Medical Sciences Program, Mt Fuji, Japan, 1974.
6. Komachi T, Iida M, Shimamoto T, Chikayama Y, Takahashi H, Konishi M, Tominaga S: Geographic and occupational comparisons of risk factors in cardiovascular disease in Japan. Jpn Circ J 35:189-207, 1971.
6a.Tillotson JL, Kato H, Nichaman MZ, Miller DC, Gay ML, Johnson KG, Rhoads GG: Epidemiology of coronary heart disease and stroke in Japanese men living in Japan, Hawaii, and California: methodology for comparison of diet. Am J Clin Nutr 26:177-184, 1973.
7. Prior IAM, Evans JG, Harvey HPB, Davidson F, Lindsey M: Sodium intake and blood pressure in two Polynesian populations. N Engl J Med 279:515-520, 1968.
8. Adlin EV, Middle CM, Channick BJ: Dietary salt intake in hypertensive patients with normal and low plasma renin activity. Am J Med Sci 261:67-71, 1971.
9. White HS: Inorganic elements in weighed diets of girls and young women. J Am Diet Assoc 55:38-43, 1969.
10. Abdulla M, Jägerstad M, Svensson S: Kostundersökning med dubbelportionsteknik bland pensionärer i Dalby — natrium och kalium. In: Steen B, Svanborg A (eds) Nordisk Gerontologi. Förhandlingar från Andra Nordiska Kongressen i Gerontologi i Göteborg, 1975. Södertälje: Astra, 1976, p 251.

11. Hankin JH, Huenemann R: A short dietary method for epidemiologic studies. I. Developing standard methods for interpreting 7-day measured food records. J Am Diet Assoc 50:487-492, 1967.
12. Hankin JH, Reynolds WE, Mogen S: A short method for epidemiologic studies. II. Variability of measured nutrient intakes. Am J Clin Nutr 20:935-945, 1967.
13. Hankin JH, Stallones RA, Messinger HB: A short dietary method for epidemiologic studies. III. Development of questionnaire. Am J Epidemiol 87:285-298, 1968.
14. Dahl LK, Love RA: NaCl intake as related to human hypertension. Fed Proc 15:513-523, 1956.
15. Palmero HA, Caeiro A: Epidemiology of hypertension in Cardoba, Argentina. Part II. Blood pressure as a function of body weight, salt consumption and heredity. Medicina (B Aires) 31:404-416, 1971.
16. Swaye PS, Gifford RW, Berrettoni JN: Dietary salt and essential hypertension. Am J Cardiol 29:33-38, 1972.
17. Dawber TR, Kannel WB, Kagan A, Donabedian RK, McNamara PM, Pearson G: Environmental factors in hypertension. In: Stamler J, et al (eds) The epidemiology of hypertension. New York: Grune and Stratton, 1967, pp 255-282.
18. Dahl LK: Sodium intake of the American male: Implications on the etiology of essential hypertension. Am J Clin Nutr 6:1-7, 1958.
19. Kirkendall WM, Connor WE, Abboud F, Rastogi SP, Anderson TA, Fry M: The effect of dietary sodium chloride on blood pressure, body fluids, electrolytes, renal function, and serum lipids on normotensive man. J Lab Clin Med 87:418-434, 1976.
20. Baldwin D, Alexander RW, Warner Jr EG: Chronic sodium chloride challenge studies in man. J Lab Clin Med 55:362-375, 1960.
21. Lee DH: Terrestrial animals in dry heat: Man in the desert. In: Dill DB, et al (eds) Handbook of physiology. Section 4: Adaptation to the environment. Baltimore: Williams and Wilkins, 1964, pp 551-582.
22. Guyton AC: Textbook of medical physiology. Philadelphia: WB Saunders, 1966.
23. Goodhart RS, Shils ME: Modern nutrition in health and disease, 5th edn. Philadelphia: Lea and Febiger, 1973.
24. Geigy scientific tables, 7th edn. Basel: Geigy, 1970.
25. Mickelsen O, Makdani D, Gill JL, Frank RL: Sodium and potassium intakes and excretions of normal men consuming sodium chloride or a 1:1 mixture of sodium and potassium chlorides. Am J Clin Nutr 30:2033-2040, 1978.
26. Grand RJ, Sant'Agnese PA di, Talamo RC, Pallavicini JC: The effects of exogenous aldosterone on sweat electrolytes. I. Normal subjects. J Pediatr 70:346-356, 1967.
27. Langford HG, Watson RL: Electrolytes, environment and blood pressure. Clin Sci Mol Med 45:111-113, 1973.
28. Marr JW: Individual dietary surveys: purposes and methods. World Rev Nutr Diet 13:105-164, 1971.
29. Kesteloot H, Park BC, Lee CS, Joossens JV: An epidemiological survey of blood pressure and sodium excretion in Belgium and Korea. Circulation [Suppl] 55 and 56:III-44, 1977.
30. Vestergaard P, Leverett R: Constancy of urinary creatinine excretion. J Lab Clin Med 51:211-218, 1958.

31. Paterson N: Relative constancy of 24-hour urine volume and 24-hour creatinine output. Clin Chim Acta 18:57-58, 1967.

32. Scott PJ, Hurley PJ: Demonstration of individual variation in constancy of 24-hour urinary creatinine excretion. Clin Chim Acta 21:411-414, 1968.

33. Edwards OM, Bayliss RIS, Millen S: Urinary creatinine excretion as an index of the completeness of 24-hour urine collections. Lancet 2:1165-1166, 1969.

34. Stanbury SW, Thomson AE: Diurnal variations in electrolyte excretion. Clin Sci 10:268-293, 1951.

35. Wesson LG: Electrolyte excretion in relation to diurnal cycles of renal function. Plasma electrolyte concentrations and aldosterone secretion before and during salt and water balance changes in normotensive subjects. Medicine (Baltimore) 43:547-592, 1964.

36. Mills JN: Human circadian rhythms. Physiol Rev 46:128-171, 1966.

37. Wisser H, Doerr P, Stamm D, Fatranska M, Giedke H, Wever R: Tagesperiodik der Ausscheidung von Elektrolyten, Katecholaminmetaboliten und 17-Hydroxy-corticosteroiden im Harn. Clin Wochenschr 51:242-246, 1973.

38. Widdowson EM, McCance RA: Use of random specimens of urine to compare dietary intakes of African and British children. Arch Dis Child 45:549-552, 1970.

39. Dauncey MJ, Widdowson EM: Urinary excretion of calcium, magnesium, sodium and potassium in hard and soft water areas. Lancet 1:711-715, 1972.

40. Moore M, Burgess R, Volosin K, Buckalew Jr V: Spot urinary sodium/creatinine ratio predicts previous day's 24-hour sodium excretion in young essential hypertensives. Prev Med 8:200, 1979.

41. Fukase M: Nutritional improvement for stroke prevention (Abstr). In: Postcongress Satellite Meeting of the 8th World Congress of Cardiology, Matsue, Japan. 1978.

42. Zorab PA, Clark S, Harrison A: Creatinine excretion. Lancet 2:1254, 1969.

43. Curtis G, Fogel M: Creatinine excretion: Diurnal variation and variability of whole and part-day measures. A methodological issue in psychoendocrine research. Psychosom Med 32:337-350, 1970.

44. Langford HG, Watson RL, Douglas BH: Factors affecting blood pressure in population groups. Trans Assoc Am Physicians 81:135-146, 1968.

45. Watson RL, Langford HG: Usefulness of overnight urines in population groups. Pilot studies of sodium, potassium, and calcium excretion. Am J Clin Nutr 23:290-304, 1970.

46. Langford HG, Watson RL: Electrolytes and hypertension. In: Paul O (ed) Epidemiology and control of hypertension. New York: Stratton International Medical, 1975, pp 119-128.

47. Pietinen PI, Findley TW, Clausen JD, Finnerty Jr FA, Altschul AM: Studies in community nutrition: estimation of sodium output. Prev Med 5:400-407, 1976.

48. Pietinen PI, Wong O, Altschul AM: Electrolyte output, blood pressure, and family history of hypertension. Am J Clin Nutr 32:997-1005, 1979.

49. Froment A, Milon H, Vincent M, Dupont J-C, Dupont J: La pression artérielle chez l'enfant d'âge scolaire. Relation avec quelques variables. Bull INSERM 25:1237-1248, 1970.

50. Lucas CP, Ocobock RW, Sozen T, Stern MP, Haskell WL, Holzwarth GJ, Wood PDS, Farquhar JW: Disturbed relationship of plasma-renin to blood pressure in hypertension. Lancet 2:1337-1339, 1974.

51. Puska P, Tuomilehto J, Salonen J, Neittaanmäki L, Mäki J, Virtamo J, Nissinen

A, Koskela K, Takalo T: Changes in coronary risk factors during comprehensive five-year community programme to control cardiovascular diseases (The North Karelia Project). Br Med J 2:1173-1178, 1979.
52. Liu K, Stamler J, Dyer A, McKeever J, McKeever P: Statistical methods to assess and minimize the role of intra-individual variability in obscuring the relationship between dietary lipids and serum cholesterol. J Chronic Dis 31:399-418, 1978.
53. Jacobs Jr DR, Anderson JT, Blackburn H: Diet and serum cholesterol. Do zero correlations negate the relationship? Am J Epidemiol 110:77-87, 1979.
54. Meneely G, Battarbee HD: High sodium-low potassium environment and hypertension. Am J Cardiol 38:768-785, 1976.

3. ELECTROLYTES AND CREATININE IN MULTIPLE 24-HOUR URINE COLLECTIONS (1970–1974)*

J.V. Joossens, J. Claessens, J. Geboers, and J.H. Claes

The main goal of this study is to report the variability between and within persons of 24-h urine constituents. It was undertaken in order to learn about the number of individual samples necessary to characterize a person. Similar previous investigations [1] were limited to blood pressure and to four 24-h urine samples in males (sodium and creatinine only).

Only few aspects of the relationship of urinary sodium and potassium with blood pressure will be dealt with here, since this topic will be extensively covered in the comparison of the data of this study with those from Korea [2].

The reliability and the reproducibility of the home-reading technique for the measurement of blood pressure, as used here, has been established not only over short periods of time, but also after two years [3].

Another aspect of this study deals with the parameters influencing urinary electrolytes and creatinine.

1. METHODS

Because of the necessity to get ten 24-h samples, it was impossible to use a random population sample. Therefore 'normal' volunteers were recruited from different population groups living in Leuven and surroundings:

1) academic, nursing, and laborer personnel of the University Hospital,
2) teachers from different schools,
3) religious communities, and
4) a small residential area, Diependaal, near Leuven.

All volunteers were working regularly and were not under treatment for any chronic disease, especially not for high blood pressure. When, however, a higher blood pressure was detected in a volunteer after entering the study, he would remain in the group.

* Supported by grants from NFWO, Brussels.

H. Kesteloot, J.V. Joossens (eds.), Epidemiology of Arterial Blood Pressure, 45–63.

In total, 300 persons, 133 males and 167 females, participated. They all delivered the ten desired 24-h urine samples. The study lasted from the end of 1970 until 1974.

The volunteers were instructed to read their blood pressure at home [3] four times a day during the day of the urine collection, namely (a) in the morning in the supine position in bed, (b) ±10 min after rising, in the standing position, (c) in the evening before retiring, in the standing position, and (d) in the evening, in the supine position in bed.

The 3-l plastic containers, used for urine sampling, contained 10 ml of glacial acetic and a knife point of powdered thymol, both pro analysi. This was added in order to prevent bacterial or fungal growth and also to prevent precipitation of calcium and magnesium. The mean daily temperature (C°), as measured in Uccle (situated ±25 km from Leuven), was noted on the day of the urine collection. All participants were given careful oral and printed instructions on how to collect 24-h urine samples.

The blood pressure readings and the urine collections were performed on ten nonconsecutive days with at least a five-day interval inbetween. The data-gathering period ranged from three months to two years. The mean interval between the first and the tenth collections amounted to 137 days in males and 143 in females.

The participants were allowed to collect the 24-h urine on the day they preferred, the reason for this being that urinary sodium excretion has a time lag of about two days in normal subjects; 679 samples from men and 878 from women were collected on weekdays; 651 and 792, respectively, were obtained during the weekend.

In total, 3000 24-h urine collections and 12,000 blood pressure readings were performed. Sodium and potassium were determined by standard flame photometry, and calcium by EDTA titration [4], after removal of phosphates [5]. Magnesium was analysed by atom absorption spectrophotometry (with $LaCl_3$ precipitation of sulfates and phosphates) and creatinine on a Technicon Autoanalyser I [6, 7].

Some of the results will be compared with data (population A2 + A3 = A2, 3) [8] by using only one casual blood pressure reading and one 24-h urine collection (males, $n = 1114$, females, $n = 412$). These subjects were also living in Leuven and surroundings and were studied between 1968 and 1969. They belonged to similar age groups, the average social class, however, was sowewhat lower. Multiple linear regression was performed with stepwise downward regression until all regression coefficients were at least significant with $P < 0.05$. The mean value of ten observations of each variable was used for computation ($n = 133$ or 167). In order to test the linearity of the independent variables, powers 1 to 5 of the variable minus the mean value were added for sodium, potassium, age, weight, and height. The results of these

Table 1. Average values from ten 24-h urine collections and 40 blood pressure home readings: mean in 133 males.

	Mean	SD	SE	% Variat. coeff.	Min. value	5th perc.	95th perc.	Max. value
Sodium (mmol/24 h)	184	45	3.9	24.2	35	116	253	303
Potassium (mmol/24 h)	77	15.4	1.3	20.1	32	51	103	126
Calcium (mmol/24 h)	6.4	1.86	0.16	29.0	3.1	3.7	9.5	12.4
Magnesium (mmol/24 h)	4.4	0.87	0.075	19.7	2.8	3.0	5.7	8.1
Creatinine (g/24 h)	1.83	0.27	0.023	14.8	0.99	1.41	2.21	2.46
Height (cm)	174	6.4	0.56	3.7	156	163	185	189
Weight (kg)	75	10.8	0.94	14.3	54	58	93	102
Age (years)	39.3	11.0	0.96	28.1	21	23	58	66
Systolic blood pressure	121	12.6	1.1	10.4	98	104	143	183
Diastolic blood pressure	78	8.6	0.74	10.9	63	65	94	103

Table 2. Average values from ten 24-h urine collections and 40 blood pressure home readings: mean in 167 females.

	Mean	SD	SE	% Variat. coeff.	Min. value	5th perc.	95th perc.	Max. value
Sodium (mmol/24 h)	153	44	3.4	28.7	59	86	236	314
Potassium (mmol/24 h)	65	12.5	0.97	19.2	31	46	87	112
Calcium (mmol/24 h)	5.3	1.56	0.12	29.2	2.0	3.3	7.9	10.7
Magnesium (mmol/24 h)	3.8	0.74	0.057	19.3	1.7	2.9	5.2	6.8
Creatinine (g/24 h)	1.28	0.20	0.016	15.8	0.82	0.97	1.62	2.00
Height (cm)	161	6.4	0.49	3.9	145	150	171	176
Weight (kg)	61	8.2	0.64	13.6	42	48	77	84
Age (years)	40	12	0.95	30.5	19	22	61	80
Systolic blood pressure	115	13.9	1.07	12.1	91	97	142	164
Diastolic blood pressure	73	8.4	0.65	11.5	54	59	87	98

Table 3. Individual observations.

	Males (n = 130)				Females (n = 170)			
	SD	% variat. coeff.	Min. value	Max. value	SD	% variat. coeff.	Min. value	Max. value
Sodium (mmol/24 h)	68	37.0	20	579	60	39.3	16	453
Potassium (mmol/24 h)	23	29.5	6.7	181	19	29.4	15	187
Calcium (mmol/24 h)	2.5	38.9	0.90	18.6	2.1	39.9	0.87	18.2
Magnesium (mmol/24 h)	1.3	29.6	1.2	15.4	1.1	29.7	0.66	12.3
Creatinine (g/24 h)	0.40	21.8	0.48	3.88	0.29	22.9	0.22	3.37
Systolic blood pressure	13	10.8	94	190	14.4	12.6	86	180
Diastolic blood pressure	9	11.6	57	106	8.9	12.2	48	111

Table 4. Significant correlation coefficients ($P<0.05$ or less): males $n = 133$.

	K	Ca	Mg	Creat.	Height	Weight	Social class	Age	SBP	DBP
Na (mmol/24 h)	0.27	0.27	0.26	0.21	—	—	0.21	—	—	—
K (mmol/24 h)		—	0.38	0.51	—	0.20	—	—	—	—
Ca (mmol/24 h)			0.26	0.27	—	—	—	—	—	—
Mg (mmol/24 h)				0.30	—	—	—	—	—	—
Creatinine (g/24 h)					0.32	0.55	-0.18	-0.25	—	—
Height						0.38	-0.19	-0.23	—	—
Weight							-0.21	—	0.28	0.30
Social class (I – V)								—	—	—
Age									0.48	0.48
Systolic blood pressure										0.76

Mean daily temperature was not significantly related to any variable.

Table 5. Significant correlation coefficients ($P<0.05$ or less): females $n = 167$.

	K	Ca	Mg	Creat.	Height	Weight	Social class	Mean $r°$	Age	SBP	DBP
Na (mmol/24 h)	0.48	0.24	0.37	0.43	0.16	0.27	0.18	-0.27	—	—	0.18
K (mmol/24 h)		0.27	0.41	0.54	0.29	0.29	—	—	—	—	—
Ca (mmol/24 h)			0.38	0.22	—	0.16	—	—	—	—	—
Mg (mmol/24 h)				0.34	0.16	0.26	—	—	—	—	—
Creatinine (g/24 h)					0.46	0.42	-0.16	—	-0.26	-0.16	—
Height						0.33	-0.33	—	-0.30	0.24	0.26
Weight							—	—	0.19	—	—
Social class (I – V)								—	—	—	—
Mean $r°$									-0.44	-0.23	-0.34
Age										0.52	0.57
Systolic blood pressure											0.67

Table 6. One-way analysis of variance.

Variable	Males				Females			
	S^2a $df=1197$	S^2r $df=132$	Ratio $\dfrac{S^2a}{S^2r}$	Number k of samples required for $P>0.95$	S^2a $df=1503$	S^2r $df=166$	Ratio $\dfrac{S^2a}{S^2r}$	Number k of samples required for $P>0.95$
Sodium (mmol/24 h)	2947.99	1987.25	1.484	14	1880.54	1917.74	0.981	9
Potassium (mmol/24 h)	306.66	238.39	1.286	12	236.01	156.66	1.507	14
Calcium (mmol/24 h)	3.072	3.462	0.887	8	2.364	2.424	0.976	9
Magnesium (mmol/24 h)	1.049	0.757	1.386	13	0.837	0.550	1.522	14
Creatinine (g/24 h)	0.0947	0.0732	1.293	12	0.0498	0.0408	1.222	11
Systolic blood pressure	17.04	158.06	0.108	1	19.02	192.07	0.099	1
Diastolic blood pressure	10.69	73.55	0.145	1	10.95	70.09	0.156	1

S^2a is the intraindividual variance, S^2r is the interindividual variance and df = degrees of freedom. For estimation of k, see text.

computations will be provided only if they markedly and significantly increased the value of the correlation coefficient. Multiple correlation using powers of variables is the best technique to ascertain significant nonlinearity and at the same time to quantify the effect of nonlinearity.

The one-way analysis of variance directly provided the intraindividual variance S^2a and the interindividual variance S^2r and was calculated according to the method described by Wonnacott and Wonnacott[9]. The number of samples necessary to limit the reduction of the real correlation coefficient, e.g., between blood pressure and urinary sodium, was estimated according to the method described by Liu et al.[1]. This reduction of the value of the real correlation coefficient is due a.o. to the intraindividual variation of, for example, sodium in 24-h urine specimens. The number of required samples (k) to limit the diminution to less than 100 $(1-p)$ percent, with $0 < p < 1$, can be estimated from $k = p^2 / (1-p^2) \times S^2a/S^2r$.

2. RESULTS AND DISCUSSION

The mean values and other parameters of the variables are listed in Tables 1 and 2 ($n = 133$ or 167). The values obtained from the total 1330 or 1670 observations are listed in Table 3. The significant simple correlations are given in Tables 4 and 5. The analysis of variance together with the number of

Table 7. Observed minimum and maximum of average values of one urine sample (out of ten) or of four blood pressure readings.

	Males ($n = 133$)		Females ($n = 167$)	
	Minimum	Maximum ±SE	Minimum	Maximum ±SE
Sodium (mmol/24 h)	174.0 ±5.5 (9)	193.8 ±5.6 (5)	149.0 ±4.5 (3)	155.7 ±4.8 (2)
Potassium (mmol/24 h)	74.1 ±1.9 (9)	79.2 ±2.2 (3)	64.3 ±1.6 (10)	66.4 ±1.5 (3)
Calcium (mmol/24 h)	6.19±0.19 (2)	6.66±0.21 (7)	5.25±0.16 (3)	5.45±0.16 (7)
Magnesium (mmol/24 h)	4.31±0.11 (8)	4.48±0.13 (3)	3.74±0.08 (3)	3.97±0.10 (6)
Creatinine (g/24 h)	1.77±0.034 (8)	1.86±0.035 (7)	1.25±0.021 (5)	1.31±0.027 (3)
Systolic blood pressure	120.9 ±1.1 (4)	121.9 ±1.2 (1)	113.6 ±1.07 (6)	115.8 ±1.15 (1)
Diastolic blood pressure	78.0 ±0.82 (7)	79.0 ±0.81 (1)	72.6 ±0.67 (10)	73.5 ±0.73 (1)

The number in brackets indicates the number of the sample where the minimum or maximum was observed.

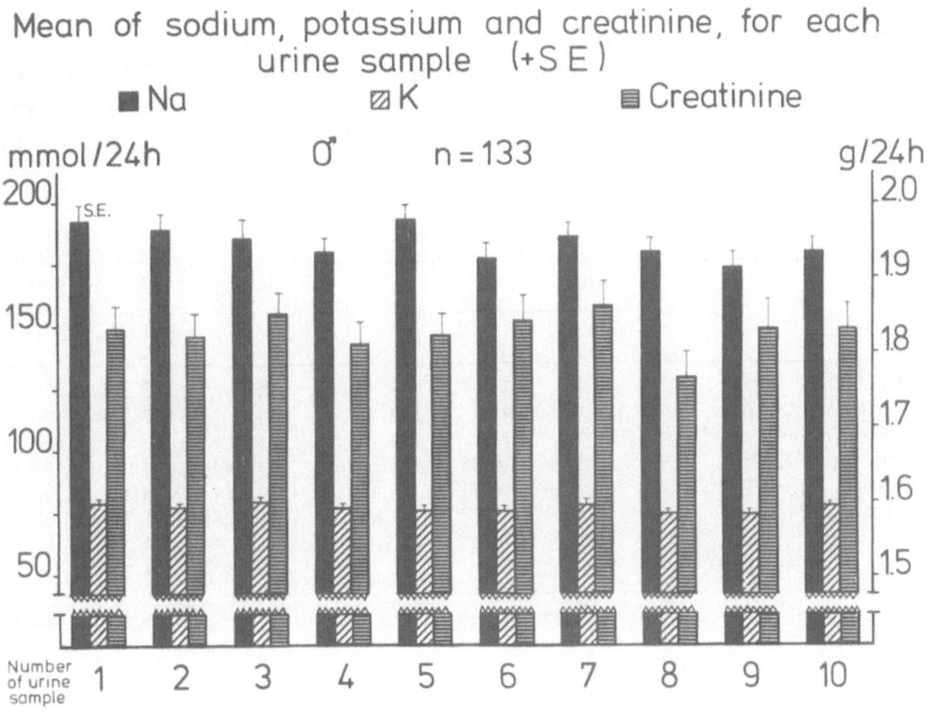

Figure 1. The first and second bar refer to sodium and potassium, respectively, with the left-hand scale; the third one is from creatinine with the right-hand scale.

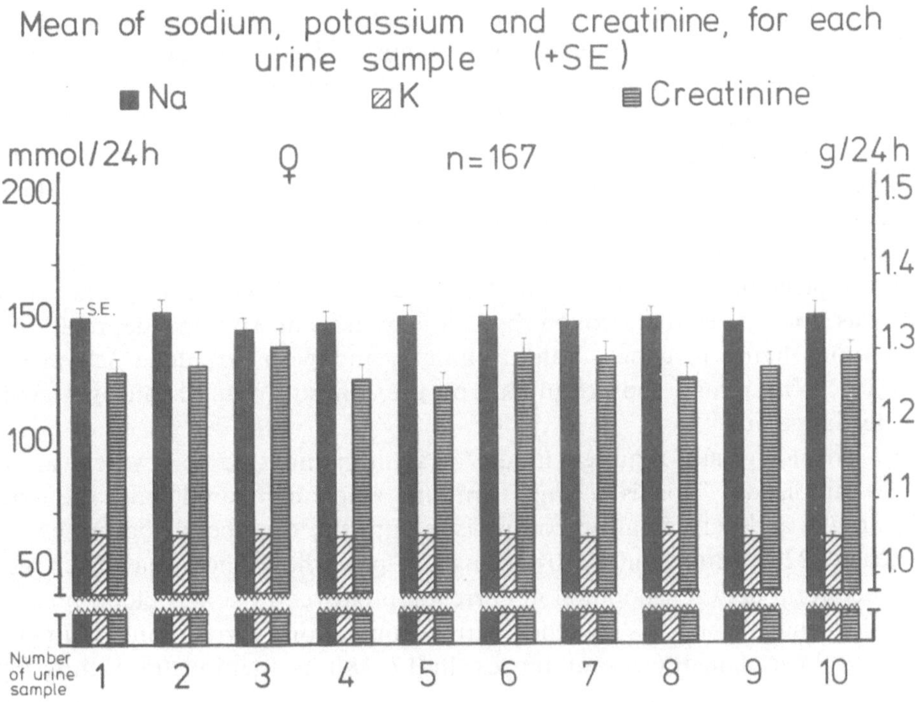

Figure 2. See text in Figure 1.

required samples is given in Table 6. The range of mean urinary electrolytes and creatinine excretion and blood pressure in ten groups of only one urine sample is listed in Table 7 and illustrated for each sample in Figures 1 and 2. The reproducibility of values from small groups of several individuals while using means of ten samples is given in Table 8.

Table 8. Mean values of terciles according to date of entry in the study.

	Males			Females		
	I	II	III	I	II	III
n Individuals	45	44	44	56	55	56
Sodium (mmol/24 h)	166	193	194	146	152	160
Potassium (mmol/24 h)	79	77	74	64	66	66
Calcium (mmol/24 h)	6.34	6.25	6.66	5.47	5.54	5.02
Magnesium (mmol/24 h)	4.52	4.22	4.48	3.84	3.84	3.85
Creatinine (g/24 h)	1.86	1.82	1.80	1.28	1.34	1.22
Systolic blood pressure	119	124	121	114	114	116
Diastolic blood pressure	77	81	78	74	71	73

Each individual value was the average of ten values for urine samples and 40 for blood pressure.

2.1. Sodium

The frequency distributions of sodium and creatinine are presented in Figure 3. The 24-h sodium excretion is most likely an important population health parameter [10–13]. It is almost equal to the intake of sodium, since the kidney carefully monitors the sodium balance (see discussion in [14]). A minute error would result in either a positive or negative sodium balance, both being most dangerous situations. The only other source of sodium loss is by perspiration of through the feces. This is in general only a small percentage of the total intake. The mineral content of the perspiration adapts itself to the total intake of sodium. This had already been shown 30 years ago [15] and was more recently proven by the absence of sodium deprivation in populations living in a hot, humid climate, and with no added salt in their food [16]. With a high sodium intake, on the contrary, loss of salt by sweating can be dangerous.

The physiologically required intake of sodium must be somewhere around 10–30 mmol/day. This is a small amount when compared with the actual daily intake and very small in comparison with the total body sodium content of nearly 2200 mmol for a 70-kg man. Up to now there has been good evidence for a between-population correlation between Na and blood pressure. This has not been so for the within-population correlation. Numerous attempts have failed (see references in [17, 18]) to demonstrate this. This

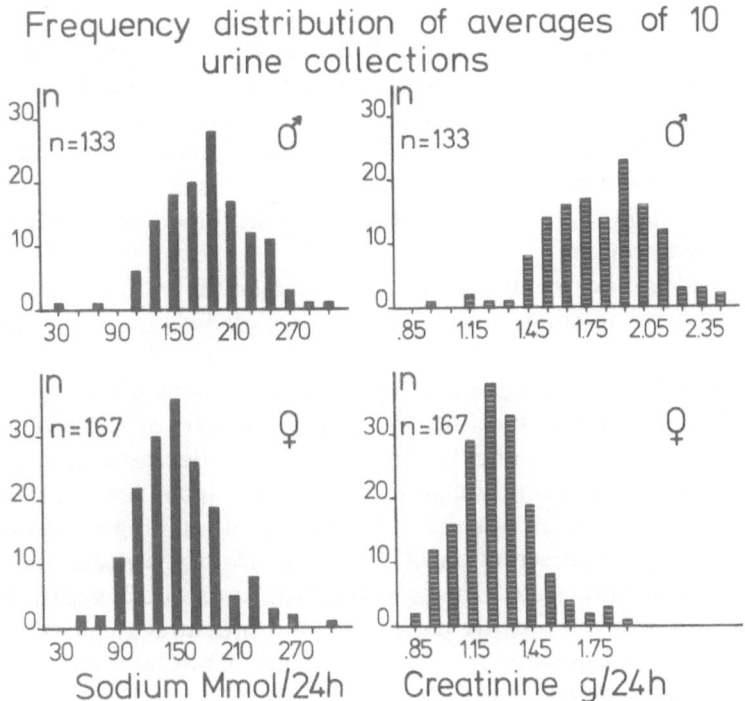

Figure 3.

situation exists also for serum cholesterol in relation to saturated fat intake. It must, however, be realized that a within-population zero correlation for a given parameter is no proof against a possible causal relation [19].

Many factors may confound the within-population salt–blood pressure relationship:

1) The measurement of blood pressure, although technically simple, has a great within-person variability due to neurohumeral factors and to the disturbing influence of the observer [20]. This influence is sharply reduced by the multiple home-reading technique used in this study.
2) Repeated measurements over time show, in general, a downward trend, indicating that the first readings were too high as in the Framingham study; again this was not observed with the home-reading technique [3].
3) Salt intake measured by 24-h urine excretion has a huge variation coefficient, due to real differences in day-to-day salt intake and to spurious ones resulting from under- or overcollection of 24-h samples (Tables 1–3 and 6). In western populations, the real range of salt intake between persons, if it could be measured by continuous monitoring, is probably not as large as suggested by the collection of one 24-h sample. In this study, the variation

coefficient in a single person ranged between 11% and 50% in males and between 8% and 55% in females. In a group of individuals giving each one sample, it was around 36% in males and 40% in females; for the same group with the average of ten samples, it dropped to 24% in males and 29% in females. The real range of variation of the independent variable, in casu salt, must be smaller than the observed one, making it difficult to prove a relation with the dependent variable (blood pressure) through the regression technique.

4) Many studies have been performed with relatively small groups, although some studies utilizing large groups have failed to prove the association [21].

5) The values of sodium excretion measured in a given period, even using ten or more samples, are probably not representative of the average lifetime salt intake. In some countries, an unconscious decrease in salt intake has been documented, as in Belgium [22, 23], in Japan [24], and in Switzerland [25]. This probably results from the use of cooling techniques instead of salting for the preservation of food, and from the decreasing consumption of bread, lard, salted meat, salted fish, and salted vegetables.

6) People with an even slightly elevated blood pressure frequently lower their salt intake, which results in a negative relationship between blood pressure and sodium excretion.

7) The most important confounding factor is probably the genetic one. The salt hypothesis states that salt is a necessary condition for essential hypertension, but not a sufficient one. Genetic factors may be active here, making people resistant to salt intake. This point has been conclusively proved in rats [26]. Ten Berge-Van der Schaaf [27] has shown a significant relation of urinary sodium with blood pressure in a group of schoolchildren, when their mothers were hypertensives, but not in the others.

In this study a positive and independent (independent of weight, age, height, and powers of these values) relation between sodium excretion and blood pressure was found under certain conditions only [2]. It can be noted that the variation coefficient of sodium was higher in females. The main reasons for the partial failure are probably factors 3) and 5)–7). The most important relations between sodium excretion and other factors are given in Table 9 for males, females, and both sexes together. Creatinine in 24-h urine is by far the most potent factor, but is different between sexes; then comes social class, age, and environmental temperature. Weight is a much weaker determinant.

The combined data of both study groups and of both sexes ($n = 1826$, Table 9) showed an independent sex difference of 42 mmol/24 h for urinary sodium, when the other factors such as urinary creatinine, social class, sex,

Table 9. Determinants of 24-h urinary sodium (mmol): significant multiple regression coefficients ± standard deviation.

Variable	This population (1970–74) (mean of 10 samples)		Population A2, 3 (1968–69) (unique sample)		Total group [c]
	♂	♀	♂	♀	♂+♀
$n =$	133	167	1114	412	1826
Creatinine (g/24 h)	50.0 ±14.2	101.5 ±14.3	67.7 ±4.0	101.7 ±8.0	83.1 ±4.3
Creatinine x sex[a]					−15.4 ±4.1
Social class	10.8 ± 3.3	8.2 ± 2.4	6.2 ±1.5	b	6.6 ±1.1
Age	0.69± 0.34		0.32±0.16	b	0.47±0.12
Environmental temperature C°		−2.71± 0.71	−0.59±0.28		− 0.56±0.21
Weight			0.41±0.18		0.31±0.14
Group[a]					− 5.4 ±1.8
Sex[a]					20.8 ±5.9
Constant factor	40.0	24.4	25.1	27.1	2.16
Multiple correlation coefficient	0.37	0.56	0.51	0.53	0.58

[a] Sex = +1 for males and −1 for females; group = +1 for this study and −1 for population A2, 3.

[b] Social class was nearly significant with a regression coefficient of 6.6±3.4; for age this amounted to 0.56±0.33.

[c] The total group was also checked for factors such as weight and age and powers of up to 5 of these factors, plus the same factors multiplied by +1 in males and −1 in females. None of these was significant except the first power of age and weight.

Table 10.

	n	Sodium	Potassium	Calcium	Magnesium	Creatinine	SBP	DBP
Mean values from males								
Weekdays	679	176.2	75.5	6.32	4.38	1.788	123.2[a]	79.6
Weekend	651	177.1	73.8	6.10	4.17	1.862	119.8[a]	77.6
Mean values from females								
Weekdays	878	172.9	74.5	6.04	4.36[a]	1.257	115.1	73.2
Weekend	792	167.7	71.7	5.87	4.25[a]	1.305	113.8	72.6

All electrolytes were corrected for creatinine; for males $\dfrac{\times 1.77}{\text{obs. creat.}}$; for females $\dfrac{\times 1.77}{\text{obs. creat.} + 0.3}$; electrolytes in mmol/24 h, creatinine in g/24 h.

[a] Significant difference $P < 0.05$, between the mean values obtained the weekdays ($n = 5$) and those obtained during the weekend ($n = 2$). SBP = systolic blood pressure; DBP = diastolic blood pressure.

age, weight, and environmental T° were accounted for. There was an independent significant difference of about 11 mmol/24 h between the A2,3 group from 1968–69 and the one from 1970–74. This is probably related to the secular downward trend of sodium intake since the introduction of the refrigeration technique [22–25]. Although the influence of weight on sodium excretion is weak, there was a positive independent association in the total group and in males from the A2,3 group. A higher weight associated with higher sodium excretion could provide at least a partial explanation of the obesity–hypertension relationship. The independent and negative relationship of sodium with environmental temperature amounts to 0.6 mmol less for each increase of 1 °C. Of course this could be higher in countries where more extreme temperatures are noted.

The influence of the day of the week is given in Table 10. There was no significant difference between the mean values of urinary electrolytes (corrected for creatinine) and creatinine collected on weekdays and during the two days of the weekend, except for magnesium from females. It can, however, be noted that in general creatinine content has a tendency to be slightly higher during weekends, whereas the opposite is true for electrolytes 7 times out of 8. Liu et al. [1] observed a 5% – 10% lower excretion of sodium during

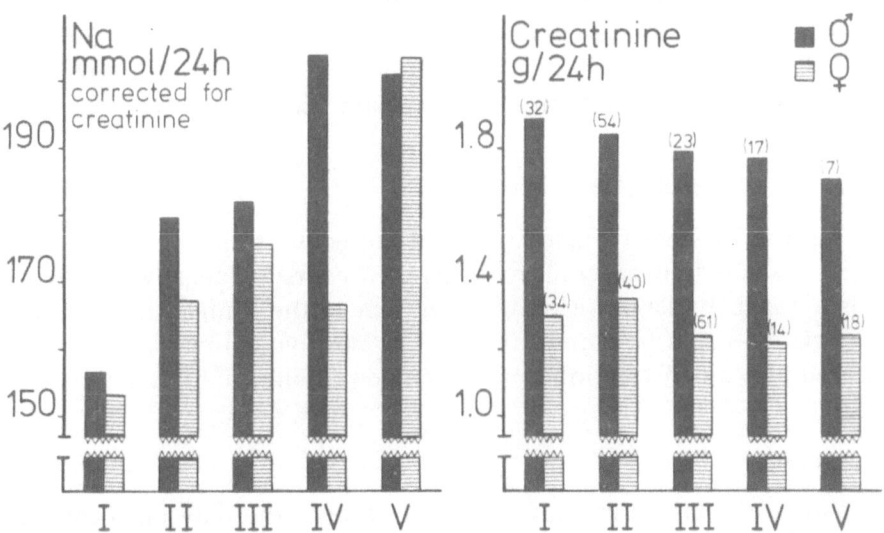

Figure 4. Total number is 133 for males and 167 for females. Each value of sodium and creatinine is the mean of *n* average values of 10 samples; *n* is indicated for creatinine only at the top of each bar between brackets and is identical for the respective value of sodium. Sodium is corrected for creatinine (see text).

weekends, which seems larger than the differences observed here (0% in males and 3% in females). No significant difference was observed between the mean values observed during weekdays and during weekend for age, height, weight, and systolic and diastolic blood pressure, except for males where a 3.4-mm lower systolic blood pressure was observed during the weekend. Since the data from urine collections during the weekend are sufficiently representative of the population values, this practice can be recommended with safety.

Figure 4 illustrates the importance of social class on sodium excretion. The significant relationship between social class and sodium excretion can be deduced from the fact that cheap food is general heavily salted, e.g., bread, cheese, prepared meat, smoked meat and fish, and lard. This kind of food is generally used by the lower socioeconomic classes. It gives an explanation for the existing relation between social classes and blood pressure [28] and stroke mortality [29]. Those findings, because of the possible relation between salt intake and stomach cancer]30], are also consistent with the observed social-class gradient in stomach cancer [31, 32].

2.2. Potassium

Experimental [33] and epidemiological evidence [2] shows that potassium may be important. The only important, significant relationship was with creatinine and weight (in males and females, separately), but the fact that the correlation with weight was no longer significant when creatinine was included as a second independent variable indicates a spurious association. There was an indication of a higher potassium excretion with higher social classes.

2.3. Calcium and magnesium

Urinary calcium has been singled out as a protective factor against hypertension [34]. This could not be confirmed here. Of course, a negative result never excludes a possible relation, it only shows that in the sample under study no such association could be demonstrated. The positive correlation with weight disappeared also when creatinine was included in the multiple regression.

2.4. Creatinine

The importance of creatinine lies in the fact that is the only practical way to test the accuracy of the urine collection in a group. For this reason, the multiple regression analysis of creatinine on its most important factors was studied and the results compared and combined with previous findings in 1526 persons where only a single 24-h urine sample was taken.

Figures 5 and 6 make it possible to estimate 24-h creatinine in both sexes, knowing weight, age, and height. Weight is by far the most important factor. From the combined data of both sexes, it can be derived that for equal weight, height, and age, there still subsists a difference in creatinine excretion between males and females. As best estimate up to now, a difference of 0.3 g/24 h can be taken.

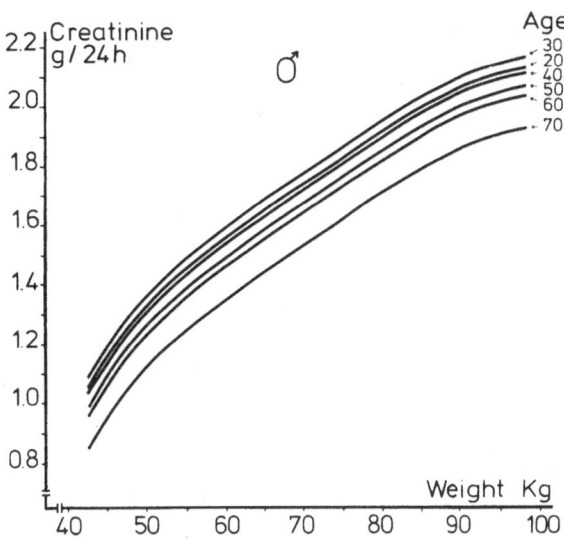

Figure 5. Urinary creatinine in males in function of weight and age for a given height of 175 cm and an average social class II. Notice that excretion at age 30 is higher than at age 20 or 40. This figure was obtained from multiple polynomial regression with $n=1826$, resulting from the combination of 300 values from this study and 1526 from population group A2,3 (see text). The regression equation is valid for both sexes and given in Figure 6.

Using the same equation (see Fig. 6) the mean creatinine excretion was estimated from data of age, weight, height, sex, and social class, as given by Simpson[35] in New Zealand. For the total group of males, 1.78 g/24 h was calculated versus an observed one of 1.82 g; for the total group of females, this was 1.28 g and 1.28 g, respectively.

In several 24-h specimens over- and undercollection is quite frequent (Table 3). This can at least partially be prevented by using more samples (Tables 1 and 2).

Creatinine is lower in lower social classes even when taking into account all other factors. This can be a real difference, but the odds are that less careful collection in certain groups also contributes to the difference.

60

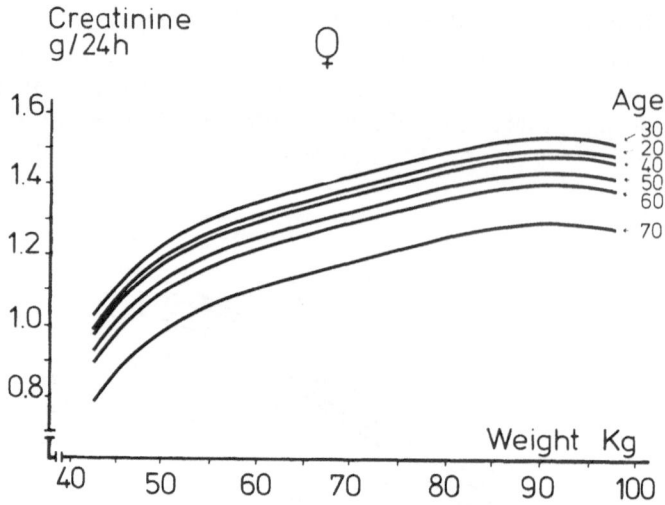

Figure 6. As in Figure 5, but now for females and a given height of 160 cm, with W = weight in kg, A = age, H = height in cm, SC = social class, ΔW = weight $-$ 69.563, ΔA = age $-$ 37.3028, and Sex = $+1$ in males and -1 in females.
The regression equation equals: Urinary creatinine g/24 h = 0.34 + 0.012739 W + 0.0053669 ΔW $\times$ Sex + 0.14642 $\times$ Sex $-$ 0.00000027811(ΔW)^4 + 0.0000000033894(ΔW)^5 $-$ 0.0061216 A + 0.000012985 (ΔA)^3 $-$ 0.000000400166 (ΔA)^4 + 0.0036177 H $-$ 0.01935 SC.
Total R = 0.61.

3. SUMMARY

Ten 24-h specimens of urine in 133 males and 167 females were analyzed for sodium, potassium, calcium, magnesium, and creatinine. Blood pressure was measured four times by using the home-reading technique on the day of urine collection. In total, 3000 24-h urine samples were analyzed together with 12,000 blood pressure readings.

The day of the urine collection (weekday or weekend) was noted and so was the average temperature of that day in Uccle.

A significant independent contribution of sodium to blood pressure was found under certain conditions only. The reasons for the lack of within-country correlations between both parameters have been discussed. Age, weight, sex, and environmental temperature (in females only) were the other parameters to influence blood pressure.

The day-to-day variability of constituents of 24-h urine collections can be very large. From an analysis of variance, it was determined that 9–14 24-h samples were needed to characterize an individual in terms of average electrolytes and creatinine excretion with $P>0.95$. One-day blood pressure recording (mean of four values) with the home-reading technique was enough to characterize a given person.

A single 24-h urine specimen is enough for mean population studies. When, for example, a standard error of about 3 mmol Na/24 h is satisfactory, a sample size of about 500 people is recommended.

Differences between electrolytes and creatinine from 24-h urine obtained on weekdays and during weekends are small. There is even an indication that samples are more complete on weekends. Therefore weekend collection is advised for population studies.

Urinary sodium is independently and positively determined by urinary creatinine, sex, social class (higher in lower classes), age and weight, and negatively by environmental temperature. The association with social class is important in relation to the existing blood pressure gradient among those classes. The association with weight can provide a partial explanation of the obesity–hypertension relationship.

Urinary creatinine is independently and positively related to weight, sex, height, and negatively to social class. Between 24 and 35 years, age is not important. Urinary creatinine excretion is lower outside those age limits.

Graphs are provided to estimate the creatinine excretion of a population, when the previously mentioned variables are known. They can be used to get an idea about the completeness of the collected specimens. Although morning specimens can be used to learn about local gradients of salt intake, this is not recommended for international comparisons.

For comparisons between countries, it is strongly advised to standardize the sodium and potassium excretion against an arbitrarily selected value of creatinine. In our studies this has been 1.77 g creatinine for males (mean of study A2,3).

$$\text{standardized Na} = \frac{\text{observed Na} \times 1.77}{\text{observed creatinine in g/24 h}}$$

The same factor can be used for females, but the standardized value is then overestimated. To correct this, an alternative formula can be used for females.

$$\text{standardized Na} = \frac{\text{observed Na} \times 1.77}{\text{observed creatinine (g/24 h)} + 0.30}$$

When the influence of age, social class, height, and weight has been removed, 0.30 g creatinine is the independent difference between sexes.

62

REFERENCES

1. Liu K, Cooper R, McKeever J, McKeever P, Byington R, Soltero I, Stamler R, Gosh F, Stevens E, Stamler J: Assessment of the association between habitual salt intake and high blood pressure. Am J Epidemiol 110:219-226, 1979.
2. Kesteloot H, Park BC, Lee CS, Brems-Heyns E, Claessens J, Joossens JV: A comparative study of blood pressure and sodium intake in Belgium and in Korea. In this book, chapter 28.
3. Joossens JV, Brems-Heyns E, Claessens J: The value of home blood pressure recordings. A tool for epidemiological studies. In: Kesteloot H (ed) Methodology and standardisation of non-invasive blood pressure measurement in epidemiological studies. Brussels: CRM/CREST, 1976, pp 51-68.
4. Holtz A, Seekles L: Direct titration of calcium in bloodserum. Nature 169:870-871, 1952.
5. Horner W: The determination of calcium in biological material. J Lab Clin Med 45:951-957, 1955.
6. Jaffé M: Über den Niederschlag, welchen Picrinsäure in normalen Harn erzeugt und über eine neue Reaktion des Kreatinins. Z Physiol Chem 10:391-400, 1886.
7. Chasson A, Grady H, Stanley M: Determination of creatinine by mean of automatic chemical analysis. Am J Clin Pathol 35:83-88, 1961.
8. Joossens JV, Willems J, Claessens J, Claes JH, Lissens W: Sodium and hypertension. In: Fidanza F, Keys A, Ricci G, Somogyi JC (eds) Nutrition and cardiovascular diseases. Rome: Morgagni Edizioni Scientifiche, 1971, pp 91-110.
9. Wonnacott TH, Wonnacott RJ: Introductory statistics, 3rd edn. New York: John Wiley and Sons, 1977.
10. Dahl LK: Salt and hypertension. Am J Clin Nutr 25:231-244, 1972.
11. Freis ED: Salt, volume and the prevention of hypertension. Circulation 53:589-595, 1976.
12. Joossens JV, Brems-Heyns E: Cerebrovasculaire sterfte, maagkankersterfte en zoutverbruik. Tijdschr Soc Geneeskd 53:530-542, 1975.
13. Joossens JV: Dietary salt restriction. The case in favour. Proc R Soc Med (in press) 1980.
14. Pietinen P, Tuomilehto J: Estimating sodium intake in epidemiological studies: review and results of methodological pilot study in Finland. In this book, chapter 2.
15. Conn JW: The mechanism of acclimatization to heat. Adv Intern Med 3:373-393, 1949.
16. Oliver WJ, Cohen EL, Neel JV: Blood pressure, sodium intake and sodium related hormones in the Yanomamo Indians, a 'no-salt' culture. Circulation 52:146-151, 1975.
17. Joossens JV: Salt and hypertension, water hardness and cardiovascular death rate. Triangle 12:9-16, 1973.
18. Simpson FO: Dietary salt restriction. The case against. Proc R Soc Med (in press) 1980.
19. Jacobs DR, Anderson JT, Blackburn H: Diet and serum cholesterol: do zero correlations negate the relationship? Am J Epidemiol 110:77-87, 1979.
20. Armitage P, Rose GA: The variability of measurements of casual blood pressure. Clin Sci 30:325-335, 1966.

21. Simpson FO, Waal-Manning HJ, Bolli P, Phelan EL, Spears GFS: Relationship of blood pressure to sodium excretion in a population survey. Clin Sci Mol Med 55:573S-575S, 1978.
22. Joossens JV: De epidemiologische betekenis van het keukenzout. In: Gerlings PG, Birkenhäger WH, Van Es JC, Joossens JV (eds) Het Medisch Jaar 78. Utrecht: Bohn, Scheltema and Holkema, 1980, pp 17-31.
23. Kesteloot H, Vuylsteke M, Costenoble A: Relationship between blood pressure and sodium and potassium intake in a Belgian male population group. In this book, chapter 20.
24. Komachi Y, Shimamoto T: Salt intake and its relationship to blood pressure in Japan. Present and past. In this book, chapter 24.
25. Société des salines suisses du Rhin réunis: La situation actuelle du sel iodé en Suisse. Schweizerhalle, Switzerland, 1980.
26. Dahl LK, Heine M, Tassinari L: Effects of chronic salt ingestion. J Exp Med 115:1173-1190, 1962.
27. Ten Berge-Van der Schaaf J: Onderzoek naar het verband tussen bloeddruk en zoutverbruik bij kinderen. Thesis, Groningen, 1979.
28. Kesteloot H, Van Houte O: An epidemiological survey of arterial blood pressure in a large male population group. Am J Epidemiol 99:14-29, 1974.
29. Howard J, Holman BL: The effect of race and occupation on hypertension mortality. Milbank Mem Fund Q 48:263-296, 1970.
30. Joossens JV: Stroke, stomach cancer and salt. A possible clue to the prevention of hypertension. This volume, chapter 30.
31. Clemessen J: Statistical studies in malignant neoplasms.   Munksgaard, 1965.
32. Stukonis M, Dahl R: Gastric cancer in man and physical activity at work. Int J Cancer 4:248-254, 1969.
33. Meneely GR, Battarbee HD: High sodium–low potassium environment and hypertension. Am J Cardiol 38:768-785, 1976.
34. Langford HG, Watson RL: Electrolytes, environment and blood pressure. Clin Sci Mol Med [Suppl 1] 45:111S-113S, 1973.
35. Simpson FO, Nye ER, Bolli P, Waal-Manning HJ, Goulding AW, Phelan EL, Hamel FA de, Stewart RDH, Spears GFS, Leek GM, Stewart AC: The Milton Survey, Part 1. General methods: height, weight and 24-hour excretion of sodium, potassium, calcium, magnesium and creatinine. NZ Med J 87:379-382, 1978.

4. RECOMMENDATIONS OF THE WORKING GROUP ON THE METHODOLOGY AND STANDARDIZATION OF NON-INVASIVE BLOOD PRESSURE MEASUREMENT IN EPIDEMIOLOGICAL STUDIES *

H. KESTELOOT and J.V. JOOSSENS

The recommendations of the working group on the methodology and standardization of non-invasive blood pressure measurement are presented in addition to the proposals made by the American Heart Association [1] and the World Health Organization [2]. The primary goal is to standardize the methodology of blood pressure measurement in order to assure a maximum of comparability between different epidemiological studies.

1. NECESSARY INFORMATION ABOUT THE POPULATION GROUP STUDIED

1.1. Minimum requirements

1) General description of the population group examined (e.g. rural or citadine, industrial or farmer, etc.)
2) Way in which the population group was obtained (e.g. by random sampling or not, voluntarily or compulsory)
3) Minimum anthropometric data: age, height, weight, sex, and heart rate.

1.2. Optional data

1) Social class, graded 1–4, both for level of education and level of income (1—highest class)
2) Marital status (married, single, or divorced)
3) Number of children
4) Number of subjects taking medication against hypertension
   — type of medication
     – diuretics
     – ganglion blockers
     – centrally acting drugs
     – beta-receptor blockers

---

* Workshop organized in Leuven, Belgium, on 6–7 December 1974, by CRM (Chairman: Prof. Dr. H. Kesteloot).

H. Kesteloot, J.V. Joossens (eds.), Epidemiology of Arterial Blood Pressure, 65–68.

5) Arm circumference at mid-cuff place
6) For women
   — pregnant or not
   — taking anticonceptional pills or not

2. METHODOLOGY OF BLOOD PRESSURE MEASUREMENT

2.1. General requirements

1) The blood pressure values should be recorded to the nearest 2 mmHg.
2) The time of the day when the blood pressure measurement is made should be recorded (in view of the large differences that can occur between morning and evening values).
3) Record whether the blood pressure was obtained in the sitting, lying or standing position.
4) Record whether as a part of the examination a venous puncture was performed. The blood pressure measurement should be made before the venous puncture. The examination procedure, of which the blood pressure measurement is a part, should be specified.
5) Describe the type of device used for measuring blood pressure. Aneroid manometers should be checked regularly.
6) The blood pressure should be measured during one continuous deflation, and be measured twice. The number of measurements made should be specified, and the time interval between measurements should be recorded.
7) Both phase 4 and 5 of diastolic blood pressure should be recorded.
8) The qualifications of the person recording blood pressure should be given (e.g. doctor, nurse, technician). The blood pressure should preferably be recorded by a trained nurse or technician. The recording observer should be given a code number, in order to be able to check the results obtained by each observer.
9) Information should be given about the training program for observers. Theoretical information should be given to the observers making the blood pressure measurements in order to help them understand the procedure. The observers should learn to locate the cubital artery.

2.2. Physical aspects

— A cuff size of 14×40 cm is considered optimal. The minimum cuff size should be 12×28 cm (values for adults).
— The rubber bag should be applied firmly.

— For practical reasons, the self-adhesive type of wrapping is preferred.
— The most important frequencies of the Korotkoff sounds are situated below 100 Hz, and this should be taken into account.

3. SPECIAL RECOMMENDATIONS

— The working group strongly feels that home recording of blood pressure seems to be of special value for epidemiological surveys. This problem should be studied further.
— The possible value of automatic devices for recording blood pressure in epidemiological surveys should be evaluated.

4. PROPOSAL FOR STANDARDIZATION OF HOME BLOOD PRESSURE READINGS

4.1. Conditions of blood pressure (BP) measurement (for subjects working at night)

1) Recumbent in the morning before rising
2) Standing 5–10 min after rising in the morning
3) Standing in the evening just prior to retiring
4) Recumbent after 5–10 min bed-rest

4.2. Methodology of home BP

1) Cuff around left upper arm (right in the left-handed subjects)
2) Position of the arm: cuff at heart level
3) Cuff to be used: specially designed for ego-reading in order to enable an easy application
4) Use phase 5 for diastolic BP
5) Read to nearest even number
6) Measure during preferably seven consecutive days (or at least three working days); indicate the non-working days with an S on the daily form

4.3. Training for home BP reading

1) During the training session in BP reading before the test week, patients are instructed to measure phase 5
2) The recommendations proposed by the other subcommittee could be followed here

68

4.4. Desirable additional information on home BP reading

— Identification
— Sex
— Birth date
— Weight (according to WHO criteria)
— Height (according to WHO criteria)
— Correction of the cuff used when tested against Hg manometer
— Standardized casual reading (see section 2)
— Heart rate: recumbent in the morning by the patient (optimal)
— Circumference of left upper arm (optimal)
— Social class (optimal)
— 24-Hour urinary sodium and creatinine excretion (optimal)
— Questionnaire on drug intake and past medical history (optimal)
— Blood sample (optimal)
— ECG (optimal)
— Urine for albumin (optimal)

4.5. Criteria for the selection of participants (optimal)

1) Exclusion criteria for home BP reading
   — treated hypertensives (excluded after questionnaire)
   — subjects unable to work
   — subjects unable to read BP within 10 mmHg of trainer for both SBP and DBP
   — presence of any serious illness, now or in the recent past, known to influence BP
2) Selection criteria
   — preferably random sample of population
   — if not, specify the selection

REFERENCES

1. Kirkendahl WM, Burton AC, Epstein FH, Freis ED: Recommendations for human blood pressure determination by sphygmomanometers. Report of subcommittee of the postgraduate education committee. *American Heart Association. Circulation* 36:980, 1967.
2. WHO expert committee on arterial hypertension and ischaemic heart disease. WHO Tech Rep 231, 1962.

PART TWO

EPIDEMIOLOGY AND BLOOD PRESSURE IN CHILDREN

5. IMPORTANCE OF BLOOD PRESSURES IN CHILDREN
Distribution and measurable determinants

G.S. BERENSON, A.W. VOORS, and L.S. WEBBER

There is a growing realization that essential hypertension in the adult is a disease which likely has its onset in childhood [1, 2]. At present, however, little is known about pediatric essential hypertension and the early natural history of this disease. Comprehension of the evolution of primary hypertension from youth until the disease state becomes recognizable in adulthood is important to our goal of trying to prevent this major cardiovascular problem. In the United States, hypertension is the second most common cardiovascular disease, and its importance is compounded by its role in accelerating coronary artery disease. Further, hypertension is a more severe disease with a greater morbidity and mortality in the black population of this country than in whites. Evidence indicates familial aggregation of hypertension; therefore, occurrence in parents might signal a tendency toward hypertension in children of affected families and, when combined with observations at a young age, may provide an indication of future hypertensive disease.

It is generally recognized that the current high incidence of coronary heart disease and cerebrovascular accidents is in part caused by essential hypertension. There is also increasing evidence that control of hypertension will reduce morbid events related to hypertension, namely, cerebrovascular accidents and congestive heart failure [3]. It is logical then to assume that prevention of these serious complications would be even more successful if hypertension could be controlled in its early phases.

Several studies have now recorded indirect blood pressure measurements in large numbers of children by using both the school [4] and a physician's office setting [5]. These studies have attempted to stimulate physicians' interest in obtaining blood pressures in children as part of routine examinations, and investigators' interest in exploring mechanisms accounting for the variability of blood pressure levels in children.

Several areas need consideration in the study of blood pressures in children. These include methods of indirect blood pressure measurement to obtain reproducible and representative levels, an appreciation of the blood pressure changes over time as the child grows, the relationship of blood pressure as a risk factor for cardiovascular disease to other risk factor variables, and what observations can be made on large populations of free-living children that

H. Kesteloot, J.V. Joossens (eds.), Epidemiology of Arterial Blood Pressure, 71–97.

might give clues to subtle mechanisms operative in the development of hypertension. With a better understanding of these areas, it will become easier to determine what 'normal' arterial blood pressures may be in childhood, or conversely, what is abnormal, and how high blood pressure levels in children may rationally be prevented.

Table 1. Suggested methods to decrease measurement error of blood pressure observations.

INSTRUMENT

Maintenance. Check the functioning of blood pressure instruments at regular intervals, and perform required maintenance [6].

Adjust mercury. In case the amount of mercury in the sphygmomanometer reservoir needs adjustment, use a plastic syringe or a medicine dropper and add mercury [6].

Recalibrate aneroid manometer. Recalibrate the aneroid manometer frequently with a mercury column. A reserve manometer is useful.

Correct cuff bladder size. A choice of rubber cuff bladder sizes is needed. Use the widest size that fits the particular arm. Each bladder should have sufficient length for its width. These precautions will help avoid excessively high pressure readings [7, 8].

Application of cuff to arm. When using the instrument, apply the deflated rubber bladder and cuff evenly and snugly around the arm, in order to avoid excessively high pressure readings [9].

Stethoscope acoustics. Use either a bell stethoscope without diaphragm or an electronic transducer with amplification of the 10–80 Hz band in order to increase the audibility of the crucial low-frequency components of the Korotkoff sounds. These are weak in young children [10, 11].

EXAMINER

Audiometric testing. Perform audiometry tests on examiners of blood pressures. Avoid selection of examiners with impaired hearing in the frequency range of the Korotkoff sounds.

Self-instruction. Acquire instructional audio tape of normal Korotkoff sounds [12, 13] to avoid misinterpreting sounds.

Split stethoscopes. Examiners can be compared to each other by observing blood pressure readings on a subject at the same time.

Auscultatory pause. Avoid misdiagnosis of an auscultatory pause through proper inflation techniques; include pulse palpation.

Venous engorgement. Avoid softness of the Korotkoff sounds due to venous engorgement of the lower arm by elevating the arm, exercising the forearm muscles, repositioning the arm, and rapidly reinflating the cuff bladder.

Avoid parallax. Maintain eye level at the mercury meniscus or with the aneroid needle, in order to avoid misreading due to parallax.

Hydrostatic pressure error. Keep the patient's brachial artery at the heart level in order to avoid bias in pressure measurement due to the weight of the blood.

Child diastolic pressure. The 4th Korotkoff phase in measuring the diastolic pressure of children is recommended.

EXAMINEE

Urinary bladder pressor effect. Urge child to void before blood pressure is measured. An elevation of blood pressure can be caused by distension of the urinary bladder [14].

Child apprehension. Efforts should be made to reduce apprehension. Keep the examination nonthreatening by removing objects associated with pain and discomfort. Demonstrate the measurement procedure ahead of time. Take multiple measurements interspaced by 1-min or 2-min pauses. Use a female examiner in a relaxed environment, if possible.

Intrasubject variability. Take several measurements and base level on measurements taken at serial examinations. This will avoid misdiagnosis due to the variability of the child's pressure.

---

1. METHODS FOR OBTAINING VALID AND REPRODUCIBLE INDIRECT BLOOD PRESSURE MEASUREMENTS

1.1. Instrumentation

The mercury sphygmomanometer is considered the general reference standard instrument due to its wide use by physicians. For children five years of age and older, we found that the sphygmomanometer in conjunction with a bell stethoscope is acceptable for routine use. Care should be taken to see that the instrument is in proper working order (Table 1)[6–14]. The reservoir of the mercury sphygmomanometer should have the proper amount of mercury or the aneroid manometer routinely standardized [6]. The instrument should be placed at eye level to avoid misreading due to parallax, with a good light source. A relaxed atmosphere is necessary, perhaps with a nurse as the blood pressure examiner. We, as others, observed that the examiner has an effect on blood pressure levels, and hence a low-keyed female nurse is perhaps preferable as an examiner.

In younger children, several disadvantages to the mercury sphygmomanometer were noted. Audible Korotkoff phases were difficult to distinguish because of the reduced intensity of the sounds, although the 4th phase seems to be most reliable for diastolic measurement [15]. Low-frequency 'sounds' from the artery under the cuff are not audible with the stethoscope [10, 11]. Overreadings may result due to the relative narrowness of the rubber cuff bladder because of the need to leave space at the elbow skin crease for the stethoscope, or due to a short bladder that incompletely surrounds the arm. In our studies, the Infrasonde (Marion Scientific Corp., Costa Mesa, California) Seemed to work best for children aged five years or younger. Reasonable systolic, but somewhat low diastolic, blood pressures can be obtained with the aid of a low-frequency transducer [16, 17].

1.2. Cuff size

We recommend using cuffs large enough to cover at least two-thirds of the arm and encircle the circumference of the arm [7–9]. The standard Baumanometer cuffs (W.A. Baum Co., Inc., Copiague, New York) are now available with calibrations to warn the physician when the arm circumference is too large for the cuff size. We recommend using the 'adult-size' cuff *below* the 'acceptable range' as printed on the cuff, but switching to the 'large adult-size' as soon as the calibration is *within* the 'acceptable range' (Table 2). The Infrasonde provides an 'adult-size' cuff which we found satisfactory, provided that sponge rubber is adapted around the transducer to equalize a localized pressure on the arm exerted by the instrument [17]. Selection of the bladder

Table 2. Cuff size by right upper arm circumference and length (in cm) for use with the mercury sphygmomanometer, Bogalusa Heart Study, Bogalusa, LA.

Length (cm) [a]	Circumference (cm) [b]		
	≤27	27 – 29	≥30
≤21	Small	Small	Medium
22 – 27	Medium	Medium	Adult
28 – 31	Medium	Adult	Adult
≥32	Medium	Adult	Large
Cuff	Dimensions of bag (in cm)		
Small	6.98 × 12.06		
Medium	9.52 × 21.59		
Adult	12.06 × 22.22		
Large	15.2 × 33 [c]		

[a] Acromio-olecranon distance as measured by caliper (anthropometer).
[b] Measured halfway between acromion and olecranon.
[c] Length may be slightly larger depending on the manufacturer of the large cuff.

sizes for the mercury sphygmomanometer cuff was based on arm measurement criteria recommended by Karvonen et al.[18], Simpson et al.[19], and King[7], but with the restriction that commonly available bladders were used and that shorter arms required a narrower cuff in order to leave room for the stethoscope at the elbow skin crease[8].

1.3. Automatic instruments

In a large survey and even in selected office settings, automatic instruments can be used for recording indirect blood pressures[20]. Such factors as observer bias, examiner fatigue, and prolonged observer training can be eliminated. In addition, some instruments provide a permanent record in the form of a graph, disk, or print.

We used several methods for examining various automatic instruments[21]. The *Graeco-Latin square* design is particularly useful since it allows the examination of the instruments in a controlled design. Implementation of such a design requires proper function of instruments, n^2 examinations to measure the blood pressure of n examinees with n instruments and n observers during n time periods. Effects on the blood pressure levels due to the subjects, performance of the observers, instruments, and time are thus accounted for in the analysis.

We also tested the instruments in a *field* setting. The reproducibility and validity of observations in the field are important in collecting data for epidemiologic studies. In field studies, consideration must be given to randomization schemes for instruments, examiners, and subjects. Subtle differences can be detected only through many observations.

In our study of school-aged children, indirect blood pressures were measured both by the mercury sphygmomanometer and by the Physiometrics automatic blood pressure recorder (USM-105 Sphygmetrics, Woodland Hills, California) that records on a paper disk.

1.4. Observer training

Periodic training of blood pressure observers is essential in an epidemiologic survey (Table 1). Audiometry testing for hearing defects should be given before allowing an observer to record blood pressures. Various prerecorded tapes and motion pictures are available for instructional purposes [12, 13]. The examiner should be instructed to elevate the child's arm, reposition the cuff if necessary, and rapidly inflate the cuff bladder in order to reduce venous engorgement of the lower arm. The brachial artery should be kept at heart level.

In addition, the use of split stethoscopes enabling two observers to record the blood pressure on one subject at the same time is a very effective training technique. Two mercury columns can be joined to the cuff bladder so that each observer can independently record the blood pressure. Based on serial readings of several subjects, we were able to rank the observers. If one observer's readings deviate significantly, then that observer can be identified, retrained, or shifted to other duties.

For most automatic instruments, less rigorous observer training is necessary. In some cases, the difficulty may not be in the use of the instrument, but in the interpretation of a permanent record. The records can be read by a number of individuals in a Latin-square design for testing their record-reading capability and reproducibility [21]. Subtle differences may require retraining of observers or revision of the protocol for correct interpretation of records.

As a research program, all of these measures were used in the Bogalusa Heart Study to decrease the measurement error in the recording of indirect blood pressures. We observed a measurement error of about 5 mmHg for systolic and approximately 5 mm for 4th phase diastolic blood pressures.

1.5. Choice of diastolic phase

We were unable to obtain consistently reproducible results in children with the 5th Korotkoff phase [15]. The 5th phase values were about 19 mmHg less than the 4th phase values, and in about 6% of the children no discrete 5th phases were recorded since sounds persisted to 0 mmHg. Some studies have suggested that 4th phase measurements may more closely approximate intraarterial pressures. Although our observers obtained reasonably reproducible results for both phases, they were more consistent in obtaining 4th phase values. Recording both 4th and 5th phases is recommended since 5th phase, as the diastolic measurement, is often used in adults [22].

1.6. Relaxed children

The setting in which the children are examined determines, in part, their blood pressure. The environment should be nonthreatening, the child should be informed exactly about the blood pressure measurement in advance, and the child should have urinated before the examination [14].

1.7. Repeated measurements

In order to ensure a relaxed state and to avoid the influence of recording fluctuations of blood pressure, repeated measurements should be taken during the examination. In our research study, three measurements by each of three nurses were taken. Two used the mercury sphygmomanometer and one used the Physiometrics instrument [23]. The recording of three readings by one or two nurses in an office setting would offer a good approximation of a child's relaxed pressure for comparison to those obtained in the Bogalusa Heart Study rather than those that might be obtained by a physician in a more hurried manner.

Blood pressure levels obtained in the Bogalusa Heart Study were much lower than those reported by the Task Force Report [24], but were quite similar to those levels reported by Goldring et al. [25] earlier (see discussion below).

2. EPIDEMIOLOGIC OBSERVATIONS ON BLOOD PRESSURE RELATED TO EARLY ESSENTIAL HYPERTENSION

2.1. Distribution of blood pressure and relation with other characteristics

Two questions were posed with respect to essential hypertension in the general population of pediatric age:

1) What is the mean level and distribution of blood pressures in black and white children of various ages?
2) How does the blood pressure level relate to height and weight in children?

For these purposes, the Bogalusa Heart Study observed blood pressures of children from an entire geographic community, namely, Bogalusa, Louisiana, with a total population of approximately 22,000. For approximately 4200 children, ages 3–14 years, we recorded age, race, sex, height, weight, arm measurements, triceps skinfold thickness[26], hemoglobin[27], serum lipids and lipoproteins[28, 29], the result of a brief physical examination by a physician[30], and blood pressure[16, 23].

2.2. Blood pressure measurements in an epidemiologic survey

Each day of the study, some 25–40 children were examined. Blood pressures were recorded at the end of the examination sequence. The children were encouraged to void before the blood pressures were measured, and volunteer workers guided them through a designated random sequence for examination. Children of preschool age were accompanied by their parents, and were held by their parents during the blood pressure measurement, where a concerted effort was made to keep the children relaxed. For each child, the blood pressure was determined by three trained observers in randomized sequence, each observer independently measuring three consecutive blood pressures per child. Under quiet conditions, in a screened-off corner, observers recorded the 1st and 4th Korotkoff phases to determine the right arm blood pressure while each child was seated. The 5th phase was also recorded with sphygmomanometer readings, but these readings were less consistent and are not part of this report. Care was taken to cover the brachial artery with the center of the rubber bladder. Physiometrics disks were read blindly by the same observer throughout the entire study period.

2.3. Observations of blood pressures in children

Comparative measurements of blood pressure levels in several surveys of children are of interest and indicate the need for attention to methodology. Figure 1[25, 31–35] compares mean systolic and diastolic (4th phase) levels of blood pressure on the mercury sphygmomanometers, by age, as measured by our study (Bogalusa) with similar studies published by others. Our values are considerably lower, and reached near-basal levels. Such levels are helpful in following blood pressures of children as they grow, and are more predictive of future hypertension than 'casual' blood pressure levels[36, 37], as reported in the Task Force Report[24].

Selected percentile levels of blood pressure on the Physiometrics, by age, are presented in Figure 2. The 95th percentile for blacks was higher than for whites. For mercury sphygmomanometer readings, the differences were smaller, although racial differences were still noticeable. This racial difference

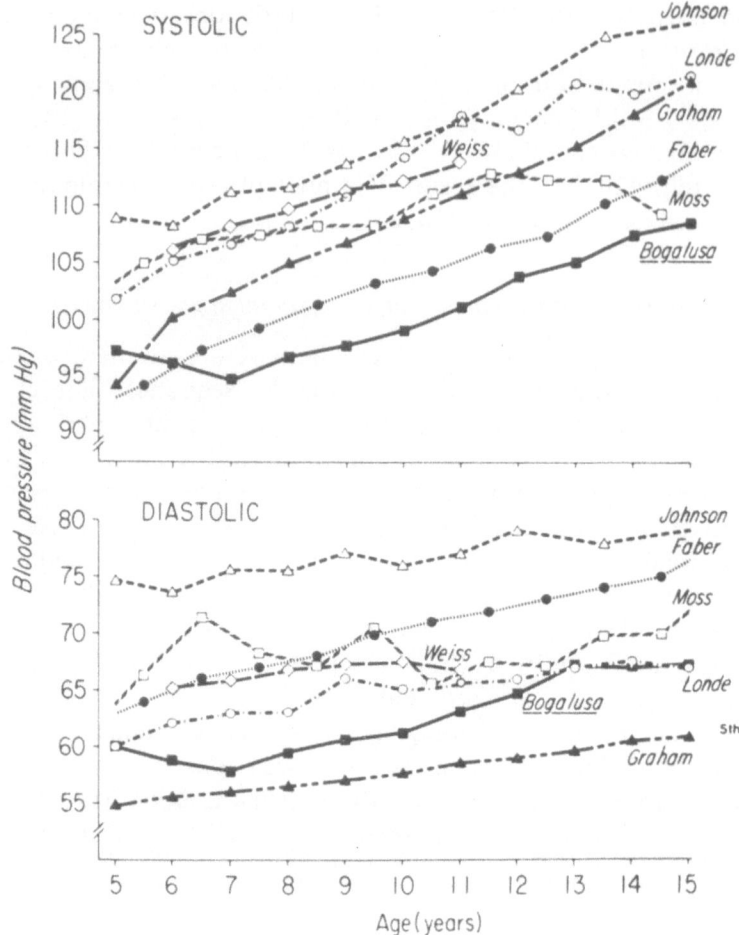

Figure 1. Comparison of indirect blood pressure measurements of white school children, by age, among selected studies in the literature. Graham used the 5th Korotkoff phase for determining diastolic pressure. The other studies used either 4th or a combination of 4th and 5th Korotkoff phases. By permission of the American Heart Association, Inc. Circulation 54:319-327, 1976.

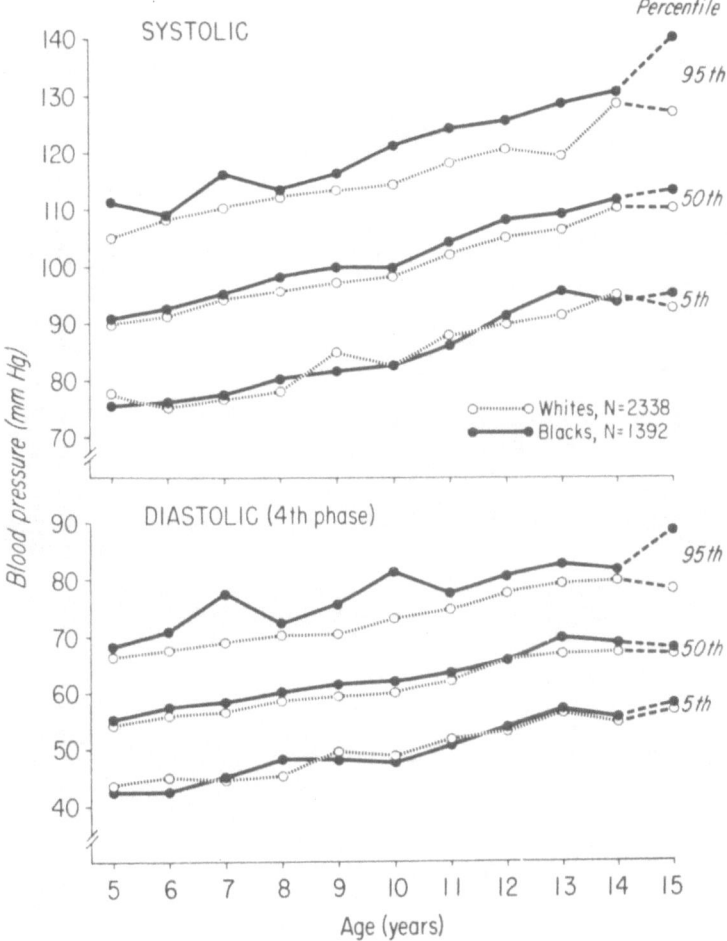

Figure 2. Percentiles of Physiometrics instrument blood pressures in school children, by age and race. By permission of the American Heart Association, Inc. Circulation 54:319-327, 1976.

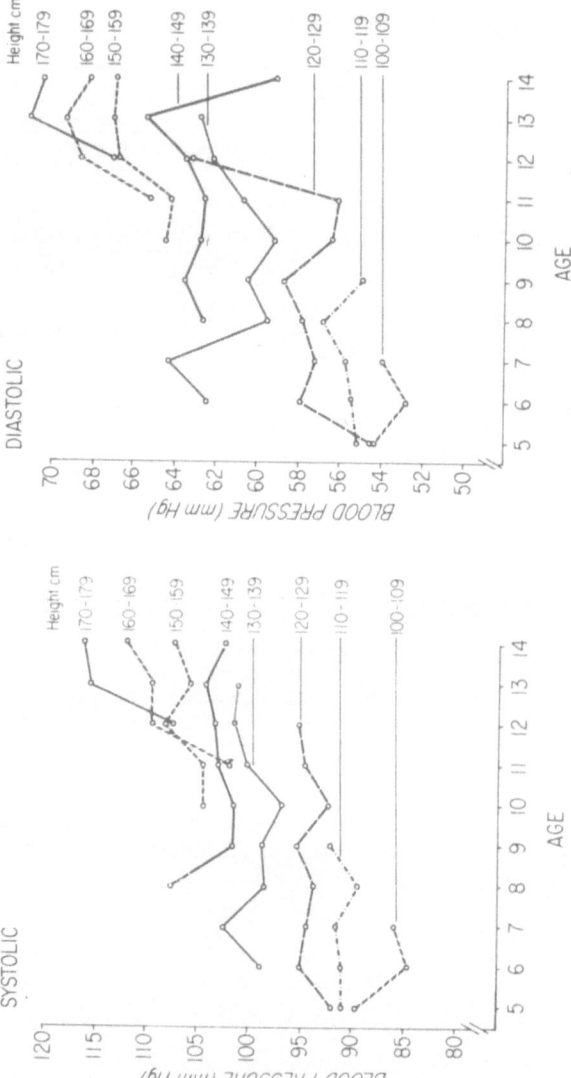

Figure 3. Mean blood pressures measured on 3478 school-aged children by Physiometrics® instrument, by age, for each 10-cm height interval. Similar information was obtained for blood pressures measured by mercury sphygmomanometer. Samples sizes <3 omitted. By permission Am J Epidemiol 106:101-108, 1977.

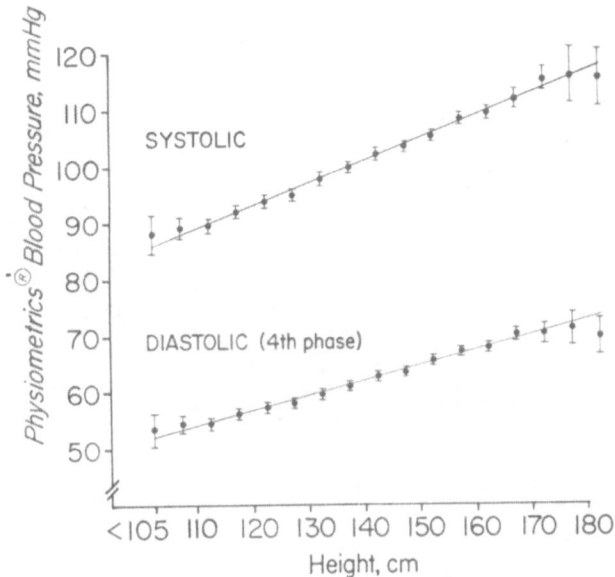

Figure 4. Blood pressure by height intervals. The linear regression line of blood pressure (measured by automatic infrasonic instrument) is superimposed on height-specific blood pressure distributions. Observation on each child ($n = 3517$; age 5–14 years) represents mean of three readings. In 33 of 34 instances, the $\pm 2\,$SE intervals bracketed the linear regression lines. By permission Cardiovasc Med 3:911–918, 1978.

is well known in adulthood related to higher morbidity from hypertension in the black adult population, but has not been noted in children before.

When children were grouped by body height, these height-specific groups did not show the usual positive correlation between age and blood pressure (Fig. 3)[38]. There was an almost perfectly linear relationship between height and blood pressure (Fig. 4), and similarly between log weight and blood pressure. Other studies[31, 39–45] found that the rise in blood pressure with age terminated abruptly when adult stature was reached (Fig. 5). This consti-

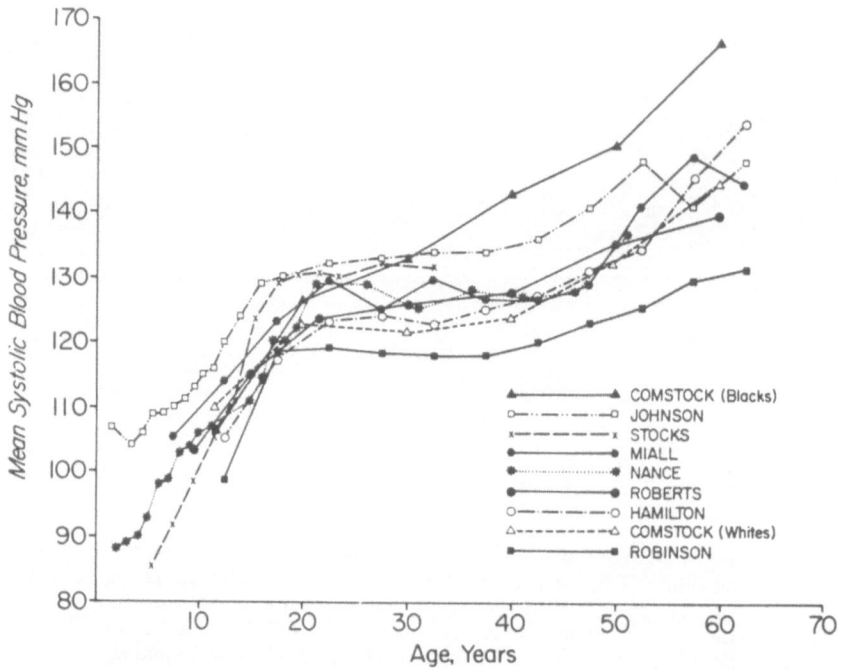

Figure 5. Relationship between blood pressure and age in populations containing both children and adults. In all surveys, a distinct change in age trend of systolic pressures from increasing to horizontal levels occurs at the age of incipient adult stature (age 18–20 years). Later in life, the blood pressure rise follows an almost exponential pattern. These data show findings for male subjects; female subjects show similar changes. By permission Cardiovasc Med 3:911–918, 1978.

tutes a strong indication in favor of body size as a blood pressure determinant.

Selected percentiles of blood pressure recorded by an infrasonic instrument on preschool-aged children and by mercury sphygmomanometer on school-aged children were expressed by height (Fig. 6). These grids could be used as normative values in judging observations on individual children, but only if blood pressures are taken with exactly the same methodology.

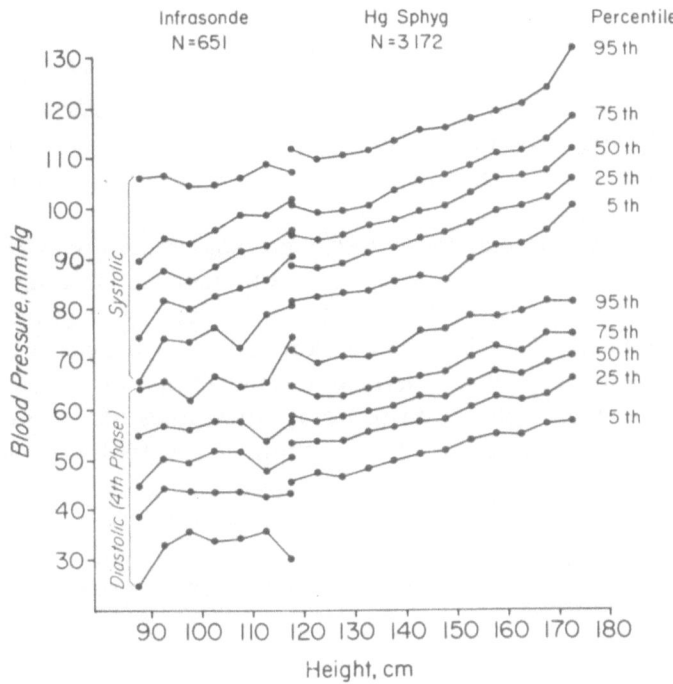

Figure 6. Selected percentiles of blood pressure as measured by Infrasonde and mercury sphygmomanometer, by age, in children $2\frac{1}{2}$–14 years of age. By permission Cardiovasc Med 3:911–918, 1978.

These observations emphasize the importance of careful attention to the methods used in obtaining blood pressures, especially in children. Reproducible observations are helpful in following children as they grow and develop stature. Further, values obtained by a similar protocol as used in large surveys to obtain percentile distributions for a population can be used to evaluate high levels in a single child.

3. PERSISTENCE OF BLOOD PRESSURE LEVELS (TRACKING) OVER TIME

If prevention of essential hypertension is to be successful, then the disease process must be attacked in its early phase. Consequently, it is important to determine whether blood pressure levels track in children, as they do in adults [46]. Tracking may be defined as the tendency for an individual's blood pressure levels, in relation to his peers, to remain in a respective range over time.

84

3.1. Observations on tracking

From September 1973 to May 1977, 872 children aged 5, 8, 11, and 14 years were examined annually in the Bogalusa Heart Study. The same detailed protocol for obtaining reproducible blood pressures, already described in this chapter, was used at each examination. Only data from the mercury sphygmomanometer are used in this presentation.

A remarkably high correlation of blood pressure readings over the three-year period is noted (Table 3). Correlation coefficients for readings from year 1 to year 2 ranged from 0.62 to 0.73 systolic and from 0.41 to 0.54 diastolic. Only a very slight drop was noted in the correlation coefficients by year 4. As a matter of fact, the correlation coefficients of readings three years apart are only slightly lower than those from some of our studies of readings 1 h apart (0.83 systolic and 0.78 diastolic) or one month apart (0.81 systolic and 0.65 diastolic) [46].

Table 3. Product moment correlation coefficients for blood pressure readings over three successive years, Bogalusa heart study, 1973 – 77.

Age (year 1)		Year 1 with		
	n	Year 2 r	Year 3 r	Year 4 r
Systolic				
5	191	0.64	0.60	0.58
8	246	0.73	0.67	0.62
11	270	0.68	0.64	0.63
14	161	0.62	0.60	0.52
Diastolic				
5	191	0.42	0.35	0.45
8	246	0.48	0.44	0.41
11	270	0.55	0.43	0.44
14	161	0.52	0.40	0.23*

* $P<0.01$; $P<0.0001$ for all other correlation coefficients.

A tendency for those children with elevated readings at one point in time to remain high is apparent. Presented in Figure 7 are the yearly systolic blood pressure distributions for 191 children five years of age initially. Although some 'regression to the mean' is noted (discussed below), many of the children tend to remain high in succeeding years. A slight improvement is noted if we use the average of two or three years to establish a base-line distribution.

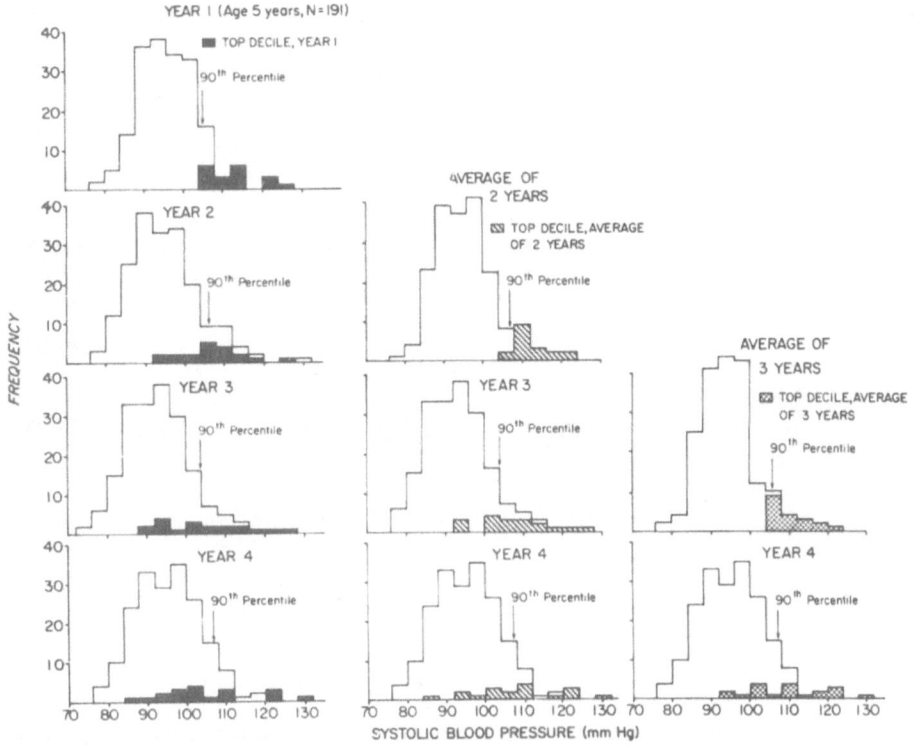

Figure 7. Systolic blood pressure distributions for 191 children, age five years initially, who were examined annually for three successive years. Shaded are the readings for those children in the highest decile during the first examination. Whether one reading, the average of two readings, or the average of three readings are used to determine the highest deciles, a remarkable persistence in levels is noted.

We can summarize this for all four age groups (Table 4). For the 85 children who were in the highest decile in year 1, some 41 (48%) remained there in year 2, while 57 (67%) were in the highest two deciles. By year 4, 28 (33%) were still in the top decile. If blood pressure readings for three years are then averaged, of the 87 who were in the top decile, 38 (44%) were in the top decile in year 4. A better persistence of ranking is noted if we restrict the selection to those children who where in the highest decile in year 1 *and* year 2 *and* year 3. Some 16 (59%) of 27 remain in the highest decile in year 4, and 21 (78%) were in the highest two deciles.

3.2. *Effect of 'regression toward the mean' on subsequent observations*

Do blood pressures in the highest decile remain high when examined one year later? In order to answer this question, adjustments have to be made for

Table 4. Number of children in highest deciles for systolic blood pressure, Bogalusa Heart Study, 1973 – 77.

Highest decile	Decile					
	Year 2		Year 3		Year 4	
n	9 + 10 n (%)	10 n (%)	9 + 10 n (%)	10 n (%)	9 + 10 n (%)	10 n (%)
Year 1 only 85	57 (67)	41 (48)	58 (68)	40 (47)	47 (55)	28 (33)
Average of 2 years 86			68 (79)	43 (50)	56 (65)	35 (41)
Average of 3 years 87					61 (70)	38 (44)
Each of 2 years 41			38 (93)	27 (66)	30 (73)	20 (49)
Each of 3 years 27					21 (78)	16 (59)

the regression toward the mean resulting from short-term variations in the blood pressure measurements on a single child. After such adjustments, we found that the mean systolic blood pressure for this group had a relative decrease of only 3.5 mm mercury, and the mean diastolic pressure only 0.5 mm mercury (Fig. 8)[47]. In all likelihood, the smallness of these changes relates to measuring relaxed children at near-basal levels. These results, as well as our analyses of tracking after three years, show that blood pressure tracks considerably better in children than has been described in the studies of others. The variability of blood pressure levels in a given individual is also important, but has to be determined by methods different from those used in our current epidemiologic study.

Repeated observations and serial blood pressure measurements over time in growing and developing children are necessary in making judgments on abnormal levels. Early diagnosis of hypertension depends on continued observations and on appreciation of levels relative to other children in the same population. Such considerations are important in attempting to define hypertension as a disease in childhood.

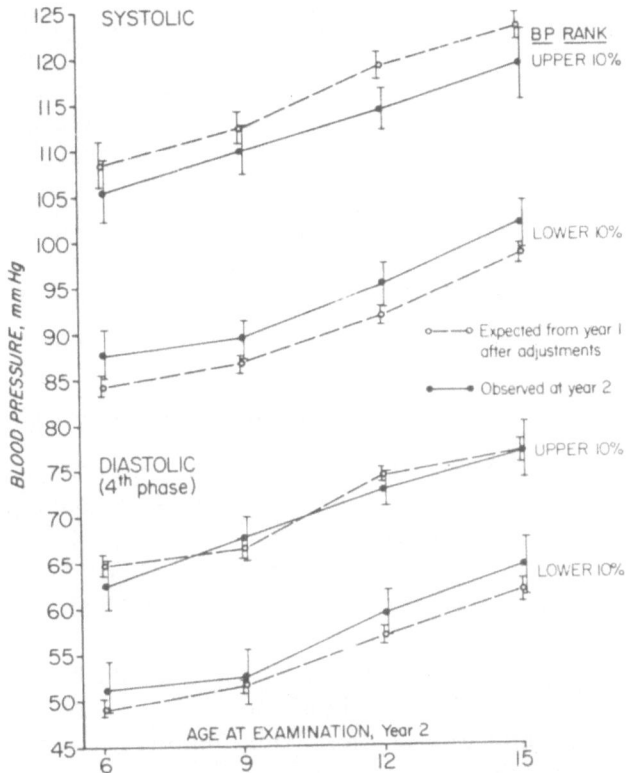

Figure 8. Comparison of blood pressure (mean ± 2 SE; $n = 1099$) expected from ideal tracking with observed reexamination after one year. Systolic and diastolic (4th phase) pressures of extreme deciles from the initial examination were 'regressed toward the mean' resulting in pressures expected for ideal tracking. Extreme deciles from initial examination were reexamined after one year to give observed values. The degree of fit is a measure of tracking. By permission Am J Epidemiol 109:320–334, 1979.

4. POTENTIAL DIFFERENCES IN MECHANISMS CONTRIBUTING TO HIGH BLOOD PRESSURES IN BLACK AND IN WHITE CHILDREN

In order to study potential mechanisms operative in hypertension prevalence, we posed two questions regarding the biracial adolescent population of our study:

1) How do blood pressure levels relate to various factors such as urine electrolytes, plasma renin, adrenergic activity, and glucose tolerance in healthy free-living children?
2) What are the potential racial differences in mechanisms contributing to essential hypertension?

As an approach to obtaining information on various factors related to the early onset of essential hypertension, multiple clinical and laboratory observations were made on a selected sample of children. In this study, racial differences were detected which could provide clues to better understanding of the greater severity of essential hypertension in black people. Certain racial differences on anthropometric, lipid, and blood pressure variables have now been noted from the cross-sectional studies [23, 26–29]. The observations indicate that in children, upper percentile blood pressure levels are higher for blacks than for whites, and that white children have more body fat and black children greater body mass [48].

4.1. In-depth study of blood pressure in a stratified sample of children

We ranked school-aged children from the cross-sectional study according to diastolic blood pressure, separately for each age-race-sex group, and sampled 100% of the extreme two percentiles and 70% of the next 4% – 9% of both upper and lower pressures. Finally, we sampled 3.5% – 8.0% of the remaining children in each age-race-sex group. Thus, 278 children were reexamined [49, 50].

On an ambulatory basis, 24-h urines were collected during the two days preceding the reexamination. The children underwent a series of procedures during an entire morning of examination. They reported fasting in the morning and were kept standing and occupied for approximately $1-1\frac{1}{2}$ h. Their urine collection bottles were received, and they were interviewed on the completeness of the urine collection and the details of their fasting. We performed a series of anthropometric measurements, obtained blood samples from each child for multiple laboratory analyses, and administered a standard oral glucose load for glucose-tolerance testing. A physician performed a physical examination to aid exclusion of children with secondary hypertension from the study. One hour after the venipuncture a second venipuncture was done, and at mid-morning a brunch was served. To further exclude secondary hypertension, a urinalysis and culture of fresh, clean, midstream urine sample were obtained. We measured blood pressure as described before, and also conducted a series of cardiovascular tests [50]. Blood samples were examined for plasma renin activity, serum dopamine β-hydroxylase, lipids and lipoproteins, electrolytes, and creatinine. Urine samples were studied for electrolytes and creatinine.

4.2. Observations on children with different levels of blood pressure

Since the frequency distribution of 24-h urine creatinine per kg body weight gives a measure of the completeness of the urine collection for boys and girls

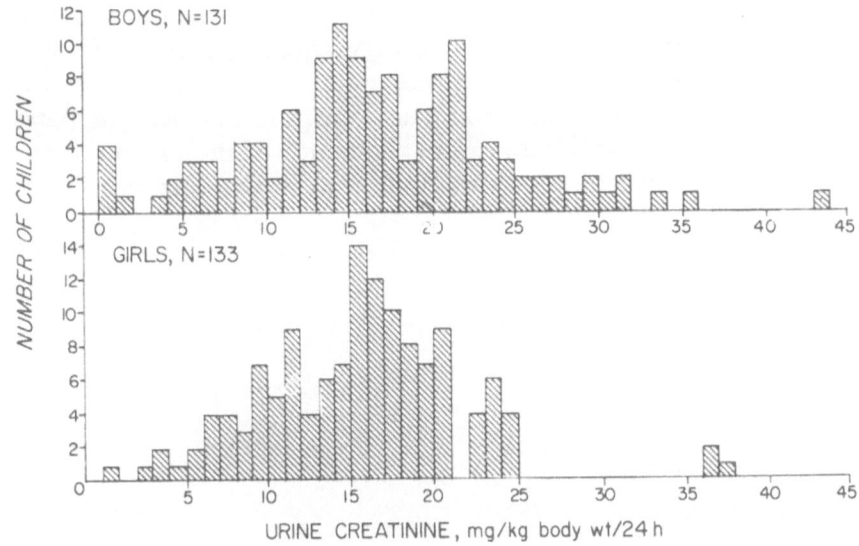

Figure 9. Relative urine creatinine excretion as expressed per kg body weight, for boys and girls (age 7–15 years), in the second 24-h period of collection. Boys tended to excrete more creatinine; no racial differences were noted. The distribution of relative creatinine excretion in the first 24-h period of collection was quite similar. By permission J Lab Clin Med 93:535–548, 1979.

(Fig. 9), we arbitrarily discarded observations for boys with values of less than 10 mg/kg and for girls with values of less than 8 mg/kg.

In the defined study sample, we found that 24-h urine sodium was higher at the older ages, but this difference disappeared after correction for body surface. There was no difference in these adjusted levels among blood pressure strata ($P > 0.05$). In the high blood pressure strata for the black children, there was a positive association between 24-h urine sodium and blood pressure as measured on that day, adjusting for body surface.

Table 5. 24-h urine sodium and potassium by race and blood pressure stratum in children, aged 7–15 years, Bogalusa Heart Study, 1975–76 ($n = 249$).

Electrolyte	Race	Blood pressure stratum		
		Low	Medium	High
		meq (mean ±2 SE)		
Na⁺	White	106 ± 13	98 ± 17	109 ± 14
	Black	97 ± 12	103 ± 17	115 ± 18
K⁺	White	39 ± 4	34 ± 7	42 ± 7
	Black [a]	26 ± 3	27 ± 4	29 ± 5

[a] $P < 0.0001$.

90

The 24-h excretion of potassium was lower in blacks than in whites (Table 5). In a 50% random sample of all 10-year-old children in the entire Bogalusa study population, we conducted 24-h dietary recalls one year previously [51]. In this earlier study, we could not detect racial differences in potassium intake. Therefore, the urinary potassium difference in the present study may indicate actual racial differences in renal electrolyte reabsorption at the molecular level.

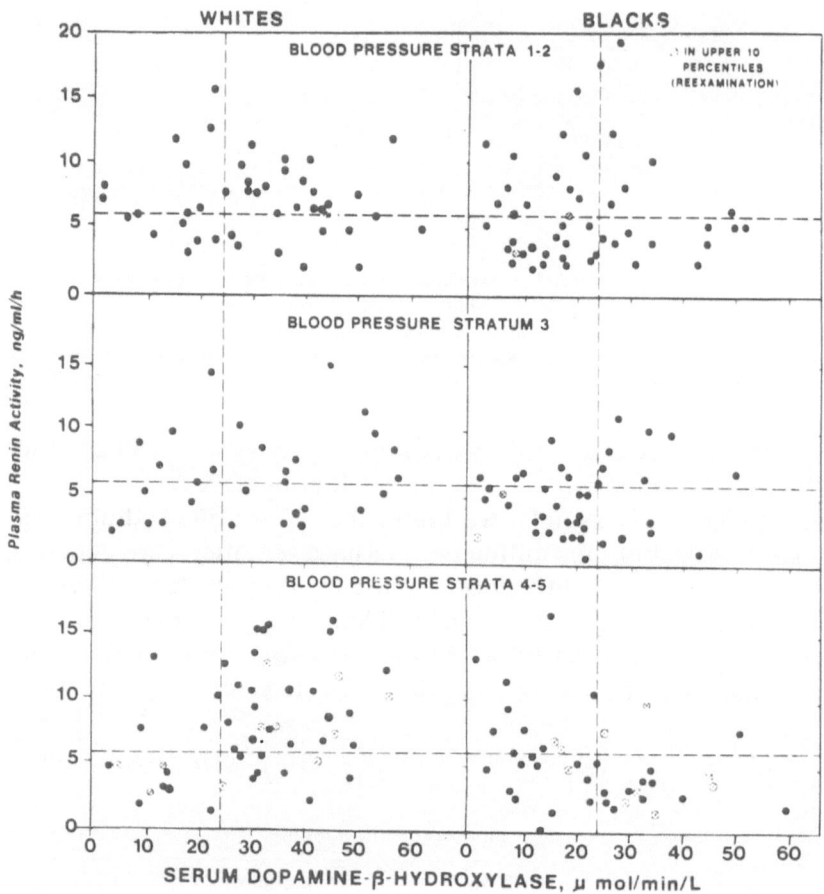

Figure 10. Scattergram of plasma renin activity by serum dopamine β-hydroxylase, by race and by blood pressure stratum. Median values for the combined children are represented by dotted lines. The preponderance of children with combined high renin and high DβH, expected in the high blood pressure strata, is lacking among the blacks. Children whose diastolic mercury sphygmomanometer pressure (4th phase) as measured during reexamination was in the upper 10% of his (her) age (age 7–15 years) and race group are marked open circles. They conform to the above conclusions. By permission Science 204:1091–1094, 1979.

White children had higher levels of plasma renin activity than blacks ($P < 0.0001$), and the differences tended to be larger in the high blood pressure strata and at older ages. Plasma renin values plotted by 24-h urine sodium separately by blood pressure stratum and by race clearly showed the racial difference in renin levels in the high blood pressure strata.

Serum dopamine β-hydroxylase was much greater for whites than for blacks (Fig. 10)[50].

In the relaxed-sitting position, the children ranked on the average exactly as expected from the stratum according to which they were selected; however, in a resting-supine position and under upright stressed conditions, the black boys from the high blood pressure stratum showed the highest systolic levels (for resting-supine measurements, see Fig. 11). For these boys, there

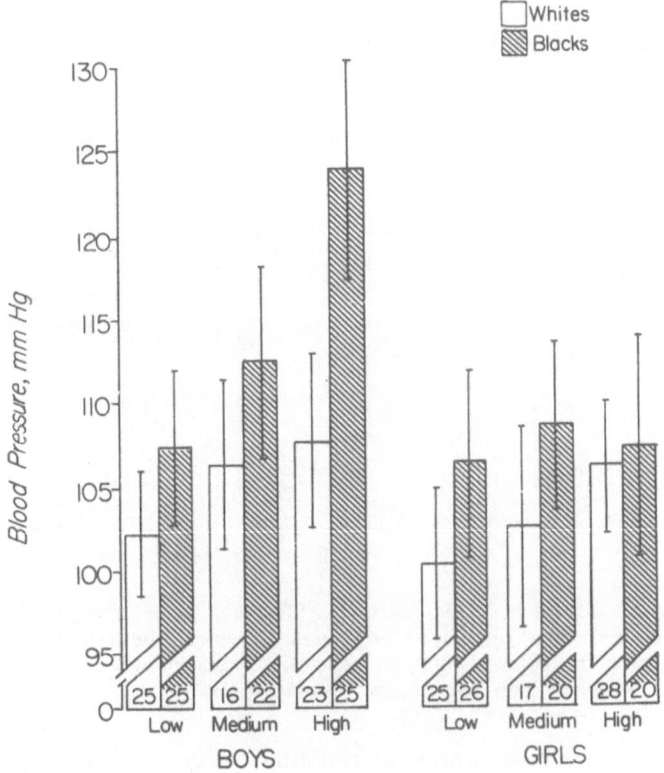

Figure 11. Resting supine systolic blood pressure (mean ± 2 SE) as measured by the Whittaker Sphygmostat (Waltham, Massachusetts), by race, sex, and blood pressure stratum in children (age 7–15 years). Only black boys showed a significant ($P < 0.005$) positive trend over the blood pressure strata. A similar pattern was seen under upright stressed conditions for the three response tests. The Bogalusa Heart Study, 1975–76.

92

was a statistically significant negative correlation between plasma renin and all resting and stressed systolic pressures, except the resting pressure on the Physiometrics.

Supine-resting heart rates were higher for whites than for blacks in the high blood pressure strata (controlling for sex, there was significant interaction between race and the regression of heart rate on blood pressure stratum, $P<0.0005$, Fig. 12).

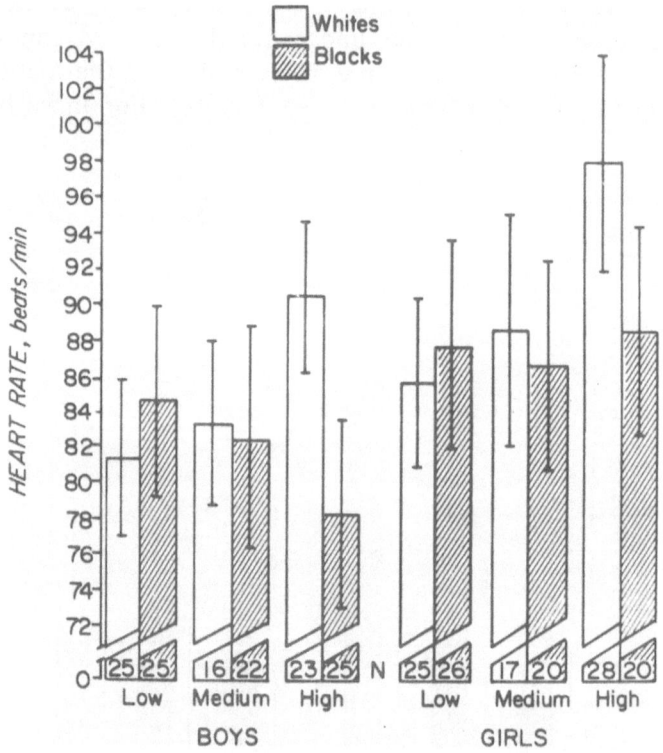

Figure 12. Resting heart rate (mean ± 2 SE) by race, sex, and blood pressure stratum. Ages ranged 7–15 years. In whites, the heart rate is increased in the high blood pressure strata. This is not the case for blacks. By permission Science 204:1091–1094, 1979.

White children, especially those in the high blood pressure strata, showed higher levels of 1-h plasma glucose. It should also be commented that we previously observed white children to have higher serum triglycerides and higher serum pre-β-lipoprotein levels than black [28, 29]. In the absence of systematic racial differences in diet, the combination of these findings points to genetic differences in the carbohydrate-lipid metabolism between the races which appear to influence blood pressure levels.

4.3. Comment

The racial differences shown here are unlikely to denote race-exclusive mechanisms. Rather, the biracial population enabled us by epidemiologic methods to discern separate mechanisms which are likely acting by subtle differences to influence blood pressure levels in the two racial groups (Table 6).

Table 6. Racial differences for high blood pressure strata of children, aged 7 – 15 years, Bogalusa Heart Study, 1975 – 76.

Characteristic	Direction	$P<$
Children with high renin and high DβH	W > B	0.0001
Correlation 24-h Na$^+$ vs blood pressure	B > W	(0.05)[a]
One hour serum glucose	W > B	0.0001
Resting heart rate	W > B	0.05
Boys' systolic pressure:		
Resting supine and under stress	B > W	0.01
Negative correlation with renin	B > W	(0.05)[a]

[a] Black children only.

To conclude the findings on the black children, the data presented here indicate beginning sodium sensitivity in black children of the high blood pressure strata and different potassium-handling mechanisms for renal potassium excretion. For the white children, particularly in the high blood pressure strata, the data presented indicate increased adrenergic reactivity, faster heart rates, and higher 1-h plasma glucose levels.

5. CLINICAL IMPLICATIONS FROM AN EPIDEMIOLOGIC STUDY OF BLOOD PRESSURE IN CHILDREN

The measurement and recording of blood pressure should be routine in the physical examination of every child. These measurements should become a basic part of the medical record, to be followed with the development and growth of the child. Although it is important to describe the distribution of blood pressures in a free-living and presumably healthy population of children, it will be more important to follow children over time and observe how blood pressure levels change in an effort to understand the early natural history of essential hypertension. Percentile charts from population studies have now been developed and can be used to follow and compare a child with the described population [52]. As discussed earlier, anthropometric measurements, height and weight, should be considered in the growing child and related to blood pressure levels. Correction for race and sex is probably not needed in the young age group, but it cannot be emphasized too strongly that when comparisons are made with population studies or when percentile charts are used as a reference to determine the need for further observation or possibly for treatment of a child, the *method* of measuring blood pressure needs to be comparable. Measurements in the Bogalusa Heart Study were made strictly according to specific guidelines and were obtained by trained examiners in an effort to observe reproducible blood pressure levels. Levels which were presumably obtained in a relaxed state have been demonstrated to be most reproducible over time. As pointed out earlier, the basal level of an individual appears potentially better than the casual level for predicting subsequent of blood pressure or later occurrence of hypertension. Since it is important to follow the change of blood pressure in an individual child over time to observe whether tracking of levels occurs within a high or low distribution, attention must be given to methods of obtaining blood pressure measurements. Since tracking does occur in children [53] and the long-term studies from Evans County [54] and on naval aviators [55] extend the period from young adulthood to a period in life when overt hypertensive disease is observed, the careful measurement of blood pressure in children may be predictive of future hypertension.

The observations showing tracking imply that hypertension originates in youth and that hypertension likely exists in a significant number of children considered healthy. With this realization, modification of life style, such as prevention of obesity and reduction of salt intake, becomes quite important for many children. The observations on racial differences suggest salt restriction, control of blood volume, and higher intakes of potassium may be more important to black children with a predisposition to hypertension. As noted by family history in both black and white children, tracking at high percentile levels demands vigorous primary and secondary therapeutic measures to reduce their levels to a lower range of blood pressure, perhaps to 75 percentiles or below. Obviously, such decisions can only be arbitrary at this time.

It does become increasingly clear that essential hypertension begins in childhood. The continued study of the onset of essential hypertension in children is needed to prevent this devastating cardiovascular disease as commonly observed in adulthood. A great deal of progress has been made in understanding hypertension in its early phases and can soon be applied to the general population of children.

Acknowledgments. The Bogalusa Heart Study is a collaborative effort of many people. We especially thank Mrs. Imogene Talley for her outstanding work as Community Coordinator and the children and parents of Bogalusa, without whom the study would not be possible. This research has been supported by funds from the National Heart, Lung, and Blood Institute of the U.S. Public Health Service, Specialized Center of Research—Arteriosclerosis (SCOR-A), HL15103.

REFERENCES

1. Voors AW, Webber LS, Berenson GS: A consideration of essential hypertension in children. Pract Cardiol 3(5):29-40, 1977.
2. Voors AW, Webber LS, Berenson GS: Epidemiology of essential hypertension in youth—implications for clinical practice. Pediatr Clin North Am 25:15-26, 1978.
3. Veterans Administration Cooperative Study Group on Antihypertensive Agents: Effects of treatment on morbidity in hypertension: II. Results in patients with diastolic blood pressure averaging 90 through 114 mmHg. JAMA 213:1143-1152, 1970.
4. National Heart, Lung and Blood Institute: Cardiovascular profile of 15,000 children of school age in three communities, 1971–1975. DHEW Publ No. (NIH) 78-1472, 1978.
5. Londe S: Blood pressure standards for normal children as determined under office conditions. Clin Pediatr 7:400-403, 1968.
6. Corns RH: Maintenance of blood pressure equipment. Am J Nurs 76:776-777, 1976.
7. King GE: Errors in clinical measurement of blood pressure in obesity. Clin Sci 32:223-237, 1967.
8. Voors AW: Cuff bladder size in a blood pressure survey of children. Am J Epidemiol 101:489-494, 1975.
9. Nuessle WF: The importance of a tight blood pressure cuff. Am Heart J 52:905-907, 1956.
10. Ertel PY, Lawrence M, Brown RK, Stern AM: Stethoscope acoustics II. Transmission and filtration patterns. Circulation 34:889-898, 1966.
11. Golden DP, Wolthuis RA, Hoffler GW, Cowen RJ: Development of a Korotkoff sound processor for automatic identification of auscultatory events—Part 1: Specification of preprocessing band pass filters. IEEE Trans Biomed Eng 21:114-118, 1974.
12. Ravin A: The clinical significance of the sounds of Korotkoff. University of Colorado School of Medicine. An audio-cassette program previously distributed by Merck, Sharp and Dohme.
13. National Medical Audiovisual Center: Practice in blood pressure readings. Bethesda, MD: National Library of Medicine. (motion picture.)
14. Pickering G: High blood pressure. London: JVV Churchill, 1966, p 38.
15. Voors AW, Webber LS, Berenson GS: A choice of diastolic Korotkoff phases in mercury sphygmomanometer of children. Prev Med 8:492-499, 1979.
16. Berenson GS, Foster TA, Frank GC, Frerichs RR, Srinivasan SR, Voors AW, Webber LS: Cardiovascular disease risk factor variables at the preschool age—The Bogalusa Heart Study. Circulation 57:603-612, 1978.
17. Voors AW, Webber LS, Berenson GS: Blood pressure of children, ages 2½–5½ years, in a total community—The Bogalusa Heart Study. Am J Epidemiol 107:403-411, 1978.
18. Karvonen MJ, Telivuo LJ, Jaervinen EJK: Sphygmomanometer cuff size and the accuracy of indirect measurement of blood pressure. Am J Cardiol 13:688-693, 1964.
19. Simpson JA, Jamieson G, Dickhaus DW, Grover RFL: Effect of size of cuff bladder on accuracy of measurement of indirect blood pressure. Am Heart J 70:208-215, 1965.

20. Labarthe DR, Hawkins CM, Remington DR: Evaluation of performance of selected devices for measuring blood pressure. Am J Cardiol 32:546-553, 1973.
21. Webber LS, Voors AW, Foster TA, Berenson GS: A study of instruments in preparation for a blood pressure survey of children. Circulation 56:651-656, 1977.
22. Kirkendall WM, Burton AC, Epstein FH, Freis ED: Recommendations for human blood pressure determination by sphygmomanometers. Circulation 36:980-988, 1967.
23. Voors AW, Foster TA, Frerichs RR, Webber LS, Berenson GS: Studies of blood pressure in children, ages 5–14 years in a total biracial community—The Bogalusa Heart Study. Circulation 54:319-327, 1976.
24. Blumenthal S, Epps RP, Heavenrich R, et al: Report of the Task Force on Blood Pressure Control in Children. Pediatrics 59:797-820, 1977.
25. Goldring D, Londe S, Sivakoff M, Hernandez A, Britton C, Choi S: Blood pressure in a high school population. I. Standards for blood pressure and the relation of age, sex, weight, height, and race to blood pressure in children 14–18 years of age. J Pediatr 91:884-889, 1977.
26. Foster TA, Voors AW, Webber LS, Frerichs RR, Berenson GS: Anthropometric and maturation measurements of children, ages 5 to 14 years in a biracial community—The Bogalusa Heart Study. Am J Clin Nutr 30:582-591, 1977.
27. Frerichs RR, Webber LS, Srinivasan SR, Berenson GS: Hemoglobin levels in children from a biracial southern community. Am J Public Health 67:841-845, 1977.
28. Frerichs RR, Srinivasan SR, Webber LS, Berenson GS: Serum cholesterol and triglyceride levels in 3,446 children from a biracial community—The Bogalusa Heart Study. Circulation 54:302-309, 1976.
29. Srinivasan SR, Frerichs RR, Webber LS, Berenson GS: Serum lipoprotein profiles in children from a biracial community—The Bogalusa Heart Study. Circulation 54:309-318, 1976.
30. Blonde VA, Frerichs RR, Foster TA, Webber LS, Berenson GS: Physician diagnosed abnormalities in black and white children in a total community. Public Health Rep 94:124-129, 1979.
31. Johnson BC, Epstein FH, Kjelsberg MO: Distributions and familiar studies of blood pressure and serum cholesterol levels in a total community—Tecumseh, Michigan. J Chronic Dis 18:147-160, 1965.
32. Graham AW, Hines EA, Gage RP: Blood pressures in children between the ages of five and sixteen years. Am J Dis Child 69:203-207, 1945.
33. Faber HK, James CA: The range and distribution of blood pressures in normal children. Am J Dis Child 22:7-28, 1921.
34. Moss AJ, Adams FH: Problems of blood pressure in childhood. Springfield: Charles C Thomas, 1962.
35. Weiss NS, Hamill PVV, Drizd T: Blood pressure levels of children 6–11 years: relationship to age, sex, race and socioeconomic status. US Vital Health Stat, Ser 11, No. 135, DHEW Publ No. (HRA) 74-1617, Public Health Service. Washington: US Government Printing Office, 1973.
36. Shock NW: Basal blood pressure and pulse rate in adolescents. Am J Dis Child 68:16-22, 1944.
37. Voors AW, Webber LS, Berenson GS: Body height and body mass as determinants of basal blood pressure in children—The Bogalusa Heart Study. Am J Epidemiol 106:101-108, 1977.

38. Voors AW, Webber LS, Berenson GS: Relationship of blood pressure levels to height and weight in children. Cardiovasc Med 3:911-918, 1978.
39. Comstock GW: An epidemiologic study of blood pressure levels in a biracial community in the southern United States. Am J Hyg 65:271-315, 1957.
40. Stocks R. In: Hamilton M, Pickering GW, Fraser Roberts JA, Sowry GSC: The etiology of essential hypertension: 1. The arterial pressure in the general population. Clin Sci 13:11-35, 1954.
41. Miall WE, Lovell HG: Relation between change of blood pressure and age. Br Med J 2:660-664, 1967.
42. Roberts J, Maurer K: Blood pressure of persons 6–74 years of age in the United States. Advance Data from Vital Health Stat, Ser 1, No. 1, Public Health Service. Washington: US Government Printing Office, 1976.
43. Hamilton M, Pickering GW, Fraser Roberts JA, Sowry GSC: The etiology of essential hypertension: 1. The arterial pressure in the general population. Clin Sci 13:11-35, 1954.
44. Robinson SC, Brucer M: Range of normal blood pressure: a statistical and clinical study of 11,383 persons. Arch Intern Med 64:409-444, 1939.
45. Gordon T, Shurtleff D: The Framingham Study—an epidemiological investigation of cardiovascular disease. Sect 29, DHEW Publ No. (NIH) 74-478, 1973.
46. Voors AW, Webber LS, Berenson GS: Time course studies of blood pressure in children—The Bogalusa Heart Study. Am J Epidemiol 109:320-334, 1979.
47. Harsha DW, Frerichs RR, Berenson GS: Densitometry and anthropometry of black and white children. Hum Biol 50:261-280, 1978.
48. Berenson GS, Voors AW, Dalferes Jr ER, Webber LS, Shuler SE: Creatinine clearance, electrolytes, and plasma renin activity related to the blood pressure of white and black children—The Bogalusa Heart Study. J Lab Clin Med 93:535-548, 1979.
49. Voors AW, Berenson GS, Dalferes Jr ER, Webber LS, Shuler SE: Racial differences in blood pressure control. Science 204:1091-1094, 1979.
50. Voors AW, Berenson GS: Cardiovascular response to rest and stress in children with high and low blood pressures. Hypertension (in press), 1980.
51. Frank GC, Berenson GS, Webber LS: Dietary studies and the relationship of diet to cardiovascular disease risk factor variables in 10-year-old children—The Bogalusa Heart Study. Am J Clin Nutr 31:328-340, 1978.
52. Berenson GS, McMahan CA, Voors AW, Webber LS, Srinivasan SR, Frank GC, Foster TA, Blonde CV: Cardiovascular risk factors in children—the early natural history of atherosclerosis and essential hypertension. New York: Oxford University Press, 1980.
53. Zinner SH, Martin LF, Sacks F, Rosner B, Kass EH: A longitudinal study of blood pressure in childhood. Am J Epidemiol 100:437-442, 1974.
54. Sneiderman C, Heyden S, Heiss G, Tyroler H, Hames C: Predictors of blood pressure over a 16 year followup of 163 youths. Circulation [Suppl 2] 54:II-24, 1976.
55. Harlan WR, Oberman A, Mitchel RE, Graybiel A: A 30 year study of blood pressure in a white male cohort. In: Onesti G, Kim KE, Moyer JH (eds) Hypertension: mechanisms and management. New York: Grune and Stratton, 1973.

6. DISTRIBUTION AND DETERMINANTS OF BLOOD PRESSURE IN FREE–LIVING CHILDREN

Results from an open population study of children aged 5–19 (EPOZ Study)

A. Hofman and H.A. Valkenburg

The growing popularity of the idea that the roots of atherosclerosis can be traced in young individuals has evoked many studies of cardiovascular risk indicators in childhood [1]. The finding of early lesions in the aorta and coronary arteries of children [2] and young adults [3] has led to the statement that atherosclerosis is a pediatric problem essentially [4]. Epidemiological research of determinants of atherogenesis in childhood can be motivated by two main objectives. Firstly, studies of the distribution and determinants of cardiovascular risk indicators can provide insight into the pathogenesis of atherosclerosis. Secondly, when atherosclerotic lesions are present in children, interventive measures implemented early in life can possibly prevent the development of atherosclerotic complications later.

With respect to blood pressure in childhood, the hypothesis has been proposed that overactivity of the sympathetic nervous system in youngsters sets the stage for hypertension in adults [5]. Furthermore, a specific hemodynamic pattern in children and young adults with raised blood pressure has been postulated, characterized by high cardiac output and normal peripheral resistance [6–10].

But before meaningful conclusions can be drawn on the development of essential hypertension in adults, the predictive value of blood pressure in childhood must be examined. Therefore a study emphasizing etiological aspects of atherosclerosis was designed to investigate the natural history ('tracking') of blood pressure and other risk indicators. The present report deals with the distribution of blood pressure in childhood, as well as with the determinants and the persistency of raised blood pressure over a short period of time. Also data on interrelations with other cardiovascular risk indicators and familial relationships of blood pressure are presented.

1. METHODOLOGY

1.1. Population

In the period between April 1975 and June 1978, the total population aged 5 or over of two districts (one rural and one urban) of a Dutch town was asked

H. Kesteloot, J.V. Joossens (eds.), Epidemiology of Arterial Blood Pressure, 99–117.

to take part in the Epidemiological Preventive Organization Zoetermeer (EPOZ). Data were collected on cardiovascular risk indicators, rheumatic and lung diseases, and urinary tract infections. Of the 13,462 persons who were invited 10,532 (78%) participated. Blood pressure was measured in 3942 children (82%) aged 5–19, out of 4806 eligible. The response rate was highest in children aged 5–9 (87%), intermediate in the age group 10–14 (84%), and lowest in 15–19 year olds (77%). The nonresponse in boys was somewhat higher than in girls, due to sex-specific differences in the age group 15–19. The primary nonresponse was about 5% higher in the rural than in the urban district.

All the children who belonged to the age- and sex-specific upper decile of the distribution of one or more of the cardiovascular risk indicators (systolic and diastolic blood pressure, total serum cholesterol, Quetelet index, and smoking habits) were selected for a tracking study. A control group was recruited at random from the remaining part of the same population. In total, 1435 children, initially aged 5–19, were selected for follow-up. The general protocol consisted of reexamination at four weeks after the initial measurement for blood pressure and cholesterol. Further on, the subjects got annual follow-up examinations for all risk indicators. Children with a blood pressure reading of 140 and/or 90 mmHg or over at the first examination round were followed for their blood pressure after 2, 4, and 26 weeks before entering the general protocol.

1.2. Methods

Blood pressure (BP) was measured in a strictly standardized protocol, using a random-zero sphygmomanometer [11], known to reduce observer bias. Two independent readings were taken, in time separated only by a count of the pulse rate. The mean of these two readings was used for BP calculation.

Eight well-trained paramedical observers measured BP on the left arm of a sitting subject, with the arm held at heart level. In general, the measurement was performed between 8 a.m. and 5 p.m., after a rest period of about 15 min in sitting position and before venipuncture.

Following published recommendations [12, 13], the largest cuff comfortably encircling the arm was used, which meant that, in general, children aged 5–9 were measured with a $23 \times 10 \, cm^2$ cuff, while for subjects aged 10 or over, a cuff of $23 \times 14 \, cm^2$ was used.

The first, fourth, and fifth Korotkoff sounds were noted. For diastolic pressure, the fifth Korotkoff sound was used in the analysis. A remarkably constant mean difference of 4 mmHg between fourth and fifth Korotkoff sounds was found in all age groups up to 65 years.

The absolute and relative measurement error was assessed from the duplicate readings. A mean absolute error of ±9.0 mmHg was found for both systolic and diastolic pressure in subjects aged 5–19. The measurement error increased with age in both sexes, and varied between observers from ±7.3 to ±11.9 mmHg.

Serum total cholesterol was measured in plasma of nonfasting subjects with a modification [14] of an automated enzymatic method according to Kageyama [15], in the laboratory of the Department of Epidemiology, which participates in the standardization program of the WHO Lipid Centre in Prague.

Uric acid was measured by using an automated enzymatic method [16] in a Technikon Auto-analyzer II.

Weight and height were estimated while the subjects were without shoes and wearing indoor clothes. Quetelet index (weight/height^2) was used as an index for relative weight.

Smoking habits were determined for subjects aged 15 or over by means of a home-filled questionnaire. Children aged 5–14 were interviewed in absence of the parents in the examination center.

1.3. Data analysis

Data analysis was performed with an IBM-370 and a PDP-11/34 computer system. Standard statistical techniques were applied, using an SPSS or a BMD package [17, 18]. The household being the sampling unit, the EPOZ project is essentially a family study and therefore, whenever possible, the parents of all examined children were also studied.

Only the 1589 families on which BP data are available for both father and mother and at least one child were used in the family analysis. In these 1589 families, age-adjusted regression coefficients of BP of the parents and of all children aged 5 or over were calculated. Data on 1346 families are available with the first child aged 5–19 years. Age-specific Pearson correlation coefficients were calculated for BP of the first child, on the one hand, and the parents and sibs, on the other.

2. RESULTS

2.1. Mean values of blood pressure

In Figure 1 and Table 1, mean values of systolic and diastolic BP are presented for boys and girls aged 5–19. Systolic BP is slightly higher in girls up to 12 years of age, but a marked difference in systolic BP appears after the age of 13, when boys have 7–10 mmHg higher systolic BP than girls. This

Table 1. Age- and sex-specific mean values ±SD of systolic and diastolic blood pressure in children aged 5–19 (n = 3924) (EPOZ 1975–78).

Age	n		Systolic BP		Diastolic BP	
	Boys	Girls	Boys m ± SD (CV%)[a]	Girls m ± SD (CV%)	Boys m ± SD (CV%)	Girls m ± SD (CV%)
5	148	151	97 ± 9 (9)	97 ± 11 (11)	61 ± 9 (15)	60 ± 9 (15)
6	153	148	99 ± 10 (10)	99 ± 11 (11)	63 ± 9 (14)	63 ± 10 (16)
7	136	138	103 ± 10 (10)	104 ± 12 (12)	64 ± 10 (16)	65 ± 12 (18)
8	140	151	103 ± 12 (12)	105 ± 12 (11)	65 ± 9 (14)	66 ± 10 (15)
9	150	146	104 ± 12 (12)	106 ± 13 (12)	64 ± 9 (14)	65 ± 11 (17)
10	132	129	108 ± 12 (11)	109 ± 13 (12)	67 ± 9 (13)	64 ± 11 (17)
11	160	131	109 ± 11 (10)	110 ± 12 (11)	65 ± 11 (17)	66 ± 10 (15)
12	150	147	111 ± 13 (12)	114 ± 14 (12)	65 ± 10 (15)	68 ± 10 (15)
13	144	141	116 ± 14 (12)	116 ± 14 (12)	66 ± 11 (17)	68 ± 10 (15)
14	127	143	118 ± 14 (12)	116 ± 12 (10)	66 ± 10 (15)	69 ± 8 (12)
15	128	127	123 ± 14 (11)	116 ± 11 (9)	66 ± 11 (17)	68 ± 11 (16)
16	106	135	125 ± 14 (11)	118 ± 12 (10)	68 ± 11 (16)	69 ± 9 (13)
17	107	115	126 ± 13 (10)	121 ± 13 (11)	70 ± 11 (16)	70 ± 10 (14)
18	85	85	129 ± 15 (12)	122 ± 14 (11)	71 ± 9 (13)	71 ± 11 (15)
19	94	77	131 ± 15 (11)	120 ± 12 (10)	71 ± 10 (14)	70 ± 10 (14)
Total	1960	1964	113 ± 16 (14)	111 ± 15 (14)	66 ± 10 (15)	67 ± 10 (15)

[a] Percent coefficient of variation.

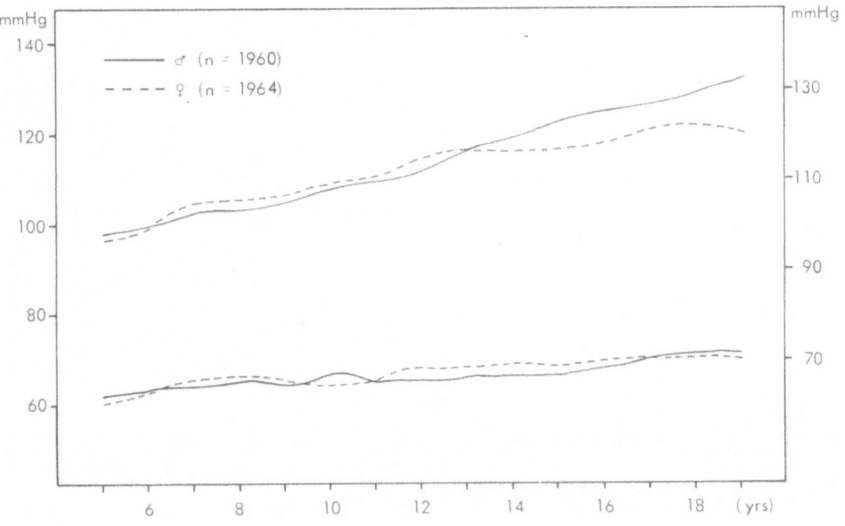

Figure 1. Age- and sex-specific mean values of systolic and diastolic blood pressure in children aged 5–19 (*n* = 3924) (EPOZ) 1975–78).

difference in systolic BP continues to exist until the end of the fourth decade, after which mean systolic BP of women increases over that of men.

No large differences in diastolic BP between the sexes are found in either children or adults. As a result of this, boys have considerably larger pulse pressures than girls between the ages of 13 and 43.

In Figure 2, the 5th, 50th, and 95th percentiles for systolic and diastolic BP versus weight are shown for both sexes. Weight was chosen as the reference variable, because it proved to be the best predictor of systolic and diastolic BP of all measured maturity indicators in this study. Besides that, it is standard practice in (school) health services to weigh children. In this presentation of percentiles, no adjustment for menarche was made. Such an adjustment would change the percentiles only slightly.

Only for systolic BP in boys is there an increase in absolute (mmHg) within-population variability, as indicated by the increasing standard deviations with age (Table 1).

When a relative measure of variability is applied (coefficient of variation), no differences in variability between the sexes and no increases with age are found. The relative variability of diastolic BP is considerably larger than that of systolic BP.

The age- and sex-specific distributions of both BP parameters are nearly normal. All distributions of systolic BP are slightly skewed to the right, while the distributions of diastolic BP are all (except the 15- to 19-year-old girls) skewed to the left.

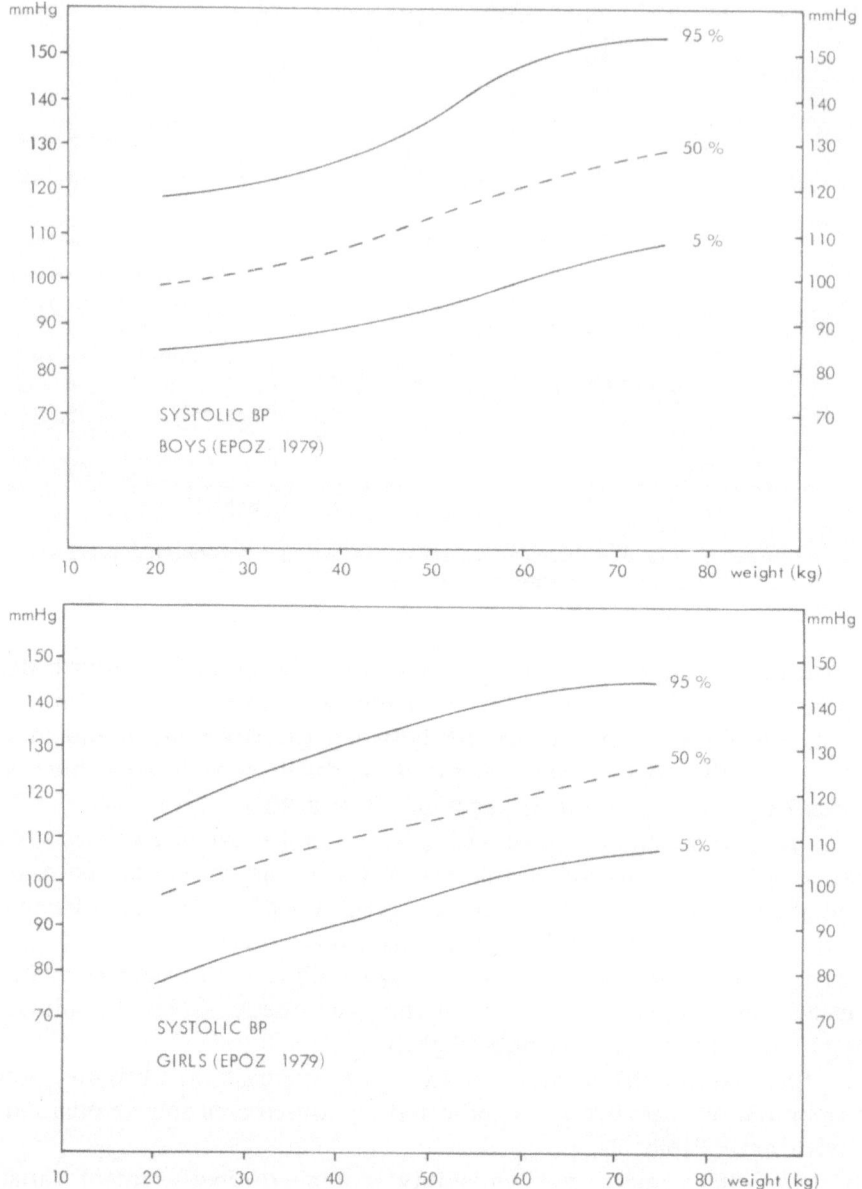

Figure 2. Systolic and diastolic blood pressure in boys and girls aged 5–19: 5th, 50th,

Children living in the rural district have higher mean systolic BP (114 vs 110 mmHg) than those in the urban district. This is true for both sexes and nearly all age groups. For diastolic BP and weight, no large differences are found between the districts.

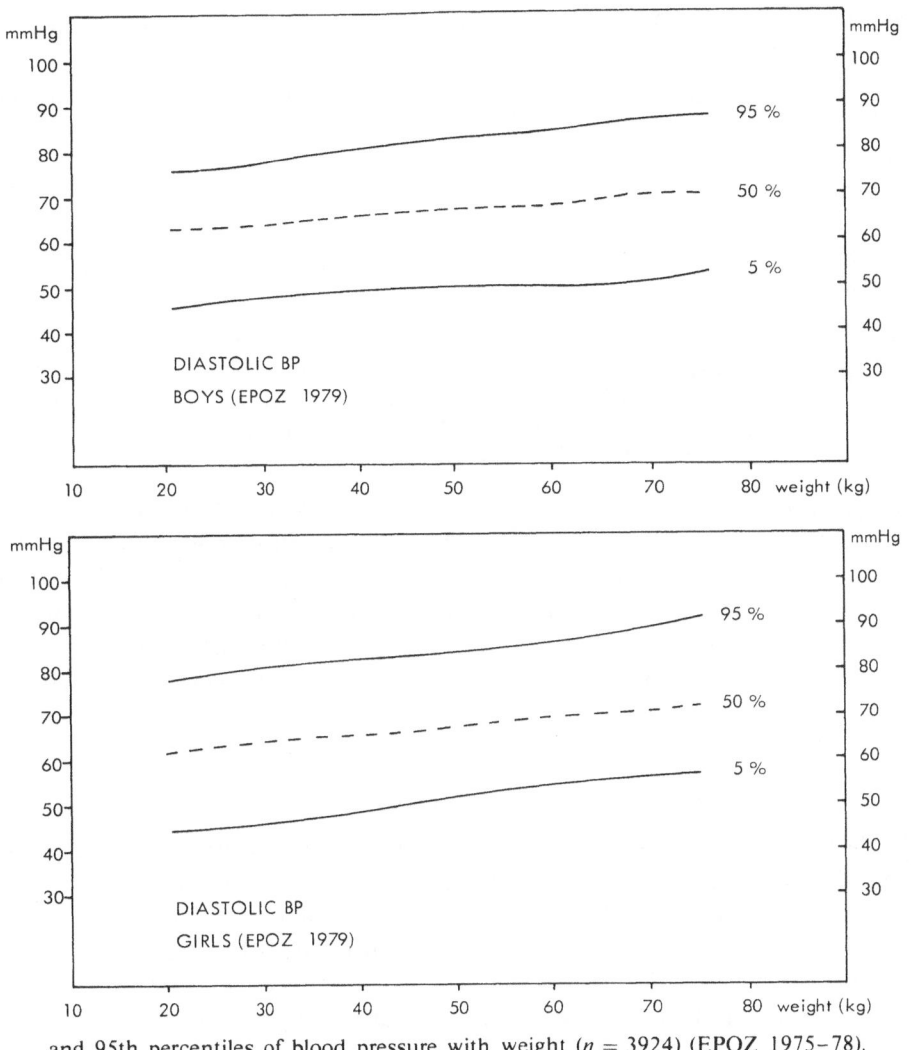

and 95th percentiles of blood pressure with weight ($n = 3924$) (EPOZ 1975–78).

2.2. Prevalence of relatively high blood pressure

In Table 2, the percentages of children exceeding certain arbitrary cutoff points are shown. The cutoff levels recommended by WHO [19] for youngsters (140/90 mmHg) and adults (160/95 mmHg) are presented. The age dependency of BP in childhood is clearly demonstrated in these data. Over 20% of the boys aged 15–19 exceed 140/90 mmHg, while only 0.3% of the 5–9 year olds do so. Of the 15- to 19-year-old girls, 8.3% have a BP reading of 140/90 mmHg or over.

Table 2. Blood pressure in children aged 5–19: percentages at various cutoff points and follow-up (*n* = 3924) (EPOZ 1975–78).

Age		Total number in study	≥140 and/or 90 %	≥160 and/or 95 %	3× ≥140/90 [a] % [b]
Boys	5–9	727	0.3	0.1	0.0
	10–19	713	5.3	0.6	0.2
	15–19	520	20.6	2.3	3.9
	Total	1960	7.5	0.8	1.1
Girls	5–9	734	0.8	0.1	0.0
	10–14	691	2.9	0.3	0.3
	15–19	539	8.3	0.9	0.6
	Total	1964	4.4	0.4	0.3

[a] Three times consecutively ≥140 and/or 90 mmHg within a month.
[b] Total number corrected for loss at follow-up.

For an impression of the persistency of raised BP in childhood, the percentage of children who exceed 140/90 mmHg in all of three consecutive readings is also presented in Table 2. This criterion (or the 95th percentile) is sometimes advocated to define 'persistent hypertension' in childhood [13, 20]. Nearly 4% of the boys and 0.6% of the girls aged 15–19 had a BP level above 140/90 mmHg in all of three consecutive measurements, performed within a month.

2.3. Interrelations of cardiovascular risk indicators

Interrelations between various cardiovascular risk indicators were estimated by calculation of age-adjusted standardized regression coefficients of systolic and diastolic BP with total serum cholesterol, Quetelet index, and smoking habits (Table 3). Except for systolic with diastolic BP (0.52), the age-adjusted regression coefficients are very small. The positive association between serum total cholesterol and diastolic BP (0.13) is statistically significant with respect to this sample size, while the other smaller coefficients are not.

Table 3. Interrelations of cardiovascular risk indicators in children aged 5–19: age-adjusted standardized regression coefficients between blood pressure, cholesterol, smoking, and Quetelet index (*n* = 3924) (EPOZ 1975–78).

	Diastolic BP	Total cholesterol	Smoking habits [a]	Quetelet index [b]
Systolic BP	0.52	0.06	0.04	−0.01
Diastolic BP		0.13	0.04	−0.02
Total cholesterol			0.05	−0.02
Smoking habits				−0.02

[a] 3-Point scale: smoked never, in the past, now.
[b] Quetelet index = weight/height ^{2}.

2.4. Family analysis

Age is an important confounding variable in the relationship between BP of the parents and of their children. Therefore, overall age-adjusted (parent-child) regression coefficients were calculated. Between parents, a regression coefficient of 0.15 (systolic BP, $P<0.001$) and 0.11 (diastolic BP, $P<0.001$) is found. Overall age-adjusted father-child and mother-child regression coefficients are 0.13 ($P<0.001$) and 0.11 ($P<0.001$), respectively, for systolic BP. For diastolic BP, these overall coefficients are 0.11 ($P<0.001$) for both parent-child relations.

Table 4. Correlation coefficients between systolic and diastolic blood pressure of the first child with parents and siblings in three age groups (EPOZ 1975–78).

First child	Father	Mother	Second child	Third child
Systolic BP				
5–9 years	0.11[a] (417)	0.15[c]	0.40[c] (225)	0.34[a] (38)
10–14 years	0.17[b] (459)	0.26[c]	0.34[c] (422)	0.27[c] (172)
15–19 years	0.14[c] (470)	0.12[b]	0.25[c] (388)	0.16[b] (233)
Diastolic BP				
5–9 years	0.07 (417)	0.22[c]	0.17[b] (225)	0.29[a] (38)
10–14 years	0.17[c] (459)	0.26[c]	0.19[c] (422)	0.12 (172)
15–19 years	0.12[b] (470)	0.11[b]	0.21[c] (388)	0.11[c] (233)

[a] $P<0.05$;
[b] $P<0.01$;
[c] $P<0.001$.

Table 4 presents the various parent-sib and sib-sib correlations for both pressure parameters in three age groups. For the first child, the correlation with maternal BP is slightly larger than with BP of the father. No clear relationship with age of the first child can be shown except that the age group 10–14 years shows the largest coefficients. In general, the coefficients with siblings decrease with increasing difference in rank order. For systolic pressure, the magnitude of sib-sib correlations decreases with increasing age of the first child. This pattern is less clear for diastolic pressure, and the coefficients are not so large as for systolic BP.

2.5. Determinants of blood pressure

Correlation coefficients between systolic and diastolic BP and some anthropometric variables are presented in Table 5. All measured indicators of growth and physical maturity (age, height, weight and Quetelet index) have correlation coefficients with systolic BP of 0.5–0.6 and with diastolic BP of

Table 5. Correlation coefficients [a] of systolic and diastolic blood pressure with some variables, in children aged 5–19 (*n* = 3914) (EPOZ 1975 – 78).

	Systolic BP	Diastolic BP
Age	0.55	0.22
Sex	0.05	−0.03
Height	0.60	0.24
Weight	0.64	0.27
Quetelet index	0.55	0.25
Triceps skinfold [b]	0.16	0.08
Pulse rate	0.11	0.11

[a] Pearson test;
[b] *n* = 2523.

0.2–0.3. The only exception is the skinfold above the triceps muscle as measured by caliper, which has very small coefficients with both systolic and diastolic BP (0.08–0.16). The magnitude of these coefficients can be partly explained by mutual interrelations. Therefore, a stepwise multiple regression analysis was performed with systolic and diastolic BP as dependent variables.

Table 6. Stepwise multiple regression of systolic and diastolic blood pressure in children aged 5–19 (*n* = 3914) (EPOZ 1975–78).

Independent vars	Systolic pressure Regression coefficients		Diastolic pressure Regression coefficients	
	Unstandardized	Standardized	Unstandardized	Standardized
Weight (kg)	0.58	0.60	0.19	0.31
Pulse rate (/30 s)	0.56	0.27	0.23	0.17
Sex [a]	2.24	0.07	−0.35	−0.02
Age (years)	0.29	0.08	0.27	0.01
Smoking habits [b]	−0.71	−0.04	−0.35	−0.03
Height (cm)	0.30	0.04	0.12	0.00
Intercept (mmHg)	54.12		47.96	
Cumulative R^2	0.47		0.10	

[a] 0 = girls, 1 = boys;
[b] 3-Point scale: never smoked, in the past, now.

Table 6 shows that by entering weight, pulse rate, sex, age, smoking habits, and height into the equation, 47% of systolic variability and only 10% of diastolic variability can be explained in youngsters aged 5–19. By far, the most important determinants of both BP parameters are *weight* and *pulse rate*. Weight has a standardized regression coefficient of 0.60 with systolic BP, and of 0.31 with diastolic BP. Pulse rate is also positively associated with systolic and diastolic BP, having standardized coefficients of 0.27 and 0.17, respectively.

Parental blood pressure levels are positively associated with BP of their children, but the independent contribution is small as compared with weight and pulse rate. No relation between BP in children and the *profession* or *educational level* of their fathers is found in the multiple regression analysis.

Age per se, expressed by its linear term, makes only a very small independent contribution in explaining the variability of BP in childhood.

Smoking is negatively associated with both BP parameters. The standardized regression coefficients are small (-0.04 with systolic and -0.03 with diastolic BP) although statistically significant.

Of 526 girls aged 15–19 years from whom this information was obtained, 140 (26.6%) were using *oral contraceptives*. Pill users have significantly higher systolic (123 vs 118 mmHg) and diastolic (71 vs 69 mmHg) BP than nonusers. In a multiple regression analysis (Table 7), women taking oral contraceptives have 0.93 mmHg higher systolic BP than women of the same weight, pulse rate, smoking habits, and age, but not taking the pill.

Table 7. Stepwise multiple regression of systolic blood pressure in women aged 15–19 ($n = 526$) (EPOZ 1975–78).

Independent vars	Cumulative R^2	Regression coefficients	
		Unstandardized	Standardized
Weight (kg)	0.12	0.52	0.35
Pulse rate (/30 s)	0.23	0.52	0.33
Smoking habits[a]	0.23	-1.33	-0.09
Oral contraceptives	0.24	0.93	0.06
Age (years)	0.24	0.36	0.05
Height (cm)	0.24	0.10	0.01
Intercept		55.45	

[a] 3-Point scale: never smoked, in the past, now.

The age-adjusted regression coefficients between *uric acid* and systolic and diastolic BP are 0.13 and 0.05, respectively. Uric acid makes no statistically significant contribution to the multiple regression analysis.

2.6. 'Tracking' of blood pressure

For the analysis of 'tracking' of BP, the children in the control group were randomly supplied with a proportional number of children from the group in the upper decile of risk indicators, to provide a representative sample of the

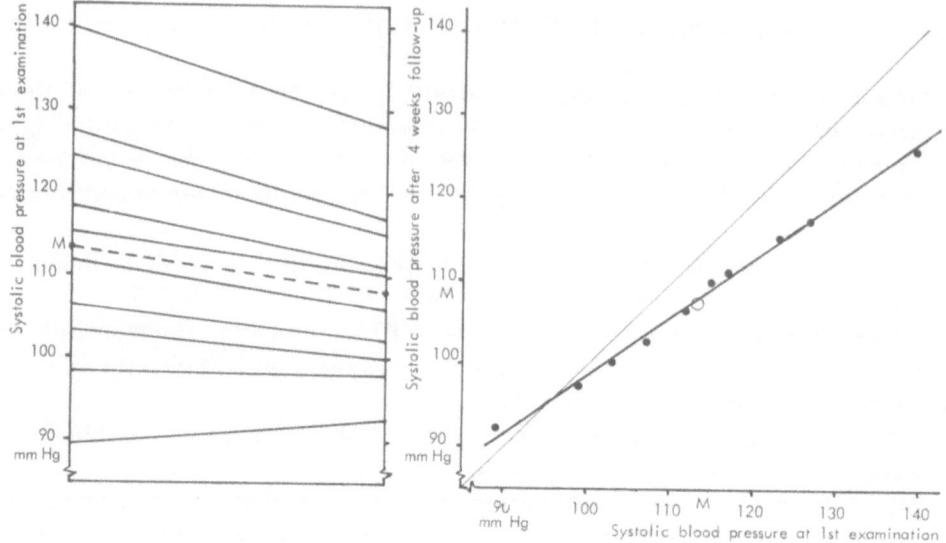

Figure 3. Systolic blood pressure at first examination and at follow-up after four weeks in a sample from the total initially examined population of children aged 5–19: mean values per decile at first examination and after 4 weeks (*n* = 435) (EPOZ 1975–78).

total population of children initially examined. In Figure 3, the mean values for systolic BP in the ten deciles at first examination and at follow-up at four weeks are presented. The overall mean value decreased from 113 mmHg to 108 mmHg, and a clear regression toward the mean is depicted. The regression line plotted in the right-hand part of Figure 3 presents no evidence for curvilinearity.

The variability of BP over time is also illustrated in Table 8. Tracking correlations are presented for the values at first examination and those at four-week follow-up. The correlation coefficients are larger for systolic than for diastolic BP (for the total group: 0.68 vs 0.41). The coefficient of pulse rate for the total group is 0.51.

Table 8. Tracking correlations [a] between initial examination and four-week follow-up in controls (*n* = 435) (EPOZ 1975–78).

Age	*n*	Systolic BP	Diastolic BP	Pulse rate
5– 9	139	0.53	0.48	0.42
10–14	159	0.55	0.34	0.48
15–19	137	0.63	0.31	0.54
Total	435	0.68	0.41	0.51

[a] Pearson test.

3. DISCUSSION

The *response rates* in various investigations of BP in childhood depend largely on the age of the subjects. In primary school children, the response rates are over 85% in most studies in the USA [21–25] as well as Europe [26–28]. By contrast, in adolescents and young adults, the response rates are below 80% in general [29–31]. The age-specific response rates in the EPOZ study reflect this general pattern.

In our tracking study in a rural and in an urban district, we have to cope with a very mobile study population. Although the results of follow-up can be influenced by this phenomenon, this is not the case for the prevalence data as presented in this paper. In our experience, home visits, with a personal approach to persuade youngsters to participate in the study, are very effective.

For systolic BP, a clear increase of *mean values* with age occurs in both sexes. The dissociation of mean values between the sexes after 13 years of age has been observed in various studies [21–24, 26] and can be explained only partly by weight differences. Its relevance is that during the 'incubation period' of atherosclerosis, males have higher BP levels than females, combined with higher mean values of total cholesterol and body mass index [32].

The comparison of our findings with other studies is hampered severely by differences in sampling frame, procedures, and methods. To exclude some dissimilarities, we compared our results with other open population studies only. Mean values of systolic BP were found to be higher in Tecumseh [21] and in the National Examination Survey [23, 24], about the same in Muscatine [29], and lower in whites in Bogalusa [22]. After correction for different definitions of diastolic BP, all American studies, except the National Examination Survey, found lower diastolic BP. Various school-based studies in European countries (UK, Ireland, Greece, FRG, GDR, Austria, Switzerland, and The Netherlands) [26–28, 31, 33–36] show large differences in mean values. Relatively high levels of systolic BP were found in Greece [36] and Austria [33], and low values in the UK [26] and Holland [27]. The gradient between the same age and sex group in these different studies is 15–20 mmHg. Unfortunately, the degree to which these differences are due to methodological dissimilarities cannot be estimated.

The within-population *variability* differs between both pressure parameters; diastolic BP having larger standard deviations. In both sexes, the variance of systolic BP increases with age. This phenomenon is more distinct for boys. The larger absolute variability in boys has been implicated in the origin of essential hypertension [20] and has been interpreted as an argument for the existence of a hyperkinetic phase in early essential hypertension.

However, when a measure of relative variability is used—the coefficient of variation—no clear difference in variability is found between the sexes. Hence, the increasing variability with age and the differences between the sexes, as reported above and in other studies, seem to be associated with higher mean values of systolic BP, and not with increasing variability per se. Mean values of diastolic BP increase only slightly with age, and no changes in absolute diastolic variability with age can be observed. This also supports the view that age is not related with BP variability per se.

As far as the *determinants* of BP are concerned, there is little doubt about the great importance of *genetic factors* [38]. This point has been stressed in particular by elegant adoption studies [39, 40], which indicate that about half of the variability of BP in children is genetically determined.

In our study as well as in others [41], there is a striking resemblance between the sex- and age-specific curves of mean systolic BP and mean uric acid values, especially in younger ages. Since mean values of uric acid are merely the result of endogenously determined factors, this is likely to be an expression of the impact of genetic factors. Our family analysis shows essentially the same pattern as reported from other investigations [21, 37, 42].

Weight has been reported from most other studies as being a very important independent variable in the explanation of BP variability in childhood. In relation with BP, it seems to be the best predictor of maturity [22, 37]. Age per se is unimportant in relation with BP.

Pulse rate is an important determinant of systolic and diastolic BP in this study and in others [30]. There are several possible explanations for this finding. Firstly, the association between pulse rate and BP can be an expression of excitation during the (first) BP examination. The fact that pulse rate makes an independent contribution to the explanation of systolic variability at the follow-up examination after four weeks, which is of about the same magnitude as of the first examination, contradicts this explanation. Secondly, it has been postulated that this association is a result of a hyperkinetic response of BP in childhood, which characterizes an early stage in essential hypertension. Published [43] and still unpublished data from a case-referent study of hemodynamic variables in our follow-up cohort do not support this hypothesis.

Smoking and the use of *oral contraceptives* have small and inverse effects on systolic BP. In the regression analysis, increased systolic BP is associated with the use of the pill, and with nonsmoking. Although the regression coefficients are small, these findings probably are important because of the short period of usage of the pill and the smoking of cigarettes in this age group.

A potentially important variable, currently under study in the same population of children, is *sodium intake* and its influence on the natural history of BP, and on the changes in BP values over time.

The study of the *natural history* of BP in adults as well as in children has gained much interest [44]. In 'tracking studies' devoted to this subject, the relative position of an individual in the distribution of BP is studied over time. In this way, an impression of the persistency of BP elevation can be obtained. In adults, correlation coefficients of about 0.6–0.7 have been found in various studies [45, 46]. In children, the situation is less clear. Some investigators reported tracking correlations in youngsters of 0.4–0.5 [46–48], while others found considerably smaller coefficients, varying from 0.2 to 0.4 [49–51].

In this paper, only data on short-term follow-up (after four weeks) are presented. Correlation coefficients of 0.7 for systolic BP and 0.4 for diastolic BP were found. Preliminary analysis of our data on longer follow-up periods shows coefficients of about 0.5 for systolic BP and 0.2 for diastolic BP, after two and three years of follow-up in children aged 5–19 [52]. The findings of regression toward the mean and decrease of mean BP after four weeks of follow-up are as expected. In this relatively short period of follow-up, the decreasing effect of the growing familiarity with the examination on mean BP level is more important than the process of maturation, which tends to increase BP over time.

The regression line of systolic BP, as shown in Figure 3, is linear, even in the highest deciles of BP levels. This linear regression in a nonintervened population is important for the interpretation of effects of interventive measures in hypertensive adults. When the same pattern of regression holds true for the adult population, the effect of intervention can be estimated by comparing the linearly extrapolated regression line from normotensives with the regression line obtained from hypertensives receiving therapy.

4. CONCLUSIONS

1) Persistently elevated BP is not uncommon in childhood, especially in boys aged 15–19.
2) There is no evidence for the increase in relative variability of BP with increasing age. Furthermore, in this respect there are no differences between the sexes and the BP parameters.
3) Mean systolic BP increases with age in both sexes. The increase is more marked in boys after 13 years of age, when a considerable dissociation between the sexes in mean systolic BP emerges. In both sexes, diastolic BP increases only slightly with age.
4) Weight, pulse rate, and parental BP levels are the most important determinants of BP in childhood. In a multiple regression analysis, a relatively

large part of systolic variability and only a small part of diastolic variability can be explained.

5) Smoking and the use of oral contraceptives have small, but independent, contributions in explaining systolic BP variability. Smoking is negatively associated and the use of oral contraceptives is positively associated with systolic BP.

6) 'Tracking' correlations of BP over a brief follow-up period (four weeks) are 0.68 for systolic BP, 0.41 for diastolic BP, and 0.51 for pulse rate. There is a clear regression toward the mean. Preliminary data about longer follow-up periods support the hypothesis of tracking of systolic BP.

7) The regression of BP at follow-up examination on the level at the initial examination is linear in the total population of nonintervened children.

Acknowledgments. We are grateful to all of the children and their parents who are participating in the EPOZ study. We thank Dr. F.N. Groustra, Ria Rijneveldshoek and through her all co-workers in the EPOZ examination center, and Inge Werdmuller, Liesbeth Pijl, Nannie Dijkstra, Jolanda Bekker, Leo Muller, and Bram van Laar for their enthusiasm and their skilful contributions to data gathering and analysis. This part of the EPOZ study has been supported by grants from the Dutch Prevention fund and the Dutch Health Organization TNO. EPOZ Progress Reports are available on request from the Department of Epidemiology, Medical Faculty, Erasmus University, P.O. Box 1738, Rotterdam, The Netherlands.

REFERENCES

1. Berenson GS: Risk factors in children—the early natural history of atherosclerosis. In: Schettler G, Goto Y, Hata Y, Klose G (eds) Atherosclerosis IV. Berlin: Springer, 1977, pp 489-497.
2. Strong JP, McGill Jr HC: The pediatric aspects of atherosclerosis. J Atheroscler Res 9:251-265, 1969.
3. Enos WF, Holmes RH, Beyer J: Coronary disease among United States soldiers killed in action in Korea. JAMA 152:1090-1093, 1953.
4. Holman RL: Atherosclerosis—a pediatric nutrition problem? Am J Clin Nutr 9:565-572, 1961.
5. Brown JJ, Lever AF, Robertson JIS, Schalekamp MA: Pathogenesis of essential hypertension. Lancet 1:1217-1221, 1976.
6. Eich RH, Peters RJ, Cuddy RP, Smulyan H, Lyons RH: The hemodynamics in labile hypertension. Am Heart J 63:188-195, 1962.
7. Finkielman S, Worcel M, Agrest A: Hemodynamic patterns in essential hypertension. Circulation 31:356-368, 1965.
8. Lund-Johansen P: Hemodynamics in early essential hypertension. Thesis, Bergen, 1967.
9. Levy AM, Tabakin BS, Hanson JS: Hemodynamic responses to graded treadmill exercise in young untreated labile hypertensive patients. Circulation 35:1063-1072, 1967.

10. Tarazi RC, Dustan HP: The hemodynamics of labile hypertension in adolescents. In: Strauss J (ed) Pediatric nephrology. New York: Plenum Press, 1976, pp 97-108.
11. Wright BM, Dore CF: A random-zero sphygmomanometer. Lancet 1:337-338, 1970.
12. Report of a subcommittee of the postgraduate education committee, American Heart Association: Recommendations for human blood pressure determination by sphygmomanometers. Circulation 36:980-988, 1967.
13. Report of the Task Force on blood pressure control in children. Pediatrics [Suppl] 59:797-820, 1977.
14. Van Gent CM, Van der Voort HA, De Bruyn AM, Klein F: Cholesterol determinations. A comparative study of methods with special reference to enzymatic procedures. Clin Chim Acta 75:243-251, 1977.
15. Röslau P, Bernt E, Gruber W: Enzymatische Bestimmung des Gesamt-Cholesterins im Serum. Z Klin Chem Klin Biochem 12:226-231, 1974.
16. Gochman N, Schmitz JM: Automated determination of uric acid, with use of a uricase-peroxidase system. Clin Chem 17:1154-1159, 1971.
17. Nie NH, Hull CH, Jenkins JG, Steinbrenner K, Bent DH: Statistical package for the social sciences, 2nd edn. New York: McGraw-Hill, 1975.
18. Dixon WJ, Brown MB: Biomedical computer programs P-series. Berkeley: University of California Press, 1977.
19. WHO: Hypertension and coronary heart disease: classification and criteria for epidemiological studies. WHO Tech Rep Ser 168, 1959.
20. Kilcoyne MM, Richter RW, Alsup PA: Adolescent hypertension. I. Detection and prevalence. Circulation 50:758-764, 1974.
21. Johnson BC, Epstein FH, Kjelsberg MO: Distributions and familial studies of blood pressure and serum cholesterol levels in a total community—Tecumseh, Michigan. J Chronic Dis 18:147-160, 1965.
22. Voors AW, Foster TA, Frerichs RR, Webber LS, Berenson GS: Studies of blood pressure in children ages 5–14 years, in a total biracial community. The Bogalusa Heart Study. Circulation 54:319-327, 1976.
23. NCHS: Blood pressure levels of children 6–11 years: relationship to age, sex, race, and socioeconomic status. NCHS Vital Health Stat Ser 11 (135), 1973.
24. NCHS: Blood pressure of youths 12–17 years. NCHS Vital Health Stat Ser 11 (163), 1977.
25. Fixler DE, Laird WP, Fitzgerald V, Stead S, Adams R: Hypertension screening in schools: results of the Dallas study. Pediatrics 63:32-36, 1979.
26. Beresford SAA, Holland WW: Levels of blood pressure in children: a family study. Proc R Soc Med 66:35-37, 1973.
27. Uppal SC: Coronary heart disease risk pattern in Dutch youth. A pilot study in Westland schoolchildren. Thesis, Leiden, 1974.
28. Böthig I, Böthig S, Eisenblätter D, Weiss M, Briedigkeit W, Ulrich S, Kunick I, Teichert R, Hellmer I, Gross R, Harksen U: Der Blutdruck im Kindes- und Jugendalter. Dtsch Gesundheitswes 33:2010-2014, 1978.
29. Lauer RM, Connor WE, Leaverton PE, Reiter MA, Clarke WR: Coronary heart disease risk factors in school children: the Muscatine study. J Pediatr 86:697-706, 1975.
30. Miller RA, Shekelle RB: Blood pressure in tenth-grade students. Resutls from the Chicago Heart Association Pediatric Heart Screening Project. Circulation 54:993-1000, 1976.

31. Laaser U: Risikofaktoren bei Jugendlichen. Indikatoren des kardiovaskulären Risikos bei Schülern der Oberstufe in Köln. Fortschr Med 95:256-262, 1977.
32. Valkenburg HA, Hofman A, Klein F, Groustra FN: Een epidemiologisch onderzoek naar risico-indicatoren voor hart- en vaatziekten (EPOZ). Ned Tijdschr Geneeskd 124:183-189, 1980.
33. Marktl W, Rudas B: Screening for risks of cardiovascular disease in children. A preliminary report. Br J Nutr 35:223-227, 1976.
34. Hoffman A, Bruppacher R, Gutzwiller F, De Roche C: Blutdruck in der Adoleszenz. Helv Paediatr Acta 31:121-129, 1976.
35. Gill DG: Blood pressure in Dublin school-children. Irish J Med Sci 146:255-259, 1977.
36. Cassimos C, Varlamis G, Karamperis S, Katsouyannopoulos: Blood pressure in children and adolescents. Acta Paediatr Scand 66:439-443, 1977.
37. Holland WW, Beresford SAA: Factors influencing blood pressure in children. In: Paul O (ed) Epidemiology and control of hypertension. Stuttgart: Thieme, 1975, pp 375-386.
38. Feinleib M, Garrison RJ, Havlik RJ: Environmental and genetic factors affecting the distribution of blood pressure in children. Presented at Primary Prevention in Childhood of Atherosclerotic and Hypertensive Diseases, Chicago, 1978.
39. Biron P, Mongeau J-G, Bertrand D: Familial aggregation of blood pressure in adopted and natural children. In: Paul O (ed) Epidemiology and control of hypertension. Stuttgart: Thieme, 1975, pp 397-405.
40. Annest JL, Sing CF, Biron P, Mongeau J-G: 18th Annual conference on cardiovascular epidemiology (Abstr 110), Orlando, FL, 1978.
41. Mikkelsen WM, Dodge HJ, Valkenburg H: The distribution of serum uric acid values in a population unselected as to gout or hyperuricemia. Am J Med 39:242-251, 1965.
42. Zinner SH, Levy PS, Kass EH: Familial aggregation of blood pressure in childhood. N Engl J Med 284:401-404, 1971.
43. Hofman A, Boomsma F, Schalekamp MADH, Valkenburg HA: Raised blood pressure and plasma noradrenaline in teenagers and young adults selected from an open population. Br Med J 1:1536-1538, 1979.
44. Labarthe DR: Variation in serial blood pressure readings of individuals in a defined population. PhD thesis, University of California, Berkeley, 1974.
45. Feinleib M, Halperin M, Garrison RJ: Relationship between blood pressure and age. Regression analysis of longitudinal data. 97th Annual meeting of the American Public Health Association, Philadelphia, 1969.
46. Rosner B, Hennekens CH, Kass EH, Miall WE: Age-specific correlation analysis of longitudinal blood pressure data. Am J Epidemiol 106:306-313, 1977.
47. Jesse MJ, Hokanson JA, Klein B, Levine R, Gourley J: Blood pressures in childhood: initial recording versus one year followup. Circulation [Suppl] 53:II-23, 1976.
48. Sneiderman C, Heyden S, Heiss G, Tyroler H, Hames C: Predictors of blood pressure over 16 years follow-up of 163 youths. Circulation [Suppl] 53:II-24, 1976.
49. Zinner SH, Martin LF, Sacks F, Rosner B, Kass EH: A longitudinal study of blood pressure in childhood. Am J Epidemiol 100:437-442, 1977.
50. Clarke W, Woolson R, Schrott H, Wiebe D, Lauer R: Tracking of blood pressure, serum lipids and obesity in children: the Muscatine study. Circulation [Suppl] 53:II-23, 1976.

51. Bringgold B, Labarthe DR, Weidman WH: A re-examination of the 'tracking' hypothesis in a familial study of blood pressure. Circulation [Suppl] 53:II-24, 1976.
52. Hofman A, Valkenburg HA: Distribution and tracking of risk-indicators for cardiovascular diseases in an open population of children aged 5–19 (EPOZ study) (Abstr 16). Trans Eur Soc Cardiol 1, 1979.

PART THREE

EPIDEMIOLOGY OF BLOOD PRESSURE IN ADOLESCENTS AND CHILDREN

7. BLOOD PRESSURE DISTRIBUTION AND DETERMINANTS IN A SAMPLE OF ADOLESCENT AND ADULT BELGIAN POPULATION

Results of the Belgian Hypertension Committee Epidemiological Survey 1973–1977

J.C. DEMANET, K. SAMII, G. RORIVE, Y. MAUS, E. COUSSAERT, and P. SMETS

When, a few years ago, the Belgian Hypertension Committee sponsored an epidemiological study regarding the hypertension in the belgian population, a few reports had already been published, giving some information on the blood pressure (BP) distribution in this country; however, they all concerned limited categories of people, such as selected professional groups [1, 2] or selected age classes [1]. The aim of the project, which has now been put to an end, was to explore a cross-section of the belgian population, as representative as possible of every age, professional and social class. It was not conceived as a very large survey, including the recording of casual BP in tens of thousands of people, but was elaborated to measure very carefully the BP of a relatively limited sample of persons in good condition of rest, taking time to make several determinations, and to record much information concerning their medical history, symptoms, medications, habits, origin, professional occupation, and place of residence.

1. PROCEDURE: EXAMINATION OF THE SUBJECTS

Working teams were constituted, comprising a doctor and a female technician well trained for indirect BP determination.

Each individual was allowed to rest in the lying position in a quiet room for 10 min, after which four consecutive BP determinations were recorded (two at each arm) by the technician, with a standard mercury manometer (Erkameter) and a cuff 14 cm wide. The pulse rate, arm circumference, height, and weight were also recorded.

The second part of the examination consisted of an interview by the doctor, which enabled the documentation of (a) a possible familial history of hypertension, (b) the values of eventual previous determination of BP, and (c) in case of established hypertension, its eventual treatment at the time of the screening. This interview also concerned the smoking habits of the subjects, their possible ingestion of contraceptive pills, their place of residence (city or suburbs), and their professional occupation. They were finally asked if they complained of certain symptoms: headache, nervousness, palpitations, chest pain, or other.

H. Kesteloot, J.V. Joossens (eds.), Epidemiology of Arterial Blood Pressure, 121–144.
Copyright © 1980 Martinus Nijhoff Publishers bv. The Hague/Boston/London. All rights reserved.

122

2. CONSTITUTION AND CHARACTERISTICS OF THE SAMPLE

In order to include in the sample people of all ages (excluding children under 10 years old), of both sexes, and of different social and professional categories, the examination procedure was carried out in different environments. Mainly employees and workers of official administrations, department stores and factories, university students, schoolchildren, and boarders of homes for the aged were involved. Some people were also examined at home, but this procedure proved difficult and time-consuming, and was abandonned.

Between 1973 and 1977, a total of 6584 persons were included in the study, comprising 3483 males and 3101 females. Ages ranged from 10 to 98 years; the distribution in the sample of the different age classes is given in Table 1.

Table 1. Number of persons in the different age groups per sex.

Age group (years)	Males	Females
10–19	1019	657
20–29	919	628
30–39	463	521
40–49	475	696
50–59	352	375
60–69	157	76
70–99	98	146
Total	3483	3101

The numerical importance of these age classes decreases from the youngest to the oldest, but this may be considered favorably, since the incidence of hypertension greatly increases with age.

The distribution of the main professional categories in this population sample is given in Table 2. The proportions of these categories in the sample

Table 2. Professional categories in the total sample (in % per sex).

	Males (100%)	Females (100%)
Schoolchildren and students	39	20
Blue-collar workers	34	13
White-collar workers (employees, clerks, executives)	22	60
Retired	5	7

are grossly comparable with the situation of the Belgian population. The main discordance would be the small participation of the category of independent workers (farmers, housewives, tradesmen, liberal professions). A few of them are included in the 'white collar' category. Table 3 gives the distribution of

Table 3. Origin (birthplace) and place of residence categories (in % of total population and of age and sex groups).

	% of total population	Males (in % per age group)			Females (in % per age group)		
		10–19 years	20–49 years	≥50 years	10–19 years	20–49 years	≥50 years
Origin (birth)							
Brabant	26	29	22	47	18	22	41
Flemish	9	6	9	10	7	9	9
Walloon	52	54	48	35	62	60	43
Foreign	13	11	21	8	13	9	7
Residence							
City	58	59	49	63	56	58	77
Suburb	14	14	14	10	14	18	13
Country	28	27	37	27	30	24	10

124

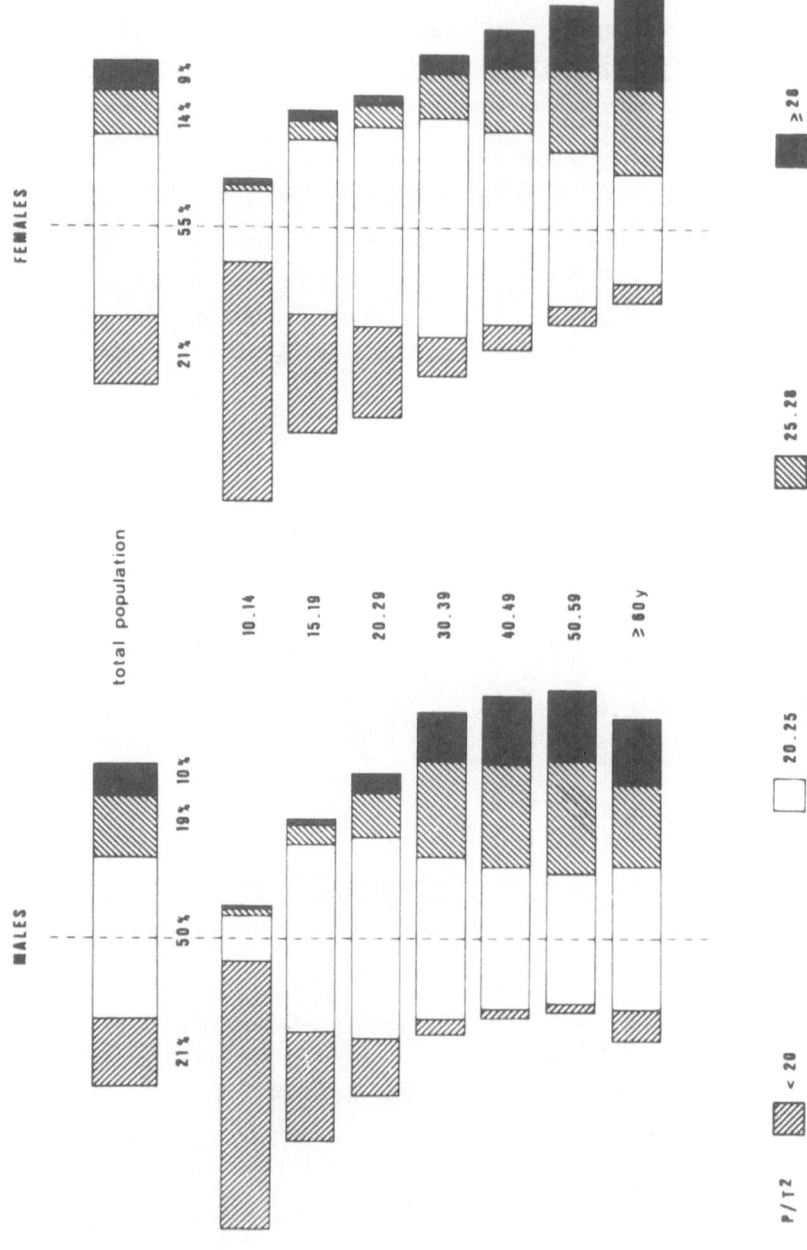

Figure 1. Percent distribution of the population in four arbitrary categories of weight based on the Quetelet index (P/T²). For both sexes, the distribution is given for the total sample and for each age class.

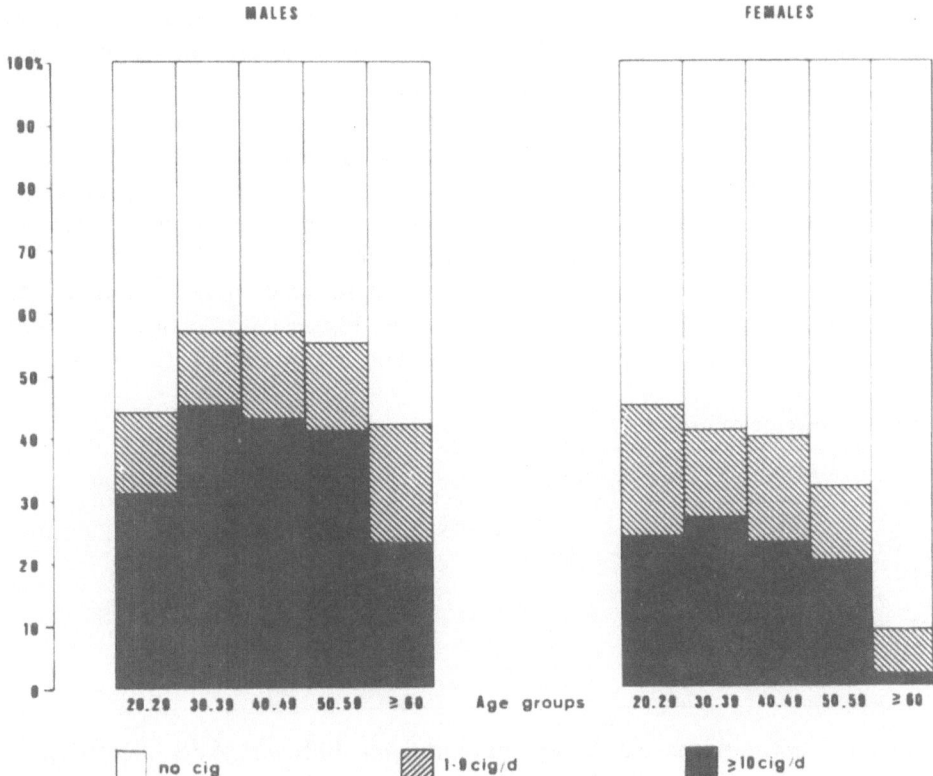

Figure 2. Percent distribution of the adult males and females in three categories of cigarette consumption (nonsmokers, light smokers, and heavy smokers).

the sample in categories of origin (defined as the place of birth) and of place of residence.

As the inquiry was realized by two groups, one in Liège and one in Brussels, people born in the Walloon provinces and in the province of Brabant are best represented, while the Flemish provinces are poorly represented. Foreigners living in Belgium are numerous in the sample (13%), but this is little in excess of the actual situation (8%). Residence distribution in the sample is in good accordance with the high urbanization level of the Belgian population.

In order to dispose of a parameter, i.e., the relative weight of each person studied, the Quetelet index of weight was chosen. This index is the weight in Kilograms divided by the square of the height in meters (P/T^2). Arbitrarily, the sample has been divided in four categories of weight index (Fig. 1): (a) 'thin' persons, with a ratio less than 20, (b) 'normal' persons, with a ratio between 20 and 25, (c) 'stout' persons, with a ratio between 25 and 28, and (d) 'obese' persons, with a ratio of more than 28. These limits, when applied

126

to all males in the sample, gave the proportion of, respectively, 21% thin, 50% normal, 19% stout, and 10% obese persons, and an approximately equivalent distribution in the female category (Fig. 1).

The relative proportions of these weight categories in the different age classes are shown in Figure 1 for both sexes. One sees that the tendency to become overweight appears early in life in men as compared with women, but decreases after 60 years, though women tend toward overweight slowly with aging, but continue to do so after the age of 60.

The cigarette consumption is more important in adult males (more than 20 years) than in females; Figure 2 shows that the highest proportion of smokers may be found in men aged between 30 and 60 years. Table 4 lists the

Table 4. Cigarette consumption as a function of age in adolescents.

Age group (years)	Males (in % per age group)			Females (in % per age group)		
	no cig	1–9 cig/day	≥10 cig/day	no cig	1–9 cig/day	≥10 cig/day
10–11	98	2	0	96	4	0
12–13	97	3	0	95	5	0
14–15	87	12	1	76	19	5
16–17	74	16	10	63	26	11
18–19	63	17	20	65	21	14

proportions of the same categories (nonsmokers, light smokers, heavy smokers) in the adolescents ranked in five age groups. It is interesting to note that girls seem to start smoking earlier than boys, and that boys become heavier smokers than girls only after 18 years.

The consumption of contraceptive pills by women between 20 and 50 years old is given in Table 5. As can be seen, it involves only about 20% of the women in these age categories as a whole.

Table 5. Oral contraceptive consumption (females aged 20–50 years).

Age group (years)	No. of persons	% on contraceptives
20–29	621	26
30–39	517	21
40–49	679	13

3. INTERPRETATION OF BP RECORDS

The four BP determinations obtained in each person studied were recorded using the first Korotkoff sound for the systolic value and fifth (last sound) for the diastolic value. The mean of the four determinations was calculated for the systolic and diastolic BP and these mean values were considered as representative for each individual in further analyses.

Every adult (aged more than 20 years) with a BP of less than 140/90 mmHg and without history of previously elevated BP was considered as normotensive (NL), irrespective of his age. All adults who fell out of these

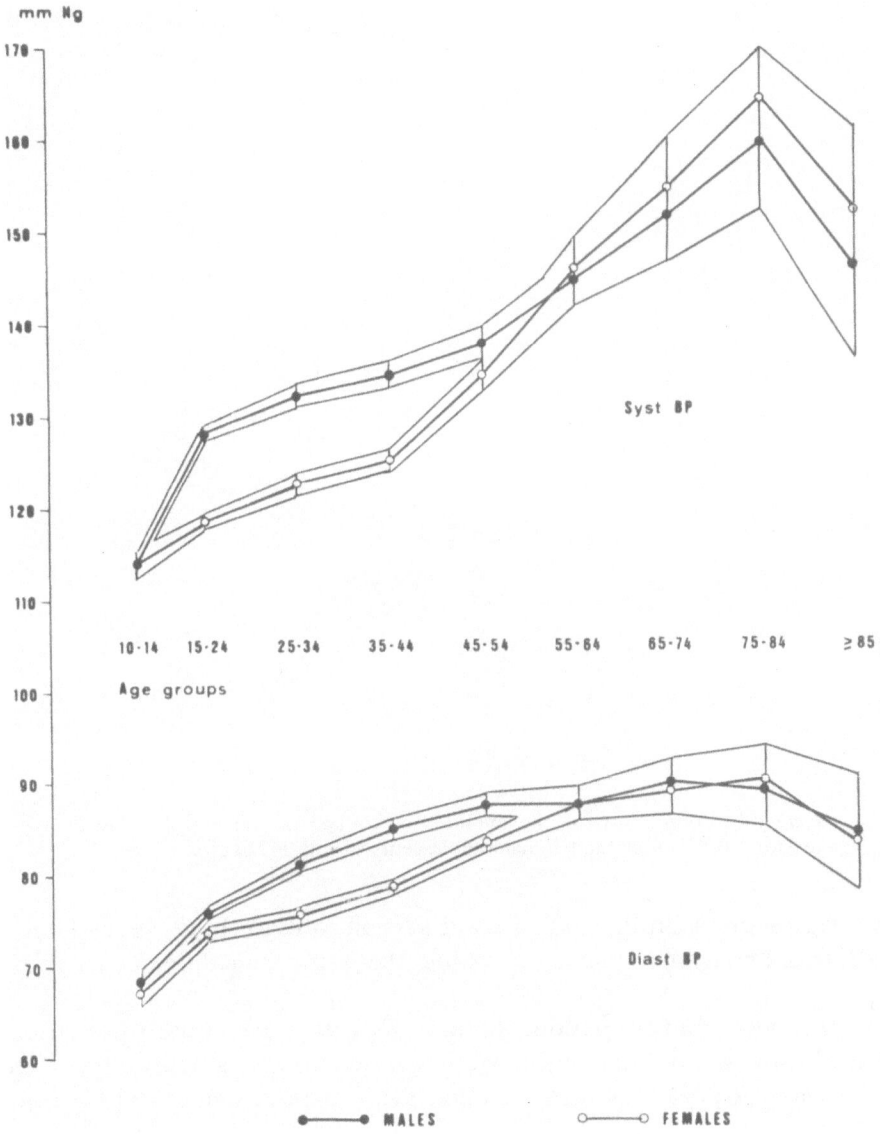

Figure 3. Comparison of the evolution with age of the systolic and diastolic BP in males and females (all ages) (mean ± 2 s/√n).

128

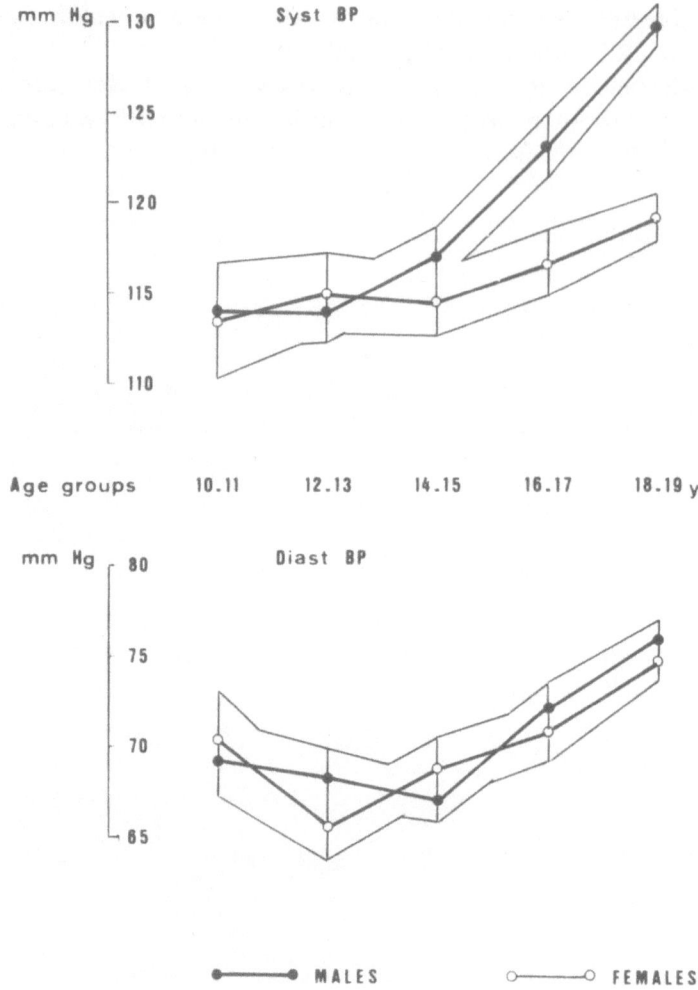

Figure 4. Comparison of the evolution with age of the systolic and diastolic BP in male and female adolescents (mean ± 2 s/√n).

criteria were seen again during a second session, one to three weeks later, and the BP was determined again by using the same schedule as at the first visit.

After this second examination, the persons with a BP equal to or in excess of 160/95 mmHg on both visits were considered as actually hypertensive (HT). In this category was also included every person treated with drugs for hypertension at the moment of the screening, irrespective of his BP.

All other conditions were classified in a third group of borderline hypertensives (BD).

In adolescents (10–19 years old), these criteria for hypertension and borderline hypertension were not applied. They were, for further study, considered as presenting 'high level of BP' if the diastolic BP or the systolic BP (or both) were above the 90th percentile, calculated within each age group of two years (10–11 years, 12–13 years, etc.).

4. RESULTS

4.1. Evolution of BP with age

The BP values obtained during the first session in all persons screened have been studied in relation to age in both sexes. Figure 3 concerns all age groups: age classes are ten years wide, except the first one, which is five years wide. Figure 4 concerns the adolescents divided in five age classes, two years wide. As can be observed on these figures, the systolic BP of boys and girls is similar until the age of 15, afterwards the increase with age is more pronounced in males, so that the mean value remains significantly higher in males than in females up to the age of 50. Thereafter the systolic BP continues to rise in both sexes up to the age of 80, but the BP tends to decrease in the eldest group.

The same pattern, but less pronounced, characterizes the evolution of the diastolic BP, with a similar difference between sexes for the age groups of 20–50 years.

4.2. Prevalence of hypertension: relationships with age, with hypertension in relatives, and with symptoms

The percentage of NL, BD, and HT in each age class is given in Table 6 for adult males and females. The increase in prevalence of both BD and HT is highly significant in men and in women as well.

Table 6. Prevalence of hypertension (HT) and borderline hypertension (BD) in the different age and sex classes (adults).

Age group (years)	Males (in % per age class)			Females (in % per age class)		
	HT	BD	NL	HT	BD	NL
20–29	7	20	73	2	7	91
30–39	10	26	64	5	13	82
40–49	18	26	56	12	21	67
50–59	24	26	50	21	30	49
60–69	36	32	32	35	35	30
≥ 70	40	38	22	51	37	12

130

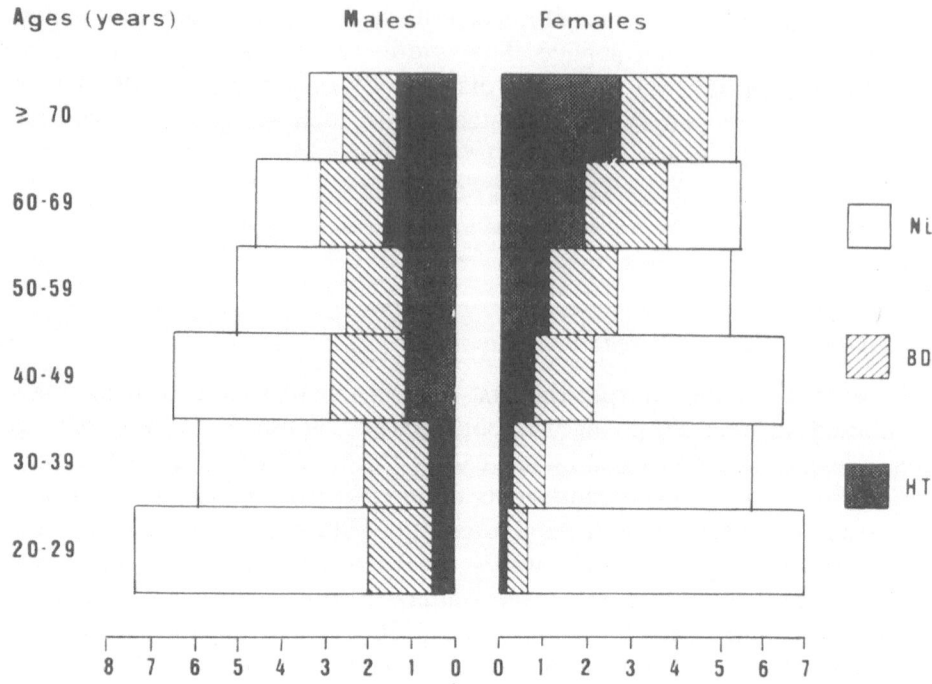

Ages (years)   Males   Females

≥ 70

60-69

50-59

40-49

30-39

20-29

NL

BD

HT

8 7 6 5 4 3 2 1 0   0 1 2 3 4 5 6 7

Figure 5. Tentative estimation of the total number of hypertensives (HT) and borderline hypertensives (BD) in the actual Belgian adult population, in 100.000 inhab. (total male and female
inhabitants by age classes as published for 1973 by the Belgian National Institute of Statistics).

Based on these percentages by age classes, a tentative estimation of the
actual number of BD and HT in the total adult Belgian population is shown
in Figure 5. If we now suppose as a principle that a regular medical follow-up
would be advisable for BD as well as HT aged less than 50 years, but would
be limited to HT for persons aged more than 50 years, the total number of
persons to consider for medical supervision because of high BP in Belgium
should be about 1,100,000 men and 950,000 women, which together represent

Table 7. Comparison of the proportion of hypertension in the relatives of normal (NL), borderline
(BD), and hypertensive (HT) adults.

| | % With hypertension in relatives | |
	Males	Females
NL	19	34
BD	23	41
HT	24	42
x^2	$P < 0.05$	$P < 0.01$

more than 20% of the population of the kingdom (a little less than 10,000,000 people).

Table 7 compares the proportion of persons who know that some of their relatives are hypertensive. For both males and females, this proportion is significantly different in NL, BD, and HT, but the difference is not very important. It must be outlined that women of all groups gave much more positive answers to that question than did men. This indicates that women are generally better informed about the medical state of their family, but also questions the reliability of this kind of information.

Table 8 compares the percentage of persons affected by two very common symptoms, headache and nervousness, in function of their BP status, all age groups taken together. There is a clear and highly significant higher prevalence of both symptoms in HT, although both are very frequent in normotensive persons, especially women.

Table 8. Prevalence of symptoms 'headache' and 'nervousness': Comparison of HT, BD, and NL (adults).

	Males				Females			
	% in HT	% in BD	% in NL	x^2	% in HT	% in BD	% in NL	x^2
Headache	19	15	12	$P < 0.001$	37	26	26	$P < 0.001$
Nervousness	45	42	34	$P < 0.001$	60	54	45	$P < 0.001$

4.3. Other determinants of hypertension

To study the influence of weight status on the prevalence of hypertension, independently of the factor age—weight tends to increase with age (Fig. 1) —the proportions of NL, BD, and HT have been compared in the four categories of weight (as mentioned above) within each age class in adult males and females. The results of this analysis are given in Figures 6 and 7. A very strong increase in the prevalence of hypertension is observed with increasing weight index, within each category of age and in both sexes. In males, the weight could be a determinant of hypertension as strong as age, if one considers that the prevalence of HT and BD is even higher in obese men aged 20–29 than in thin men aged more than 60 years.

In adolescents, a direct relationship can also be found between weight index and BP status, as indicated in Figure 8. Each 2-year-wide age class has been divided in two groups of weight, based on the value of individual Quetelet index. In each group, the dividing point was chosen so that the heaviest category would constitute about 20% – 30% of the total. The proportion of

132

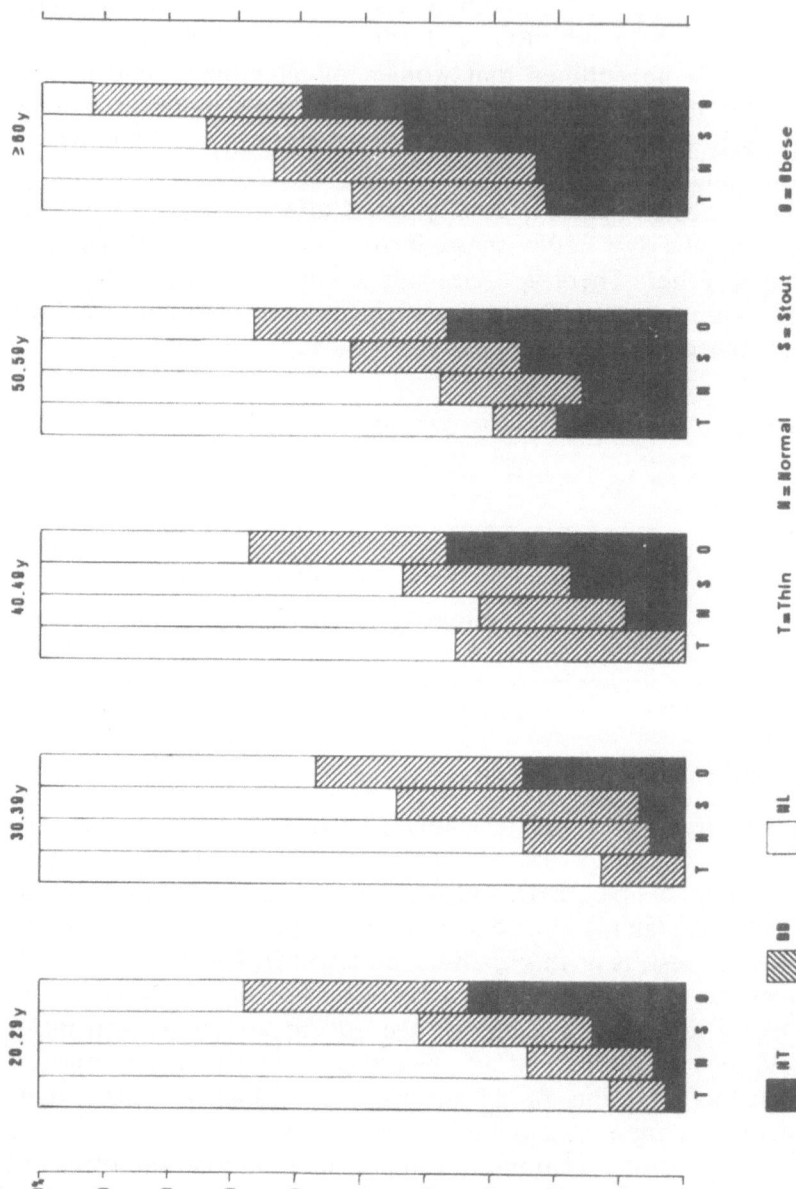

Figure 6. Percent distribution of normotensives (NL), borderline hypertensives (BD), and hypertensives (HT) in five age classes, each divided in four categories of weight based on the Quetelet index (adult males).

133

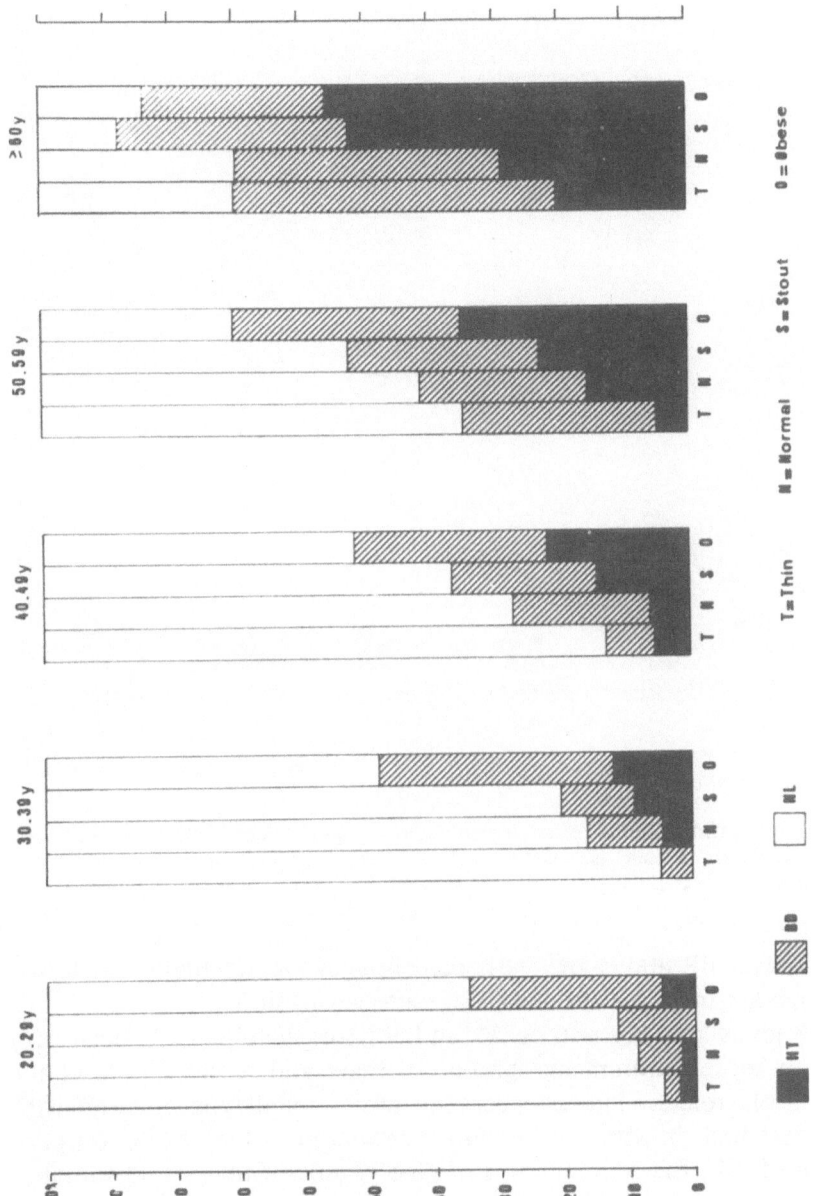

Figure 7. (cf. Fig. 6). Adult females.

134

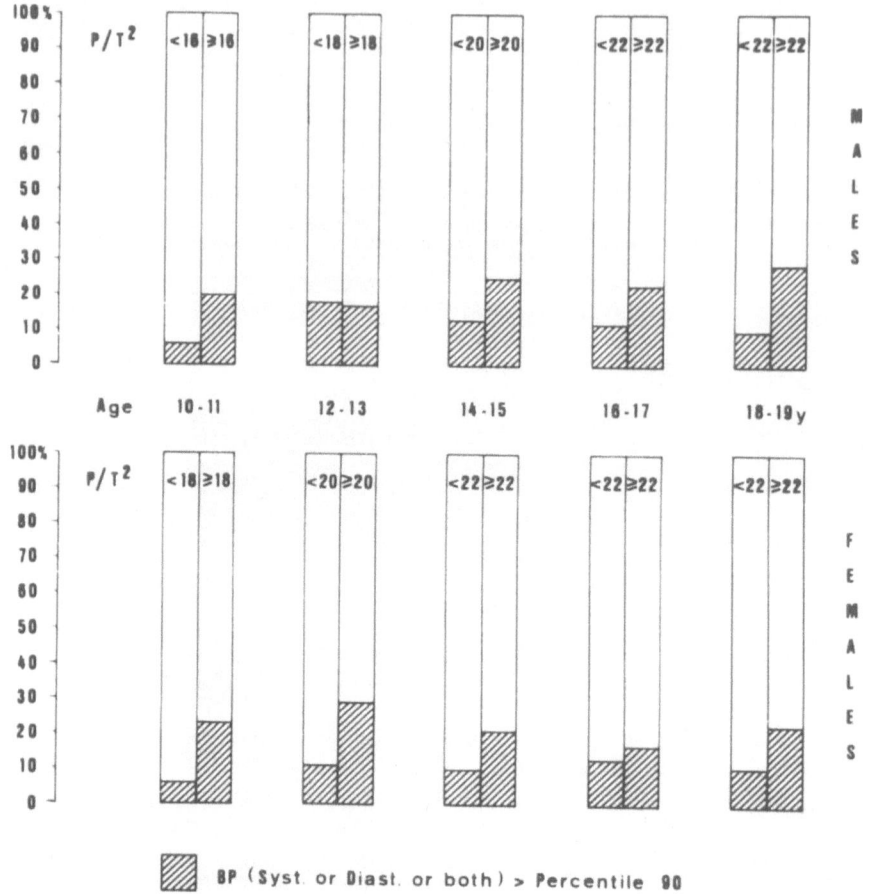

Figure 8. Percent distribution of adolescents with a high BP (above 90th percentile) in the different male and female age classes, each divided in two categories of weight based on Quetelet index (P/T²).

subjects with a BP above the 90th percentile is clearly higher in four of the five age groups in boys, and in all age groups in girls.

Table 9 gives the percentiles 50 and 90 for systolic and diastolic BP as observed in these different age groups of male and female adolescents.

The possible relationship between the professional type and the BP status was also studied in the active adult population. Figure 9 compares the prevalence of NL, BD, and HT in four age groups of males and females, each divided in two professional categories: white-collar and blue-collar workers. The increasing prevalence of HT and BD with age is again very clear, contrasting with the absence of any influence of the type of profession on BP status.

135

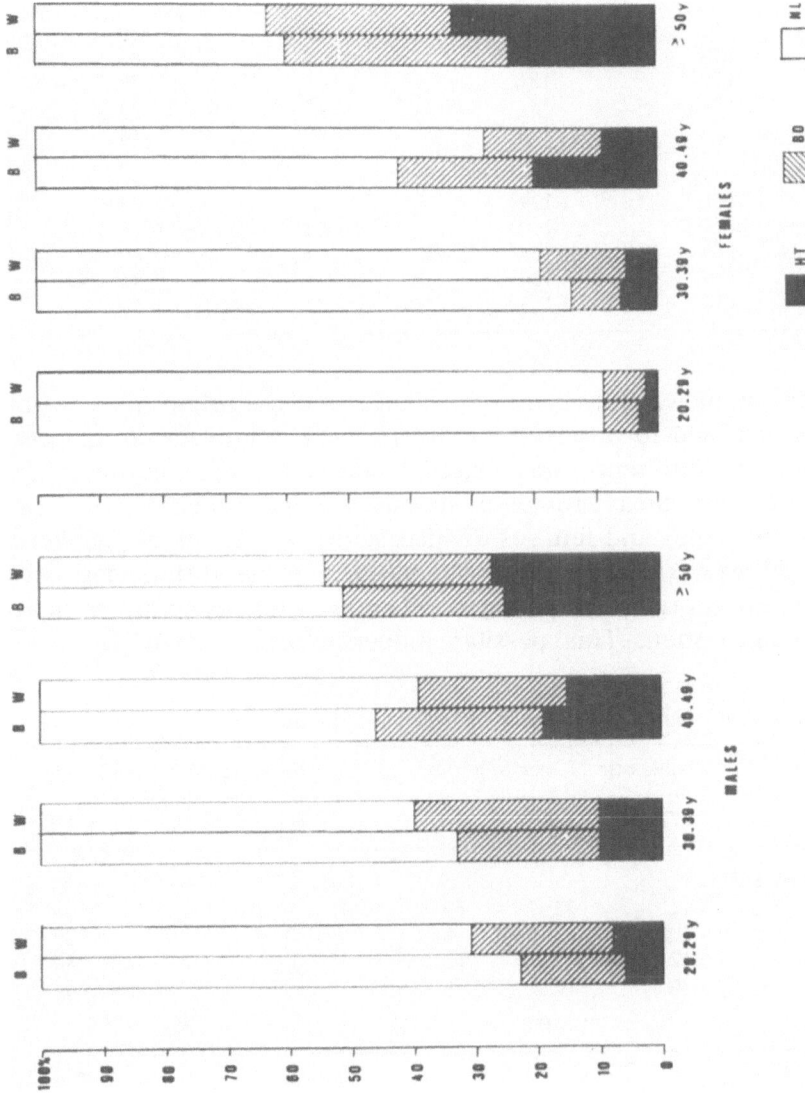

Figure 9. Percent distribution of normotensives (NL), borderline hypertensives (BD), and hypertensives (HT) in four age classes of active adult males and females, each divided in two professional categories: blue-collar (B) and white-collar (W) workers.

Table 9. Percentile values for systolic and diastolic BP in adolescents.

	Systolic BP (mmHg)		Diastolic BP (mmHg)	
	Percentile 50	Percentile 90	Percentile 50	Percentile 90
Males (years)				
10–11	113	126	70	80
12–13	111	128	69	80
14–15	117	131	68	79
16–17	124	137	72	83
18–19	130	146	77	88
Females (years)				
10–11	111	129	70	83
12–13	114	130	66	77
14–15	113	128	69	80
16–17	116	130	70	80
18–19	118	133	73	85

Two other parameters, the place of residence and the origin (place of birth), have also been tested for a possible influence on HT prevalence. Concerning the residence, no difference was detected between people living in urban, suburban, or country areas. Table 10 analyses the prevalence of NL, BD, and HT in the adult males and females divided in two categories of age: less and more than 50 years. The χ^2 analysis indicates some differences between persons of different origins, in young men and aged women, but not in young women and aged men. This possible influence of origin on BP was not

Table 10. Influence of origin on prevalence of hypertension (adults).

Origin	Males (in % per origin)			Females (in % per origin)		
	HT	BD	NL	HT	BD	NL
Age group 20–49 years						
Brabant	12	23	65	9	15	76
Flemish	10	22	68	7	14	79
Walloon	12	27	61	6	14	80
Foreign	6	16	78	7	9	84
χ^2		$P < 0.01$			NS	
Age group $\geqslant 50$ years						
Brabant	31	32	37	37	35	28
Flemish	35	24	41	30	32	38
Walloon	25	30	45	24	27	49
Foreign	33	22	45	29	47	24
χ^2		NS			$P < 0.01$	

Table 11. Analysis of variance (SPSS, Vogelback computing center, Northwestern University, option 9).

| | Males | | Females | |
	Syst BP	Diast BP	Syst BP	Diast BP
Significance of *F*				
Source of variation				
Age	NS	0.001	NS	0.001
Age squared	0.002	0.001	0.001	0.001
Weight index	0.001	0.001	0.001	0.001
Arm circumference	0.001	0.001	0.05	NS
Pulse rate	0.001	0.001	0.001	0.001
Cigarette consumption	NS	NS	NS	NS
Origin	NS	NS	NS	NS
Residence	NS	NS	NS	NS
Observator	NS	NS	NS	NS
Contraceptive pills	—	—	0.053	0.058
Multiple correlation coefficient squared				
	0.256	0.211	0.312	0.238
Partial regression coefficients (*β*) (mmHg)				
Weight index (1 unit)	0.495	0.352	1.237	0.762
Arm circ. (1 cm)	0.298	0.150	0.119	NS
Pulse rate (1 b/min)	0.319	0.132	0.294	0.120

confirmed in a more sophisticated statistical analysis including all age classes, presented in Table 11.

From this analysis of variance of the systolic and the diastolic BP in both sexes, taking into account different parameters, presented as continuous variable (age, weight index, arm circumference, and pulse rate) or not (cigarette or contraceptive consumption, residence, place of birth, and the technician measuring BP) the following conclusions may be drawn:

1) The proportion of the total variation between individual BP values is but very partially explained by these parameters all together, this proportion comprising 21% – 31% of the total variation, as indicated by the values of the squared multiple correlation coefficients.

2) Significant sources of variation of the BP may be found in the age and in the weight index as demonstrated above, but also in the arm circumference and in the pulse rate. The main increases in BP to be expected from the increase of one unit of weight index, arm circumference, or pulse rate, are indicated at the bottom of the Table 11 (partial regression coefficients).

3) Other possible sources of variation (cigarette consumption, origin, residence, and observer) have no significant effect on systolic or diastolic BP in either males or females.

138

4) The consumption of oral contraceptives is affected by a value of F, which is at the limit of statistical signification. This possible increase in BP with contraceptive consumption is also illustrated in Figure 10, showing a small increase in the prevalence of HT in women consuming 'the pill' in two age classes. These differences however, are not significant in the χ^2 test.

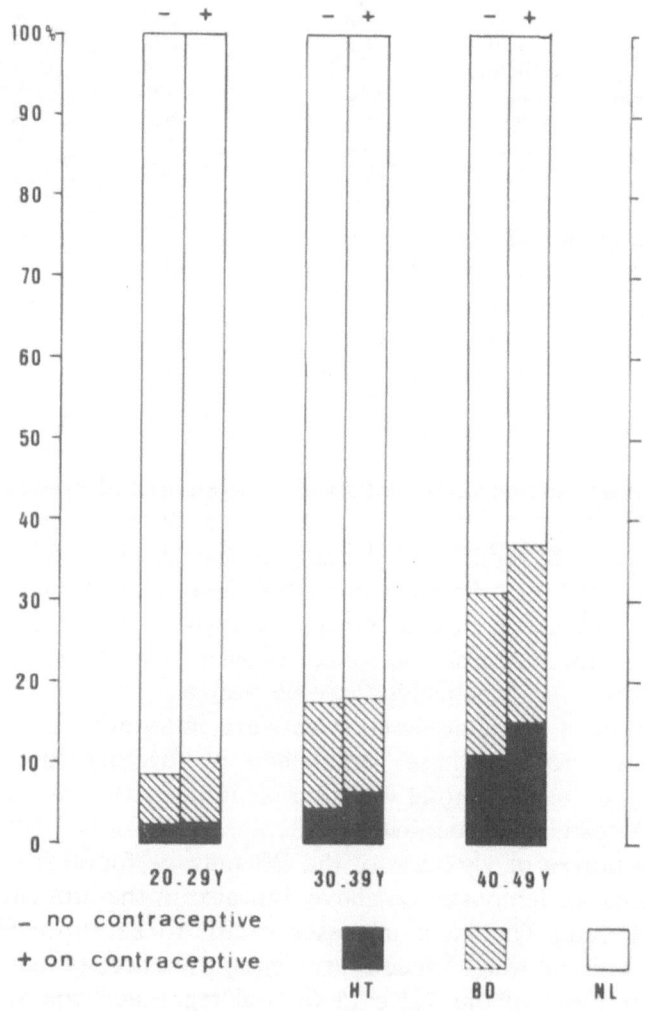

Figure 10. Percent distribution of **NL**, **BD**, and **HT** in three age classes, each divided in women consuming oral contraceptives or not.

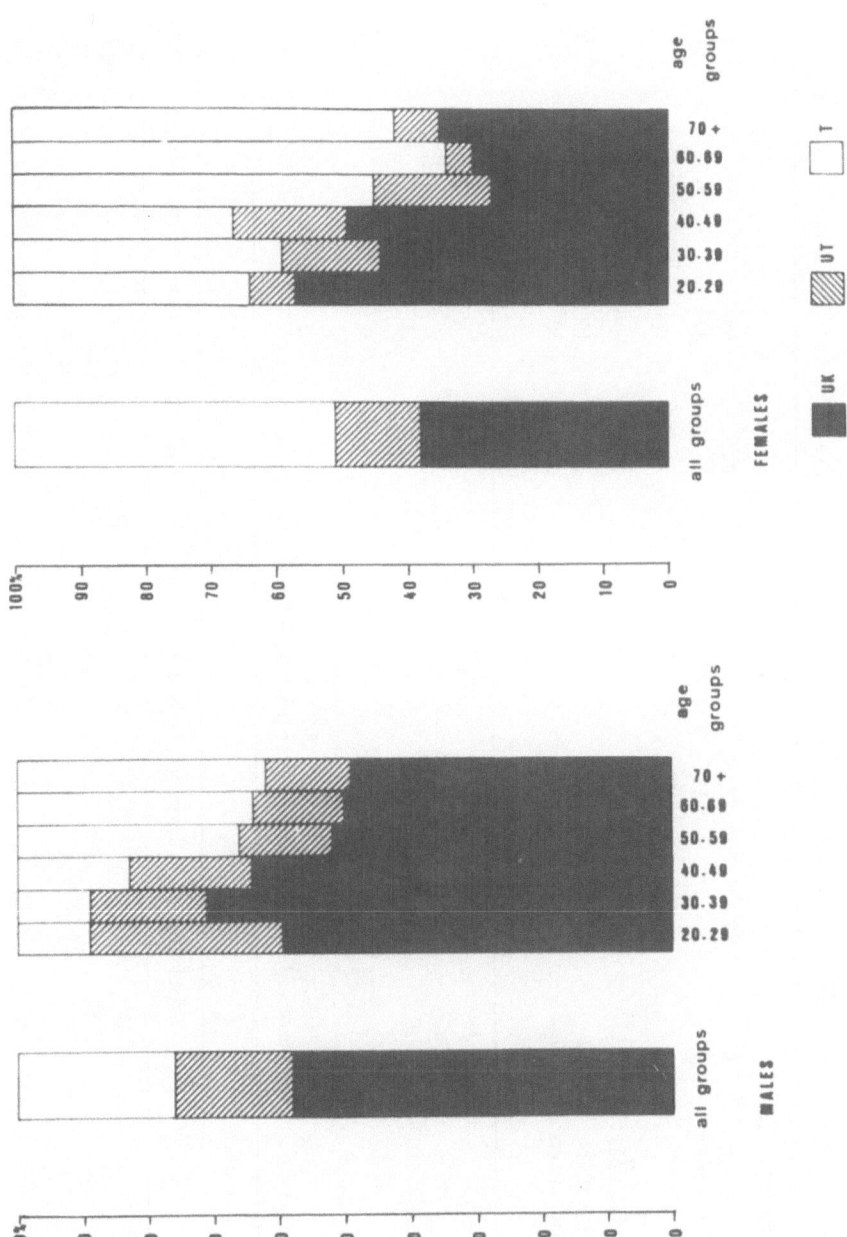

Figure 11. Percent distribution of three subgroups: unknown HT (UK), untreated HT (UT) and treated HT (T) in hypertensive males and females taken all together or divided in age classes.

Table 12. Influence of professional category on the type of hypertension (adults).

	Males				Females			
	No. of HT	% Unknown	% Untreated	% Treated	No. of HT	% Unknown	% Untreated	% Treated
Age group 20 – 49 years								
Blue collar workers	101	63	25	12	44	59	9	32
White collar workers	93	67	18	15	76	42	20	38
x^2		NS				NS		
Age group $\geqslant$ 50 years								
Blue collar workers	57	47	16	37	27	19	22	59
white collar workers	60	55	10	35	57	30	16	54
x^2		NS				NS		

Table 13. Influence of origin (place of birth) on the type of hypertension (adults).

Origin	Males				Females			
	No. of HT	% Unknown	% Untreated	% Treated	No. of HT	% Unkown	% Untreated	% Treated
Brabant	140	59	13	28	128	41	9	50
Flemish	36	45	33	22	28	29	11	60
Walloon	160	62	15	23	123	39	17	44
Foreign	39	51	34	15	23	26	17	57
x^2		$P < 0.05$				NS		

4.4. *Partition of hypertensive subjects into treated and untreated*

It is well known that a large proportion of hypertensive subjects are not aware of their elevated BP (unknown HT), or know this ailment but are not under medical treatment for it (untreated HT). Figure 11 shows the partition of the adult hypertensives (HT) of the sample studied into three subgroups: treated HT, untreated HT, and unknown HT.

It is apparent that the proportion of unknown HT is larger in men than in women, and inversely that the proportion of treated HT is much larger in women (about 50%) than in men (less than 25%). The effect of age on this partition in subgroups is also very clear from Figure 11. In both sexes, a clear-cut difference exists between subjects less than 50 and more than 50 years old. This difference, characterized by an important increase in the proportion of treated HT in older persons, is statistically highly significant in the χ^2 test.

Two other parameters possibly influencing this partition of hypertensive persons in subgroups were also studied. The influence of professional category is shown in Table 12. Because of the difference related to age, two age classes have been considered. In neither of them, in either sex, were any differences demonstrated between blue-collar and white-collar workers. Finally, the influence of origin (place of birth) on the partition in subgroups of the hypertensive persons is analyzed in Table 13. The χ^2 analysis indicates no significant difference between groups of origin for women, but differences at the limit of significance for men. Any further interpretation of these possible differences is difficult.

5. DISCUSSION

The sample studied here comprises 6584 persons living in Belgium, the great majority of whom were examined at their place of work. To what extent is this sample representative of the actual Belgian population? All age categories of both sexes have been involved, and a large-scale weight index has been observed. Although some discordance with the reality exists in the sample concerning the different professional categories and the low proportion of persons from the Flemish provinces, these discordances have little effect, if any, on the BP characteristics of the sample, as it has been demonstrated by multiple regression analysis that the parameters 'origin' and 'profession' have no influence on BP values. Without reaching the accuracy of a sample constituted at random, based, for example, on electoral listings, but much more difficult to manage, the sample that has been realized in this study enables a quite good estimate of the BP distribution in the Belgian population.

The BP determination based on four measurements after 10 min of rest, the second determination of BP required before assigning any person to the HT group, constitutes more strict and severe criteria compared with most other studies of this type. Taking this in consideration, the estimated frequency of HT in the population has probably not been overestimated, and consequently is notably lower than the values published in similar studies in other countries [3–5]. This study also draws attention to the large proportion of borderline hypertensive subjects, who may constitute the part of the population especially at risk for cardiovascular events, and toward which the problem of preventive measures to be eventually taken remains open to discussion. The estimated values of prevalence of HT and BD in the total population of Belgium are given only as indicative, but this evaluation may serve as a basis for the estimation of its medical implications, at a time when the cost of health becomes tremendous for state budgets.

Estimation of HT in childhood and adolescence remains a difficult problem. It now seems clear that the limits of normal BP used and recommended in adults do not fit and there has been a consensus on the use of percentile values calculated for consecutive age classes. We used the 90th percentile, as did Londe and Goldring [6] and recommended by others [7], because it seems in closer agreement with the percentile value of 140/90 mmHg, which is considered as the upper limit of normal in young adults. Table 9 lists the 90th percentiles that we observed in our five age classes of adolescents. For practical purposes, we suggest that they be simplified as follows: 130/80 mmHg as the upper limit for 10- to 18-year-old girls and for 10- to 16-year-old boys. After 18 for girls and after 16 for boys, the 140/90 mmHg limit used in young adults may be appropriate. All boys and girls regularly exceeding these values of BP must remain under periodic medical control and probably may benefit from some preventive measures such as sodium reduction in alimentation, weight control if overweight, and avoidance of cigarette smoking [8].

Different determinants of BP have been studied. The increase of BP with age is very clearly illustrated in Figures 3 and 4. These results are in complete agreement with curves published elsewhere, e.g., in the USA [9, 10]. The weight index is also a strong determinant of BP in every age class, and is relevant to the many reports indicating that weight reduction in obese hypertensives may be sufficient to control BP elevation [11]. The effect of the arm circumference is also established, independently of the weight increase that often determines it. Its effect on the BP is more marked in males than in females, although the effect of weight is more pronounced in the latter, as indicated by the partial correlation coefficients (Table 11). The heartbeat frequency also appears as a determinant of the BP in this study. This underlines the probable role of emotional factors intervening at the moment of BP determination and stimulating autonomic regulation of heart rate, cardiac output, and BP. It may especially concern mild and borderline HT [12].

The study of subjective symptoms classically related to hypertension, such as headache and nervousness, confirms the existence of a strong relationship between them and elevated BP. However, these symptoms are very common in nonhypertensive subjects, and the increase of their prevalence related to hypertension is relatively modest. Therefore, their value in predicting hypertension and as screening indicators is extremely limited.

The partition of hypertensive persons in treated and untreated HT indicates a clear-cut difference between males and females, and between younger and older people. Male sex and youth are factors mostly related to unknown and untreated hypertension. As this study has pointed out the relatively high prevalence of HT in young men, the question arises as to how to improve this situation. Psychological dispositions of young men against a state of rejected ailment possibly plays a role in this situation, but the attitude of the medical corps may also be questioned. The reverse psychological attitude of patients and doctors in front of hypertensives over 50 probably contributes to the change observed.

6. SUMMARY

A cross section of the Belgian population, comprising about 6600 persons of both sexes, aged from 10 to 98 years, of different professional occupations, places of residence, and origin, was studied for blood pressure (BP) distribution and for prevalence of hypertension (HT). The BP was recorded four times after 10 min while the subjects were in the supine position, and the mean of the four determinations was used for further analysis. Regression curves for systolic and diastolic BP in function of age classes were obtained for males and females. In adults, three categories of BP were defined (hypertensives, borderline hypertensives, and normotensives), based on BP limits as recommended by WHO (140/90 and 160/95 mmHg), obtained at two different sessions of BP measurements. In adolescents, high BP was defined as values in excess of the 90th percentile for each age class.

The prevalence of hypertension increases strongly with age as well as with the weight index of the subjects. Other significant determinants of BP were arm circumference in males and pulse rate in both sexes. Inversely, place of residence, place of birth, cigarette consumption, and observers were not related to the value of BP.

An estimate of the total number of hypertensives in Belgium has been possible on the basis of this screening. The proportion of treated versus untreated hypertensions is lower in the young than in the elderly, and lower

144

in males than in females; thus a real effort must still be made to improve the detection and treatment of hypertension in men under the age of 50.

Acknowledgments. On behalf of the Belgian Hypertension Committee, we wish to express our gratitude to the public and private establishments, the schools and care centers, that authorized our survey on their personnel, students, or boarders.

We are particularly grateful to the Universities of Brussels and Liège, the CPAS of Brussels and Liège, the 'Centres de Contacts de la Ville de Bruxelles,' the school medical inspection services of the cities of Brussels and Liège, and the following enterprises: Bon Marché (Liège), Tihange Nuclear Plant, Grand Bazar (Liège), Innovation (Liège), Forges de Clabecq, SAFAK (Sclessin), Sarma-Penney (Brussels), and Usines Henricot (Court St-Etienne).

We also gratefully acknowledge all the persons who contributed in different ways to this survey: enterprise managers, doctors of work medical services, school medical inspection services or homes for the elderly, as well as the doctors, nurses, secretaries, and technicians of our team.

We address our thanks to the Professors Colinet, Geubelle, and Welsch; to Doctors Bovy, Charlier, Cordier, Fassotte, Franckson-Devogel, Hassanzadeh, Henuzet, Kunstler, Mawet, Mottard, Muller, Odio, Roggen, Shita, Taeymans, and Van Roy; to Mr. Busieaux and Mr. Lekaemen; and to Mrs. Bertrand-Verleye, Dubois-Saenen, Sanioura-Cherain, Toussaint-Jaradin, and Yerna.

This study was made possible through a grant from Merck, Sharpe and Dohme.

REFERENCES

1. Kornitzer M, Demeester M, Delcourt R, Goossens A, Bernard R: Enquête cardio-vasculaire prospective dans une population sélectionnée. Résultats de l'enquête initiale. Acta Cardiol 26:285-343, 1971.
2. Kesteloot H, Van Houte O: An epidemiologic survey of arterial blood pressure in a large male population group. Am J Epidemiol 99:14-29, 1974.
3. Lellouch J, Richard J-L: La pression artérielle d'une population masculine active. Etude épidémiologique de 19.714 sujets. Presse Med 79:1749-1751, 1971.
4. Escher M, Heyden S, Christeller S, Gasser JP, Keller H, Ramsler L, Geel O: Hypertonie, Nikotinabusus, Hypercholesterinämie und Übergewicht bei Schweizer Mannern 1973. Schweiz Med Wochenschr 104:1423-1428, 1974.
5. Hawthorne VM, Greaves DA, Beevers DG: Blood pressure in a Scottish town. Br Med J 1:600-603, 1974.
6. Londe S, Goldring D: High blood pressure in children: problems and guidelines for evaluation and treatment. Am J Cardiol 37:650-657, 1976.
7. McLain LG: Hypertension in childhood: a review. Am Heart J 92:634-647, 1976.
8. Blumenthal S: Precursors in childhood of primary hypertension in the adult. Ann NY Acad Sci 304:28-32, 1978.
9. Stamler J, Stamler R, Riedlinger WF, Algera G, Roberts RH: Hypertension screening of 1 million Americans. Community Hypertension Evaluation Clinic (CHEH) programs, 1973–1975. JAMA 235:2299-2306, 1976.
10. Task Force on Blood Pressure Control in Children. National Heart, Lung and Blood Institute and National High Blood Pressure Education Program. Pediatrics 59:797-819, 1977.
11. Tobian L: Hypertension and obesity. N Engl J Med 298:46-48, 1978.
12. Julius S, Shork MA: Predictors of hypertension. Ann NY Acad Sci 304:38-52, 1978.

8. CARDIOVASCULAR RISK FACTORS IN THE ADOLESCENT POPULATION OF COLOGNE

Stability over one year and tendencies towards aggregation

U. LAASER and A. SCHÜTT

Morbidity and mortality in the western world are dominated by cardiovascular diseases. For the Federal Republic of Germany, only about two-fifths of the total mortality can be attributed to other causes, mainly cancer [1]. Whereas in spite of limited success with regard to a few tumors like Hodgkin's lymphoma, cancer mortality in general could not be reduced convincingly [2], e.g., in the United States mortality from myocardial infarction has declined since the late 1960s [3]. Concomitant changes in smoking and eating behavior as well as the extensive detection of elevated blood pressure in the population [4–6] are likely to be associated with this development. However, although cardiovascular risk factors are known in adult populations that enable the prediction of the occurrence of cardiovascular events with high probabilies [7], intervention studies—designed to achieve a decline of sequelae of atherosclerosis by minimizing its known risk factors—have provided so far only intermediate, limited [8] or doubtful [9] results. A promising approach lies therefore in studies undertaken in order to enlighten the early genesis and the dynamics of precursors of atherosclerosis in childhood and youth. The World Health Organization, trying to coordinate such undertakings, has recently [10] enumerated their objectives as follows (shortened):

1) The distribution of risk factors of atherosclerosis in the young.
2) Their relation to parental risk factors.
3) Their relation to parental disease.
4) The determinants of their formation and evolution.
5) Their geographic and sociocultural variation.
6) Possible measures of early intervention.
7) The effectiveness of early intervention in preventing the development of risk factors or in reducing their levels if elevated.

The Cologne study, begun in December 1974 [11], follows these lines.

H. Kesteloot, J.V. Joossens (eds.), Epidemiology of Arterial Blood Pressure, 145–162.

1. DESIGN OF THE STUDY

The first cross-sectional survey comprising the adolescent school population of Cologne was carried out from December 1974 to February 1976 in order to determine blood pressures, heart rate, total cholesterol, serum uric acid, postprandial blood glucose, body mass index, and smoking behavior. Variables like arm circumference, sibling status, social status, drug intake (especially hormonal contraception), family history, and personal history as well as several vegetative complaints have been recorded additionally. Rescreening of a large part of this population took place a year later including data on alcohol consumption and—in a subpopulation—on HDL-cholesterol. The third follow-up is scheduled for 1979/80.

1.1. Sampling area and study population

At the beginning of the study, 32 regular high schools (Gymnasien) and 18 vocational schools (Berufsschulen)[12] existed in the urban area within the administrative boundaries valid as of 28 November 1972. Due to lack of transportation, six high schools and one vocational school—all in the eastern part of the city—had to be excluded from the study. Two other high schools not yet fully established in autumn 1974 could not be taken into consideration. Within the remaining 41 eligible schools, the target population comprised the three—only occasionally four—upper grades. Sometimes, final examination procedures reduced participation rates for the highest grades, thus the age groups of 15 and 19 years are underrepresented in the study population. With regard to high-school pupils, the investigation aimed at a total population sample.

The large number of pupils in vocational schools (almost 30,000) demanded an appropriate reduction of the sample size. This was achieved by random sampling of one-tenth of the complete list of vocational school classes; 6302 pupils or 76.4% of the eligible total (8252) were finally examined. About one year later, 3004 (81.4%) of 3692 eligible adolescents still at their schools had been reexamined.

1.2. Examination procedure

The examination team, usually of four female medical technicians and occasionally student workers supervised by a physician, screened up to three classes of about 25 pupils per morning. After a short general instruction, the questionnaire 'to the parents' (disease history, social status), handed out some days before via the teaching personnel, was recollected. The participants received a second questionnaire 'to the pupils' asking for smoking habits and vegetative complaints.

They completed the latter form in a waiting area (or preferably in a waiting room). Thereafter, they entered a first examination room for the measurement of blood pressure and related variables. Then they moved into a second separate room for the measurement of height and weight, and the collection of capillary blood from the fingertip. The blood samples enabled the determination of blood glucose, total cholesterol, and (if sufficient in quantity) of serum uric acid. Because the majority of this population were minors, venous blood sampling would have required written parental consent very likely being associated with organizational difficulties and reduced compliance. Similarly, a demand for fasting would have been difficult to realize. In case of pathological results, the pupils were advised to see their family physician. Some of the pupils with repeatedly elevated blood pressures or other pathological features were investigated in the medical outpatient department of the University of Cologne.

2. METHODS OF MEASUREMENT

2.1. Measurement of blood pressure and heart rate

Blood pressures were measured twice with the subject in the sitting position according to a protocol proposed by the Committee on Medical Research and Public Health of the European Communities [13], which integrates also the regulations of the American Heart Association [14]. The instrument of preference was the Mark-IV sphygmomanometer [15], otherwise a standard device (Erkameter). Details on the training of observers by tape [16] and film [17] have been published previously [18]. The repeated application of the testing sequences on the tape enabled the calculation of coefficients of variation (CV) for the entire observer group throughout two years: 1.6%/systolic, 2.6%/diastolic 4th phase, and 1.5%/diastolic 5th phase. The corresponding accuracies for the means of the observer group were −0.9%, 2.1%, and 1.2%. For the film, the total intraobserver error expressed as CV of the entire group (seven observers) was 1.5%/systolic, 2.9%/diastolic 4th phase and 2.7%/diastolic 5th phase. 'Cologne validation [18]' of the film was computed from the observer means for the single sequences.

For the presentation of the diastolic pressures, usually the 4th phase is adopted. In some analyses, 'blind' measurements with the Mark-IV device are used exclusively because of their higher quality [19, 20]. The standard cuff size was 12.5×28.0 cm (maximum arm circumference encountered 39 cm, mean for males 26.5 ± 2.4 cm). Great care was taken to standardize the measurement situation in the schools as far as possible and to code all variables known to influence the measurement (e.g., locality, date, time, room temper-

148

ature, observer, apparatus, arm circumference, fasting state, heart rate). The Cologne protocol, in German, is available upon request. Capillary blood was taken after the measurement of blood pressure in a separate room. The heart rate was taken between the two blood pressure measurements by starting a stopwatch at a first palpated pulse wave and stopping it after 15 s.

2.2. Anthropometric measurements

The measurement of weight, height, and arm circumference followed the instructions as provided by WHO [21], with some minor modifications.

Biochemical parameters. Capillary blood from the fingertip was centrifuged on the day of collection and stored at $-22\,^{\circ}$C.
Glucose. Analysis of a hemolysate by the hexokinase technique [22]: accuracy $\pm 0.5\%$ (precinorm S 110 mg/dl), CV day-to-day below 2%.
Cholesterol. Analysis of serum by the enzymatic catalase or CHOD-PAP method [23]: accuracy $\pm 1.5\%$ (Precilip 131–138 mg/dl, extralaboratory control by Deutsche Gesellschaft für Klinische Chemie), CV day-to-day below 2.5%.
Uric acid. Analysis of serum (if quantities sufficed) according to Kageyama [24]: accuracy below 2.5% (Precilip 3.96–4.01 mg/dl, extralaboratory control as above), CV day-to-day 5.6%.

2.3. Questionnaires

With few exceptions the self-administered questionnaires contained 'closed' questions. The testing of repeatability in a subpopulation of 147 pupils [25] revealed an average of 88.4% for identical answers. The coefficient of correlation for the numerical item of smoking cigarettes was 0.87.

2.4. Collection and analysis of data

The forms designed for this study contain the whole set of coded data. After punching, the data were controlled and analyzed by use of the Statistical Package for the Social Sciences (SPSS), implemented on the CDC CYBER 76, University of Cologne.

3. METHOD OF ANALYSIS

Epstein and Eckoff had already shown in 1967 [26] that even small differences in means and standard deviations may account for rather large differences in prevalence. Even this is more valid when prevalences are computed for skewed probability distributions. In addition, biological risk parameters usually follow continuous distribution functions without any jumps, which might indicate a 'natural' borderline between normal and pathological values.

For these reasons, we prefer to define risk situations by means of selected percentiles. The calculation of these percentiles by using empirical frequency distributions seems to be more feasible than calculation of quantiles by using means and standard deviations. In most cases, the underlying assumption of normal distribution is not fulfilled.

Usually the 90th or 95th percentile is employed to define the upper 10% or 5% as potentially pathological. However, for the analysis carried out here, we chose the 80th percentile as the artificial limit. The reason for that was simply to obtain sufficiently large sample sizes in the so-defined high range.

The argument might be based upon the steadily increasing cardiovascular 'risk' attributed to the parameters in question in almost all epidemiological studies and upon the a.m. continuous distribution functions, which theoretically enables the drawing of limits at any point of the distribution.

For the analysis of risk factor aggregation, we applied the 'analysis of configuration frequencies' ('Konfigurationsfrequenzanalyse') developed by Krauth and Lienert [27]. This multivariate nonparametric technique compares observed frequencies of combinations of elevated risk parameters (configuration) with the frequency that could be expected in case of mutual independence of risk variables. This expected frequency is computed by using estimations of the 'risk' probabilities (beyond the 80th percentile). The latter are obtained from the marginal distributions and differ slightly from the theoretical value (0.20) due to the discrete character of measurement and analysis.

The deviation of observed from expected frequencies of certain configurations can be measured by chi^2. However, this value should not be used in testing hypotheses, because the total number of degrees of freedom for analysis is less than the number of possible configurations. In any way high values of chi^2 indicate certain types of configurations that may be investigated further.

Configurations might be ranged according to absolute or expected frequencies, according to chi-square values, or to configuration orders (number of positive, i.e., elevated, variables). An extended analytical capacity is provided by the technique of hierarchical configuration analysis: this means stepwise elimination of that specific variable or factor, which contributes least to the total chi-square or demonstrates the smallest association effect to the other variables.

4. RESULTS

In order to facilitate comparisons with other populations and methodological approaches, the figures given in Table 1 were derived from variables refined as much as possible, i.e., only blind measurements of blood pressure, exclusion of adolescents on antihypertensive medication, exclusion of fasting glucose values, and cases of juvenile diabetes mellitus. As there are only very small variations according to type of school [28], except for smoking, we consider the two school populations (high schools and vocational schools) as one homogeneous population, although sampled in a different way (see above design of the study). Similarly, the influence of age on the variables seems to be relatively unimportant (see Table 2) and therefore might enable the integration of the whole adolescent age range into one class of 15–19 years. The smoking habit requires only standardization taking into account type of school and age.

Considerable sex-dependent differences can be demonstrated for blood pressures (males higher than females), especially in the systolic phase, total serum cholesterol (females higher than males), uric acid (males higher than females), and smoking (males higher than females). With the exception of cholesterol, males have higher risk factors than females. This does not necessarily mean that they are really at higher risk—with the likely exception of smoking cigarettes. The differences between sexes are small or negligible for heart rate, blood glucose, and body-mass index. The identical or even a little higher heart rates of girls might be used as an argument against a possible interaction between the usually feminine observers and male pupils.

For rescreening and control of cardiovascular risk factors in adolescence, we tend to recommend the limits given in Table 1, if our methodology is employed. These limiting values are based upon our results, which are to a certain degree representative for Cologne and probably other metropolitan areas in northern Germany. They attempt to balance the clinical relevance, the feasibility of the method in a routine setting, and the capacity of the health care system. Also, existing international agreements had to be taken into account. Consequently, for blood pressure we adopted the cutoff value of WHO [29], although the range for girls of 140/90 mmHg might be too tight. On the other hand, the upper limit of 130 mg/dl for blood glucose [30] is recommended for the fasting state. Thus the percentage of values 'truly' exceeding this threshold might be even smaller than the 1.8% or 1.0%, respectively, given in Table 1. With regard to smoking, it is questionable to indicate borderlines above zero in so far as the smoking of cigarettes in general is undesirable. Low consumption rates might be considered just as an early stage of later high consumption [31].

The above-mentioned balance with regard to estimates of the limit can be approached, for the moment, only on empirical grounds. Definite decisions depend on the determination of the actual cardiovascular risk associated with such levels in youth. These are to be expected as results of ongoing prospective studies, covering broad age spectra [10]. Means differ from medians given in Table 1, depending on skewness of the distribution with an excess at the right tail. This applies especially to systolic blood pressure, serum cholesterol, and blood glucose.

A general overview of the correlations between risk variables is given in Table 2. The calculation of the correlation coefficients is based on the complete sample. Any refinements, be it exclusion of certain diseases or methodological considerations, have been relinquished. The Pearson correlation coefficients are generally low and quite unaffected by factors associated with maturation, i.e., height and age. Correlations in the order of $r = 0.3$ exist between the variables systolic blood pressure, diastolic blood pressure, heart rate, and body-mass index, respectively. Smaller correlations (about 0.15) exist for systolic blood pressure vs cholesterol, vs glucose (females only), and vs

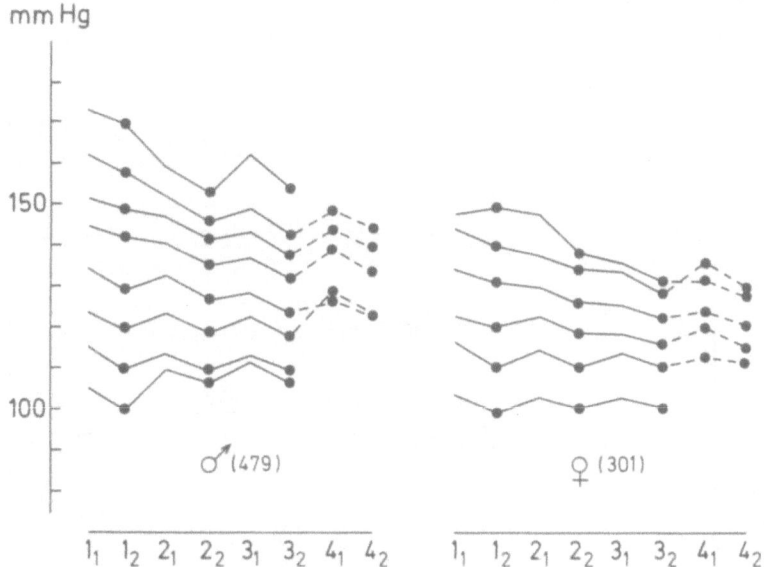

Figure 1. Comparison of classified systolic blood pressure means (participants of control measurements only). Cologne 1975/76.

For a total of 780 adolescents (mainly aged 15–19 years), two follow-up measurements of blood pressures were realized a few days after the initial screening; about one year later, an additional measurement was taken (reduced N). At each occasion (1, 2, 3, 4) the blood pressure has been measured twice (indicated as 1_1, 1_2, 2_1, ...). The classification is based upon the second measurement at the first occasion (initial screening, 1_2), the width of classes is 10 mmHg (e.g., 135–144, etc.).

Table 1. Prevalence (according to 'clinical' cutoff values), mean and standard deviation, and percentile values of risk variables for adolescents 15–19 years old (Cologne).

Risk variable	Unit	Mean +	SD	Percentiles			Cutoff value of prevalence (≥)	Prevalence (%) above cutoff value
				50th	80th	90th		
MALES								
Systolic blood pressure	mmHg	123	13	122	134	139	140	9.1
Diastolic (4th) blood pressure	mmHg	69	11	69	78	82	90	1.9
Heart rate	b/min	81	14	80	92	100	104	8.2
Body-mass index	kg/m²	21.2	2.6	20.7	22.8	24.2	23.0	19.0
Cholesterol	mg/dl	159	33	156	182	199	220	3.3
Uric acid	mg/dl	5.2	1.1	5.1	6.0	6.6	7.0	5.4
Glucose postprandial	mg/dl	96	13	94	104	111	130	1.8
Smoking	cig/day	12*	8	10*	19*	20*	10	34.3
FEMALES								
Systolic blood pressure	mmHg	114	11	113	124	128	140	1.8
Diastolic (4th) blood pressure	mmHg	65	10	65	74	77	90	0.7
Heart rate	b/min	84	14	84	96	104	104	10.8
Body-mass index	kg/m²	20.9	2.5	20.5	22.6	23.8	23.0	17.0
Cholesterol	mg/dl	170	33	168	194	214	220	5.0
Uric acid	mg/dl	4.0	1.1	4.0	4.7	5.3	7.0	1.3
Glucose postprandial	mg/dl	93	13	92	102	108	130	1.0
Smoking	cig/day	9*	7	8*	15*	19*	10	20.1

* Nonsmokers excluded.

Table 2. Correlation coefficients (Pearson) between various risk variables (see Table 1: variables and units) and between measurements approximately one year apart (1st screening vs 2nd screening): adolescents aged 15–19 years (Cologne).

Variables	Syst BP	Diast BP	Heart rate	Body mass	Cholest	Uric acid	Gluc pp	Smoking	Age
Systolic BP	—	0.30	0.29	0.28	0.13	...	...	...	0.14
Diastolic BP	0.40	—	0.10	0.15	...	...	...	...	0.14
Heart rate	0.39	0.17	—	...	0.11	...	0.14	...	...
Body-mass index	0.21	0.11	...	—	...	0.17	...	...	0.15
Cholesterol	...	...	...	...	—	—	...	...	...
Uric acid	...	...	...	0.14	...	—	...	...	...
Glucose postprandial	0.11	...	0.18	...	...	...	—	—	...
Smoking	...	...	...	...	...	...	—	—	...
Age	...	0.10	...	...	...	...	...	...	—
1st vs 2nd screening	0.61	0.38	0.48	0.88	0.58	—	0.19	0.76	—

Right upper triangle: males; left lower triangle: females; 1st screening vs 2nd screening, both sexes combined; coefficients lower than 0.10 are indicated by 3 points (...).

age (males only). Concerning age, similar correlations are revealed for diastolic blood pressure.

Much higher correlation coefficients, however, were shown between measurements of the first and of the second survey one year later, with an astonishingly high reproducibility for systolic blood pressure, cholesterol, and heart rate (last line, Table 2). Uric acid was not determined at the second screening.

This reproducibility or maintenance of measurement levels over time was shown especially well for blood pressures and heart rate. These hemodynamic parameters have been measured not only during the second survey one year later, but also about one and two weeks after the first screening. The subpopulation additionally controlled in this way was selected according to certain cutoff values (males = 140/80 and females = 130/75 mmHg, diastolic 5th phase in this case; based upon the preliminary results of the study in 1975 [11]), but included also a normotensive group of adolescents. Figure 1 shows clearly the phenomenon of regression to the mean, although this seems to be more apparent for the high than for the low levels. On the other hand, the second and third controls are almost identical with the levels one year later.

Most important, however, is the observation that the arithmetic means of classified measurements (classes 10 mmHg wide and overlapping the zero terminal digit) generally do not cross (two exceptions in the dotted right parts of Fig. 1). The classification was based upon the second of two measurements at the first occasion being lower than the first measurement at each occasion and level. A similar pattern of evolution over time is revealed for diastolic pressures and even heart rates. Accordingly, predictive values (true positives over positives and true negatives over negatives) from one measurement to the next are higher for normotensives staying normotensive (over 0.90) than for hypertensives staying hypertensive above the defined limits (over 0.50).

Having established a certain degree of stability of risk variables over time and knowing about correlations among these variables, the question arises as to whether an accumulation of elevated parameters can be observed in certain persons and what the stability of such accumulations over time will be. Table 3 indicates that 75% of those with one elevated risk variable had one or more variables in the high range a year later. More than one-fourth of those with 5–6 'risks' in 1975 had still 5–6 'risks' in 1976.

The analysis of configuration frequencies [27] enables the comparison of the observed frequency of occurrence for each combination of elevated risk parameters (configuration) with the frequency to be expected in the case of mutual independence of variables. This frequency is computed according to the binomial model by using estimations of the risk probabilities from the marginal distributions (see above: method of analysis). Thus, 1066 pupils in a

155

Table 3. Relative stability (in %) of the aggregated occurrence of risk variables elevated beyond the 80th percentile value (age- and sex-specific): adolescents aged 15 – 19 years (Cologne).

No. of aggregations	2nd Screening					
1st Screening	0	1-6	2-6	3-6	4-6	5-6
0	51	49	16	3	1	0
1	25	75				
2	11	89	52			
3	9	91		33		
4	2	98			35	
5-6	0	100				27

Risk variables: systolic blood pressure diastolic 4th phase blood pressure, heart rate, body-mass index, cholesterol, glucose postprandial, and smoking (an accumulation of 7 risks in one person was not observed).

population of 4820 can be expected to be free of any risk; however, 1269 have been observed, corresponding to an observed–expected ratio of 1:2. This relation increases considerably for higher degrees of accumulated risk and reaches, e.g., for the occurrence of six parameters above the 80th percentile in one person, an index value of 7.9 (both sexes).

For 3069 pupils, all eight risk variables could be determined, including uric acid; 79 (2.6%) of them carried elevated risks in more than four parameters, but only 29 (0.9%) were expected. To estimate the amount that each parameter contributes to risk aggregation, the frequencies of occurrence for each variable in the risk range were counted in this subpopulation (Table 4). Systolic blood pressure, body-mass index, and cholesterol seem to contribute the most. However, variables with a relatively small contribution as, for example, cigarette consumption occur more than twice as often as expected (in case of a selection procedure unrelated to smoking for these 79 adoles-

Table 4. Contribution of single risk variables to total aggregation in adolescents with more than 4 risk variables (out of 8) elevated beyond the 80th percentile value (age- and sex-specific): adolescents aged 15 – 19 years (Cologne).

Variables	Cases observed	% of sum	Observed/ expected
Systolic BP	65	82.3	3.2
Body-mass index	61	77.2	3.0
Cholesterol	56	70.9	2.8
Diastolic 4th BP	54	68.4	2.7
Smoking	48	60.8	2.4
Glucose	47	59.5	2.3
Heart rate	46	58.2	2.3
Uric acid	43	54.4	2.1
Total with more than 4 'risks'	79	100.0	2.7

156

Table 5. Hierarchical configuration-frequency analysis for 8 risk variables in adolescents of Cologne 1975/76 (total $\chi^2 = 1264.1$). The indicated χ^2-values should not be interpreted as a criterion of significance, rather as indicating the degree of deviation of observed from expected frequencies of aggregations. The total χ^2-value is least reduced, if uric acid is eliminated, namely to 1079.3. The smallest contributor to this amount is glucose, thus this variable is eliminated next, etc. Below the underlined remaining chi-square-values the configuration with the largest contribution to the total remaining chi-square is indicated, i.e. after the elimination of uric acid it is the configuration 12347 with a chi-square of 127. The complete configuration should be written as 1234-070 standing for syst. BP, diast. BP, heart rate and cholesterol elevated; uric acid eliminated; glucose normal; body-mass index elevated; smoking 'normal' (i.e., below the 80th percentile for smokers).

No. of variables eliminated	Syst. BP (1)	Diast. BP (2)	Heart rate (3)	Cholest. (4)	Uric acid (5)	Glucose (6)	BMI (7)	Cig./day (8)	df
1 (5)	409.9	593.4	641.0	808.6	$\underline{1079.3}$ 12 347 = 127	908.9	622.1	899.8	120
2 (6)	288.7	590.2	571.5	489.9	—	$\underline{924.9}$ 12347 = 148	687.7	895.0	57
3 (4)	215.3	472.7	536.4	$\underline{866.4}$ 123 = 171	—	—	583.2	769.8	26
4 (8)	138.4	446.2	489.3	—	—	—	683.3	$\underline{792.4}$ 123 = 288	11
5 (7)	90.1	404.7	438.0	—	—	—	$\underline{651.7}$ 123 = 300	—	4
6 (2)	40.2	$\underline{314.1}$ 13 = 211	276.2	—	—	—	—	—	1

cents, who did not smoke, about 20%, i.e., only 16 pupils were to be expected).

If, by means of configuration-frequency analysis, those variables are subsequently excluded that contribute the least to total aggregation, so-called 'types' and 'antitypes' can be identified. From the chi-square values remaining after stepwise exclusion of parameters, almost identical configurations (types) predominate.

These are (reading Table 5 from the bottom to the top), in the first line, systolic blood pressure and heart rate (type 13) to which diastolic blood pressure is added next (type 123). This remains the leading configuration throughout several hierarchical orders until on the lowest levels—elimination of uric acid and glucose only—cholesterol and body-mass index are associated (type 12347).

5. DISCUSSION

Comparing epidemiological studies, especially in terms of prevalence [26], demands reference to the methodology. As described earlier [18], international standards could be introduced only for blood pressure measurements by use of a standard tape [16]. In spite of this, the comparison with the literature reveals a considerable amount of agreement. As stated elsewhere [11], systolic blood pressures in Cologne occupy a middle position. Diastolic values are rather low in Cologne. This seems to be due to the standard tape used as discussed already elsewhere [18]. The studies in which the tape was not used for observer training [e.g., 32] show much higher diastolic levels, especially if diastolic values were defined by using the 4th phase (because of the fact that the interpretation of muffling as the criterion for the 4th phase is strongly affected by the tape training [18]) or if no precise definition at all was given. On the other hand, our diastolic levels are rather high compared with other investigators employing the standard tape. This corresponds more or less to the positive deviation of our observer group from the standard, reading 2–3 mmHg higher than the validating expert group.

Although the heart rates might be slightly overestimated, an average of 81 beats/min for males and 84 beats/min for females indicates a certain degree of excitation probably due just to the fact of being medically examined but compare, e.g., Watson and Lowrey [35], who indicate 82 beats/min for this age group. This assumption is supported by the relatively high differential pressure of about 57 mmHg for boys and 51 mmHg for girls. We hold the view [33] that a certain excitation of adolescents might be helpful to select those on prospective risk of hypertension and cardiovascular morbidity.

With regard to height, weight, and body-mass index, our data are almost identical with those from Oslo [34]. Near identity can also be shown for height between males of our study compared with results from mustering recruits [36] from North Rhine–Westphalia with a mean of 178 cm. The same report demonstrates differences of an order of 3 cm between northern and southern Germany and between metropolitan and rural areas, as well as between higher and lower educational levels. According to these differences, our population should fall into the top range, which in fact it does. Similar values have been published by Luyken and de Wijn [37] for 17- to 19-year-old boys, in the Netherlands and in the U.S.A. The averages of 177 and 176 cm for height and 70 and 71 kg for weight result in a BMI of approximately 22.3 and 22.9, respectively. This seems to indicate a little higher prevalence of adiposity than in Cologne. The average BMI values found by Bruppacher [38] for the Basle Adolescent Study again agree with those given for Cologne (19.5 and 20.2, respectively, for Basle boys and girls 14–16 years old). Height and weight are lower than in Cologne due to the younger age spectrum and possibly due to the north-south gradient.

With regard to cholesterol, several studies are comparable to the Cologne study. Especially the values from the Tecumseh study [39], with a mean of 166 mg/dl for boys and 173 mg/dl for girls (both sex groups 15–19 years old) fit our data very well. These values were determined by use of the Abell-Kendall method, which was the reference method for the enzymatic determination employed in Cologne [23]. Also very similar values have been reported from the Basle study [31] with means of 164 and 176 mg/dl, respectively. The data from the Bogalusa study [40], 154 and 162 mg/dl, respectively (here only 13- to 14-year-old white children), are somewhat lower, although the sex differential has been already established (nonexistent before puberty). The mean level of 182 mg/dl for the entire Muscatine population [41] is difficult to interpret because of lack of information on methodological validation. The authors, on the basis of their data, postulate no interpretable differences between age groups or sexes.

Very scarce information only is found in the literature on uric acid and blood glucose levels of adolescents. In the Evans County study [42], the mean values of uric acid, 5.9 and 4.0 mg/dl, respectively, for 15- to 24-year-old whites, are somewhat higher than ours. However, their values were determined by the method of Caraway, which is difficult to compare with our procedure. In Tecumseh [43], 5.4 and 4.2 mg/dl, respectively, were found for males and females by use of an enzymatic method. This is really very close to our results (see means listed in Table 1).

As the differences of population means with regard to fasting vs nonfasting glucose values were only 1.9 mg/dl for males and 3.7 mg/dl for females, the data from Cologne (97% postprandial) might be well comparable to preprandial data; but lacking appropriate information, we are unable to compare the postprandial blood glucose levels with those from other studies in adolescents.

A very limited comparison might be based on our findings in 19 adolescents (i.e., 0.3%) between 15 and 19 years old, having a history of diabetes mellitus according to the questionnaire [44]. Our prevalence of 0.3% compares with 0.14% at the age of 16 in the NCDS study [45] or with roughly 0.35%, as reported by Wadsworth and Jarrett [46] and by North et al. [47]. Based on our records, girls seem to be less affected (0.1%) than boys (0.5%). This difference between the sexes cannot be explained satisfactorily as yet. The observed difference is also described for younger children [48], but this seems to relate to growth-dependent variations (susceptibility to viral infections, antagonism of estrogens, and growth hormone on insulin).

If one accepts the limits used in Table 1 as possibly bearing on later risk, the females seem to be little affected, with the exception of the variables cholesterol, overweight, and smoking. Adolescent males, however, carry considerable risk with regard to systolic blood pressure, cholesterol, uric acid, overweight, and smoking. For both sexes, smoking is the most prominent and most influential of all possible juvenile risk factors, wherever an intelligent threshold might be established. From our investigation, despite of all educational efforts, the prevalence of smoking in adolescents is not decreasing. A very early survey conducted in Cologne [49] in 1950, looking only at vocational pupils, revealed 35% smokers regardless of sex in the age group of 17 vs 62% in this age group in 1975 [25]. Malhotra [50] confirms in a recent review that more than one-half of the adolescent population in middle Europe smoke cigarettes. More or less three-fourths have experience with nicotine abuse.

The stability, for example, of blood pressure measurements over time has been well documented as tracking phenomenon [51], although not in terms of predictability as we did [33]. To our knowledge, Lauer et al. [41] are the only ones so far who looked into cumulative phenomena with regard to the upper ranges of risk variables. They have already stated that the gross correlation coefficients were disappointingly low, but found that, for example, 17.7% of children in the upper decile of relative weight had cholesterol values above the 90th percentile, instead of the expected 10%. For comparison, the coefficient of correlation between relative weight and cholesterol in the Muscatine study [41] was only 0.04, i.e., negligible. Our analysis confirms the assumption of Lauer et al. of an increasing tendency for aggregation in the higher-risk ranges. Even in adult studies, the influence of risk levels upon the degree of association between risk variables has rarely been analyzed so far. The so-called types emerging from our analysis indicate a dominating influence of systolic blood pressure and heart rate, supposingly an equivalent of sympathetic stimulation. Thus the leading position of the type 13 (Table 5) standing for systolic blood pressure and heart rate elevated exclusively might also be interpreted as the early hyperkinetic state in the genesis of hypertension [52].

160

This interpretation is even more convincing if one takes into account the different order of importance of the various risk variables, as is indicated in Table 4 for a subpopulation of adolescents with more than four elevated risk parameters. In this subgroup, with a possibly elevated cardiovascular risk, body-mass index takes second place after systolic blood pressure; diastolic blood pressure ranges considerably higher (4th position) than heart rate (7th position). Thus it might be that in advanced cases—if one interprets a high degree of accumulation of risk factors in a temporal way, i.e., as advanced—the hyperkinetic, sympathicosensitive state has developed into a phase characterized by increased vessel resistance being expressed as increased contribution of diastolic pressure to total aggregation of risk variables. Interestingly also body mass seems to play a much more important role in this 'high-risk' group than in the general population that we analyzed by means of the analysis of configuration frequencies (Table 5). The high-risk population as selected in Table 4 was too small to be subjected to this multivariate technique.

In summary, by taking stability over time and degree of accumulation of risk factors into account, high-risk groups can be defined in adolescents justifying intensive control and probably intervention. The number of endangered adolescents in this sense is considerably greater than expected from the isolated occurrence of elevated risk parameters alone. Thus 2.6% carry more than four risks out of eight if the sex-specific 80th percentile is taken as limit. Prospective cardiovascular risk and the potential for intervention need to be determined in follow-up studies[10].

REFERENCES

1. Statistisches Bundesamt: Statistisches Jahrbuch 1978 für die Bundesrepublik Deutschland. Stuttgart: Kohlhammer, 1978.
2. Wiernick PH (ed): Symposium on advances in treatment of cancer (Foreword). Med Clin North Am 61:943, 1977.
3. Wiernick PH (ed): Present trends in mortality in the age group 35–64 in selected developed countries between 1950 and 1973. WHO Q 31, 1978.
4. USDHEW: The Surgeon General's Report on Smoking and Health 1979 (in press).
5. Schettler G, Greten H: Koronare Herzkrankheiten: Entwicklung in der Bundesrepublik Deutschland und in den USA. Dtsch Aerztebl 40:2263, 1978.
6. Laaser U, Schwartz FW, Schütt A: Sind Früherkennung und Frühbehandlung der Hypertonie in der Bundesrepublik Deutschland erreichbar? Med Welt 28:1550, 1977.
7. Kannel WB, McGhee D, Gordon T: A general cardiovascular risk profile: the Framingham study. Am J Cardiol 38:46, 1976.
8. Borhani NO: Primary prevention of coronary heart disease: a critique. Am J Cardiol 40:251, 1977.
9. Mann GV: Diet-heart: End of an era. N Engl J Med 297:644, 1977.

10. World Health Organization: WHO/ISFC meeting on precursors of atherosclerosis in children, Geneva, 1978. CVD 78, 1978.
11. Laaser U, Meurer KA, Kaufmann W: Untersuchung zur Epidemiologie der juvenilen Hypertonie in Köln. Verh Dtsch Ges Inn Med 81:1715, 1975.
12. Laaser U, Meurer KA, Kaufmann W: Informationen zum Übergang auf die städtischen, weiterführenden, allgemeinbildenden und beruflichen Schule-Bildungswege. Ed. Dept. of School Administration of Cologne, January, 1974.
13. European Community, Medical Research Council (CRM/CREST): Methodology and standardisation of non-invasive blood pressure measurement in epidemiological studies. Biol Sci EUR 5544e, p 93, 1976.
14. Kirkendall WM, Burton AC, Epstein FH, Freis ED: Recommendations for human blood pressure determination by sphygmomanometers. Committee of the American Heart Association. Circulation 36:980, 1967.
15. Rose GA, Holland WW, Crowley EA: A sphygmomanometer for epidemiologists. Lancet 1:296, 1964.
16. Rose GA: Standardisation of observers in blood pressure measurement. Lancet 1:673, 1965.
17. Institut für den Wissenschaftlichen Film, Nonnenstieg 72, D-3400 Göttingen. Catalogue no. W 1044, Blood pressure readings.
18. Laaser U: Methodik und Qualitätskontrolle der indirekten Blutdruckmessung. Z Kardiol 67:460, 1978.
19. Eilertsen E, Humerfelt S: The observer variation in the measurement of arterial blood pressure. Acta Med Scand 184:145, 1968.
20. Kanto S, Winkelstein Jr W, Sackett DL, Ibrahim MA: A method for classifying blood pressure. Am J Epidemiol 84:510, 1966.
21. Rose GA, Blackburn H: Cardiovascular survey methods. WHO Monogr Ser 56:94, 1968.
22. Schmidt FH, Dahl K v, Heidrich P, Stork H: Enzymatic determination of triglycerides in blood serum and blood glucose by automated methods. Organisation des Laboratoires — Biologie prospective. IIe Colloque de Pont-à-Mousson. Paris: L'expansion Scientifique Française, 1972, p 121.
23. Stähler F, Munz E, Kattermann R: Enzymatische Bestimmung von Gesamt-Cholesterin im Serum, Richtigkeit und Methodenvergleich. Dtsch Med Wochenschr 100:876, 1975.
24. Kageyama N: A direct colorimetric determination of uric acid in serum and urine with uricase-catalase system. Clin Chim Acta 31:421, 1971.
25. Roegele F: Eine Untersuchung über die Verbreitung des Risikofaktors Zigaretten-Rauchen bei 15–19 jährigen Berufs- und Gymnasialschülern in Köln 1974–1976. Europäische Hochschulschriften VII/20. Frankfurt: Peter Lang, 1979.
26. Epstein FH, Eckoff RD: The Epidemiology of high blood pressure — geographic distributions and ethiological factors. In: Stamler J, et al. (eds) The epidemiology of hypertension. New York: Grune and Stratton, 1967.
27. Krauth J, Lienert GA: Die Konfigurationsfrequenzanalyse (KFA) und ihre Anwendung in Psychologie und Medizin. Freiburg: Karl Alber, 1973.
28. Laaser U, Schütt A: The cardiovascular risk-profile of adolescents in Cologne: a representative study including 6302 pupils. Z Kardiol 67:837, 1978.
29. World Health Organization: Arterial hypertension and ischaemic heart disease. WHO Tech Rep Ser 628:8, 1978.
30. Gutsche H, Schirop T, Buschmann E: Blutzucker- und Seruminsulinverlauf beim oralen Glukosetoleranztest. Dtsch Aerztebl 52:3513, 1975.

162

31. Sieber M, Angst J: Zur Epidemiologie des Zigaretten-, Drogen- und Alkoholkonsums bei jungen Männern. Schweiz Med Wochenschr 107:1912, 1977.
32. Kilcoyne MM, Richter RW, Alsup PA: Adolescent hypertension. I. Detection and prevalence. Circulation 50:758, 1974.
33. Laaser U: Risikofaktoren bei Jugendlichen. Fortschr Med 95:256, 1977.
34. Brundtland GH, Liestöll K, Wallöe L: Height and weight of school children and adolescent girls and boys in Oslo 1970. Acta Paediatr Scand 64:565, 1975.
35. Watson EH, Lowrey GH: Growth and development of children, 5th edn. Chicago: Year Book Medical, 1967.
36. Statistische Kurzinformation aus dem Sanitäts- und Gesundheitswesen der Bundeswehr, Institut für Wehrmedizinalstatistik und Berichtswesen, Bundesministerium der Verteidigung, Bonn, 1975.
37. Luyken R, Wijn JF de: Body fat and muscle tissue in dutch adoelscent boys and young adult men, assessed by anthropometry. Nutr Metab 12:121, 1970.
38. Bruppacher R: Zur Ernährung der Adoleszenten. In: Bruppacher G, Ritzel G (eds) Zur Ernäherungssituation der schweizerischen Bevölkerung. Bern, 1976.
39. Johnson BC, Epstein FH, Kjelsberg MO: Distributions and familial studies of blood pressure and serum cholesterol levels in a total community — Tecumseh, Michigan. J Chronic Dis 18:147, 1965.
40. Frerichs RR, Srinivasan SR, Webber LS, Berenson GS: Serum cholesterol and triglyceride levels in 3,446 children from a biracial community: the Bogalusa Heart Study. Circulation 54:302, 1976.
41. Lauer RM, Connor WE, Leaverton PE, Reiter MA, Clarke WR: Coronary heart disease risk factors in school children: the Muscatine study. J Pediatr 86:697, 1975.
42. Klein R, Klein BE, Cornoni JC, Maready J, Cassel JC, Tyroler HA: Serum uric acid. Its relationship to coronary heart disease risk factors and cardiovascular disease, Evans County, Georgia. Arch Intern Med 132:401, 1973.
43. Mikkelsen WM, Dodge HJ, Valkenburg H: The distribution of serum uric acid values in a population unselected as to gout or hyperuricemia. Am J Med 39:241, 1965.
44. Laaser U: Kardiovaskuläre Risikomerkmale bei großstädtischen Adoleszenten: Die epidemiologische Langzeitstudie in Köln. Habilitationsschrift, Universität Köln, 1979/80.
45. Calnan M, Peckham CS: Incidence of insulin-dependant diabetes mellitus in the first sixteen years of life. Lancet 1:589, 1977.
46. Wadsworth MEJ, Jarrett RJ: Incidence of diabetes in the first 26 years of life. Lancet 2:1172, 1974.
47. North Jr AF, Gorwitz K, Sultz HA: A secular increase in the incidence of juvenile diabetes mellitus. J Pediatr 91:706, 1977.
48. North Jr AF, Gorwitz K, Sultz HA: Sex and juvenile diabetes (Editorial). Br Med J 1:594, 1977.
49. Kaiser K: Über den Nikotinverbrauch der Schüler der Kölner männlichen Berufsschulen. Oeff Gesundheitsdienst 13:169, 1951.
50. Malhotra MK: Tabakabusus bei Jugendlichen. Fortschr Med 96:32, 1978.
51. Zinner SH, Martin LF, Sachs F, Rosner B, Kass EH: A longitudinal study of blood pressure in childhood. Am J Epidemiol 100:437, 1974.
52. Sannerstedt R, Sivertsson R, Lundgren Y: Hemodynamic aspects of the early stages of human arterial hypertension. In: Rorive G, et al. (eds) The arterial hypertensive disease. New York: Masson, 1976.

9. HYPERTENSION AND ITS DISTRIBUTION IN PRAGUE

H. Geizerová, J. Widimský, Z. Piša, J. Hurych, Z. Hejl, and H. Pistulková

In Czechoslovakia, the diseases of the cardiovascular (CV) system are responsible for almost 50% of all deaths (561.1/100,000 in 1976), and are still the leading cause of mortality[1]. Between 1968 and 1976 mortality from CV disease (ICD, 1966: 390–458) exhibited a moderate upward trend from 504.8/100,000 to 561/100,000, which is an increase of about 11.3%.

However, during the past decade, the pattern of specific CV mortality has changed. Mortality from chronic rheumatic heart disease has decreased by

Table 1. Mortality in Czechoslovakia (ICD), deaths per 100,000 population.

ICD disease	1968	1969	1970	1971	1972	1973	1974	1975	1976	1977	1978
390–458	504.8	541.7	556.1	563.3	546.3	567.8	572.7	569.3	561.0	851.4	847.6
400–404	19.5	17.2	15.2	14.7	11.0	10.1	10.5	8.9	9.0	10.5	10.7
410–414	229.0	252.7	261.8	272.3	259.9	269.8	271.9	274.4	272.5	423.0	418.1
420–429	36.5	35.3	30.7	25.8	21.0	20.4	19.4	17.0	17.3	26.1	23.7
430–438	142.0	154.0	165.1	170.2	176.5	186.8	188.2	191.3	190.8	291.5	294.9

ICD: international classification of diseases.

Table 2. Mortality — ICD diagnosis: 410+411+412.

	Men in Czechoslovakia: 35-69 years of age							
	35-39	40-44	45-49	50-54	55-59	60-64	65-69	Total
1971	143	369	810	767	1717	2910	3650	10,480
1972	166	324	723	944	1467	2862	3534	10,133
1973	148	379	707	1084	1320	2829	3652	10,200
1974	167	375	686	1338	1094	2813	3654	10,228
1975	188	355	702	1356	1123	2693	3614	10,131
1976	169	317	700	1292	1352	2517	3783	10,216
1977	165	318	739	1355	1648	2225	3936	10,512
1978	157	363	710	1370	1937	2015	3791	10,466
Total	1303	2800	5786	9506	11,658	20,837	29,614	82,366

ICD: international classification of diseases,
    410 : acute myocardial infarction,
    411 : other forms of acute of subacute ischaemic heart disease,
    412 : chronic ischaemic heart disease.

H. Kesteloot, J.V. Joossens (eds.), Epidemiology of Arterial Blood Pressure, 163–171.
Copyright © 1980 Martinus Nijhoff Publishers bv, The Hague/Boston/London. All rights reserved.

38.5%, mortality from ischaemic heart disease has increased by 19% and mortality from hypertension has decreased by 53.8%, and mortality from acute CV diseases has increased by 34.4% (Tables 1–3). Cardiovascular disease ranks as one of the most frequent causes of invalidism in the CSSR, accounting for almost 40% of full and 22% of partial disability. Retirement due to hypertension (ICD, 1966:400–4) decreased by about 51.1% from 1968 to 1977.

Table 3. Mortality — ICD diagnosis: 410+411+412.

| | Women in Czechoslovakia: 35-69 years of age | | | | | | | |
	35-39	40-44	45-49	50-54	55-59	60-64	65-69	Total
1971	16	57	146	194	510	1186	2130	4251
1972	16	48	107	214	398	1120	2039	3956
1973	20	61	131	223	268	1130	2041	3883
1974	15	55	104	281	312	1156	2041	3981
1975	24	41	103	256	318	1071	2122	3952
1976	15	49	121	274	379	1074	2154	4079
1977	18	44	121	226	389	731	2084	3622
1978	19	40	118	295	516	766	2079	3837
Total	143	395	950	1963	3090	8234	16,688	31,571

ICD: international classification of diseases,
   410 : acute myocardial infarction,
   411 : other forms of acute or subacute ischaemic heart disease,
   412 : chronic ischaemic heart disease.

These data show that CV disease is one of the most important problems for the Czechoslovakian health service. Therefore an epidemiological survey of middle-aged men was performed in Prague by the Institute of Clinical and Experimental Medicine. The population samples were selected from among all men aged 50–54 and 60–64 in one Prague district (No. 2) from which statistically representative samples were selected. The data are presented in Table 4. In the first stage of our study (1963–1964), research was aimed at obtaining data on the prevalence of ischaemic heart disease (IHD) and arterial hypertension (HT).

After choosing the random samples, we examined 93.6% and 89% of men aged 60–64 and 50–54, respectively, in the original samples. The examination was carried out by means of the standard procedure recommended by the WHO [8], and the diagnosis of IHD was based on the following criteria:

1) Symptoms of angina pectoris (AP), assessed on the basis of a standardized questionnaire developed by WHO experts [8].

Table 4. Acute myocardial infarction in Prague-2, according to AMI registers of the WHO, Geneva.

A. Annual incidence (per 1000 population) of AMI including reinfarctions

Age	20-39	40-44	45-49	50-54	55-59	60-64	65-69
M	0.3	1.8	3.4	7.5	11.5	12.3	17.2
F	0.0	0.1	0.4	1.2	1.5	3.4	6.2

B. Incidence of AMI — 1st attacks only

Age	20-39	40-44	45-49	50-54	55-59	60-64	65-69
M	0.3	1.3	2.3	5.1	6.8	7.6	10.2
F	0.0	0.1	0.2	0.8	0.9	2.7	4.4

2) A history of possible myocardial infarction, according to the question-naire [8].
3) Electrocardiographic (ECG) changes indicative of the presence of IHD. A 12-lead ECG record was made with subjects at rest in the supine position. The findings were analysed using the Minnesota Code [8].

Every respondent was included in one of the following three categories:

1) *No signs of IHD.*
2) *Possible IHD.* This category included subjects with intermittent claudication [8] or with ECG evidence of possible ischaemic changes. (Minnesota Code: I-3; IV-1,2; V-1, 2, 3, i.e. moderate Q-wave changes, St-segment depressions, and inverted T waves).
3) *Probable IHD.* This group includes those persons who had AP or a history of pain evaluated as being compatible with possible myocardial infarction or showing probable ECG signs of ischaemic lesions (Minnesota Code: 1-1, 2, or VII-1, i.e. severe Q-wave changes or left bundle branch block).

The main prevalence of probable and possible IHD, AP, IM and ECG ischaemic changes is shown in Table 5.

Figures 1 and 2 show the frequency distribution of systolic and diastolic blood pressure among the respondents of our samples. The mean values for systolic and diastolic blood pressures are presented in Table 6, which shows that the two age groups exhibit a fairly similar frequency of hypertension, i.e. 16.7% of the men aged 60–64 vs 17.4% of those aged 50–54.

Table 5. Ischaemic heart disease (IHD) men 60–54 and 50–54 years of age — Prague-2.

Men — Prague-2		Age	
		60–64 (n = 443) in %	50–54 (n = 400) in %
IHD	Probable	31.4	18.0
	Possible	30.5	8.7
AP		19.4	11.0
AMI		10.6	5.5
ECG	Probable	11.8	5.0
	Possible	43.5	13.0

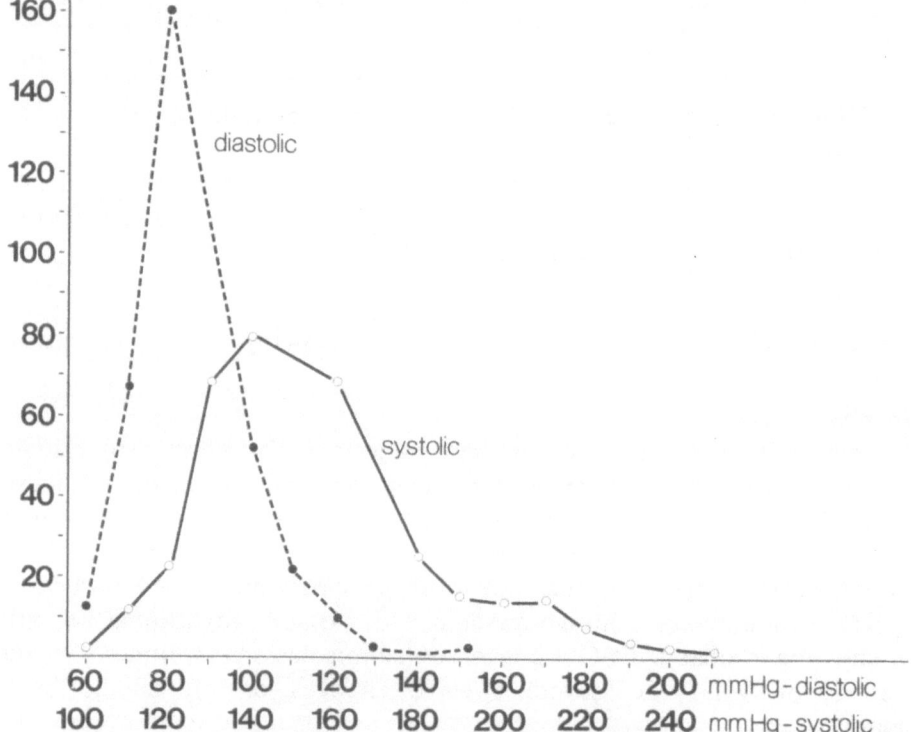

Figure 1. Distribution curves of systolic and diastolic blood pressure values: men 60–64 years of age — Prague-2.

Systolic hypertension alone (≥160 mmHg) was more frequent (35.1%) in the older age group (60–64) than in the males ten years younger (50–54) (2.3%), which is most probably among others a sign of the process of ageing.

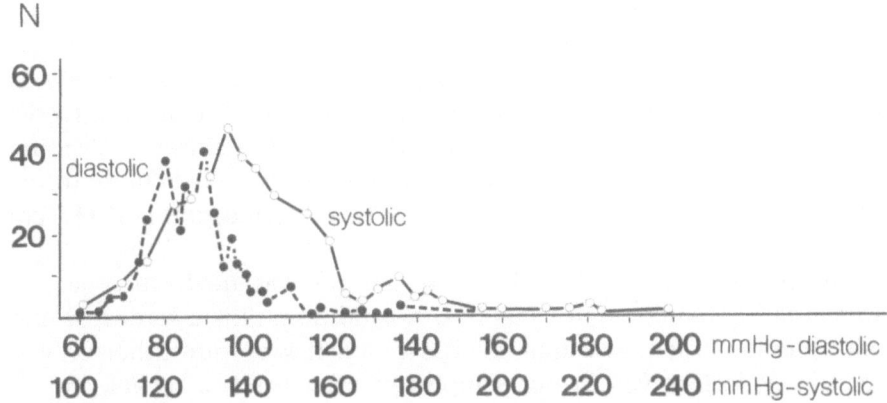

Figure 2. Distribution curves of systolic and diastolic blood pressure values: men 50–54 years of age — Prague-2.

Table 6. Blood pressure values: men 60–64 and 50–54 years of age — Prague 2.

Men — Prague-2 Blood pressure (mmHg)	Age	
	60–64 ($n = 443$)	50–54 ($n = 400$)
$\bar{x}$ Systolic ± SD	154.8 26.1	139.8 19.7
$\bar{x}$ Diastolic ± SD	85.8 13.2	89.6 11.1
≥ 95 Diastolic only (%)	19.9	5.5
≥ 105 Diastolic only (%)	8.1	2.5
≥ 160 Systolic only (%)	35.1	2.3
≥ 160/95 Both systolic/diastolic (%)	16.7	17.4

Statistically significant correlations between hypertension and IHD diagnosis ($P < 0.001$) have been found in the 50- to 54-year-old men, but not in men 60–64 years old. It is speculated that younger hypertensive men are more jeopardized by IHD manifestation and therefore their hypertension has a poorer prognosis.

In the course of a current National Multifactorial Primary Preventive Study on Myocardial Infarction and Stroke started in another Prague district two years ago, we detected hypertension (defined as BP 160/95 mmHg or more) in 19.8% ($n = 5395$) of men aged 40–50 years [7]. According to the preliminary results, hypertension was statistically significantly less common in men with higher education (19.2%); compared with men with the lowest degree of education (23.3%), hypercholesterolaemia, smoking and overweight were also less frequent. This may be interpreted as an indication that persons with higher education are generally better informed and more readily adopt primary preventive measures, i.e. they smoke less, and watch their daily caloric intake and body weight. This most probably influences their blood pressure values and serum cholesterol levels. Even though still preliminary, the results support the hypothesis that the population at large would benefit from prevention of IHD risk factors through effective health education and HT control programmes.

After detecting elevated BP values, an attempt was made to secure information about the patient's previous health conditions, his awareness, and the results of previous medical examinations, if any. It was found that only about 15% of the hypertensives in our samples of men aged of 60–64 and 50–54 years knew about their condition and, of these, only 10% were adequately treated and underwent regular check-ups. These data reflect the situation in the CSSR in 1960–1965. The same information, but obtained in 1974–1977 from a group of men aged 40–50, shows a much better situation. About 46% of all the men with elevated blood pressure values were aware of their hypertension and 62% of these men were under proper medical care.

Long-term prognosis of juvenile hypertension has been the object of many studies, but its cause is still unknown. A longitudinal study of juvenile hypertension made it possible to re-examine 73% of the individuals of a group of young hypertensives ($n = 96$) from Prague, who were investigated at this department 20 years ago at the age of 14–30 (arterial BP 170/100 mmHg or higher)[9]. Interestingly, 35.5% had a normal BP without any treatment during the intervening years; 40.2% had the same level of HT; 5.7% had higher BP levels, but without any new organic changes; and 1.5% had the same BP as 20 years earlier, but, unlike then, they were on medication. Only 17.1% of the patients showed convincing evidence of progression of the disease, i.e. new organic changes. The prognosis of moderate hypertension in adolescence significantly correlated with (a) occurrence of HT in the parents, (b) longevity of the parents, and (c) the initial BP values. There were no correlations between the prognosis and obesity, weight gain in the past 20 years, heart rate, smoking, alcohol intake, physical activity, or living standard of the given individual.

The results therefore enable the conclusion that juvenile HT does not necessarily indicate a poor prognosis and persist into middle age. Juvenile hypertension should, however, be kept under control, and checked at regular intervals.

Our interest has focussed not only on adult but also on childhood hypertension, because knowledge of its prevalence is indispensable if hypertension is to be detected early, defined exactly and treated properly in the population. The population of one Prague district was therefore screened for prevalence of hypertension. The criteria for hypertension were set arbitrarily at 130/80 and 135/80 mmHg in children aged 6–11 and 12–19 years, respectively. These values were found acceptable for the identification of potential hypertensives. These or higher pressures were found in 0.5%–3.4% of the subjects examined (Table 7).

Table 7. Blood pressure: children 6–19 years of age — Prague.

Children of both sexes		Percentage children exceeding a given blood pressure in mmHg							
Age	*n*	Systolic		Diastolic		Both			
		130	135	80	85	135/80	140/80	145/80	145/85
6–11	2152	2.7	—	1.6	—	—	0.6	—	—
12–15	8168	—	2.8	—	—	2.0	—	0.5	—
16–19	3155	—	3.4	—	2.4	—	—	—	0.4

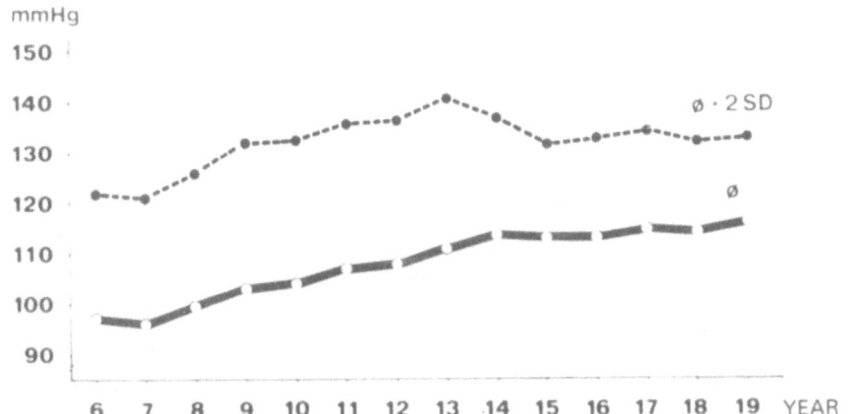

Figure 3. Distribution curves of systolic blood pressure values: girls 6–19 years of age —Prague.

The distribution curves of systolic and diastolic blood pressures of boys and girls from Prague are presented in Figures 3–6.

Children with elevated BP values in the group aged 11–15 years were given a questionnaire about their familial and personal history and life regimen, and were invited for clinical and laboratory tests. Compared with controls, these children exhibited a statistically significant higher frequency of diseases, obesity and inappropriate life regimen, and their parents were hypertensive.

Because of the complexity of the CV problem, the Czech Ministry of Health decided, in accordance with the WHO recommendations, that a CVD

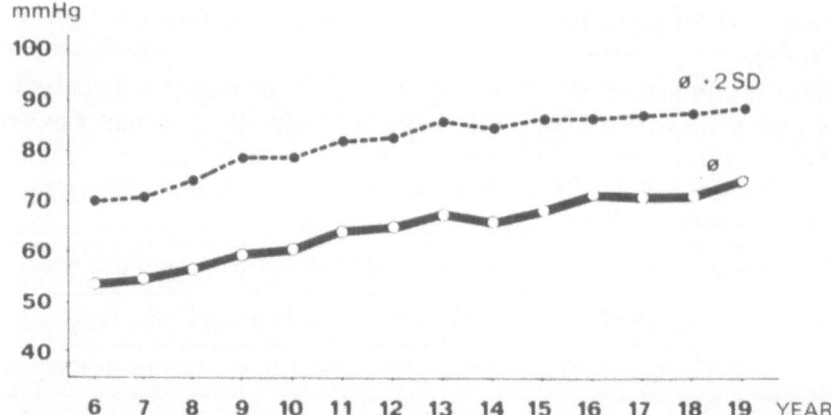

Figure 4. Distribution curves of diastolic blood pressure values: girls 6–19 years of age — Prague.

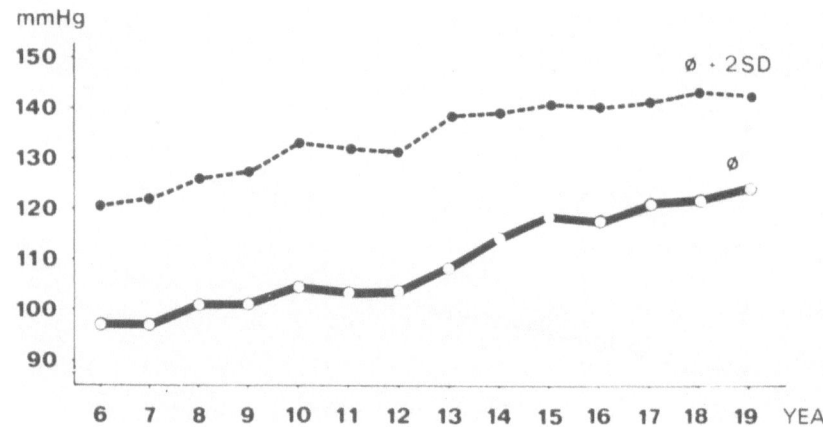

Figure 5. Distribution curves of systolic blood pressure values: boys 6–19 years of age — Prague.

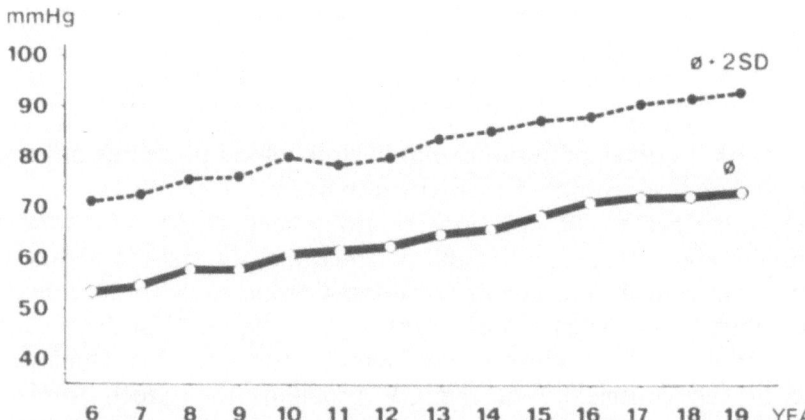

Figure 6. Distribution curves of diastolic blood pressure values: boys 6–19 years of age — Prague.

Community Control Programme be one of the priorities of the health policy [11]. Responsible for the coordination of the CV programme is the Department of Preventive Cardiology at the Ministry of Health of the CSSR [11, 12]. A nationwide Hypertension Control Programme has been prepared and carried out in selected model areas in CSSR. All these activities are conducted at the level of the existing system of general medical-care and oncological centres.

REFERENCES

1. Stat Annu Rev CSSR, 1977.
2. Fodor J, Hejl Z, Kohout M, Šantrůček M, Vavřík M, Weber K: The prevalence of ischaemic heart disease and the distribution of blood pressure in a population sample of males, aged 60–64 years, in a city district of Prague. J Atheroscler Res 4:161-164, 1966.
3. Geizerová H, Grafnetter D, Hejl Z, Widimský J, Šantrůček M: Prevalence of IHD in an urban population of males aged 50–54 years. Rev Czech Med 19:159-165, 1973.
4. Geizerová H, Widimský J, Hejl Z, Petržílková Z, Šantrůček M, Janda J, Grafnetter D, Stolz I: Angina pectoris and middle-aged man. Cor Vasa 19:428-436, 1977.
5. Geizerová H, Grafnetter D: Predictability of ischaemic heart disease in men aged 50–57 years. Rev Czech Med 20:96-106, 1974.
6. Geizerová H., et al.: Some risk factors of IHD in the Prague male population. Cor Vasa 17:81-88, 1975.
7. Geizerová H, Widimský J: Problems in prevention of IHD. Cor Vasa 18:119-128, 1976.
8. Rose GA, Blackburn H: Cardiovascular survey methods. WHO Monogr Ser 56, 1968.
9. Widimský J, Jandová R: Long-term prognosis of juvenile hypertension. Cor Vasa 19:299-309, 1977.
10. Pistulková H, Bláha J, Škodová I: Prevalence of hypertension in children and adolescents. Cor Vasa 18:237-240, 1976.
11. Píša Z, Hurych J: Situace a perspektivy kontroly kardiovaskulárních onemocnění v ČSR. Cesk Zdravotnictví 22:147-155, 1974.
12. Hurych J: Present position in the control of major cardiovascular diseases in Czechoslovakia — progress report. Meeting on comprehensive cardiovascular community control programmes, 12 Dec, Geneva, 1975.

PART FOUR

BLOOD PRESSURE DISTRIBUTION IN ADULTS

10. EPIDEMIOLOGY OF ARTERIAL BLOOD PRESSURE IN PORTUGAL

J. Pereira Miguel and F. de Pádua

The recognition of arterial hypertension as a frequent condition in the western countries and a major risk factor for stroke led to the first studies on the epidemiology of arterial blood pressure in Portugal in the early 1970s, and research has continuously progressed.

This paper reviews available information on mortality statistics, population surveys, studies of the determinants of the disease and community control programmes. On the whole, arterial hypertension has emerged as a very common disease in the Portuguese population but, hopefully, controllable and preventable.

1. MORTALITY STATISTICS

Judging from national mortality statistics, hypertensive disease is not a frequent cause of death among the Portuguese: it accounts for less than 2% of all deaths. Hypertensive disease death rates increase with age, mainly after 55, and males have higher death rates at all age groups (Table 1).

On the other hand, stroke, a disease known to be strongly associated with high blood pressure, is the leading cause of death in the Portuguese popula-

Table 1. Cardiovascular mortality in Portugal — 1975 [a].

Cause of death [b]		Age groups (years)					
		25 —	35 —	45 —	55 —	65 —	75 +
Hypertensive	(M)	1.6	2.5	7.8	36.9	104.6	258.7
diseases	(F)	0.6	2.0	4.2	16.2	65.7	255.8
Ischaemic heart	(M)	5.5	25.9	87.6	229.6	576.3	1184.6
disease	(F)	2.7	8.1	25.8	84.5	291.9	912.7
Cerebrovascular	(M)	3.1	21.6	86.1	372.1	1224.8	4052.9
disease	(F)	3.7	12.9	60.2	218.1	875.4	3573.7

[a] World Health Statistics (WHO). Death rates specific for sex and age, per 100,000 population.
[b] ICD 'A' List, 1965.

H. Kesteloot, J.V. Joossens (eds.), Epidemiology of Arterial Blood Pressure, 175–185.

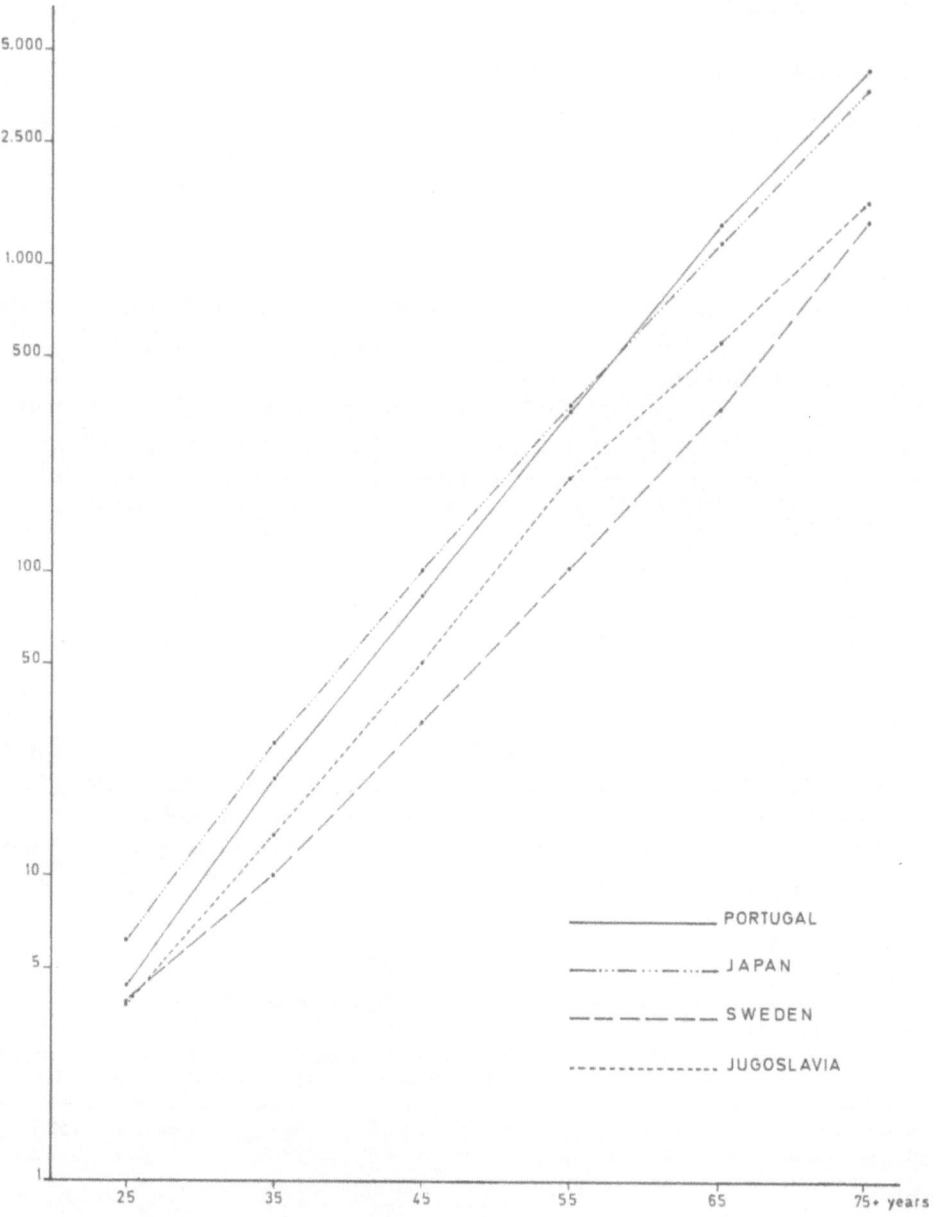

Figure 1. Cerebrovascular disease (A85), death rates per 100,000 population, males, 1974. From World Health Statistics Annual (WHO).

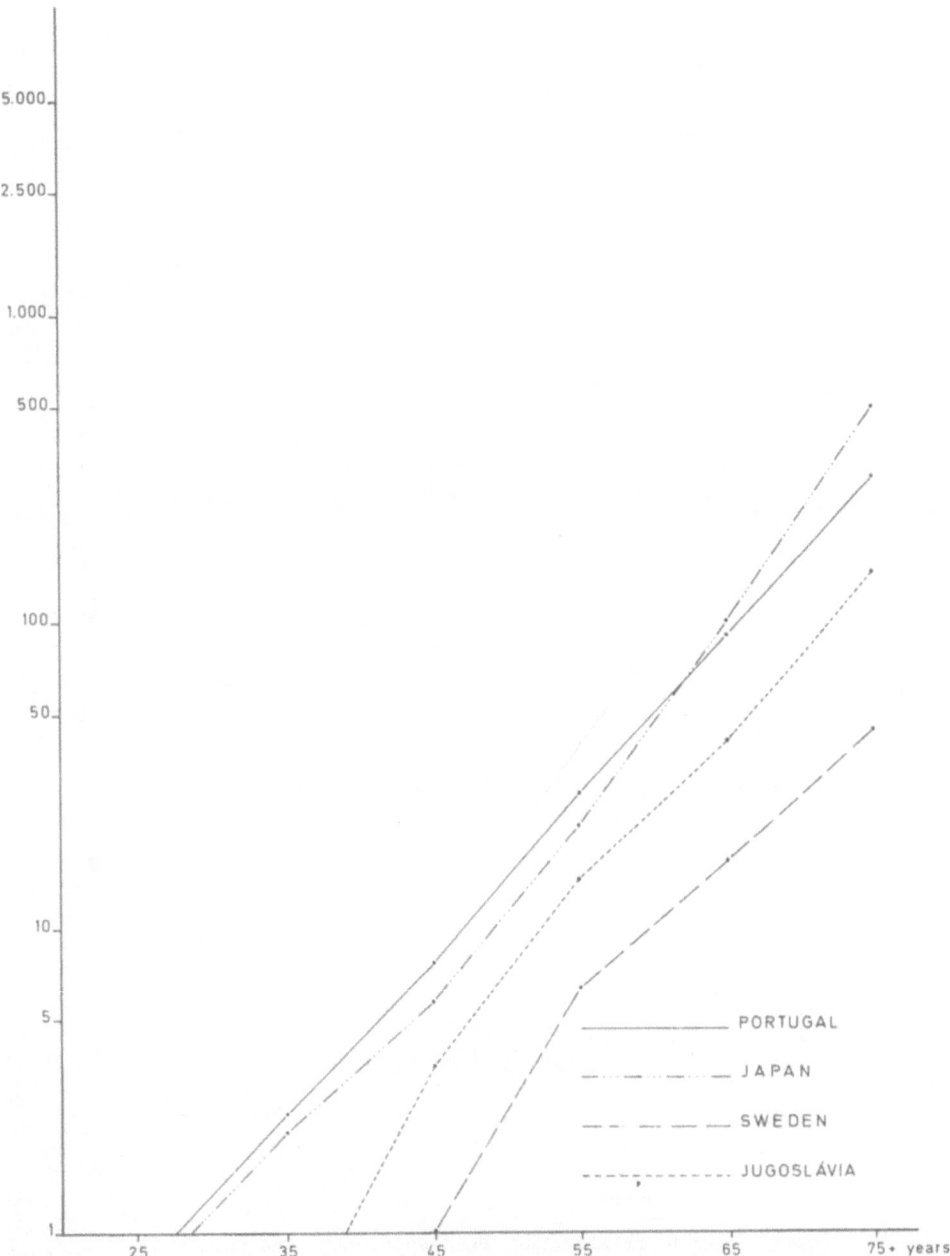

Figure 2. Hypertensive diseases (A82), death rates per 100,000 population, males, 1974. From World Health Statistics Annual (WHO).

178

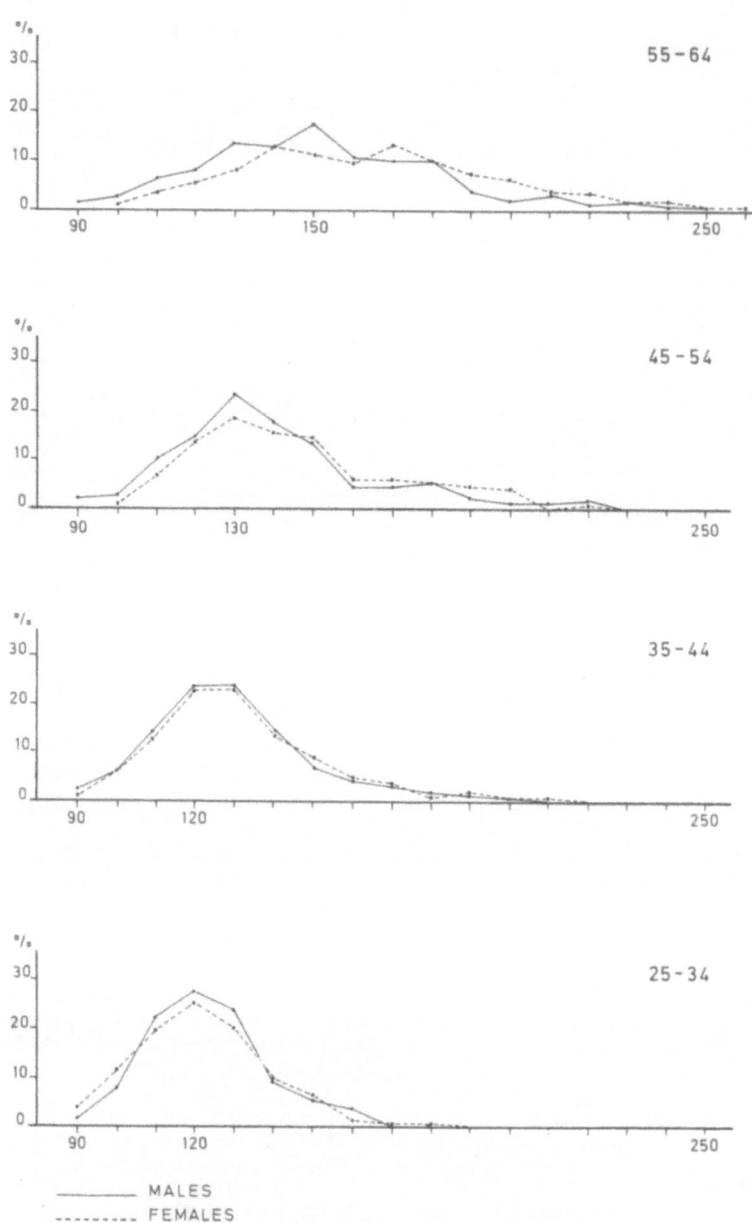

Figure 3. Systolic blood pressure distribution, males and females.

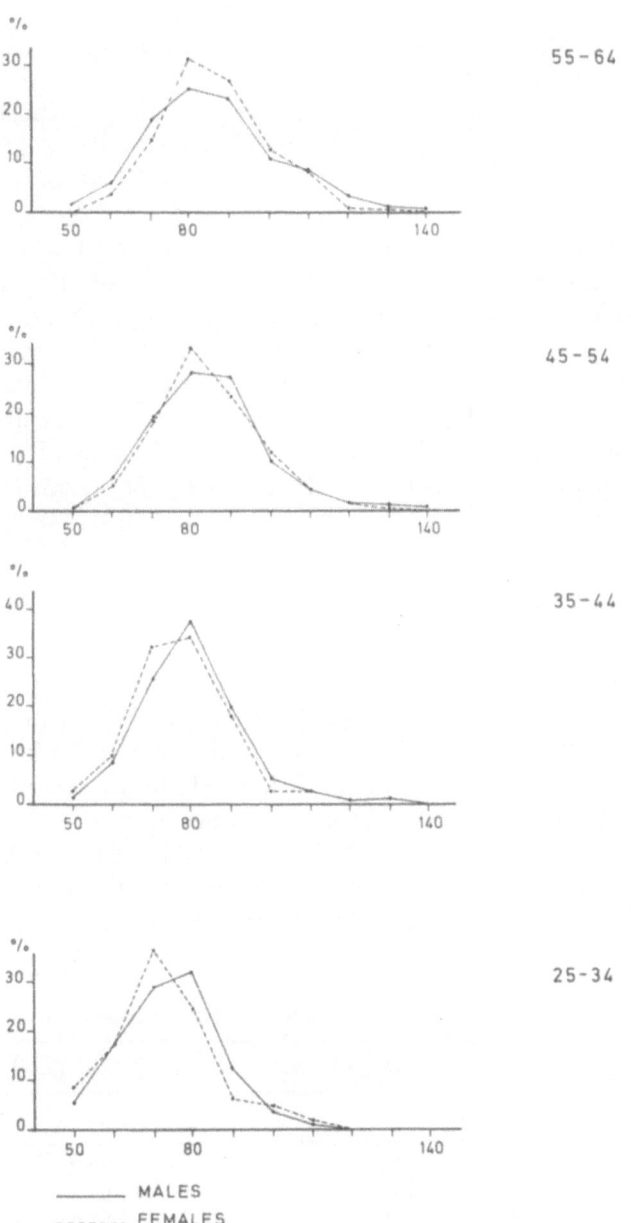

Figure 4. Diastolic blood pressure distribution, males and females.

180

tion. Cerebrovascular disease death rates are far above those for hypertensive
disease at all age groups (Table 1), and show a steep increase with age. Males
have higher death rates than females.

Death rates for ischaemic heart disease are similar to those for stroke
among males below age 55. Thereafter among males and, at all age groups,
among females, ischaemic heart disease always ranks second as cause of
death.

This pattern of cardiovascular mortality is the reverse of what is generally
found in most western countries. And, regarding stroke, Portuguese death
rates are close to Japan's or even higher in the older age groups (Fig. 1)[1]. It
is interesting to note on international comparisons that however suspicious
hypertensive disease death rates might be considered, the relative positions of
Portugal and Japan versus Jugoslavia (a country of similar health indicators)
and Sweden (known for a high coronary disease incidence) in relation to
stroke still remain much the same in relation to hypertension (Fig. 2).

2. POPULATION SURVEYS

Although several small surveys have been made in many areas, no single
study can be said to be representative of the blood pressure distribution in the
general Portuguese population. The best approximation may be a survey in
random population samples covering 2300 individuals in several districts [2].
Data from this study show mean blood pressure to rise with age in both
sexes, systolic blood pressure showing the steepest increase (Table 2). Blood
pressure distributions tend to be skewed to the right with advancing age (see
Figs. 3 and 4). Females have higher systolic blood pressures than males over

Table 2. Blood pressure distribution in samples of the Portuguese population.

Sex	Age groups	n	Systolic		Diastolic [a]	
			$\bar{x}$	SD	$\bar{x}$	SD
Males	25–34	215	125.8	15.0	77.7	12.1
	35–44	281	131.8	18.8	82.8	12.1
	45–54	272	141.4	23.8	87.6	14.6
	55–64	281	154.0	27.9	88.8	15.7
Females	25–34	227	125.2	16.6	75.7	14.0
	35–44	299	133.7	19.8	80.9	11.3
	45–54	289	149.3	26.7	87.1	12.9
	55–64	267	167.7	32.5	89.6	12.8

[a] 5th phase.

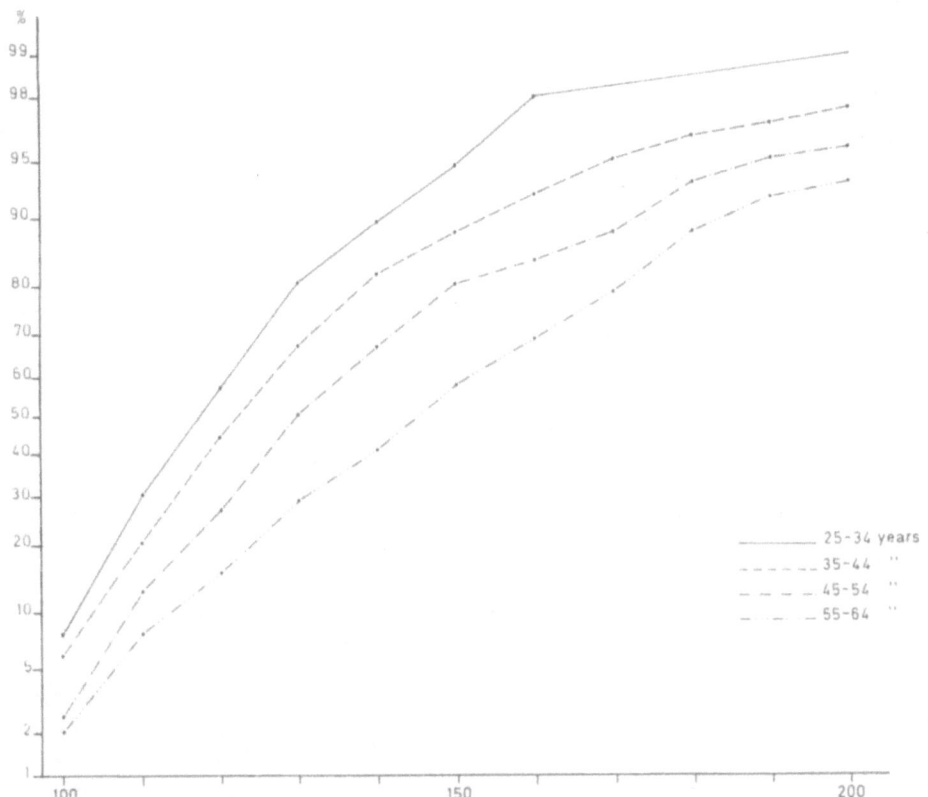

Figure 5. Systolic blood pressure, cumulative frequencies (probabilistic scale), males.

age 45 (see Figs. 5 and 6). Detailed distribution data are given in the Appendix.

When WHO hypertension criteria were used in the same survey 25.8% of the males and 30.3% of the females aged 30–64 were found to be in the hypertensive range. A larger survey covering 29,949 general practitioners' patients aged 40–64 found a higher rate, 41% [3]. Data from the first of these two surveys indicated that less than half of the hypertensives were aware of their high blood pressure, less than half of these were being treated, and only a few were adequately controlled (see Fig. 7).

3. PREVENTION AND CONTROL

These epidemiological observations have produced considerable interest on the primary prevention of hypertension as well as on its control in the community. Since salt is widely used among the Portuguese population and

182

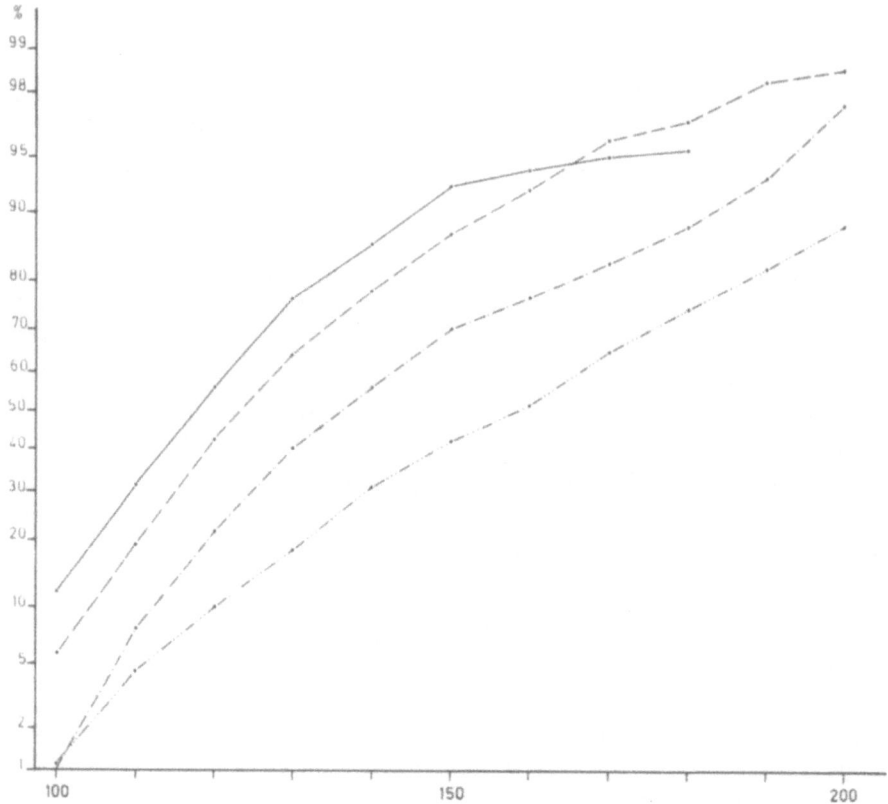

Figure 6. Systolic blood pressure, cumulative frequencies (probabilistic scale), females.

its influence on blood pressure is universally accepted, the salt hypothesis is currently being studied.

The first urine samples obtained on 107 men and 122 women selected at random revealed that they excreted high amounts of sodium (men 278 ± 123 and women 312 ± 129 mmol/24 h), approximately 16.7 g/24 h for men and 18.8 g/24 h for women. Both values have been standardized to an excretion of 1.77 g creatinine. Salt content in bread—the staple of the diet in rural areas—has also been determined. The values obtained, in the range of 7.8 and 12.6 g NaCl/kg, qualify Portuguese bread as rather salty [4].

But, while the salt hypothesis, however promising, deserves further population experiments, attempts at hypertension community control have been made as a part of a WHO programme in the field. Musgueira, a peripherical district of Lisbon with nearly 10,000 inhabitants has been the intervention community. Detection, treatment and follow-up activities have been based on a hypertension register now covering nearly 600 patients. Data on the feasi-

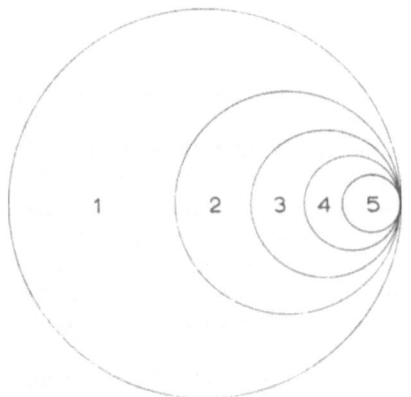

Figure 7. Hypertension in samples from the Portuguese population, ages 25–64.

1 Screened population (100%)
2 Hypertensive (31% of 1)
3 Aware (44% of 2)
4 Being treated (49% of 3)
5 Adequately controlled (32% of 4; 6.7% of 2)

bility and efficacy of this model are still subject to evaluation under WHO auspices.

On the other hand the newly born Portuguese Heart Foundation is spreading voluntary agencies throughout the country which are intended to help screen and control high blood pressure. This action is further supported by a health education campaign on cardiovascular prevention through the television network. The real value of these actions in the national fight against hypertension is still open to debate.

4. CONCLUSION

Taking altogether the scanty information on the epidemiology of blood pressure in the Portuguese, it may be said that blood pressure is generally similar to that in most western countries, and that the prevalence of hypertension seems higher than in the majority of them. The relationship between blood pressure and the high stroke rate in Portugal, which has almost no parallel in Europe, remains to be more clarified. Other unknown factors may also play an important role.

For the explanation of the blood pressure distribution and the frequency of hypertension, the salt hypothesis may prove to be valid, but still needs further study. Attempts at hypertension community control are in their first stages and need careful evaluation.

Acknowledgments. The authors wish to express their gratitude for the support received from Instituto Nacional de Saúde (Lisbon), World Health Organization (CVD Unit, Geneva) and Merck, Sharp and Dohme (Lisbon), which made several of the above-mentioned investigations possible.

Studies on salt excretion and salt content in bread were done with the collaboration of Professor J.V. Joossens (Academisch Ziekenhuis Sint-Rafaël, Leuven, Belgium) to whom the authors also wish to express their gratitude.

184

REFERENCES

1. Miguel JP, Matsuzaky T, Hatano S, Pádua F de: Epidemiology of cardiovascular diseases in Portugal and Japan (in preparation).
2. Miguel JP, Costa FL, Caiado JF, Nunes AC, Rocha EC, Pádua JP, Ladeira S, Fort C, Pádua F de: Hipertensão e Medicina Comunitária — novas perspectivas sobre o problema português. In: Costa JF Nogueira da, Ranchod R (eds) Hipertensão Arterial e Prevenção das Doenças Cardiovasculares. Lisbon: MSD, 1976, pp 51-62.
3. Costa J Nogueira da, Costa F Leal da, et al: Rastreio de hipertensão arterial. Inquérito com a colaboração de clìnicos gerais. In: Costa JF Nogueira da, Ranchod R (eds) Hipertensão Arterial e Prevenção de Doenças Cardiovasculares. Lisbon: MSD, 1976, pp 13-38.
4. Forte JG, Miguel JP, Pádua F de: O Sal na prevenção primária da Hipertensão Arterial — primeiras indicações sobre o seu possível interesse na situação portuguesa. In: Costa JF Nogueira da (ed) Actas do III Simpósio de Hipertensão Arterial. (in press) 1980.

Appendix

Blood pressure frequency distributions in samples from the Portuguese population

Diastolic BP (mmHg)	Age groups							
	25 – 34		35 – 44		45 – 54		55 – 64	
	n	%	n	%	n	%	n	%
MALES								
50– 59	11	5.2	3	1.1	1	0.4	4	1.4
60– 69	36	17.1	23	8.2	18	6.6	17	6.0
70– 79	61	28.9	71	25.3	52	19.1	53	18.9
80– 89	67	31.8	104	37.0	77	28.3	72	25.6
90– 99	26	12.3	56	19.9	74	27.2	65	23.1
100–109	7	3.3	14	5.0	27	9.9	31	11.0
110–119	2	0.9	7	2.5	13	4.8	25	8.9
120–129	0	0.0	1	0.4	5	1.8	10	3.6
130–139	0	0.0	2	0.7	3	1.1	3	1.1
140–149	0	0.0	0	0.0	2	0.7	1	0.4
FEMALES								
50– 59	20	52.6	7	18.4	1	2.6	0	0.0
60– 69	39	17.2	28	9.4	15	5.2	10	3.7
70– 79	83	36.6	95	31.8	55	19.0	40	15.0
80– 89	65	24.7	101	33.8	96	33.2	84	21.5
90– 99	13	5.7	53	17.7	68	23.5	72	27.0
100–109	10	4.4	7	2.3	35	12.1	35	13.1
110–119	3	1.3	7	2.3	12	4.2	22	8.2
120–129	0	0.0	0	0.0	6	2.1	2	0.7
130–139	0	0.0	0	0.0	1	0.3	2	0.7
150 +	1	0.4	0	0.0	0	0.0	0	0.0

Appendix (continued)

Blood pressure frequency distributions in samples from the Portuguese population

Systolic BP (mmHg)	Age groups							
	25 – 34		35 – 44		45 – 54		55 – 64	
	n	%	*n*	%	*n*	%	*n*	%
MALES								
90– 99	4	1.9	6	2.1	5	1.8	3	1.1
100–109	17	7.9	17	0.6	7	2.6	6	2.1
110–119	48	22.3	42	14.9	27	9.9	18	6.4
120–129	59	27.4	66	23.5	40	14.7	22	7.8
130–139	50	23.3	65	23.1	63	23.2	37	13.2
140–149	19	8.8	41	14.6	47	17.3	35	12.5
150–159	11	5.1	18	6.4	35	12.9	48	17.1
160–169	7	3.3	11	3.9	11	4.0	30	10.7
170–179	0	0.0	8	2.8	12	4.4	27	9.6
180–189	0	0.0	4	1.4	13	4.8	27	9.6
190–199	0	0.0	2	0.7	5	1.8	10	3.6
200–209	0	0.0	1	0.4	2	0.7	4	1.4
210–219	0	0.0	0	0.0	2	0.7	7	2.5
220–229	0	0.0	0	0.0	3	1.1	2	0.7
230–239	0	0.0	0	0.0	0	0.0	3	1.1
240–249	0	0.0	0	0.0	0	0.0	1	0.4
250–259	0	0.0	0	0.0	0	0.0	1	0.4
FEMALES								
90– 99	9	4.0	3	1.0	0	0.0	0	0.0
100–109	27	11.9	17	5.7	3	1.0	3	1.1
110–119	46	20.2	40	13.4	20	6.9	9	3.4
120–129	57	25.1	69	23.1	40	13.8	15	5.6
130–139	45	19.8	67	22.4	54	18.7	22	8.2
140–149	22	9.7	41	13.7	46	15.9	34	12.7
150–159	15	6.6	28	9.4	42	14.5	30	11.2
160–169	3	1.3	14	4.7	18	6.2	26	9.7
170–179	2	0.9	11	3.7	18	6.2	36	13.5
180–189	1	0.4	3	0.1	16	5.5	25	9.4
190–199	0	0.0	4	1.3	14	4.8	20	7.5
200–209	0	0.0	1	0.3	12	4.2	17	6.4
210–219	0	0.0	1	0.3	0	0.0	9	3.4
220–229	0	0.0	0	0.0	3	1.0	9	3.4
230–239	0	0.0	0	0.0	3	1.0	3	1.1
240–249	0	0.0	0	0.0	0	0.0	5	1.9
250–259	0	0.0	0	0.0	0	0.0	2	0.7
260 +	0	0.0	0	0.0	0	0.0	2	0.7

11. SCREENING OF HYPERTENSION IN A LARGE FRENCH PROFESSIONAL GROUP *

J.L. RICHARD, C. BLOCH, M.T. GUILLANNEUF, and J. LELLOUCH

Many studies have pointed out the high prevalence of hypertension in industrialized populations and the low proportion of patients aware of their disease, under adequate treatment and with satisfactory control [1–3]. An asymptomatic disease during the longest part of its evolution does not really incite the patients to visit their doctors before complications ensue. Thus, systematic screening of hypertension seems to be a reasonable and presumably efficient public health measure [4, 5]. Such a screening aims at classifying individuals as hypertensive or normotensive from one or more blood pressure values, but raises difficult and as yet unsolved problems, particularly on account of the great variability of blood pressure readings [6]. The present study gives the data observed during a systematic screening of hypertension in a large professional Parisian population.

1. MATERIALS AND METHODS

1.1. Materials

The subjects are the male personnel of a large Parisian administration: 15,661 subjects were studied. Their distribution according to age, between 20 and 59 years, is shown in Table 1. Very few subjects were older than 55, retirement age in this group with few exceptions.

Table 1. Numbers of subjects by age.

Age (years)	<25	25–29	30–34	35–39	40–44	45–49	50–54	≥55	Total
Numbers	1086	2495	1959	2362	1732	4043	1808	176	15,661

* Groupe d'Etude sur l'Epidémiologie de l'Athérosclérose (GREA); with the participation of INSERM (U-169 and Equipe de Recherche Cardiologie), and Préfecture de Paris (Direction Départementale de l'Action Sanitaire et Sociale); and with the help of the 'Ministère de la Santé et de la Sécurité Sociale.'

H. Kesteloot, J.V. Joossens (eds.), Epidemiology of Arterial Blood Pressure, 187–205.

These civil servants were given a systematic examination at the rate of 35 persons per morning. The subjects younger than 45 or older than 55 were examined every third year, but between 45 and 54 years the examination was annual. The results presented here concern all subjects examined at least once during three consecutive years; for the persons aged between 45 and 54, only one exam was considered.

1.2. Methods

The examination was conducted with the subjects fasting in the morning and included, in particular, a venous puncture, an electrocardiogram and a clinical exam by a cardiologist, with a blood pressure reading. Two other blood pressure measurements were made by technicians on subjects sitting in a comfortable armchair and in a room isolated from any outer disturbance; two consecutive measurements (first and second measures of reference) were made: the first after a 5-min complete rest, and the second during the following 5 min, according to the protocol of the Hypertension Community Control Program coordinated by the World Health Organization (WHO). Each measurement was made by a different technician uninformed of the other values. The reading was made with a mercury sphygmomanometer by using an auto-adhesive 14-cm-wide cuff totally encircling the arm.

The technicians underwent a collective training program to learn a standardized technique. The instrument, the arm and the heart of the subject were at the same level. The cuff was applied to the arm, its lower edge on a horizontal line located 2 cm above the bend of the elbow. It was progressively inflated with simultaneous auscultation of the humeral artery and taking of the radial pulse, until it reached a value located 20 mm above that corresponding to the disappearance of arterial sounds. The deflation was to be very slow and regular: the systolic blood pressure was measured after two successive sounds were heard and the diastolic at the disappearance of the Korotkoff sounds (phase 5). The measure was expressed in millimeters and rounded off to the closest even figure. According to the WHO criteria, hypertension is defined as blood pressure on both reference measurements equal to or greater than 150 and/or 90 mm before 30 and 160 and/or 95 mm after that age [7].

2. RESULTS

2.1. Variations of blood pressure values with age

Table 2 gives, by five-year age groups, the mean blood pressure and the standard deviation of the first measure of reference. The systolic blood pres-

Table 2. Mean systolic (SBP) and diastolic blood pressure (DBP) with standard deviation (SD) by age (first reference measurement).

Age (years)	SBP (mmHg)	SD	DBP (mmHg)	SD
<25	124.4	11.5	66.0	10.3
25–29	124.6	11.9	68.8	10.3
30–34	124.7	11.6	71.6	10.4
35–39	125.5	13.2	74.3	10.8
40–44	126.5	14.4	76.2	11.3
45–49	124.7	15.6	79.1	9.8
50–54	126.9	17.7	80.0	10.0
⩾55	146.3	21.7	81.7	11.9

sure did not increase much with age until 50 years, whereas the diastolic blood pressure increased linearly. The dispersion of values increased regularly from 20 to 59 years for the systolic values while it was, at all ages, of the same order for the diastolic values.

Table 3 gives the percentage by age of subjects with blood pressure equal to or above some cutoff points. These percentages increased markedly with age. Systolic values equal to or greater than 140 mm and diastolic levels of 80 mm or more (lower limits of borderline hypertension) were found in a rather important proportion of the population.

Table 3. Percentage by age of subjects with blood pressure equal to or above cutoff points.

Age (years)	Systolic blood pressure							Diastolic blood pressure			
	140	150	160	170	180	190	200	80	90	100	110
<25	9.6	1.8	0.2	0	0	0	0	9.6	1.7	0	0
25–29	9.8	2.4	0.7	0.2	0.2	0	0	15.3	2.0	0.1	0.1
30–34	10.1	2.6	0.7	0.1	0.1	0	0	21.5	4.3	0.4	0.1
35–39	12.0	4.1	1.9	0.7	0.3	0.2	0.1	31.3	8.7	1.1	0.2
40–44	14.8	5.6	2.8	1.3	0.7	0.3	0.1	38.5	10.4	2.0	0.3
45–49	14.4	6.5	2.8	1.4	0.7	0.3	0.2	53.0	15.6	3.1	0.8
50–54	19.1	9.6	5.1	2.2	1.0	0.4	0.2	56.3	19.9	3.9	0.8
55–59	57.9	40.0	29.0	13.0	8.0	5.1	2.2	55.7	25.0	6.8	1.7

2.2. First and second measures of reference and prevalence of hypertension

Table 4 gives the mean systolic and diastolic pressures and the prevalences measured with the first or second measures of reference; moreover are given the prevalences, taking into account the subjects who were considered hypertensive at both the first and the second measures, and the prevalence of hypertension at only one of the two readings. This last figure gives an estimation of *labile hypertension*.

Table 4. Mean blood pressure and prevalence of hypertension at screening during first and second measurements.

Age (years)	Systolic blood pressure		Diastolic blood pressure		Prevalence			
	First	Second	First	Second	First	Second	First and second	First or second
<25	124.4	123.7	66.0	65.5	3.2	1.7	0.9	3.0
25–29	124.6	124.0	68.8	68.1	4.0	3.5	2.1	3.3
30–34	124.7	124.1	71.6	71.3	1.9	1.6	0.9	1.6
35–39	125.5	124.8	74.3	74.1	3.7	3.1	2.0	2.8
40–44	126.5	125.4	76.2	76.0	6.1	4.8	3.8	3.3
45–49	124.7	123.8	79.1	79.8	5.7	7.2	4.0	4.9
50–54	126.9	128.1	80.0	81.4	8.2	10.6	5.5	7.8
≥55	146.3	144.9	81.7	80.4	31.8	27.3	23.9	11.4

The mean blood pressures and the prevalences observed during each reading were very close, but the prevalences were, at all ages, noticeably reduced when both measures were simultaneously taken into account. Hence many subjects reached or exceeded the hypertension limits at only one of the two measures; labile hypertension thus defined concerned 4% of this population.

The prevalences increased with age after 30, but the higher rates measured before this age were linked with the specific criteria used to define hypertension in young people. Very high rates were found in the subjects older than 54, but the limited sample size requires that these rates be interpreted with caution.

2.3. Treatment and control of hypertension in a professional group

Table 5 gives, by age, the total prevalence of hypertension in this group, taking into account medication and control of hypertension among treated patients. Defined as controlled was any treated patient who was not in fact

Table 5. Prevalence of hypertension in a professional group.

Age (years)	Screening Hypertensive		On treatment and controlled	Total prevalence
	Not on treatment	On treatment and not controlled		
	(1)	(2)	(3)	(1 + 2 + 3)
<25	0.9	0	0	0.9
25–29	2.1	0.1	0.2	2.4
30–34	0.8	0.1	0.3	1.2
35–34	1.9	0.1	0.5	2.5
40–44	3.4	0.4	0.7	4.5
45–49	3.5	0.5	2.1	6.1
50–54	4.5	1.0	2.8	8.3
55–59	21.0	2.8	4.0	27.8
20–59	2.8	0.4	1.1	˙4.3

screened as hypertensive after the two measures of reference. These subjects were combined with those screened as hypertensive to determine the total prevalence of hypertension. Among the individuals found to be hypertensive, some were being treated (noncontrolled hypertensives). Considering these different groups, the total prevalence of hypertension varied from 0.9% below 25 years to 8.3% between 50 and 54; it rose to 27.8% in the age range 55–59 and represented 4.3% of the whole population.

Table 6 considers the effects of treatment on hypertension according to age. The prevalence of treated hypertension was low until age 40, but afterward

Table 6. Treatment of hypertension.

Age (years)	Prevalence of hypertension on treatment	Percentage of treated patients among all hypertensives	Percentage of controlled hypertensives	
			Among treated hypertensives	Among all hypertensives
<25	0	0	—	0
25–29	0.3	11.9	85.7	10.2
30–34	0.4	30.4	71.4	21.7
35–39	0.6	22.0	84.6	18.6
40–44	1.1	25.6	65.0	16.7
45–49	2.6	42.5	80.9	34.4
50–54	3.8	41.3	60.6	33.0
55–59	6.8	24.5	58.3	14.3

increased rapidly to 6.8% between 55 and 59 years. The proportion of treated hypertensives among all hypertensives increased with age from about 12% at 25–29 years to about 42% at ages 45–54. But the higher percentage of treated patients between 45–54 years could have been related to the annual screening exam in these particular age groups.

At all ages, a high proportion of treated hypertensives, about 60% – 80%, had at least one blood pressure reading lower than the cutoff values defining hypertension. Because of the moderate proportion of hypertensives who were treated, only small percentages (10% – 35%) of the hypertensive population were controlled.

Table 7. Hypertension in a professional group: screening, treatment, and control.

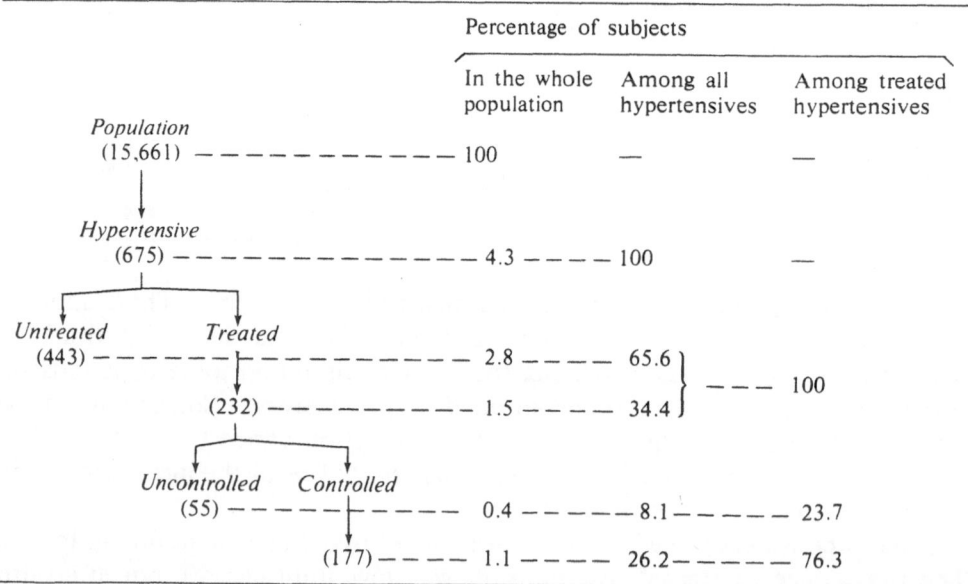

Table 7 summarizes in percentages the previous findings for the whole group. Definite hypertension concerned 675 individuals or 4.3% of the whole population. Two-thirds of these (65.6%) did not receive any treatment, but more than three-quarters of the treated hypertensives (76.3%) seemed to have an effective therapy, at least judging from their blood pressure values.

Table 8 gives an evaluation of three different levels of the health system in this group. The effects of screening are estimated by the percentages of nontreated or noncontrolled hypertensives who were detected: 3.2% of that population, or 73.8% of all hypertensives. The effects of medical care can be evaluated by the proportion of hypertensives who were actually treated (34.4%). The effects of the treatment of hypertension on blood pressure values can be estimated by the proportion of controlled hypertensives (76.3%) among the patients.

Table 8. Evaluation of hypertension screening and care.

1. SCREENING				
	Population	Total hypertensive	Untreated or uncontrolled hypertensive	
	15,661	675	498	$\begin{cases} 498/15661 = 3.2\% \\ 498/675 \quad = 73.8\% \end{cases}$

2. CARE SYSTEM		
	Total hypertensive	Treated hypertensive	
	675	232	$\begin{cases} 232/675 \quad = 34.4\% \end{cases}$

3. TREATMENT		
	Treated hypertensive	Controlled hypertensive	
	232	177	$\begin{cases} 177/232 \quad = 76.3\% \end{cases}$

2.4. Rough estimation of the health problem among males younger than age 60 in France

In Table 9 are given, by age, percentages and absolute numbers of men in France, between 20 and 59 years, who could be affected by different types of hypertension. These numbers are calculated by applying the prevalences observed in the present study to the actual French male population in each age group. The large numbers involved with the problem must be emphasized.

Table 9. Estimation of the numbers of subjects (percentage) with high blood pressure in the French male population 20–59 years old.

Age (years)	Permanent hypertension [a]	Untreated or uncontrolled hypertension [b]	Labile hypertension [c]	Borderline hypertension [d]		Male population [e]
				Systolic ≥140 mm and <160 mm	Diastolic ≥80 and <100 mm	
20–24	19,000 (0.9)	19,000 (0.9)	64,000 (3.0)	200,000 (9.4)	204,000 (9.6)	2,127,530
25–29	54,000 (2.4)	50,000 (2.1)	75,000 (3.3)	206,000 (9.1)	344,000 (15.2)	2,264,060
30–34	19,000 (1.2)	14,000 (0.9)	26,000 (1.6)	150,000 (9.4)	337,000 (21.1)	1,594,795
35–39	39,000 (2.5)	31,000 (2.0)	44,000 (2.8)	157,000 (10.1)	469,000 (30.2)	1,553,940
40–44	75,000 (4.5)	63,000 (3.8)	55,000 (3.3)	199,000 (12.0)	605,000 (36.5)	1,657,915
45–49	101,000 (6.1)	67,000 (4.0)	81,000 (4.9)	193,000 (11.6)	830,000 (49.9)	1,663,055
50–54	130,000 (8.3)	86,000 (5.5)	122,000 (7.8)	219,000 (14.0)	821,000 (52.4)	1,567,415
55–59	370,000 (27.8)	232,000 (23.9)	111,000 (11.4)	281,000 (28.9)	475,000 (48.9)	971,880
20–59	707,000 (5.3)	562,000 (4.2)	578,000 (4.3)	1,605,000 (12.0)	4,085,000 (30.5)	13,400,590

[a] Subjects found hypertensive at two reference measures or treated for hypertension (total prevalence).

[b] Numbers included in permanent hypertension: subjects found hypertensive at two reference measures with and without treatment.

[c] Subjects found hypertensive at one reference measure only.

[d] First reference measure only.

[e] Census 1975.

Table 10. Mean systolic (S) or diastolic (D) blood pressure in some recent population studies.

Age (years)	Present study S	D	Lyon [15] Pop. 1 S	D	Pop. 2 S	D	Kesteloot [14] S	D	Kulbertus [19] S	D	Heller [20] S	D	US: NHS [13] S	D	Napier [17] S	D	Bourke [11] S	D	CHEC [12] S	D	Eilertsen [10] S	D
15–19	—	—	126.0	65.1	125.5	69.0	129.1	74.1	—				—		—		—		115.9	70.0	121.5	68.5
20–24	124.4	66.0	130.6	70.7	125.8	69.7	131.7	74.9			—		123.7	76.4	—		—				127.5	74.9
25–29	124.6	68.8	130.4	73.0	126.8	72.9	132.5	75.9	129.9	77.3			125.2	80.8	126.4	75.9	127.9	75.2	128.5	77.9		
30–34	124.7	71.6	130.8	75.4	127.8	75.6	132.8	77.5	131.7	81.5												
35–39	125.5	74.3	131.7	76.9	129.0	78.3	133.8	79.0					127.0	84.2			131.3	81.5	130.2	81.3	128.5	78.9
40–44	126.5	76.2	133.6	79.2	130.8	80.4	135.4	80.5	133.8	82.3	135.1	82.4			130.4	82.2	136.2	85.6	134.0	83.9	132.9	83.8
45–49	124.7	79.1	136.3	81.2	134.1	83.3	137.5	82.1	137.3	85.0	138.5	84.2	134.7	87.5	137.7	86.8						
50–54	126.9	80.0	139.6	82.8	137.5	84.9	140.3	83.1	139.2	85.4	140.8	84.6					143.4	88.3	140.2	85.3	141.0	84.9
55–59	146.3	81.7	145.7	85.2	142.0	85.1	143.8	83.6	144.9	85.5	144.9	84.9	139.6	86.4	147.6	86.0						
60–64	—	—	150.4	86.2	146.4	85.0	—	—	145.5	84.1	—	—					150.8	90.7	145.3	84.7	156.6	86.6
65–74	—	—	—	—	—	—	—	—	—	—	—	—	146.0	84.9	157.8	85.1	151.8	89.7	148.8	82.9	—	

a Pop. 1 = intervention population; Pop. 2 = reference population.
b White males.
c ≥65 years.
d 60–69 years.

196

Table 11. Prevalence of hypertension from single readings in some recent studies.

Study [ref.] Criteria Age (years)	Present study ≥160/95 b	Lyon a Pop. 2 [16] ≥160/95 b	Kulbertus [19] ≥160/95	US:NHS [13] ≥160/95	Napier [18] ≥160/95	Bourke [11] ≥160/95	CHEC [12] ≥95	Kesteloot [14] ≥100	Heller [20] ≥100
15-19	—	—	—	—			1.3	1.5	
20-24	3.2	6.0		4.9				2.6	
25-29	4.0	8.9	8.4			6.3	5.2	2.9	—
30-34	1.9	5.0		8.2	3.6			4.1	
35-39	3.7	7.3	10.6	17.3		13.6	10.3	5.4	
40-44	6.1	11.8	12.8			23.9	15.7	7.5	
45-49	5.7	14.2	19.3	25.8	14.7			10.0	
50-54	8.2	20.7	18.5			35.9	19.3	11.0	11.2
55-59	31.8	27.5	22.5	31.1					
60-64	—	33.9	25.0		33.6 c	47.7	18.2	12.3 a	—

a Pop. 2 = reference population.
b 160/95 mm after 30 years and 150/90 mm before.
c After 59 years.
d After 55 years.

3. DISCUSSION

3.1. Blood pressure, prevalence of hypertension, and age

The data in Tables 2–4 agree with the various studies that relate an increase in the mean blood pressure with age, a linear increase for the diastolic and a curvilinear increase for the systolic with little change before 35 or 40 years [8, 9]. The increasing dispersion of the systolic values with age reflects the heterogeneity of the population with respect to the increment rate of arterial pressure over the years, so that the mean of a population varies very little in the first half of adult life although the prevalence of hypertension increases. This phenomenon is not observed for the diastolic values whose increase with age seems to involve most individuals.

The blood pressure values and especially the prevalences in the present study are lower than most of those observed elsewhere in population studies. Tables 10 and 11 show the mean blood pressures and the prevalences measured in some recent large population surveys [10–20]. But much caution is needed in interpreting the differences between populations. Many factors, especially the conditions of measurement, can influence the mean blood pressure of a group and, even more, the prevalences. Such differences have been observed in this population with different conditions of measurement [6]. A large part of such differences reflects the intraindividual variability of blood pressure. These differences can be reduced by optimal conditions and technique of measurement; it is likely that the method of measurement used in the present study is responsible for the rather low values and prevalences observed.

3.2. Distribution of the blood pressure values

Table 3 shows the high proportion of subjects who exceed the blood pressure values considered not to imply a significant deterioration in prognosis among young and middle-aged men [21, 22]. An increase in cardiovascular risk and a reduction in life expectancy are already quite clear for systolic values exceeding 140 mm and for diastolic values exceeding 80 mm.

The long-term effects of this borderline hypertension are well documented, but the practical conduct to be followed is not yet well defined [23]. The question of treatment is not resolved, but active prevention should undoubtedly constitute a reasonable alternative in these cases. In particular, the strong relation observed between weight and blood pressure at all ages in men denotes an important preventive action [24, 25]. Taking into account the high proportion of the male population concerned, such a preventive approach would be a major public health problem. Its solution seems, at least partly, to be possibly found in health education [26].

3.3. Screening: first and second measurements

The reduction of prevalences by taking into account two successive readings expresses an important intraindividual variability that interferes with an accurate evaluation of the blood pressure level of each subject. Thus a single reading overestimates the prevalence of permanent hypertension [27]. Even though the procedure of measurement used in the present study reduces this variability but cannot suppress it entirely, two successive standardized and carefully performed readings have a clear effect in reducing prevalences. Such a procedure could be recommended for different purposes but, in fact, different problems must be considered.

First, in the population studies—where distributions and prevalences are often concerned with group comparisons—the strict standardization of measurement methods with continuous training of observers is needed [28, 29]. The method proposed could be a reasonable alternative to more precise, but more time-consuming, blind or semiblind techniques.

Second, in the prediction of risk, two or more measurements can enable a better prediction of the future blood pressure level [30]. In the same way, several measurements ensure a better prediction of cardiovascular risk than a single measurement, because they enable a more precise evaluation of the individual blood pressure level, but a single casual blood pressure reading in a group already gives a good relative risk prediction [31].

Third, the problem of identifying permanent hypertensive individuals in the population for clinical examination and possible treatment is solved by the definition of strict cutoff points and, as previously, several measurements made during several examinations enable a classification of patients and give a rather good selection of hypertensive subjects, thus avoiding an excessive percentage of misclassification in the hypertensive range [32, 33]. But the percentage of false-negative cases will be increased, and only a precise cost/benefit analysis could define the best method of screening.

Fourth, the frequency of labile hypertension as defined by transient high blood pressure values, under the conditions defined in Table 4, is high. Other data from the same population or from other populations confirm the phenomenon and suggest a higher frequency of labile hypertension under certain conditions of examination and in different circumstances of daily life [6, 34]. This labile hypertension could imply a bad prognosis and raises an obvious public health problem [35], but neither the precise conditions of its screening nor the possible benefit of its treatment have as yet been defined. Obviously, further research and detailed evaluation are needed. Certainly, the diagnosis of labile hypertension needs different readings in different conditions; furthermore, its long-term prognosis and the possible benefit of its early treatment must be determined. Recording of many blood pressure values taken under

Table 12. Treatment and control of hypertension in some recent population studies.

Study [ref.]		Country	Age (years)	Criteria	Sample size	Sex [a]	Hypertensives			
							1 Prevalence (%)	2 Treated (% of 1)	3 Controlled (% of 1)	(% of 2)
Goteborg	[36]	Sweden	50–55	>175 or >115	5,223	M	18.7	36.4	15.1	41.7
CHEC	[12]	United States	20–64	≥ 95	399,552	M	20.0	53.8	37.6	69.6
Albury	[37]	Australia	50–59	≥110	1,803	M-F	21.2	59.5	43.0	82.5
Charlottes	[34]	United States	15–74	≥ 90 (<55 y) ≥100 (≥55 y)	12,371	M-F	21.0	36.6	21.8	59.7
Napier	[18]	New Zealand	40–60	≥160 – 95	1,175	M	15.4	27.0	12.1	44.8
Montreal	[38]	Canada	25–69	≥160 – 95	12,055	M-F	19.4	51.1	13.5	26.4
Baltimore	[39]	United States	30–69	≥ 95	2,069	M	38.3	45.0	26.0	57.8
Bronx	[40]	United States	Median	≥ 95	1,293	M-F	15.0	31.9	25.8	81.0
Heller	[20]	United Kingdom	40–59	≥110	8,397	M	12.0	14.8	7.0	47.3
Takala	[43]	Finland	40–64	≥160/95	1,042	M	21.1	23.5	9.5	40.3
Mayo 3 Com	[42]	United States	30–69	≥160/95	3,290	M	16.1	43.1	24.1	55.8
Indiana	[43]	United States	—	≤ 30 y >149/90 > 30 y >150/95	6,637	M-F	14.0	56.9	41.0	72.3
Kulbertus	[19]	Belgium	>35 <80	≥160/95	11,275	M	12.3	43.8	23.3	53.2
Present study		France	20–59	< 30 y ≥150/90 ≥ 30 y ≥160/95	15,661	M	4.3	34.4	26.2	76.3

[a] M, male; F, female.

various circumstances over time among large populations with good follow-up could be a useful research program and could enable a therapeutic trial.

In summary, one careful measurement could be insufficient for population studies and group comparison, but several measurements are clearly needed each time that individuals are involved in screening and diagnosis or treatment. In any case however, a careful and well-standardized method of measurement is needed.

3.4. The public health problem

The small proportion of treated hypertensives, between 20% and 30%, except for the age group 45–54, in which the proportion is a little higher, agrees with many other population studies in developed countries, which have found high proportions of undetected, untreated, and uncontrolled hypertensives. Table 12 summarizes the data of some recent studies [12, 18, 20, 36–43]. In the group of the present study, a systematic but infrequent screening does not lead to good control of hypertension. Nevertheless, the rather higher proportion of treated hypertensives within the age limits 45–54 who underwent annual examinations suggests that a continuous screening program is of some benefit in improving the treatment of hypertension in the community. But data from Table 8 clearly show what the potential benefit of an effective screening program could be: identifying three-quarters of the nontreated or noncontrolled hypertensives.

Furthermore, an obvious impediment to hypertension control is a lack of access to medical care. In fact, in the population of the present study, with a systematic screening about 80% of the people are aware of their blood pressure values. Such a high proportion agrees with this hypothesis and suggests that a screening without medical follow-up has limited efficacy.

Contrasting with the poor level of treatment in the group as a whole, individual treatment, when instituted, led to satisfactory control of hypertension in most cases. These findings show clearly that the main obstacle to effective control of hypertension in the community lies in an insufficient screening and/or an insufficient access to the medical-care system.

The findings of the present study suggest that the present health system is relatively inefficient in translating screening positives to medical-care outcome. But the weak link in this system is not yet well known. For example, in a British study, the doctors seemed responsible for the unsuccessful outcome of screening [44]; in an American study, both physicians and patients were responsible for the discontinuation of treatment [45]. Clearly, the optimal conditions of access to medical care for hypertensives must be studied, defined, and evaluated. Better access could ensure treatment for two-thirds of hypertensives, who actually do not receive therapy but need it. The benefit, in terms of percentages of treated and controlled hypertensives, suggests the efficacy of a community program as reported in various countries with very different health systems [16, 46, 47].

The number of individuals affected in the French male population represented in Table 9 is based on the hypothesis that the prevalences measured in this study could be applied to that population. This hypothesis could be severely criticized, but the calculated numbers can be reasonably accepted as a crude approximation of the extent of the problem in the population. Such an approximation illustrates clearly the quantitative importance of the hypertension health problem at the national level and should concern health authorities.

Some rather similar estimations were made from the data given by the program against hypertension under way in Lyons [48]. The expected benefit in reduction of mortality from decrease of mean blood pressure in the French population was expressed by the expected reduction of excess deaths from hypertension. An important reduction of mortality in middle-aged men could be expected to follow a modest decrease in higher blood pressure levels including mildly elevated values. Indeed, more than half of the excess deaths are due to modest increases in blood pressure, under 160 mm for systolic, thus not in the definite hypertensive range.

4. CONCLUSIONS

Undoubtedly, hypertension and even mildly elevated blood pressure are a major health problem. They are a major risk factor for all cardiovascular diseases and impair life expectancy. The effect is quantitative: risk increases regularly from the lowest to the highest blood pressure values. It is more marked among younger patients. Hypertension is one of the most prevalent chronic diseases for which medical treatment is available. The efficiency of drug therapy for severe and malignant hypertension is well established, with results demonstrating a significant reduction in cardiovascular morbidity and mortality over time [49, 50]. Recently, a randomized and controlled trial conducted in 14 varied American communities showed the ability of public health measures in identifying a high percentage of hypertensive persons in the population, and in starting a high percentage of them on long-term treatment with a significant reduction in five-year mortality, including those with values in the range of mild hypertension [51].

But the impairment of prognosis is not limited to definite clinical hypertension, and concerns many individuals with only moderate or transient elevations of blood pressure. The contribution of these subjects to the incidence of cardiovascular diseases or deaths is very impressive. Certainly the question of the benefit of treatment for these many cases of borderline or labile hypertension requires an answer. The medical literature is divided on whether treatment in such cases can lower the further incidence of permanent hypertension and be an effective preventive measure against cardiovascular diseases and death. Some large trials under way in different countries can help clinicians in the future to decide, better than they can at the present time, down to which limits high blood pressures must be treated. But looking at the relationship between mortality and blood pressure starting from the lowest values and taking into account the distribution of values in the population, a large proportion of adults could be affected in the future by active treatment of preventive measures; maybe more than 20% of the adult male population under 60.

Poor control of hypertension in the population is another public health problem that requires an answer. Systematic screening is probably not sufficiently effective. The results coming from different community control programs in different countries show their feasibility. The improvement in the health status of the population in developed countries probably requires an approach other than the traditional medical one in the prevention, detection, and early treatment of chronic and asymptomatic diseases [52, 53]. The public health problem of hypertension seems to require two different solutions: (a) the choice of the most effective sequence leading to detection, and access to health care and treatment in the context of the existing local health and medical-care system; and (b) the prevention of hypertension by hygienodietetic measures and public education. Both approaches are not mutually exclusive, but need research and evaluation before a good definition of a comprehensive public health policy can be recommended for action.

Acknowledgments. Grateful acknowledgment is extended to Mrs. Bingham and to Mrs. Zalokar for their participation in the translation and the review of the text.

REFERENCES

1. Wilber JA: The problem of undetected and untreated hypertension in the community. Bull NY Acad Med 49:510-520, 1973.
2. Sackett DL: Hypertension in the real world: public reaction, physician response and patient compliance. In: Genest J, et al. (eds) Hypertension: Physiopathology and treatment. New York: McGraw-Hill, 1977.
3. Ward GW: Changing trends in control of hypertension. Public Health Rep 93: 31-34, 1978.
4. Hypertension Study Group: Guidelines for the detection, diagnosis and management of hypertensive populations. Circulation 44:A263-A272, 1971.

5. Barlow DH, Beevers DG, Hawthorne VM, Watt HD, Young GAR: Blood pressure measurement at screening and in general practice. Br Heart J 39:7-12, 1977.
6. Richard JL, Lellouch J, Guillanneuf MT: La variabilité de la mesure tensionnelle dans un examen de dépistage systématique et ses conséquences en Santé Publique. Arch Mal Cœur 72:1128-1136, 1979.
7. Strasser T: Pilot programmes for the control of hypertension. WHO Chron 26:451-456, 1972.
8. Hamilton M, Pickering GW, Fraser-Roberts JA, Sowry GSC: The aetiology of essential hypertension. I. The arterial pressure in the general population. Clin Sci 13:11-35, 1954.
9. Miall WE, Oldham PD: Factors influencing arterial blood pressure in the general population. Clin Sci 17:409-444, 1958.
10. Eilertsen E, Humerfelt S: The blood pressure in a representative population sample. Acta Med Scand 183:293-305, 1968.
11. Bourke GJ, Cruess-Callaghan A, Hickey N, Mulcahy R, Gearty GF, Wilson-Davis K: The distribution of blood pressure in 15,171 Irish males. J Irish Med Assoc 66:346-349, 1973.
12. Stamler J, Stamler R, Ricdlinger WF, Algera G, Roberts RH: Hypertension screening of 1 million Americans. Community hypertension evaluation clinic (CHEC) program, 1973–1975. JAMA 235:2299-2305, 1976.
13. US Department of Health, Education and Welfare: Blood pressure levels of persons 6-74 years — United States 1971–1974. Vital and health statistics, ser 11, no. 203. Hyattsville, MD: National Center for Health Statistics, 1977.
14. Kesteloot H, Van Houte O: The epidemiology of arterial blood pressure. Bruxelles Med [Suppl] 29-38, 1974.
15. Groupe Coopératif Lyonnais de Lutte Contre l'Hypertension: Résultats préliminaires d'un programme de lutte contre l'hypertension dans une population occupationnelle. Colloque de l'INSERM. Epidémiologie et prévention des maladies cardiovasculaires. Paris: INSERM, 1974, pp 147-172.
16. Groupe Coopératif Lyonnais de Lutte Contre l'Hypertension: Programme lyonnais de lutte contre l'hypertension. 30 mois de fonctionnement. Arch Mal Cœur 68:119-131, 1974.
17. Christmas BW: Blood pressure levels of an urban adult New Zealand population: Napier 1973. NZ Med J 86:369-374, 1977.
18. Christmas BW, Turner AS: Prevalence of high blood pressure treated and untreated in an urban adult New Zealand population: Napier 1973. NZ Med J 86:419-423, 1977.
19. Kulbertus HE, de Leval-Rutten F, Dubois M, Petit JM: Experience with a community screening program for hypertension: results on 24,462 individuals. Eur J Cardiol 7:487-497, 1978.
20. Heller RF, Rose G, Tunstall Pedoe HD, Christie GS: Blood pressure measurement in the United Kingdom heart disease prevention project. J Epidemiol Commun Health 32:235-238, 1978.
21. Paul O: Risks of mild hypertension: a ten-year report. Br Heart J [Suppl] 33:116-121, 1971.
22. Lew E: High blood pressure, other risk factors and longevity. The insurance viewpoint. Am J Med 55:281-293, 1973.
23. Julius S, Schork MA: Borderline hypertension: a critical review. J Chronic Dis 23:723-754, 1971.

24. Tran MH, Lellouch J, Richard JL: Fat body mass. II. Its relationships with biological parameters, blood pressure and physical training in a population of 8,660 men aged 20 to 55. Biomedicine 18:499-506, 1973.

25. Ramsay LE, Ramsay MH, Hettia-Rachchi J, Davies DL, Winchester J: Weight reduction in a blood pressure clinic. Br Med J 2:244-245, 1978.

26. Levine DM, Green LW, Deeds SG, Chwalow J, Russel RP, Finlay J: Health education for hypertensive patients. JAMA 241:1700-1703, 1979.

27. Armitage P, Fox W, Rose GA, Tinker LM: The variability of measurements of casual blood pressure. II. Survey experience. Clin Sci 30:337-344, 1966.

28. Holland WW: The reduction of observer variability in the measurement of blood pressure. In: Pemberton J (ed) Epidemiology reports on research and teaching. Oxford University Press, 1962, p 271.

29. Rose GA: Standardization of observers in blood pressure measurement. Lancet 1:673-674, 1965.

30. Souchek J, Stamler J, Dyer AR, Paul O, Lepper MH: The value of two or three versus a single reading of blood pressure at a first visit. J Chronic Dis 32:197-210, 1979.

31. Gordon T, Sorlie P, Kannel WB: Problems in the assessment of blood pressure: The Framingham Study. Int J Epidemiol 5:327-334, 1976.

32. Rosner B: Screening for hypertension. Some statistical observations. J Chronic Dis 30:7-18, 1977.

33. Hypertension Detection and Follow-up Program Cooperative Group: Variability of blood pressure and the results of screening in the hypertension detection and follow-up program. J Chronic Dis 31:651-667, 1978.

34. Carey RM, Reid RA, Ayers CR, Lynch SS, McLain WL, Vaughan Jr ED: The Charlottesville blood pressure survey. Value of repeated blood pressure measurements. JAMA 236:847-851, 1976.

35. Levy RL, White PD, Stroud WD, Hillman CC: Transient hypertension. The relative prognostic importance of various systolic and diastolic levels. JAMA 128:1059-1061, 1945.

36. Wilhelmsen L: Treatment of hypertension in a Swedish community. The problem of borderline hypertension. Acta Med Scand [Suppl] 576:99-108, 1975.

37. Lovell RRH: Blood pressure in middle-aged people in Albury and Melbourne. Implications for screening. Drugs [Suppl 1] 11:2-5, 1976.

38. Shapiro M, Bleho J, Curran M, Farrell K, Klein D, Weigensberg A, Weil K: Problems in the control of hypertension in the community. Can Med Assoc J 118:37-39, 1978.

39. Apostolides AY, Entwisle G, Ovellet R, Hebel JR: Improving trend in hypertension control in a Black inner city community. Am J Epidemiol 107:113-119, 1978.

40. Wassertheil-Smoller S, Bijur P, Blaufox MD: An evaluation of the utility of high blood pressure detection fairs. Am J Public Health 68:768-770, 1978.

41. Takala J: Screening for hypertension in a middle-aged population in South West Finland. Prev Med 7:230-244, 1978.

42. Labarthe DR, Krishan I, Nobrega FT, Brennan Jr LA, Smoldt RH, Mori HD, Hunt JC: The Mayo three-community hypertension control program. I. Design and initial screening results. Mayo Clin Proc 54:289-298, 1979.

43. Servaas B, Weinberger MH: The use of multi-media motivation in enhancing compliance of hypertensives discovered at a screening operation. Am J Public Health 69:382-384, 1979.

44. Heller RF: Detection and treatment of hypertension in an inner London community. Br J Prev Soc Med 30:268-272, 1976.
45. Langfeld SB: Hypertension: deficient care of the medically served. Ann Intern Med 78:19-23, 1973.
46. Hypertension Detection and Follow-up Program Cooperative Group: Patient participation in a hypertension control program. JAMA 239:1507-1514, 1978.
47. Nissinen A, Tuomilehto J, Puska P: Follow-up of the hypertensive patients in North Karelia and some results from the hypertension register. Acta Med Scand [Suppl] 626:29-32, 1979.
48. Froment A, Milon H: Hypertension artérielle: envisager le problème médical à l'échelle de la population. Arch Mal Cœur 70:37-46, 1977.
49. Veterans Administration Cooperative Study Group on Antihypertensive Agents: Effects of treatment on morbidity in hypertension. Results in patients with diastolic blood pressures averaging 115 through 129 mmHg. JAMA 202:1028-1034, 1967.
50. Veterans Administration Cooperative Study Group on Antihypertensive Agents: Effects of treatment on morbidity in hypertension. II. Results in patients with diastolic blood pressure averaging 90 through 114 mmHg. JAMA 213:1143-1152, 1970.
51. Hypertension Detection and Follow-up Program Cooperative Group: Five-year findings of the hypertension detection and follow-up program. I. Reduction in mortality of persons with high blood pressure, including mild hypertension. JAMA 242:2562-2571, 1979.
52. Alderman MH, Schoenbaum EE: Detection and treatment of hypertension at the work site. N Engl J Med 293:65-68, 1975.
53. Rudnick KV, Sackett DL, Hirst S, Holmes C: Hypertension in a family practice. Can Med Assoc J 117:492-497, 1977.

12. EPIDEMIOLOGY OF ESSENTIAL HYPERTENSION IN YUGOSLAVIA
The Yugoslavia Cardiovascular Disease Study *

Dj. KOZAREVIĆ and D. McGEE

It has been stated that population differences may be a key factor influencing blood pressure [1]. Yugoslavia is a nation of diverse cultures. The Yugoslavia Cardiovascular Disease Study contained populations from two of these cultures. The object of the present report is to present data on blood pressure for two geographic regions of Yugoslavia. We will present data from the baseline examination, and relate baseline levels of variables to subsequent mortality. In addition we will discuss recent results from an analysis of trends in blood pressure.

1. METHODS

The Yugoslavia Cardiovascular Disease Study was conceived in 1961–63, and the initial examination of the cohort was conducted in 1964–65. The study was a cooperative venture of the Institute of Chronic Diseases and Gerontology, Belgrade, Yugoslavia; and the National Heart, Lung, and Blood Institute, Bethesda, Maryland, USA. The investigation was conducted in the communities of Tuzla in Bosnia and Remetinec in Croatia. Within each region the population could be classified as living in one of three environments: a totally urban environment, a totally rural environment, or an environment containing elements of both an urban and a rural environment ('mixed' in the following).

Tuzla is located in a mountainous region in Bosnia. It consists of a central town and a number of smaller surrounding villages. Tuzla's long history of Turkish occupation accounts for the large percentage of Moslems in the population. It is now an important mining and industrial area. Remetinec is a suburb of Zagreb, the capital of Croatia. It was never occupied by the Turks, and most of the inhabitants have Roman Catholic backgrounds. The pattern of living in Remetinec parallels that of Western Europe. Both Tuzla and Remetinec are undergoing intensive industrialization and urbanization.

* Supported by PL 480 Counterpart Funds, Research Agreement 02-001-1, NHLBI.

H. Kesteloot, J.V. Joossens (eds.), Epidemiology of Arterial Blood Pressure, 207–216.

These two culturally diverse populations allow several comparisons. Remetinec may be compared with Tuzla, and urban and rural comparisons may be made within and between these communities. Also, the Yugoslav population may be compared with the population of the Framingham Study because of the similarities in data collection and diagnostic definitions.

In Remetinec, the selected population consisted of only males 35–62 years listed in the Health Department Register, which included at least 95% of all males in this age range. In Tuzla, where no such register existed, a house-to-house survey for the purpose of developing a complete population list was conducted. By these methods, 11,933 males were identified and listed in the target population.

Through the efforts of various workers and political organizations, religious groups, health departments, and individual physicians and nurses, 6460 or 94.2% of the selected males in Tuzla and 4661 or 91.8% of the selected males in Remetinec reported for the initial examination (Table 1).

Table 1. Number of persons by area and age at exam 1 : The Yugoslavia Cardiovascular Disease Study.

	Age	Urban no.	Rural no.	Mixed no.
REMETINEC	35–39	491	439	234
	40–44	384	423	223
	45–49	190	262	107
	50–54	246	393	195
	55–59	196	419	216
	60–62	59	130	54
	Total	1566	2066	1029
TUZLA	35–39	989	766	141
	40–44	759	599	104
	45–49	379	378	40
	50–54	516	549	61
	55–59	423	503	42
	60–62	85	114	12
	Total	3151	2909	400

The Remetinec cohort was examined in the health center in Remetinec by the primary-care physicians for all the inhabitants of the area. The Tuzla cohort was examined in the clinic by a team of physicians and nurses from the Institute of Chronic Diseases and Gerontology who traveled to Tuzla especially to conduct the examinations.

Each participant received a thorough standardized cardiovascular examination. As part of the examination, three blood pressures were taken, one by a nurse and two by the examining physician. For the present report, the second reading by the physician is used. This was the last reading obtained and hence is believed to be most nearly basal. All pressures were measured on the left arm with the participant seated. A mercury sphygmomanometer with a 14-cm cuff long enough to fit the most obese arm was used. Diastolic pressure was recorded at the fifth Korotkoff phase (disappearance of sound). Much effort was extended to ensure that all methods and criteria were comparable with those of the Framingham Study [2].

All statistics presented were calculated using standard statistical methodology. Logistic coefficients were estimated using an iterative maximum likelihood approach as suggested by Walker and Duncan [3].

2. RESULTS

2.1. Level of blood pressure in the population

Table 2 presents mean level of systolic pressure at the initial examination by age and area. There is a difference of 12 mmHg between the area with the highest mean systolic pressure (Remetinec rural) and the area with the lowest mean systolic pressure (Tuzla rural). The age trends are approximately linear for each of the areas. The only exception to this linearity is the mixed Tuzla population. The noticeable departure from linearity in this population is in the

Table 2. Mean level of first examination blood pressure by age and area: The Yugoslavia Cardiovascular Disease Study.

		Systolic blood pressure						
	Age:	35–39	40–44	45–49	50–54	55–59	60–62	All ages
REMETINEC								
Urban	$\bar{x}$	132.6	135.8	139.2	144.8	149.2	150.3	138.8
	SD $(\bar{x})$	14.9	17.7	18.7	20.6	24.4	21.5	19.6
Rural	$\bar{x}$	136.7	138.4	139.6	145.5	150.5	154.9	143.0
	SD $(\bar{x})$	14.5	16.6	16.6	19.9	23.6	23.8	19.9
Mixed	$\bar{x}$	134.0	134.7	138.9	140.7	145.8	152.8	139.4
	SD $(\bar{x})$	16.0	17.7	19.6	19.2	20.2	23.7	19.5
TUZLA								
Urban	$\bar{x}$	127.0	131.0	136.8	140.8	147.6	149.3	134.8
	SD $(\bar{x})$	13.2	15.4	18.4	22.2	22.9	25.5	19.4
Rural	$\bar{x}$	123.1	125.0	129.4	132.5	138.3	142.5	129.5
	SD $(\bar{x})$	12.3	14.5	16.6	18.6	20.3	22.7	17.7
Mixed	$\bar{x}$	124.7	130.2	135.2	136.8	142.3	155.6	131.8
	SD (x)	12.0	13.4	20.7	18.7	21.4	27.5	17.6

over-60 age group. There are only 12 men in this category (Table 1) and hence this represents the most unstable estimate shown. At any age, with one exception, the mean systolic pressure in rural Remetinec is highest, while the mean systolic pressure in rural Tuzla is the lowest. Overall, the mean systolic pressures in Remetinec are higher than the mean systolic pressures in Tuzla. The urban-rural comparison is reversed for the two regions. In Remetinec the rural population has higher mean systolic pressure than the urban population, while in Tuzla the rural population has lower mean systolic pressure than the urban population.

Table 3. Mean level of first examination blood pressure by age and area: The Yugoslavia Cardiovascular Disease Study.

		Diastolic blood pressure						
	Age	35–39	40–44	45–49	50–54	55–59	60–62	All ages
REMENTINEC								
Urban	$\bar{x}$	85.7	87.6	88.9	91.5	91.2	90.3	88.3
	SD (x)	10.5	12.2	11.5	12.5	13.6	11.2	12.0
Rural	$\bar{x}$	84.7	85.8	86.2	88.6	89.4	91.5	87.3
	SD (x)	10.1	11.3	10.6	11.6	12.6	12.4	11.5
Mixed	$\bar{x}$	83.6	84.5	86.7	86.3	87.1	87.0	85.5
	SD (x)	9.8	12.2	12.4	11.4	11.6	11.8	11.5
TUZLA								
Urban	$\bar{x}$	79.5	82.7	85.0	85.6	86.8	86.2	83.1
	SD (x)	8.9	9.9	10.9	11.9	11.9	12.0	10.8
Rural	$\bar{x}$	76.6	77.6	80.3	80.2	81.7	83.1	79.1
	SD (x)	8.3	8.6	9.8	9.6	10.1	11.3	9.5
Mixed	$\bar{x}$	78.9	81.4	83.8	82.7	85.8	89.5	81.7
	SD (x)	7.4	7.4	10.6	9.3	10.7	13.4	9.0

Table 3 presents the mean level of diastolic pressure at the initial examination by age and area. As for systolic pressure, the Tuzla population exhibited the lowest mean diastolic pressure. As has been noted by the Framingham Study [4] and others, the age trend for diastolic blood pressure is not as clearly linear as was the age trend for systolic pressure.

Another characteristic known to influence blood pressure level is obesity. Table 4 presents mean level of body mass index (BMI = weight in kilograms/ square of height in centimeters). There are large differences in the level of BMI between the areas. The Tuzla rural population tends to be the least obese, while the Remetinec urban population tends to be the most obese. As has been shown by others, there is a slight tendency for level of BMI to decrease with age [4]. It is of interest that the Remetinec rural population,

Table 4. Mean level of weight-height index by area and age at exam 1: The Yugoslavia Cardiovascular Disease Study.

	Age:	Weight-height index = (weight [kg]/height ^{2} [cm]) 10000						
		35–39	40–44	45–49	50–54	55–59	60–62	All ages
REMETINEC								
Urban	$\bar{x}$	25.9	25.8	26.8	26.3	25.7	25.1	26.0
	SD (x)	3.3	3.5	3.9	4.0	4.4	3.8	3.7
Rural	$\bar{x}$	23.8	24.0	23.3	23.4	23.0	22.9	23.5
	SD (x)	3.0	3.2	2.8	3.2	3.3	2.9	3.1
Mixed	$\bar{x}$	24.8	24.9	24.6	24.5	23.9	24.4	24.5
	SD (x)	3.1	3.5	3.6	4.0	3.3	3.9	3.5
TUZLA								
Urban	$\bar{x}$	24.2	24.7	24.6	24.3	24.2	24.5	24.4
	SD (x)	3.2	3.4	3.6	4.0	4.0	4.1	3.6
Rural	$\bar{x}$	22.5	22.3	22.3	21.9	21.9	21.5	22.2
	SD (x)	2.4	2.5	2.4	2.6	2.7	2.3	2.5
Mixed	$\bar{x}$	23.3	23.3	24.5	23.1	22.1	21.4	23.2
	SD (x)	2.7	3.4	3.4	4.0	3.2	3.6	3.3

which had the highest mean levels of systolic pressure, is not the most obese of the populations.

Since the distributions of age (Table 1) and BMI (Table 4) differ in the several areas, and both affect the level of blood pressure, the level of blood pressure was compared after adjusting for both factors simultaneously. Adjustment was done using an analysis-of-covariance approach, first testing that the hypothesis of parallelism was appropriate. The results are given in Table 5. Although the magnitudes of the differences shown earlier have decreased slightly, they are in general agreement with those presented earlier (Table 2).

Table 5. Adjusted [a] mean level of systolic and diastolic blood pressure, by area: The Yugoslavia Cardiovascular Disease Study.

	Systolic pressure	Diastolic pressure
REMETINEC		
Urban	137.1	86.8
Rural	142.2	87.1
Mixed	137.5	84.6
TUZLA		
Urban	134.9	82.9
Rural	131.2	80.4
Mixed	134.1	82.7

[a] Adjusted for age and body mass index.

212

Table 6. Standardized bivariate logistic regression coefficients for the regression of specified causes of death on systolic and on diastolic blood pressure: The Yugoslavia Cardiovascular Disease Study.

Cause of death [a]	Systolic pressure		Diastolic pressure	
	β	z	β	z
All causes	0.1673	4.84	0.1895	5.35
CHD	0.4059	5.10	0.3222	3.77
Cerebrovascular	0.5796	5.94	0.6103	6.06
Cancer	−0.0768	−1.18	−0.1068	−1.57
TB	−0.2661	−1.61	−0.2216	−1.36
All cardiovascular	0.3590	7.27	0.3960	7.73
All noncardiovascular	0.0004	0.01	0.0219	0.48

[a] Coefficients with 'z' statistics greater than 1.96 are significantly different from zero.

2.2. *The impact of blood pressure on the incidence of mortality and morbidity*

It is well known that elevated blood pressure increases one's risk of mortality and morbidity from cardiovascular disease and from coronary heart disease and stroke. The relationship between blood pressure and morbidity or mortality from coronary heart disease has been documented [5]. Table 6 presents standardized logistic regression coefficients for the regression of specified end points on systolic and on diastolic blood pressure. In each case, a bivariate

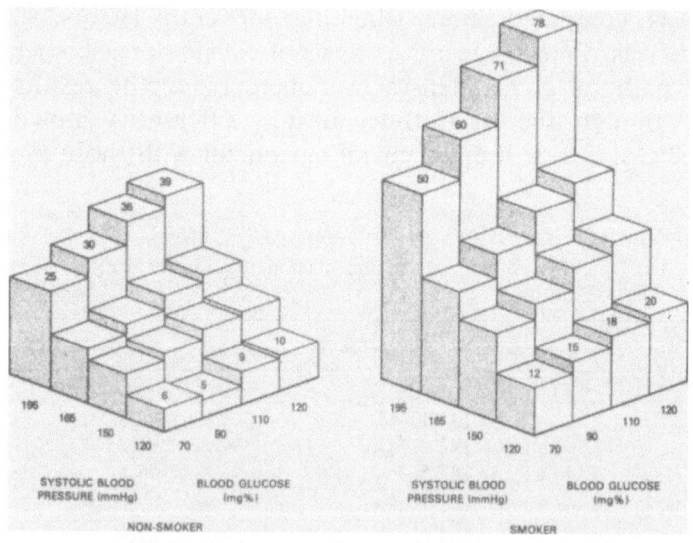

Figure 1. Probability (per 1000) of developing coronary heart disease in seven years, by smoking habit, and levels of systolic blood pressure and blood glucose: urban male, 45 years old, with serum cholesterol 260 mg%.

model (age and blood pressure) was used to control for the effect of age. For both diastolic and systolic pressure, the strongest relationship found (as judged by the size of the coefficients) was for death due to stroke. We documented no significant relationship between level of blood pressure and deaths due to noncardiovascular-renal causes. It has been hypothesized that elevated blood pressure is a risk factor for cancer mortality [6]. We do not find this to be the case, but note that the distribution of cancer sites in our population is different from that in U.S. populations [7].

While it is clear that elevated blood pressure is associated with increased risk of morbidity and mortality from cardiovascular disease, it should be emphasized that blood pressure is only one ingredient of a risk factor profile [8–10]. Figure 1 demonstrates the rise in risk associated with risk in blood sugar level for several other factors held constant. From this figure it should be clear that in Yugoslavia, as elsewhere, blood pressure is a strong risk factor, but it is best viewed in conjunction with other risk factors before assessing risk.

3. DISCUSSION

In spite of the title of this report, we have not discussed 'hypertension,' but present the actual level of blood pressure. Medical and statistical experts have pointed out the fallacy of a dichotomous approach to the study of blood pressure level and the incidence of disease [11–13]. There have generally been two situations in which the use of cutoff points to define hypertension were necessary. The first occurred when data-processing facilities were inadequate to handle large bodies of data. In this case, describing the prevalence of definite hypertension by using arbitrary cutoff points enabled a significant reduction in data-processing requirements, since the analysis could be restricted to the total number and those who meet the cutoff-point criteria. The second need occurs with controlled clinical trials. In this situation, one must select the population in which the likelihood of demonstrating successful treatment is the greatest. For practical reasons, one must define cutoff points in this instance. We were faced with neither situation, and hence have made our presentation in terms of level of blood pressure.

We noted that the blood pressure levels are generally lower in Tuzla than in Remetinec, that rural Tuzla blood pressures were slightly lower than urban Tuzla blood pressures, and that tural Remetinec blood pressures were generally higher than urban Remetinec blood pressures. We were unable to explain these differences in terms of differences in age and obesity distributions.

Numerous other differences exist between Tuzla and Remetinec, and between the urban and rural populations within these areas. There are large differences between the areas with regard to formal education. The proportion of the population without formal education is 22.4% in Tuzla. In Remetinec the proportion is 7.6%. The difference in the religious background in the two areas was noted earlier.

The occupational patterns of the population differed as well. In Remetinec, 31.1% reported being skilled or semiskilled industrial workers. Only 24% of the Tuzla cohort reported semiskilled or skilled occupations. In Tuzla, 14% of the cohort were reported to be miners. No miners were participants in Remetinec.

There are differences in diet between the areas, as exemplified by type of fat used in cooking,. In the rural Tuzla population, 24% – 30% report oil as the principal cooking fat. In Remetinec, more animal fat is used, and only 2% – 3% use oil.

All of these differences have been documented previously [2]. Their effects on blood pressure level have been explored and were published [15]. We have not been able to identify personal or environmental factors to explain the differences in blood pressure noted.

Another difference between the Tuzla and the Remetinec cohorts is in alcohol consumption. Those in the Remetinec cohort drink almost twice as much as those in the Tuzla cohort. Furthermore, it has been shown that the level of blood pressure is related to alcohol consumption [14].

Longitudinal data from the Yugoslavia Cardiovascular Disease Study [16] and from the general Yugoslavia population [17] suggest that the prevalence of hypertension is increasing within Yugoslavia. Serial data [17] suggest that the incidence of cardiovascular disease is increasing within Yugoslavia. The reasons for these increases are uncertain. There are indications that the population is becoming more obese [16], but it does not appear that the rise in blood pressure can be accounted for by rises in obesity [16].

The Yugoslavia Cardiovascular Disease Study was initiated because Yugoslavia had very low rates of coronary heart disease compared with U.S. studies [2]. We have demonstrated that Yugoslavs with elevated levels of blood pressure are at high risk for cardiovascular morbidity and mortality. Thus, the low rates of cardiovascular disease in Yugoslavia do not imply that elevated blood pressure should be considered less harmful in our population. As in previous studies, we have been unable to identify personal or environmental characteristics that explain most of the variance of blood pressure level among individuals.

Nonetheless, our study and others have pointed to new areas to be researched. Dietary sodium intake and its relationship to blood pressure level [18] needs to be explored. Such a study is now being planned as an outgrowth of our original study. We have documented that developing areas show a secular increase in the mean level of blood pressure that cannot be accounted for by changes in obesity [14]. This phenomenon needs to be documented, and, if possible, the factors bringing about this change identified. Such a study is now being planned.

Both of these studies should contribute to our understanding of regional differences in blood pressure. At present, however, we can only note that these differences exist. We cannot explain them through any of the identified correlates of blood pressure.

REFERENCES

1. Dawber T, Kannel W, Kagan A, Donabedian R, McNamara P, Pearson G: Environmental factors in hypertension. In: Stamler J, Stamler R (eds) Epidemiology of hypertension. New York: Grune and Stratton, 1967, pp 255-288.
2. Kozarevic Dj, Pirc B, Dawber T, Kahn H, Zukel W: Prevalence and incidence of coronary disease in a population study. The Yugoslavia Cardiovascular Disease Study. J Chronic Dis 24:495-505, 1971.
3. Walker S, Duncan D: Estimation of the probability of an event as a function of several independent variables. Biometrika 54:167-179, 1967.
4. Gordon T, Shurtleff D: Section 29: Means at each examination and inter-examination variation of specified characteristics: Framingham Study, Exam 1 to Exam 10. DHEW Publication no. (NIH) 74-478, 1974.
5. Kozarevic Dj, Pirc B, Racic Z, Dawber T, Gordon T, Zukel W: The Yugoslavia Cardiovascular Disease Study. II. Factors in the incidence of coronary heart disease. Am J Epidemiol 104:133-140, 1976.
6. Dyer A, Stamler J, Berkson D, Lindberg H, Stevens E: High blood pressure: a risk factor for cancer mortality? Lancet 7915:1051-1056, 1975.
7. Kozarevic Dj, Pirc B, Vojvodic N, Dawber T, Gordon T, Zukel W: The Yugoslavia Cardiovascular Disease Study. III. Death by cause and area. Int J Epidemiol 6:129-133, 1977.
8. Gordon T, Kannel W: Multiple contributors to coronary risk. Implications for screening and prevention. J Chronic Dis 25:561-565, 1972.
9. Kannel W, Dawber T: Hypertension as an ingredient of a cardiovascular risk profile. Br J Hosp Med 508-523, 1974.
10. Kannel W, McGee D, Gordon T: A general cardiovascular risk profile: The Framingham Study. Am J Cardiol 38:46-51, 1976.
11. Cornfield J: Joint dependence of risk of coronary heart disease on serum cholesterol and systolic blood pressure: a discriminate function analysis, part 2. Fed Proc 21:58-61, 1962.
12. Pickering G: Hypertension: definitions, natural histories, and consequences. Am J Med 52:570-583, 1972.
13. WHO: Arterial hypertension. Report of a WHO expert committee. Tech Rep Ser 628, 1978.
14. Kozarevic Dj, McGee D, Vojvodic N, Racić Z, Dawber T, Gordon T, Zukel W: Frequency of alcohol consumption and morbidity and mortality: The Yugoslavia Cardiovascular Disease Study. Lancet 8169:613–616, 1980.

15. Vojvodić N, Pašić I, Tešanović D, McGee D: Personal and environmental corre- lates of blood pressure. The Yugoslavia Cardiovascular Disease Study. In: Thurm R (ed) Essential hypertension. Miami: Symposia Specialists, 1979, pp 397-400.
16. Kozarevic Dj, Vojvodic N, Racić Z, McGee D: Trends in blood pressure and hypertension. The Yugoslavia Cardiovascular Disease Study. In: Thurm R (ed) Essential hypertension. Miami: Symposia Specialists, 1979, pp 49-53.
17. Kozarevic Dj: Epidemioloski aspekti arterijske hipertenzije. In: Arterijska Hiper- tenzia. Dimitrije Mihajlović, Božidar Dordević, Ivan Lambič, Dubomir Hadži Pešić Prosveta Niš Yugoslavia, 1979, pp 19-36.
18. Dawber T: Unproved hypotheses. N Engl J Med 299:452-458, 1978.

13. EPIDEMIOLOGY OF BLOOD PRESSURE IN THE GERMAN DEMOCRATIC REPUBLIC

S. Böthig and I. Böthig

Disease related to high blood pressure (BP) is an important health problem in the German Democratic Republic (GDR). The annual incidence rates of acute myocardial infarction (AMI) in Berlin/GDR are 6.3 cases per 1000 men (aged 20 years or older) and 4.2 cases per 1000 women (aged 20 years or older)[1]. Stroke occurs even somewhat more frequently than definite AMI[2]. Arterial hypertension has been coded as the direct cause of 8% of all deaths in 1973[3]. But taking into account the role of hypertension in ischaemic heart diseases, cerebrovascular diseases, and peripheral artery diseases, its real contribution to the total mortality amounts at least to one-third of all deaths. High BP causes a large proportion of hospital morbidity, sickness absenteeism, and invalidity in the country[3].

These few examples illustrate the impact of high BP on the health status of the population, but exact information on the epidemiology of hypertension and BP in general is fairly scarce in the GDR. This is mainly because cardiovascular epidemiological research work started only about ten years ago in this country. Its main results with regard to BP and arterial hypertension will be summarized in this chapter.

1. BLOOD PRESSURE IN MIDDLE-AGED MEN (EPIDEMIOLOGICAL STUDIES)

In 1968–69, three uniformly designed prospective epidemiological studies on ischaemic heart disease, arterial hypertension, and peripheral artery disease among 50- to 54-year-old men in the two city districts of Berlin-Mitte and Erfurt-Süd, and in the rural district of Pasewalk, were started[4]. The population samples, participation rates, and prevalence rates of arterial hypertension, according to the WHO-recommended definition of ≥ 160 and/or ≥ 95 mmHg, are summarized in Table 1. There are no marked differences in the prevalence rates of hypertension between the two big-city and the rural populations. Less than half of the hypertensives were aware of their illness, and only 10% – 16% of them were under regular treatment (see Table 2). Even for hypertensives with BP values ≥ 200 and/or ≥ 105 mmHg, these figures were 53% and 17%, respectively.

H. Kesteloot, J.V. Joossens (eds.), Epidemiology of Arterial Blood Pressure, 217–225.
Copyright © 1980 Martinus Nijhoff Publishers bv, The Hague/Boston/London. All rights reserved.

Table 1. Characteristics of three epidemiological studies in the GDR.

Study area	Population sample (men, 50–54 years old, born 1914–1918)	Persons examined	Participation rate (%)	Prevalence rate of hypertension (%)
Berlin-Mitte	622 Two-thirds random sample	552	89	19.0
Erfurt-Süd	309 One-third random sample	281	91	22.8
Pasewalk	191 Total population	183	96	23.5

Table 2. Degree of awareness of the illness and degree of regular treatment of the hypertensive subjects in the three epidemiological studies.

Study area	Degree of awareness of illness (% of hypertensives)	Degree of regular treatment (% of hypertensives)
Berlin-Mitte	45	9
Erfurt-Süd	31	16
Pasewalk	28	13

Within the Berlin-Mitte study, 81% of the hypertensive subjects have been clinically examined in detail and followed-up [5]. According to the findings after detailed examinations, including renovasography and kidney biopsy (if indicated), 89% had primary (essential) and 11% had renal hypertension; among them, 6% had pyelonephritis, 4% had stenosis of the renal artery, and 1% had glomerulonephritis; 41% of each were at stages I and II, and 18% at stage III of hypertension, according to the WHO definition.

The prevalence of various factors possibly related to the BP level has been analysed among the BP subgroups "hypertension" ($\geq 160/\geq 95$ mmHg), "borderline hypertension" (140–159/90–94 mmHg), and "normotension" ($< 140/ < 90$ mmHg). The following factors were found to be significantly more prevalent in the "hypertension" subgroup than in the "normotension" subgroup: overweight, impaired glucose tolerance, glucosuria, decreased urine osmolarity, proteinuria, family history of hypertension, ST depression, negative T waves in the ECG, tachycardia, left-ventricular hypertrophy in roentgenologic heart configuration, pathological eye-ground changes, increased haematocrit values, and certain psychologic characteristics (cyclothymic trait). On the other hand, there were no significant differences between the hypertensives and the normotensives with regard to the following factors: "stress" (by questionnaire), occupation, physical activity at work and in leisure time,

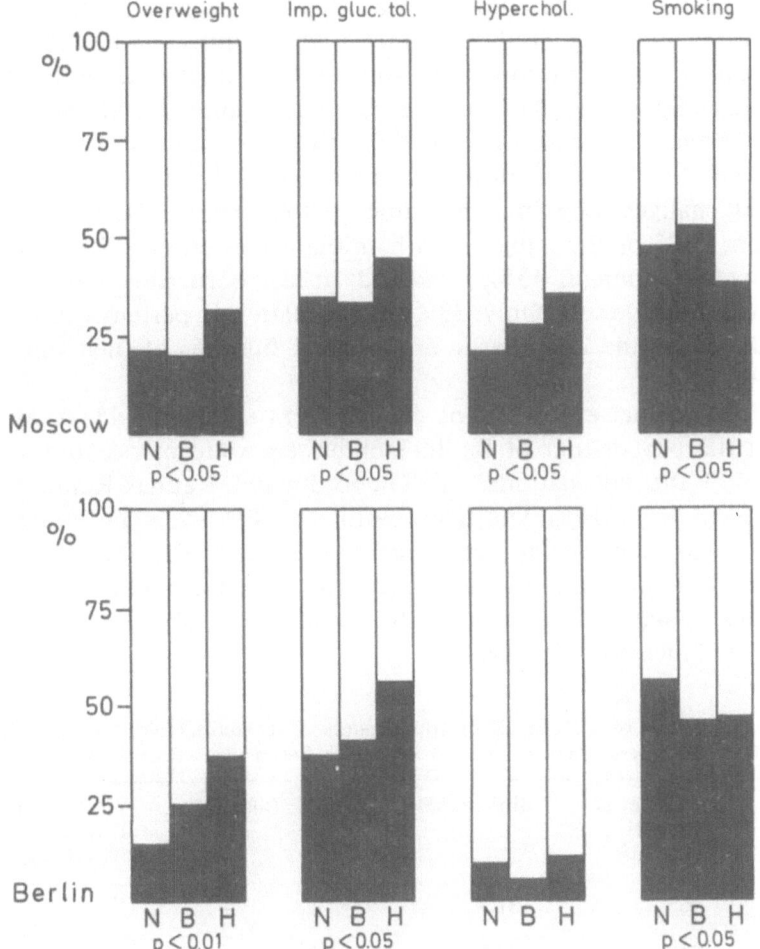

Figure 1. Prevalence rates (%) of various factors in three BP subgroups (N, normotension; B, borderline hypertension; H, hypertension) in 50- to 54-year-old men from Moscow and Berlin.

marital status, educational level, number of children, smoking habits, cholesterol level, bacteriuria, specific gravity of urine, left-ventricular hypertrophy in the ECG, vital capacity, and forced expiratory volume [6].

Some of these findings have been compared with the corresponding results of a similar study in Moscow [7] (Fig. 1). Significantly higher prevalence rates for overweight and impaired glucose tolerance and a significantly lower proportion of smokers in the hypertension subgroup as compared with the normotension subgroup were found in the Moscow as well as in the Berlin population sample.

Within the Berlin-Mitte study, out of the 156 subjects of the "borderline hypertension" subgroup (140–159 and/or 90–94 mmHg), 130 (83%) underwent a detailed clinical examination, and 99 (64% of the borderline hypertensives) were followed-up for four years. The subjects with borderline BP resembled more the hypertensives than the normotensives with regard to relative body weight, left-ventricular hypertrophy in the ECG, pathological eye-ground changes, and impaired glucose tolerance [8]. After four years of observation, 23% of the subjects with initially borderline BP values fell into the normotensive range, 43% remained in the borderline range, and 34% became hypertensives [9]. Only 33% of the latter hypertensives could have been predicted by the anamnestic and clinical findings of their initial examinations [10].

In 1974, the initial examinations of a random sample of 45- to 59-year-old men from the city district of Berlin-Lichtenberg were carried out within the framework of the international WHO-coordinated Kaunas-Rotterdam Intervention Study (KRIS) [11]. The main results on BP levels are summarized in Table 3 [12, 13]. The mean values of the systolic BP increase with age, between the older and the middle-age groups more than between the younger and the middle-age groups, whereas the mean values of the diastolic BP (fifth phase) do not increase with age.

Table 3. Mean values of systolic (SBP) and diastolic (fifth phase) blood pressure (DBP) and prevalence rates of hypertension by age groups of the Berlin-Lichtenberg Study 1974.

Age group (years)	Number of subjects examined	SBP (mmHg)	DBP (mmHg)	Prevalence rate of hypertension ($\geqslant 160/ \geqslant 95$ mmHg)
45–49	465	131.3	79.3	11.6
50–54	346	133.4	80.6	16.2
55–59	269	138.5	80.3	21.2

2. BLOOD PRESSURE IN ADULTS (SCREENING PROGRAMMES)

During the past 20 years, a number of BP screening programmes have been initiated in the GDR, predominantly in connection with the obligatory chest X-ray radiography. They will not be reviewed here because of considerable differences in the methods of BP measurement applied in these programmes. Only two projects shall be briefly mentioned as examples for the most reliable portion of these programmes: the 1970 multiphasic screening model of Sternberg [14], and the community control pilot programme of Berlin-Pankow [15].

In 1970, a multiphasic screening programme was carried out in the small town of Sternberg, county of Schwerin, in the north-west of the GDR. A random sample of 2908 persons (1730 men and 1178 women), aged between 15 and 70 years, underwent a complex screening programme. The main results of the so-called "Sternberg '70" model have been published [14]. The cardiovascular examinations constituted a part of the complex pro-gramme [16]. A member of the screening team measured the BP once every 5 mm mercury diastolic fifth phase, while the proband was in the supine position. Although problems regarding the level of standardization of BP measurement certainly exist, this project provides the only comprehensive information on mean BP values in a community of a wide age range in our country (Fig. 2). The means and standard deviations for the entire sample were 151.3 ± 24.3 mmHg for the systolic BP and 90.0 ± 13.0 mmHg for the diastolic BP.

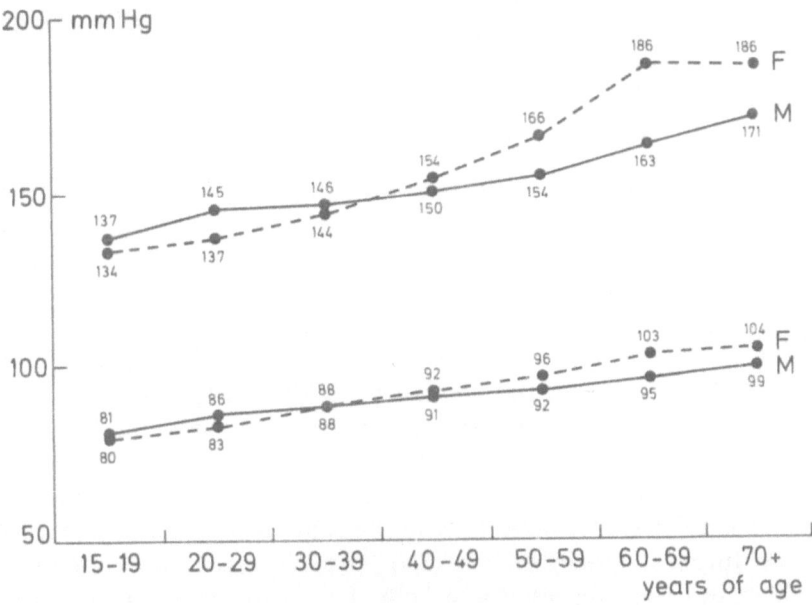

Figure 2. Mean systolic and diastolic (fifth phase) BP in males (M) and females (F) by age groups from the multiphasic screening model "Sternberg '70".

Within the framework of the international WHO-coordinated project "Community Control of Stroke and Hypertension" [17], a pilot study was started in the GDR in 1975. A random sample of 2277 men and 2817 women aged 15–59 years, from the city district of Berlin-Pankow, was examined [18]. One of the approximately 20 members of the study team measured the BP once for the proband, who was sitting; the BP was read every 2 mm mercury, diastolic fifth phase. If the values of this measurement reached or exceeded 160 and/or 95 mmHg, a second measurement was done by a different observer after about two weeks. If this second measurement showed the BP to be in this hypertensive range (according to the WHO definition), the subject was classified as hypertensive. The prevalence rates of hypertension by age and sex groups are given in Table 4. They follow the well-known course (like the means in the Sternberg '70 screening—see Fig. 2): higher in men in the younger age groups and higher in women after the 40th year of age.

Table 4. Prevalence rates (%) of hypertension ($\geqslant 160/\geqslant 95$ mmHg) by age and sex groups of the pilot study of the hypertension control programme in Berlin-Pankow 1975.

Age group (years)	Number of males examined	Prevalence rate of hypertension in males (%)	Number of females examined	Prevalence rate of hypertension in females (%)
15–19	259	6.9	271	3.3
20–24	158	8.2	196	5.1
25–29	208	14.9	211	6.6
30–34	338	19.2	401	11.2
35–39	394	15.7	471	15.3
40–44	354	16.7	374	19.5
45–49	228	20.6	303	28.1
50–54	192	21.9	337	32.0
55–59	146	29.5	253	38.7
15–59	2277	16.7	2817	18.2

3. BLOOD PRESSURE IN CHILDREN

In the GDR there is a growing interest, but so far only a few data, on BP in childhood and adolescence. In 1975, a screening study on BP in schoolchildren was carried out in the city of Halle [19]. Altogether, 967 pupils from the first to the tenth grades (7–17 years of age) were examined by two observers. The BP was measured once at the right arm of the child sitting in the class-room during a lesson of so-called "quiet work". Measurements with very high values were repeated after 1 h. Up to the third grade (10 years of age), an 8-cm-wide cuff was used; from the fourth grade on (11 years of age), a 12-cm-wide cuff was used. The diastolic BP was read at the fifth phase.

The mean BP values of the various age and sex groups are listed in Table 5. There are very small differences between boys and girls. Only from the 15th year of age do the mean systolic BP values of the boys exceed those of the girls: 9.2% of the boys and 10.1% of the girls exceeded the upper values for a "normal" BP of 135/85 mmHg up to the 12th year of age, and of 140/90 mmHg from the 13th year of age on. There seems to be no clear correlation between BP and body weight in this study [19].

Table 5. Mean and standard deviation (SD) of systolic (SBP) and diastolic (fifth phase) blood pressure (DBP) by age and sex groups in school-children; screening study, Halle, 1975.

Years of age	Children examined		Boys				Girls			
			SBP		DBP		SBP		DBP	
	B	G	Mean	SD	Mean	SD	Mean	SD	Mean	SD
7	15	22	106.3	6.7	76.3	4.9	110.2	10.7	75.2	6.3
8	52	58	110.6	9.9	75.4	7.5	110.8	10.7	76.2	5.2
9	59	40	113.1	10.7	77.0	6.4	113.9	8.8	79.1	6.3
10	49	48	113.7	9.1	77.2	6.1	114.7	10.9	79.8	5.7
11	52	57	114.9	11.0	78.5	5.6	113.9	9.6	78.5	6.5
12	46	48	113.2	11.1	71.0	10.4	114.6	10.7	73.0	11.5
13	61	43	118.6	11.8	71.0	11.7	116.2	11.9	69.0	12.4
14	58	52	119.2	12.0	75.7	7.2	123.5	11.6	73.0	8.9
15	45	40	123.0	11.8	77.0	8.5	117.3	9.8	77.4	6.1
16	42	37	123.9	8.9	77.2	6.8	119.2	13.1	78.2	5.8
17	19	19	123.5	9.7	79.2	6.1	120.9	10.4	80.5	5.6

As part of the international cooperative project "Juvenile Hypertension" (participating centres: Budapest, Moscow, Kaunas, Havanna, and Berlin/ GDR) 2154 school-children from Berlin-Pankow and 1791 school-children from Berlin-Köpenick, all born in 1964, were examined during 1977 [20]. Table 6 shows some preliminary results for the boys from the Berlin studies

Table 6. Mean values and standard deviation (SD) of systolic (SBP) and diastolic (fifth phase) blood pressure (DBP), of height and weight of 13-year-old boys from the Berlin-Pankow and Berlin-Köpenick studies 1977.

Study area	SBP ± SD (mmHg)	DBP ± SD (mmHg)	Height ± SD (cm)	Weight ± SD (kg)
Berlin-Pankow	108.8 ± 10.2	58.1 ± 10.1	155.7 ± 7.6	43.0 ± 7.8
Berlin-Köpenick	114.8 ± 11.0	62.7 ± 9.7	160.1 ± 9.7	46.9 ± 8.9

as an example. The higher values of the Berlin-Köpenick children can be explained by the fact that they were, on an average, half a year older than the Berlin-Pankow children, because the Berlin-Pankow examinations were done in the spring, but those from Berlin-Köpenick were carried out in the autumn [21]. This demonstrates the great influence of age on the BP level, particularly at around 13 years of age, a period of rapid physical and sexual maturation.

In the Berlin-Pankow part of the project, 216 children from the upper 10% of the BP distribution curves of all children examined, and 220 children as a random sample from the remaining 90% of the children, underwent a detailed medical examination [22]. It turned out that in 13-year-old children

224

from the highest decile of the BP distribution the following factors were significantly more often prevalent than in children with lower BP: higher body weight in boys and girls, higher serum uric acid levels in girls, higher degree of sexual maturity in girls, and a trend towards higher after-load blood glucose values. No significant differences were found for height and serum cholesterol for either sex, signs of sexual maturity and serum uric acid for boys, smoking habits and some qualitative urine parameters.

It is beyond the capacity of the present cross-sectional stage of the study to conclude any causal relationship from these findings. Their significance and validity with regard to the natural history of high BP in childhood will hopefully be a little more elucidated by the on-going follow-up of the two subgroups within the framework of this international cooperative project.

REFERENCES

1. Böthig S, Böthig I, Aurisch R, Breitkreuz K, Sajkiewicz K: Inzidenz und Letalität des Herzinfarktes in einer großstädtischen Population — Ergebnisse des Herzinfarktregisters Berlin-Lichtenberg. Dtsch Gesund Wesen 34:186-192, 1979.
2. Eisenblätter D, Höppner G, Böthig S, Schneider I: Herzinfarkt und Schlaganfall in der Bevölkerung der DDR — Vergleichende Ergebnisse der Herzinfarkt- und Schalganfallregister. Dtsch Gesund Wesen 30:1887-1890, 1975.
3. Akademie für Ärztliche Fortbildung der DDR: Das Gesundheitswesen der Deutschen Demokratischen Republik 1975. Berlin: Nationales Druckhaus, 1975.
4. Böthig S, Knappe J, Heine H, Anders G: Epidemiologie der Herz-Kreislauf-Krankheiten in der Deutschen Demokratischen Republik. Dtsch Gesund Wesen 27:823-829, 1972.
5. Linss G, Böthig S, Rademacher I: Die arterielle Hypertonie bei Männern mittleren Alters — Symptomatologie, Ätiologie und Schweregrad Dtsch Gesund Wesen 27:1873-1879, 1972.
6. Böthig S: Epidemiologie der Herz-Kreislauf-Krankheiten bei Männern mittleren Alters — Ergebnisse der Erstuntersuchung der Studie Berlin-Mitte. Dissertationsschrift B, Humboldt-Universität Berlin, 1974.
7. Böthig S, Metelitsa VI, Barth W, Aleksandrov AA, Schneider I, Ostrovskaya TP, Kokurina EV, Saposhnikov II, Iliushina IP, Gurevich LS: Prevalence of ischaemic heart disease, arterial hypertension and intermittent claudication, and distribution of risk factors among middle-aged men in Moscow and Berlin. Cor Vasa 18:104-118, 1976.
8. Linss G, Böthig S, Sparr KD, Fulroth H, Brennecke HJ: Borderline-Blutdruckwerte — Normotonie oder Hypertonie? 2. Mitteilung: Vergleichende epidemiologische Untersuchungen an Probanden mit Borderline-Blutdruckwerten, Hypertonikern und Normotonikern. Dtsch Gesund Wesen 29:534-539, 1974.
9. Linss G, Fulroth H, Sparr KD, Brennecke HJ, Böthig S, Günther KH: Borderline-Blutdruckwerte — Normotonie oder Hypertonie? 3. Mitteilung: Verlaufsuntersuchungen an Probanden mit Borderline-Blutdruckwerten über einen Zeitraum von vier Jahren. Dtsch Gesund Wesen 29:635-641, 1974.

10. Linss G, Günther KH, Böthig S, Brumby J, Brennecke HJ: Können Probanden mit Borderline-Blutdruckwerten, die in späteren Jahren eine Hypertonie entwickeln, bereits vorher erkannt werden? 4. Mitteilung: Eine retrospektive Betrachtung. Dtsch Gesund Wesen 29:705-708, 1974.

11. WHO Kaunas — Rotterdam Collaboration: Behavioural and operational components of health intervention programmes. Public Health Europe 2, Chronic diseases. Copenhagen: Regional Office for Europe, 1973, pp 69-79.

12. Barth W, Böthig S, Bärlehner A, Böthig I, Anders G, Miehlke G, Dübel H: Interventionsstudie Berlin — Ergebnisse der Screening- und Behandlungsphase. In: Váradi E, Berndt H, Böthig S, Eisenblätter D, Klemm P (eds) Epidemiologie nichtübertragbarer Krankheiten. Schriftenreihe der Akademie für Ärztliche Fortbildung der DDR 51, Berlin: VEB Verlag Volk und Gesundheit, 1978, pp 186-191.

13. Shkhvatsabaya IK, Metelitsa VI, Anders G, Böthig S (eds): Epidemiology of cardiovascular diseases (in Russian). Moscow: Meditsina, 1977.

14. Thiele HJ, Tredt HJ, Friedemann H (eds): Vielfachreihenuntersuchungen — Erfahrungen und Entwicklungstendenzen. Berlin: VEB Verlag Volk und Gesundheit, 1974.

15. Faulhaber HD, Böthig I, Menz M, Gohlke HR, Kahrig C, Förster R, Viergutz A, Andler S: Hypertonie-Bekämpfungsprogramm in der DDR. Dtsch Gesund Wesen 33:1537-1542, 1976.

16. Seifert A, Tiedcke H, Müller KH, Keyserlingk G von, Kirchner D, Rabenau W von, Spiegelberg E, Storm H: Epidemiologische Ergebnisse der Herz-Kreislauf-Studie im Multiphasenscreening Sternberg '70. In: Thiele HJ, Tredt HJ, Friedemann H (eds) Vielfachreihenuntersuchungen — Erfahrungen und Entwicklungstendenzen. Berlin: VEB Verlag Volk und Gesundheit, 1974, pp 351-368.

17. Strasser T: Pilot programmes for the control of hypertension. WHO Chron 26:451-455, 1972.

18. Faulhaber HD, Baumann R, Böthig I, Menz M, Gohlke HR, Schuster I, Täuscher M, Kube E: Community control programme of hypertension in a district of Berlin (GDR) (Abstr). 7th European Congress of Cardiology, Amsterdam, 1976, p 664.

19. Schwartze D, Schwartze C: Blutdruck bei Kindern und Jugendlichen — Screening-Studie Halle 1975. 1. Mitteilung: Orientierende Untersuchungen zur Normalverteilung des Blutdruckes und Hochdruckgefährdung im Kindes- und Jugendalter. Dtsch Gesund Wesen 33:2092-2095, 1978.

20. Böthig I, Böthig S, Eisenblätter D, Weiss M, Briedigkeit W, Ulrich S, Kunigk I. Teichert R, Hellmer I, Gross R, Harksen U: Der Blutdruck im Kindes- und Jugendalter — Konzeption, Organisation und Methodik einer internationalen Gemeinschaftsstudie, Ergebnisse der Pilotstudien in Berlin. Dtsch Gesund Wesen 33:2010-2014, 1978.

21. Böthig I, Böthig S, Eisenblätter D: Blood pressure in school children in Berlin/GDR. CVD Epidemiol Newslett 26, (in press) 1979.

22. Böthig I, Eisenblätter D, Weiss M, Briedigkeit W: Factors determining blood pressure in children. Second scientific meeting of the Working Group on the Epidemiology and Prevention of Cardiovascular Disease, Dublin, April 1979. Trans Eur Soc Cardiol 1:6, 1979.

PART FIVE

DETERMINANTS OF BLOOD PRESSURE
IN LOW BLOOD PRESSURE POPULATIONS

14. SODIUM HOMEOSTASIS AND LOW BLOOD PRESSURE POPULATIONS

W.J. OLIVER

Salt (sodium chloride), in respect to its dietary role in present-day societies, has been considered a necessity for health and survival [1] or, alternatively, a major determining factor in the pathogenesis of essential hypertension [2, 3]. However, this latter view is not universally shared [4, 5]. A less-polarized view is the hypothesis that essential hypertension results from a disturbance in equilibrium of activity of the sympathetic nervous system and adrenal cortex in association with an excessive sodium intake [6]. To date, the controversy continues [7].

A further point of disagreement is the distinction between *salt appetite* and *salt requirement* [2]. Although salt occupies a well-documented role in the recorded history of man, the time span of written word occupies less than a fraction of 1% of man's total history, currently estimated to be well in excess of two million years (late Pliocene Period). Even further removed in time are the evolutionary adaptations achieved by man's ancestors, other vertebrates, and lower animal forms in order to maintain a stable body content of sodium while confronted by infinitely diverse environmental conditions and food sources. A brief review of this evolutionary process can provide a potentially provocative background against which data from low-salt cultures can be considered.

1. EVOLUTIONARY ADAPTATION FAVORING SODIUM INTAKE AND CONSERVATION

The environmental conditions which probably existed and influenced the emergence of physiological mechanisms facilitating sodium intake and conservation have been described in detail by Denton [8, 9]. He theorizes that since at least the Devonian Era when the first amphibians emerged, substantial areas of the earth have been severely sodium deficient, in particular, the interior of the continents and the alpine areas. This deficiency is postulated to have had an important selection pressure upon evolutionary adaptations associated with sodium homeostasis. A deficit of sodium leads to a reduction of extracellular fluid and of blood volume, with resultant impaired circulation and reduced functional capacity for pursuit or flight. Such a deficit is greatly

H. Kesteloot, J.V. Joossens (eds.), Epidemiology of Arterial Blood Pressure, 229–241.

accentuated in response to the increased requirements of pregnancy and lactation. In the overview, one aspect of evolutionary preeminence was the ability to maintain sodium homeostasis in an environment characterized by a natural paucity of that substance.

Maintenance of sodium homeostasis, expressed in simplest terms, is the balance between intake and output. This must be tempered with the required adjustments for periods of physiologically increased needs (pregnancy and lactation) or episodes of deficiency of intake or of excessive loss (i.e., vomiting, diarrhea, sweating without acclimatization). The evolutionary components of intake and retention of sodium have been the subjects of much investigation [10].

A large body of data support the existence of a neural organization subserving behavior mechanisms leading to salt appetite in response to sodium deficiency [9]. There are two major components to this neural contribution to sodium balance: (a) recognition that a deficiency of sodium exists and (b) ability to distinguish concentrations of sodium salts in foods and liquids. The stage in evolution at which salt appetite emerged is not known. In carp, there are taste fibers which respond to varying concentrations of sodium chloride [11]. In sodium-deficient marsupials (wild kangoroos), salt appetite has been described by Abraham and colleagues [12]. In mammals, the proclivity for herbivores to seek out salt licks and other sources of high salinity is well known. In contrast, carnivorous animals obtain sufficient sodium from the meat of their prey, even if these herbivorous animals are sodium deficient. Ascending the phylogenetic scale of the primates, the majority of monkeys and higher apes are entirely herbivorous. Others are predominantly so (chimpanzees and baboons) with reported observations of occasional flesh-eating incidents. Irrespective of the precise evolutionary line by which *Homo sapiens* emerged, the available evidence is persuasive that our progenitors subsisted on a wholly, or nearly so, herbivorous diet with later, and probably, minor contributions by addition of meat [13]. It would further seem that despite the presence of taste sensation for salt, ancestors of man satisfied necessary intake of sodium without a dependence upon a mineral source of high salinity.

The conservation component for sodium balance involves principally adrenal-renal interaction. In response to a decrease in arterial perfusion pressure or a reduction in sodium concentration of the glomerular filtrate in that portion of the renal tubule adjacent to the macula densa, the renal hormone, renin, is released. In plasma, renin converts angiotensinogen to angiotensin I, which in turn is converted into angiotensin II, a highly potent vasoconstrictor and the major hormonal stimulant to the adrenal gland for secretion of aldosterone. In turn, aldosterone is responsible for maximum resorption of sodium by the renal tubular cells. Aldosterone also stimulates resorption of sodium by cells in the gastrointestinal tract, and salivary and sweat glands.

However, in the absence of disease, the kidney is the primary organ responsible for sodium homeostasis in the presence of varying levels of sodium intake.

In recognition of the major role of aldosterone in effecting maximum resorption of sodium by the kidney, and to a quantitatively lesser extent by the sweat glands and gastrointestinal tract, there has been considerable interest in the structure and secretion of the adrenal gland in lower forms of animals. The available data are included in the comprehensive review by Denton [10]. As early in evolution as the cartilagenous fish, *Elasmobranchii,* a species surviving from the Devonian era (400 million years ago), an interrenal (adrenocortical) mass of cells occurs in proximity to the kidney [14, 15]. Progressively in evolution, intrarenal cell masses are found in bony fish and amphibians [14]. In reptiles and birds, more-advanced organization of interrenal and chromaffin cells occurs, but not until the *Prototheria* (the echidna and platypus) are the chromaffin tissues aggregated at one pole of the primitive adrenal gland [16]. Commencing with marsupials, the cortical cells are arranged at the periphery of the gland and the chromaffin cells in the interior. Although appearing late in evolution, data to be described (*vide infra*) indicate that distribution of cell organization is not essential to secretion of aldosterone. Thus, a continuum of higher forms of organization of the adrenal gland parallels evolution of the vertebrates.

Measurements of secretion of hormonal substances by the primitive adrenal tissues of early vertebrates have been limited by available technology and has thwarted systematic study. Nevertheless, data of interest have been reported.

Secretion of corticosteriods has been identified in jawless vertebrates: the Atlantic hagfish (*Myxine glutinosa*) [17], the Pacific hagfish (*Polistotrema stonuti*) and a lamprey landlocked in freshwater [18, 19]. In vitro incubation of adrenal glands from dogfish, skate, and ratfish with tritiated progesterone yielded aldosterone, presumed evidence of aldosterone secretion in vivo by *Elastobranchii* [20]. In *Amphibia,* aldosterone has been demonstrated by in vitro incubation of the adrenal of the bullfrog (*Rana Catesbieana*) [21]. In both reptiles [22] and birds [23, 24], in vitro incubation of the adrenal glands leads to production of aldosterone.

The significance of the adrenal gland in maintaining sodium homeostasis has been investigated in representative species, commencing with the elasmobranch. In the torpedo, adrenalectomy is fatal in four days [25]. Following adrenalectomy in frogs (*Rana temporaria*), loss of sodium and accumulation of potassium occur [26, 27]. The effect of adrenal insufficiency upon sodium and potassium balance in mammals, including man, is well known, as is the ability of aldosterone to reduce renal excretion of sodium and to increase excretion of potassium [28].

In a wide spectrum of species existing in freshwater or in a terrestrial habitat, including freshwater eel and fish (salmon), alligators, birds, dolphin, desert mammals, and other less ambiently stressed mammals, there are similar concentrations of plasma sodium and muscle sodium [29, 30]. Considered in the overview, the data document the evolutionary nature of physiological mechanisms ensuring a constancy of extracellular composition for a spectrum of species beyond primitive forms. These protective processes are obviously well developed in man.

2. ADAPTATION OF MAN TO A SCARCITY OF DIETARY SODIUM

Survival and health of man in the absence of sources of mineral salt or substances of high salinity have been reported in numerous studies of primitive peoples. An early account of this adaptation is described in Schomburgk's 'Travels in British Guiana: 1840–1844' [31]. He noted that the Warrau Indians living on the Barima River in the interior dried meat by fire for preservation and cooked wild game 'in the blood of the animal, strongly seasoned with *capsicum.*' The latter is a variety of pepper. Other, more formal, reports of populations living with little or no mineral salt and without evidence of consequent disadvantages in health include the aboriginal ethnic groups of Szechwan Province, West China [32], the Masai of Africa [33], the North American Indians [34], the Melanesians of the New Guinea Highlands [35], the Polynesian inhabitants of the Pukapuka, an atoll in the South Pacific [36], the Chimbu of New Guinea [37], the Tilfamin people in the interior of New Guinea (who have the interesting habit of drinking opossum urine when these animals are captured and killed, perhaps a mineral source) (W. Wheatcroft, personal communication) [38], inhabitants of the Solomon Islands [39], the Tasaday of the Philippines (K. MacLeish, personal communication) and the Yanomama of South America [40].

Our studies of the Yanomama Indians living in the interior of northern Brazil and southern Venezuela document the absence of salt in the diet and an amazing ability to avidly conserve sodium to the extent of limiting 24-h urinary sodium loss to as little as 2 mg [40]. The major staples in the diet of the Yanomama are plaintains, with irregular additions of game, fish, insects, and wild vegetable foods. Analyses confirm a paucity of sodium in the nonanimal sources of food in their diet, with the highest sodium present in the cooking ashes in which the peeled plaintains and other foods are roasted (W.J. Oliver, unpublished data).

The physiological basis for successful adaptation to a life-long paucity of dietary sodium is dependent upon maximum stimulation of the sodium-conserving hormonal mechanisms—the renin-angiotensin-aldosterone sys-

Table 1. Plasma renin activity and 24-h urine excretion rates for sodium, potassium, and aldosterone in the Yanomama, a 'salt-free' culture, and in control subjects.

	Plasma renin activity (ng/ml/h)	Urinary sodium excretion (meq/24 h)	Urinary potassium excretion (meq/24 h)	Urinary aldosterone excretion (ng/24 h)
	Mean ± SD	Mean ± SD	Mean ± SD	Mean ± SD
Yanomama males	13.10 ± 14.17	1.34 ± 2.01	200.38 ± 80.17	74.52 ± 44.94
Caucasian males (controls)	4.94 ± 3.71	218.33 ± 31.78	60.33 ± 7.31	2.76 ± 1.53

tem—accompanied by maximum response of the organs responsible for resorption of sodium— kidney, gastrointestinal tract, and sweat gland. In the Chimbu of equatorial New Guinea, living on a vegetarian diet without access to salt, peripheral blood levels of aldosterone are elevated fourfold over those of other tribes having access to a Western diet [37]. In our studies [40] (Table 1). plasma renin activities were within or exceeded the range of North Americans ingesting short-term, very low (10 meq/day) sodium diets. In these same subjects, excretion rates of aldosterone were all above the upper limits found in Caucasians on a general diet with free access to salt. In plasma, aldosterone-binding globulins and free-aldosterone concentrations are both markedly increased in these same subjects, suggesting an increased peripheral activity of aldosterone at responsive receptor sites associated with sodium resorption (W. Nowaczynski, personal communication) [41]. Of interest, these same findings of increased mineralocorticoid activity have been described in *essential hypertension!* [6, 41].

It is well known that levels of sodium-associated hormones markedly increase in pregnancy [42], but this is in the presence of a usually unrestricted access to salt. A recent extension of our previous hormonal studies [42a] to pregnant Yanomama women document an even greater hormonal response of the renin-aldosterone system with levels of plasma renin activity double those observed for Yanomama males upon the same sodium-restricted diets. Similarly, the concentrations of urinary aldosterone for these pregnant women are greater than their male counterparts, and are exceedingly high in comparison to expeditionary controls. The healthy appearance of Yanomama infants and mothers (Fig. 1) does not suggest a nutritional disadvantage resulting from the limited availability of dietary sodium ion. The adult male in this society is certainly robust (Fig. 2) and displays great stamina in the long treks characteristic of this culture [43].

Of pertinence to consideration of health and reproductivity in an environment devoid of mineral salt is the fact that the area of land occupied by the Yanomama Indians has been calculated to be 2.8 times greater than 100 years ago with an associated twofold increase in the number of villages [44]. These

234

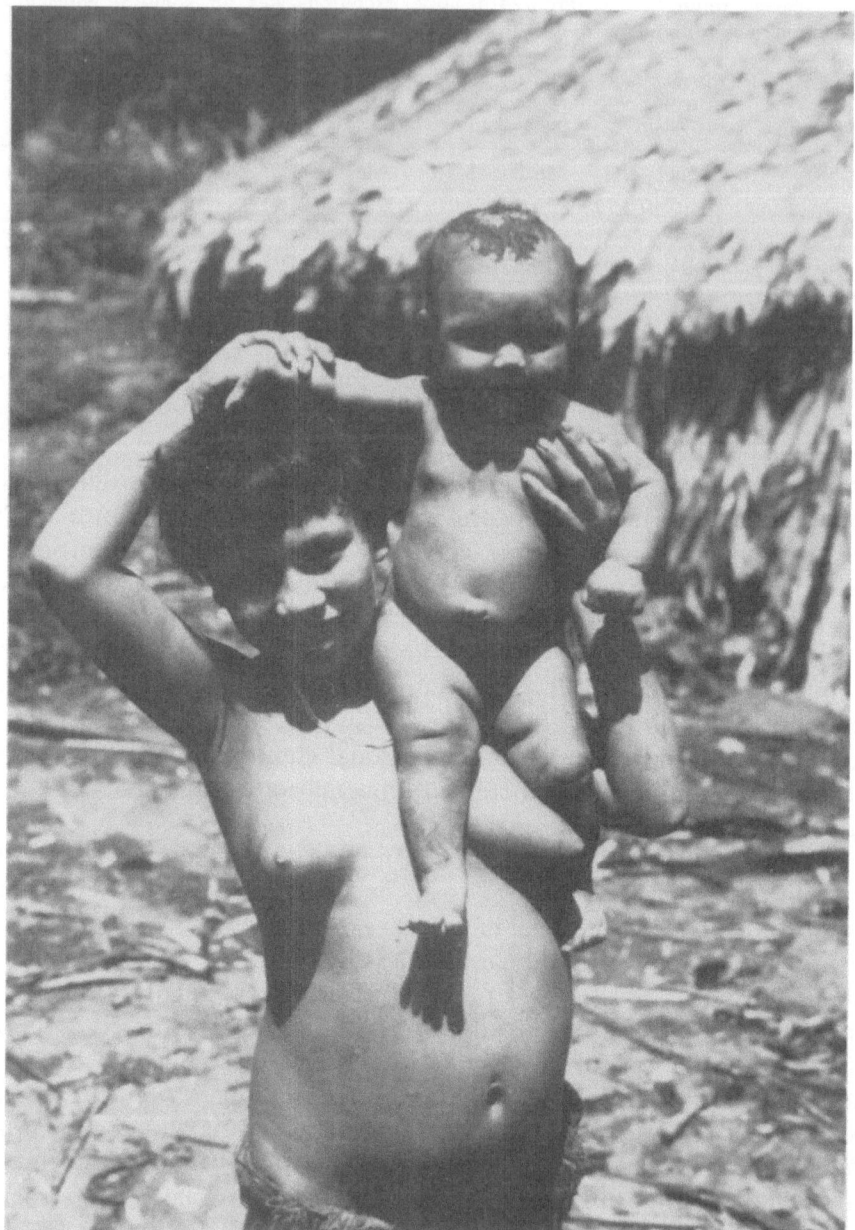

Figure 1. Yanomama mother and infant.

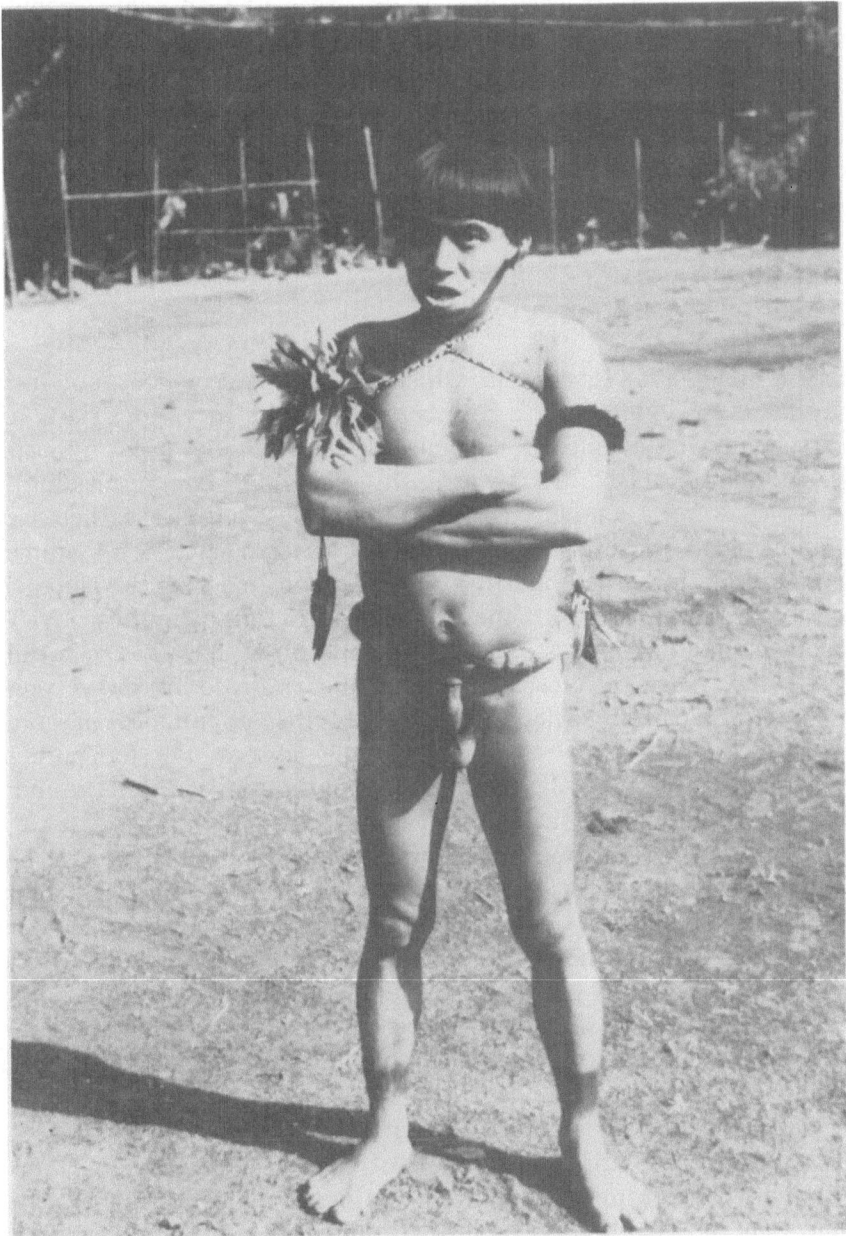

Figure 2. Yanomama warrior in his village in the northern interior of Brazil.

236

estimates of expansion are calculated to be associated an *annual* population growth rate of not less than 0.5% – 1.0%. Some data suggest the annual rate could be as high as 2% [44]. These observations suggest that for this ethnic group, at least, survival and procreation with an increase of population can occur successfully in a 'no-salt' culture. It should be noted that this increase has occurred despite the pressures of tropical disease and the high rate of homicide due to warfare [43, 45].

3. LOW BLOOD PRESSURE POPULATIONS

Discovery of population groups in which blood pressure does not increase with age has been reported for a number of societies in various parts of the world. These are well detailed in several articles and reviews (W. Wheatcroft, personal communication; K. MacLeish, personal communication) [2, 3, 32–40, 46–54]. A conspicuous characteristic of these groups is their lack of acculturation. The process of acculturation is associated with numerous changes suggested to be potential risk factors associated with development of hypertension with aging [39]. Of these, access to liberal quantities of salt and salted foods is only one, but is quite consistently observed. That man can live throughout the expected lifespan without the increase in blood pressure associated with civilized societies emphasizes the importance of studying those groups in which hypertension is virtually absent. For the purpose of this discussion, attention will be directed only upon salt intake and will exclude other potential risk factors.

Consideration of the relationship between salt intake and hypertension has been extensively discussed [2, 3, 6, 7]. Actual measurements of salt intake in low blood pressure populations are quite limited. In unacculturated groups, field conditions prevent metabolic balance studies to provide precise data. However, utilization of 24-h urinary excretion of sodium provides a reliable index of minimum salt intake [3]. Since urinary sodium–potassium ratios indicate a *trend* in intake of salt, this technique has also been used in studies of low blood pressure populations.

In studies of two populations of Polynesians, the group with the lower blood pressures had a urinary excretion of slightly greater than 60 meq of sodium per day; the group with higher blood pressures had urinary excretions of greater than 100 meq per day [36]. In Eskimos of Alaska, urinary excretion of sodium indicated an intake of slightly less than 4 g daily [3]. In !Kung bushman, urinary excretions of sodium averaged 30 meq per 24 h, suggesting an intake of less than 2 g of salt daily [48]. In a comparison between two groups of Melanesians, one living in the Highlands of New Guinea, the other in a coastal area with access to Western foods, the unacculturated group of the

Highlands had lower sodium–potassium ratios in their urine, and lower blood pressures [35]. Similar data have been described for another group in New Guinea, the Chimbu, living in a remote area when comparison of urinary ratios for sodium and potassium and of blood pressure are made with natives having some access to a European diet [37]. With progressive acculturation of tribal groups. observed increases in their blood pressure have been associated with progressive increases of urinary sodium–potassium ratios [55]. In six societies of the Solomon Islands, estimates of salt intake derived from analyses of random urine samples displayed an association of increased salt intake with increases of systolic pressure in females with age, but not in males [39]. However, there was a fall in diastolic pressure with age in males with the lower salt intake.

The association of a stable blood pressure throughout life with a low salt intake can be extended to even lower levels of intake with recent data found in our observations [40]. In our studies of the Yanomama, field conditions prevented measurements of intake. However, the impressively small quantity of 24-h urinary sodium excretion in the presence of evidence for very high activity of the hormonal system responsible for sodium conservation suggests the intake to be lower than any previously reported. A further unique finding in our studies was the levels of blood pressure maintained throughout the entire age span (Table 2). For both males and females, the systolic pressures

Table 2. Blood pressures obtained in the Yanomama Indians.

Age	No. of subjects	Systolic		Diastolic	
		Mean	SD	Mean	SD
MALES					
0–9	59	93.2	8.9	58.6	9.2
10–19	63	107.5	9.6	66.9	8.6
20–29	58	108.4	8.6	69.1	7.3
30–39	30	105.9	8.9	69.4	5.7
40–49	27	106.6	7.6	67.1	6.8
50+	7	100.0	8.2	63.7	8.1
FEMALES					
0–9	60	95.7	12.0	61.6	8.0
10–19	72	104.9	9.7	64.5	10.8
20–29	62	99.8	10.0	62.6	6.6
30–39	32	99.5	10.5	62.9	6.3
40–49	19	97.6	11.4	62.2	16.8
50+	17	105.7	17.7	64.1	7.3

From *Circulation* 52: 146–151, 1975 [40] (by permission of the American Heart Association, Inc.).

were under or slightly above 100 mm of mercury. Meneely and Dahl[3] described and depicted the correlation between intake of salt and prevalence of hypertension in five ethnic groups. The Alaskan Eskimos constituted the group of people with the lowest intake of salt, at an average of 4 g daily, and an absence of hypertension. Our data support the contention that even lower quantities of salt intake suffice for health throughout life and are associated with impressively low mean blood pressures. Among the groups considered to be 'low blood pressure populations,' mean blood pressures similar to those of the Yanomama have been reported for several. These include an aboriginal group in West China[32], 'primitives' of central Australia[53], Carajas of the Amazon basin[52], and Melanesians of New Guinea[35]. It is of interest that in other reports describing a lack of rise in blood pressure with age, the mean systolic blood pressures are in the ranges of 115–125 mm of mercury. Thus, within the societies in which mean blood pressures remain at a plateau throughout adult life, it is possible to distinguish at least two populations based upon the observed ranges in blood pressure. The data on salt intake between these two populations of societies are too scant to enable more than speculation. Certainly for the Yanomama Indians, it is evident that very low salt intake and very low mean blood pressure are correlated. Further observations are required before generalizations of this correlation can be made.

4. COMMENTARY

The prevalence of essential hypertension in civilized populations emphasizes the importance of identifying risk factors in its pathogenesis. The data reviewed in this discussion describe an association of low blood pressure throughout life with low salt intake in unacculturated societies. Published reports also document the ability of man to live in a healthy state in the absence of dietary salt. Given the efficient mechanisms for sodium homeostasis which exist in man, these data can be further interpreted to indicate that the customary salt intake of civilized people far exceeds need. Resolution must be made of the seeming paradox between the known salt appetite of man (and other animals) and the daily intake of excess salt by most people. That salt appetite is an acquired phenomenon, not a response to need, has been persuasively presented by Dahl[2]. Thus, it would seem that delineation of physiological needs for sodium by further studies in our society could result in development of dietary guidelines for maximum intake. In recognition that essential hypertension is multifactorial in origin[6, 39] dietary salt cannot be considered the sole culprit. However, reduction in intake is certainly a simple form of therapy for those in whom other risk factors are present. The difficulty will be, as for other habits, gaining compliance. The rewards well merit the effort.

5. SUMMARY

It is postulated that a severe deficiency of sodium in the environment existing over millions of years influenced and favored the evolution of efficient mechanisms for sodium homeostasis. In man, these are well developed and enable health and survival in the absence of dietary salt. Low salt intake is characteristic of societies in which increases of blood pressure do not occur with age. Based on available data, the groups with the lowest blood pressures also had the lowest intake of salt. These data from unacculturated groups may have relevance for dietary guidelines for populations in whom essential hypertension is frequent and salt intake is high.

Acknowledgments. The studies of the Yanomama Indians cited were supported in part by Department of Energy contract 77-C-02-2828 and National Science Foundation grant DEB-76-20591. My colleagues and I gratefully acknowledge use of the R/V *Alpha Helix* of the National Science Foundation during the summer of 1976. We also thank the Instituto Nacimal des Pesquisas da Amazônia and the Fundacão Nacimal do Indio for the necessary clearances.

REFERENCES

1. Kaunitz H: Causes and consequences of salt consumption. Nature (London) 173:1141-1144, 1956.
2. Dahl LK: Salt intake and salt need. N Engl J Med 258:1152-1157, 1205-1208, 1958.
3. Meneely GR, Dahl LK: Electrolytes in hypertension: the effects of sodium chloride. Med Clin North Am 45:271-283, 1961.
4. Pickering G: High blood pressure. London: J and A Churchill, 1968.
5. Dawber TR, Kannel WB, Kagan A, Donabedian RK, McNamara PM, Pearson G: Environmental factors in hypertension. In: Stamler J, Stamler R, Pullman TN (eds) The epidemiology of hypertension: proceedings of an international symposium. New York: Grune and Stratton, 1967, pp 255-288.
6. Genest J, Nowaczynski W, Boucher R, Kuchel O: Role of the adrenal cortex and sodium in the pathogenesis of human hypertension. Can Med Assoc J 118:538-549, 1978.
7. Dawber TR: Annual discourse — unproved hypotheses. N Engl J Med 299:452-458, 1978.
8. Denton DA: Sodium and hypertension. In: Sambhi MP (ed) Mechanisms of hypertension, proceedings of an international workshop conference, Los Angeles, 7–9 March 1973. Amsterdam: Excerpta Medica, 1973, pp 46-54.
9. Denton DA: The brain and sodium homeostasis. Conditional Reflex 8:125-146, 1973.
10. Denton DA: Evolutionary aspects of the emergence of aldosterone secretion and salt appetite. Physiol Rev 45:245-295, 1965.
11. Konishi J, Zotterman Y: Taste functions in fish. In: Zotterman Y (ed) Olfaction and taste. Oxford: Pergamon, 1963, p 215.
12. Abraham SF, Blaine EH, Blair-West JR, Coghlan JP, Denton DA, Mouw DR, Scroggins BS, Wright RD: New factors in control of aldosterone secretion. In: Scow RO (ed) Proceedings, IV international congress of endocrinology, Washington, DC, 1972. Amsterdam: Excerpta Medica, 1973, pp 733-739.

13. Clarke JD: The prehistory of Africa. New York: Praeger, 1970.
14. Chester-Jones I, Philips JG, Bellamy D: The adrenal cortex throughout the vertebrates. Br Med Bull 18:110-113, 1962.
15. Witschi E, Dale E: Steroid hormones at early development states of vertebrates. Gen Comp Endocrinol Suppl 1:356, 1962.
16. Wright A, Chester-Jones I, Philips JG: The histology of the adrenal gland of the prototheria. J Endocrinol 15:100-107, 1957.
17. Philips JG, Chester-Jones I, Bellamy D, Greep RO, Day LR, Holmes WGN: Corticosteroids in the blood of *myxine glutinose* L. (Atlantic hagfish). Endocrinology 71:329-331, 1962.
18. Chester-Jones I, Philips JG: Adrenocorticosteroids in fish. Zool Soc Land Symp No. 17, p 17, 1960.
19. Philips JG: Adrenocorticosteroids in fish. J Endocrinol 18:37, 1959.
20. Bern HA, Biglieri EG: Personal communication cited by Holmes WH, Philips JG, Chester-Jones I: Adrenocortical factors associated with adaptation of vertebrates to marine environments. Recent Prog Horm Res 19:616, 1963.
21. Ulick S, Solomon S: The synthesis of aldosterone from progesterone by the amphibian adrenal. J Am Chem Soc 82:249, 1960.
22. Philips JG, Chester-Jones I, Bellamy D: Biosynthesis of adrenocortical hormones by adrenal glands of lizards and snakes. J Endocrinol 25:233-237, 1962.
23. Roos R de: In vitro production of corticosteroids by chicken adrenals. Endocrinology 67:719-721, 1960.
24. Sandor T, Lamoureux J, Lanthier A: Adrenocortical function in birds: In vitro biosynthesis of radioactive corticosteroids from pregnenolone-7-H^3 and progesterone-4-C^{14} by adrenal glands of the domestic duck (*Anas platyrhynchos*) and the chicken (*Gallus domesticus*). Endocrinology 73:629-636, 1963.
25. Dittus P: Histologie und Cytologie des Interrenalorgans der Selachier unter normalen und experimentellen Bedingungen. Z Wiss Zool 154:40, 1940.
26. Chester-Jones I: The adrenal cortex. Cambridge: Cambridge University Press, 1957.
27. Gorbman A, Bein HA: Adrenal cortex and interrenal gland. In: A textbook of comparative endocrinology. New York: John Wiley and Sons, 1962, p 297.
28. Bartter FC, Casper AGT, Delea CS, Slater JDH: On the role of the kidney in control of adrenal steroid production. Metabolism 10:1006-1020, 1961.
29. Prosser CL, Kirschner LB: Inorganic ions. In: Prosser CL (ed) Comparative animal physiology, 3rd edn. Philadelphia: WB Saunders, 1973, pp 79-110.
30. Manery JF: Water and electrolyte metabolism. Physiol Rev 34: 334-417, 1954.
31. Schomburgk R: Travels in British Guiana: 1840–1844. Roth WE (trans). Georgetown: Daily Chronicle Press, 1922, pp 125-127.
32. Morse WR, Beh YT: Blood pressure amongst aboriginal ethnic groups of Szechwan Province, West China. Lancet 1:966-967, 1937.
33. Orr JB, Gilks JL: Studies of nutrition: The physique and health of two African tribes. Medical Research Council Spec Rep 155:82, London: His Majesty's stationery office, 1931.
34. Kroeber AL: Culture element distributions. XV. Salt, dogs, tobacco. Anthropol Rec 6:1–6, 1941–1942.
35. Maddocks I: Blood pressure in Melanesians. Med J Aust 1:1123-1126, 1967.
36. Prior IAM, Evans JG, Harvey HPB, Davidson F, Lindsey M: Sodium intake and blood pressure in two Polynesian populations. N Engl J Med 279:515-520, 1968.

37. Denton DA, Nelson JF, Orchard E, Weller S: The role of adrenocortical hormone secretion in salt appetite. In: Pfaffman C (ed) Olfaction and taste. New York: Rockefeller University Press, 1962, pp 535-547.

38. Wheatcroft W: Tifalmin: realms of ritual—key to a world—New Guinea. In: Grosvenor GM (ed) Primitive worlds: people lost in time. Washington DC: National Geographic Society, 1973, pp 57-83.

39. Page LB, Damon A, Moellering RC: Antecedents of cardiovascular disease in six Solomon Island societies. Circulation 49:1132-1146, 1974.

40. Oliver WJ, Cohen EL, Neel JV: Blood pressure, sodium intake and sodium related hormones in the Yanomama Indians, a 'no-salt' culture. Circulation 52:146-151, 1975 (by permission of the American Heart Association, Inc.).

41. Nowaczynski W, Kuchel O, Genest J, Parvin-Pande R, Messerli FH, Grose J, Lebel M: Further evidence of an altered aldosterone metabolism in benign essential hypertension. In: Breuer H, Hughes A, Klopper A, Conti C, Jugblut P, Lerner L (eds) Research on steroids, sixth meeting of the international study group for steroid hormones. New York: American Elsevier, 1975, pp 149-161.

42. Weir RJ, Paintin DB, Brown JJ, Fraser R, Lever AF, Robertson JIS, Young J: A serial study in pregnancy of the plasma concentrations of renin, corticosteroids, electrolytes and proteins and of haematocrit and plasma volume. J Obstet Gynaecol Br Commun 78:590-602. 1974.

42a. Oliver WJ, Neel JV, Grekin RJ, Cohen EL: A note on hormonal adaptation to stresses imposed upon sodium balance by pregnancy and lactation in the Yanomama Indians, a culture without salt. Circulation (in press).

43. Neel JV, Weiss KM: The genetic structure of a tribal population. XII. Biodemographic studies. Am J Phys Anthropol 42:25-52, 1975.

44. Neel JV: Lessons from a 'primitive' people: do recent data concerning South American Indians have relevance to problems of highly civilized communities? Science 170:815-822, 1970.

45. Chagnon NA: Yanomama: the fierce people. New York: Holt, Reinhart and Winston, 1968.

46. Murrill RI: A blood pressure study of the natives of Ponape Island, Eastern Carolines. Hum Biol 21:47-59, 1949.

47. Mann GV, Roels OA, Price DL, Merrill JM: Cardiovascular disease in African pygmies: a survey of the health status, serum lipids, and diet of pygmies in Congo. J Chronic Dis 15:341-371, 1962.

48. Truswell AS, Kenelly BM, Hansen JDL, Lee RB: Blood pressures of !Kung bushman in Northern Botswana. Am Heart J 84:5-12, 1972.

49. Evans JG, Rose G: Hypertension. Br Med Bull 27:37-42, 1971.

50. Blair-West JR, Coghlan JP, Denton DA, Funder JW, Nelson J, Scoggins BA, Wright RD: Sodium homeostasis, salt appetite, and hypertension. Circ Res [Suppl 2] 26-27:251-265, 1970.

51. Maddocks I: Possible absence of essential hypertension in two complete Pacific island populations. Lancet 2:396-399, 1961.

52. Lowenstein FW: Blood pressure in relation to age and sex in the tropics and subtropics. Lancet 1:389-392, 1961.

53. Abbie AL, Schroder J: Blood pressure in Arnhem Land Aborigines. Med J Aust 2:493-496, 1960.

54. Shaper AG: Cardiovascular disease in the tropics: III. Blood pressure and hypertension. Br Med J 3:805-807, 1972.

55. MacFarlane WV: Functional acculturation of Melanesians. I. Salts, hormones and blood changes. Abstracts of the 42nd congress of the Australian and New Zealand association for advancement of science, 1970.

15. BLOOD PRESSURE PATTERNS, SALT USE AND MIGRATION IN THE PACIFIC

I.A.M. Prior and J.M. Stanhope

Epidemiological studies of blood pressure among the differing populations in the Pacific provide a wide range of opportunities for extending knowledge of how environmental and genetic factors interact and influence the rate and extent of changes in arterial pressure with increasing age. The health consequences of hypertension and its sequelae, including stroke and coronary heart disease, constitute major problems in many developed societies yet are virtually absent from certain of the low blood pressure, low-risk populations such as have been described in Pukapuka [1, 2], the Solomon Islands [3], Fiji [4], and New Guinea [5].

The concept of primordial prevention has recently been put forward by a WHO Expert Committee and implies a need to prevent the development of abnormalities such as hypertension and coronary heart disease in those groups in whom the disorders are uncommon but may be increasing as such groups become involved in modernisation, urbanisation and migration [6].

Earlier work in the Pacific, including the studies in Rarotonga and Pukapuka in the Cook Islands [2], gave strength to the hypotheses that changes in body weight and increased salt use were important factors influencing the homeostasis of blood pressure. The demonstration that healthy people could reach old age without any increase of note in systolic and diastolic blood pressure levels was one of the most important contributions from these studies.

Recent physiological studies by Guyton [7] and others have drawn attention to the part played by increased extracellular fluid volume following increased intake of sodium chloride in the genesis of hypertension. We must recognise that in most modern societies the intake of sodium chloride greatly exceeds the requirements for it. Migrants moving from areas where salt is used less become involved in the eating patterns of the parent society and become subject to the risks of such increased exposure.

The experimental work by Dahl has established that there are strong genetic factors controlling responsiveness of rats to sodium, and salt-sensitive and salt-resistant strains have been developed [8].

It is easy to put forward a model in which similar predispositions in humans could play an important role in the setting of blood pressure levels.

H. Kesteloot, J.V. Joossens (eds.), Epidemiology of Arterial Blood Pressure, 243–262.

A possible saturation effect in most western developed societies where the sodium intake is very much greater than the requirement makes it difficult, however, to assess the strength of such a contribution in either an individual or population sample.

The Tokelau Island Migrant Study, which involves the study of non-migrants who are remaining in Tokelau and migrants who move to New Zealand, offers opportunities for further insights into these and related problems [9], The total study population in 1979 comprises 3760 subjects, almost the entire Tokelau living population, of whom 1560 are still living in Tokelau and 2200 living in New Zealand. Detailed genealogies have been built into a complex pedigree genealogical file and are enabling more critical examination of changes in blood pressure, weight and other variables, in subjects in the two environments. The relationship of dietary components, including sodium and potassium intakes and outputs to blood pressure levels, in subjects of varying degrees of relationship in the two environments may well provide further evidence on the correlation between these factors.

Migrant studies, such as the Tokelau study, with subjects living in two distinct environments provide some measure of control for genetic homogeneity and temporal changes. This, we believe, provides a quasi-experimental situation which may prove to be one of the most valuable contributions coming from the South Pacific. The need for such studies has been emphasised by Kempthorne [10]. The present report will review some of the results from the Cook Island Surveys [2, 11] carried out in 1964, and from the Tokelau Island Migrant Study which has been developed since 1966. Blood pressure patterns, habitual salt use and the concomitant factors influencing blood pressures in adults and children in the two environments will be considered.

1. METHODS

1.1. Populations and samples

1.1.1. Cook Islands. The total population of the Cook Island group in 1964 was 19,214 subjects scattered in islands over a wide area of the South Pacific. Rarotonga, the main island of the Cook group, had a total population of 9768.

The sample in Rarotonga was drawn from a household census in the main town of Avarua, of subjects who had lived for ten years or more in an urban environment. A total of 480 people aged 20 years and over were in the sample, and 98% participation of subjects was achieved.

Pukapuka is a small atoll in the Northern Cooks with a total population of

796 in 1964, of whom 100% were examined. The Cook Island Maoris are Polynesians and have historical and cultural links with the New Zealand Maori.

1.1.2. Tokelau. Tokelau is a group of three small atolls situated 480 km north of Samoa and 3600 km north-east of New Zealand. The population is predominantly Polynesian. The Tokelauan society is small, cohesive and relatively insulated from western industrial culture and consequently the island life styles and values are still very traditional.

In 1925 Tokelau became a New Zealand dependency, and in 1948 they were granted rights as New Zealand citizens, with free right of entry to New Zealand. However, little migration occurred prior to 1965. In early 1966, a hurricane devastated tree crops and the New Zealand Government set up a resettlement programme to bring migrants to New Zealand to relieve food shortages and overcrowding. Details of the research design and sampling have been published and will be briefly summarised [9].

The longitudinal survey of health and disease among Tokelauans has been conducted in New Zealand since 1967 and in Tokelau since 1968. For logistic reasons, only one of the three Tokelau atolls, Fakaofo, was surveyed in detail in 1968. The residents of the remaining two atolls, Atafu and Nukunonu, together with a small group of Fakaofo residents who had been absent at a church conference and for other reasons, were surveyed in detail in 1971. A complete survey of Tokelau was carried out in 1976.

In New Zealand, a register of government-sponsored migrant Tokelauans was commenced in 1966. From 1971, self-sponsored and family-sponsored migrants, direct from Tokelau and indirect after some years of residence in Samoa, were also included in the register. Three surveys of all registered Tokelauans in New Zealand have been held in 1967–70, 1972–74 and in 1975–77.

1.2. Tokelau census data

1.2.1. Tokelau. In 1968, the total population of the three atolls was 1750: 906 adults aged 15 years and over, and 744 children under 15. In 1971, the total population was 1639: 877 adults aged 15 years and over, and 762 children under 15. In 1976, the total population was 1558: 835 adults aged 15 and over, and 723 children under 15.

1.2.2. Tokelauans in New Zealand. In 1966, there were approximately 600 Tokelauans in New Zealand, based on national census data. In December 1973, the total on the register was 1961: 1014 adults aged 15 years and over, and 947 children under 15. In 1977, the register was updated and the total was 2534: 1250 adults aged 15 years and over, and 1284 children under 15.

1.3. Participation

Participation in Tokelau has been approximately 98% in successive surveys, while in New Zealand it has been approximately 94% in the two major rounds of examinations. This report will compare the findings in the Tokelau 1971 survey and the New Zealand 1972–74 survey. The children's results will be based on the examination in Tokelau in 1976 and in New Zealand in 1975 of those under 15 years of age.

1.4. Blood pressure and anthropometric measurements

In the Cook Island survey, sitting blood pressures were taken by a physician using a standard sphygmomanometer and recording fourth phase as the diastolic pressure. Since 1968, random-zero muddler sphygmomanometers have been used in the Tokelau study to measure the sitting blood pressures, taking fourth phase as the diastolic pressure. Since 1970, the mean of two measurements, one by a physician and one by a research assistant, have been used [12]. The methods used in these studies have been detailed in previous publications and essentially follow the recommendations of WHO [13].

1.5. Urinary electrolyte estimations

Details of the methods and results of the 24-h collections and casual urinary sodium concentrations in the Cook Islands [2] and for the 1968 Tokelau survey have been published [9]. Estimations of the urinary sodium and potassium electrolytes, uric acids and creatinines were carried out on frozen aliquots in the unit laboratory. Urinary electrolytes were estimated on an EEL flame photometer, and uric acids and creatinines by auto-analyser methods [9].

In Tokelau in 1968, two consecutive 24-h collections were obtained from 204 adults, and single 24-h collections from 154 subjects. In 1971, multiple collections were made in subsamples on up to five separate occasions.

The means have been taken for each subject in order to reduce the intra-individual variation and get a better measure of habitual sodium and potassium intake. A total of 513 subjects collected 24-h samples during the two visits, 1968 and 1971; 31% had one, 53% had two, 4% had three, 3% had four and 3% had five collections.

1.6. Early morning urinary specimens

Samples of the first urine specimens passed on awakening were collected from 354 males and 461 females in Tokelau in 1971, and from 527 males and 427 females in New Zealand in 1972-74, and used for estimating the sodium and potassium concentrations.

2. STATISTICAL METHOD FOR BLOOD PRESSURE REGRESSION

The regression of systolic and fourth-phase diastolic blood pressures with selected variables was examined for each sex separately. The selected variables were examination history, age, Quetelet index, serum cholesterol and uric acid concentrations, whole blood haemoglobin concentration, duration of stay in New Zealand, and place of examination.

Examination history was classified as to whether the subject's blood pressure was being recorded by the survey team for the first time or not. Age was recorded in years. A quadratic term was included to allow for a non-linear relationship between blood pressure and age.

Time in New Zealand was recorded as the time from first arrival to examination in years. Subjects examined in Tokelau were scored zero.

Place of examination was classified as New Zealand or Tokelau.

Nature of examination was classified as full medical/anthropometric or abbreviated, but was not found to relate significantly to either blood pressure in either sex, and was dropped from analysis.

Packed cell volume was found to relate less significantly to blood pressure than did haemoglobin concentration, and non-significantly when haemoglobin concentration was taken into account. Accordingly, it was dropped from analysis.

As a measure of the comparative strength of relationship between each selected variable and blood pressure, a standardised increment of blood pressure associated with each selected variable was calculated, as the change in blood pressure associated with a one-standard-deviation increase in the selected variable. Since age included a quadratic term, the one-standard-deviation interval chosen was equally distributed about the mean age.

Urinary Na and K and Na/K ratio in 24-h and early morning specimens were correlated with systolic and diastolic blood pressures, both before and after adjustment for the selected variables. The regression coefficients obtained by multiple regression analysis were used in this adjustment.

2.1. Blood pressure and social interaction

The administration of sociological questionnaires to adult Tokelauans in New Zealand in 1972–73 enabled the development of a social interaction score for each subject. The questionnaires measured the extent to which subjects in New Zealand were still involved with Tokelauans in social interactions, church, leisure and work, and the extent to which they had moved into a non-Tokelauan or New Zealand (NZ) network.

The basic hypotheses being tested related to the way in which involvement in NZ society and social patterns for which they had not been accustomed or prepared during childhood would initiate neurohumoural changes raising blood pressure. Involvement in a primarily Tokelau environment in NZ was thought likely to protect or cushion subjects to a much greater degree and so lessen the effect on blood pressure. Details of the questionnaires and methods of analysis and results have been published [14].

2.2. Tokelau children's studies

The blood pressures being reported in this chapter were measured by the one observer during examinations in 1975 in New Zealand and in 1976 in Tokelau. The pressures were taken using a random-zero sphygmomanometer after a period of 3–4 min sitting in a quiet room. Cuff sizes were chosen to fit comfortably, according to the size of the arm. In this report, adjustments were made according to cuff size to conform with previous studies [15]. Heights, weights and anthropometric measurements were taken in a standard method.-

3. RESULTS

3.1. Cook Island survey

The 1964 studies in Rarotonga and Pukapuka showed considerable differences between the groups in blood pressure, weights, 24-h urinary sodium output and casual urinary sodium concentrations. The Pukapukans showed only a minor increase in blood pressure with age in contrast to the Rarotongans where a much steeper rise occurred in both men and women. A comparison of the systolic and diastolic blood pressures by sex and age is shown in Figure 1. The mean weights of Rarotongans were much greater than those of the Pukapukans for both men and women, and are shown in Figure 2.

The mean 24-h sodium outputs were 62 meq ± 7 SE and 64 meq ± 7 SE for men and women in Pukapuka compared with 114 meq ± 9.9 SE and 102 meq ± 9 SE in Rarotonga. The urine volumes were higher in Pukapuka than in Rarotonga [2]. The mean casual urinary sodium concentrations by sex

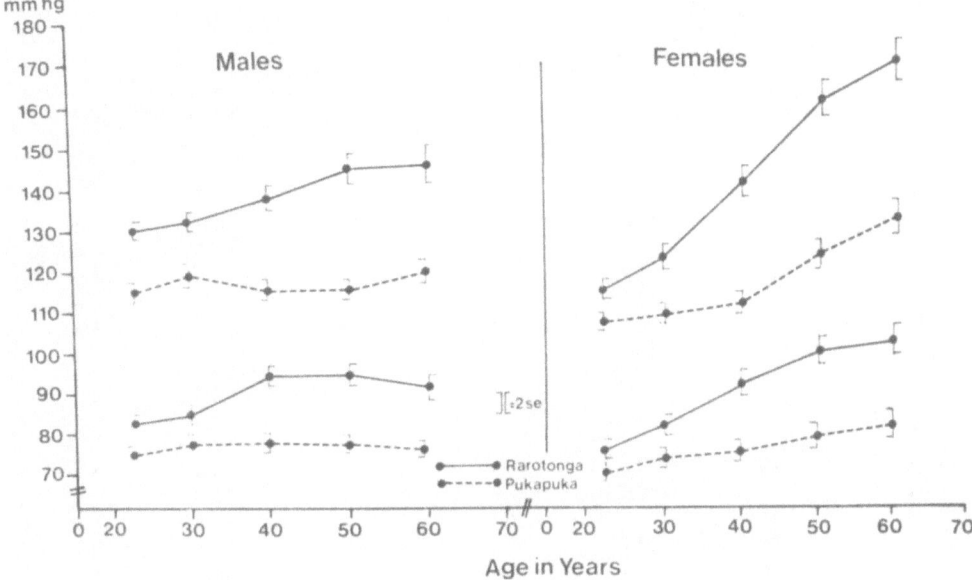

Figure 1. Mean systolic and diastolic blood pressures in Rarotonga and Pukapuka by age and sex.

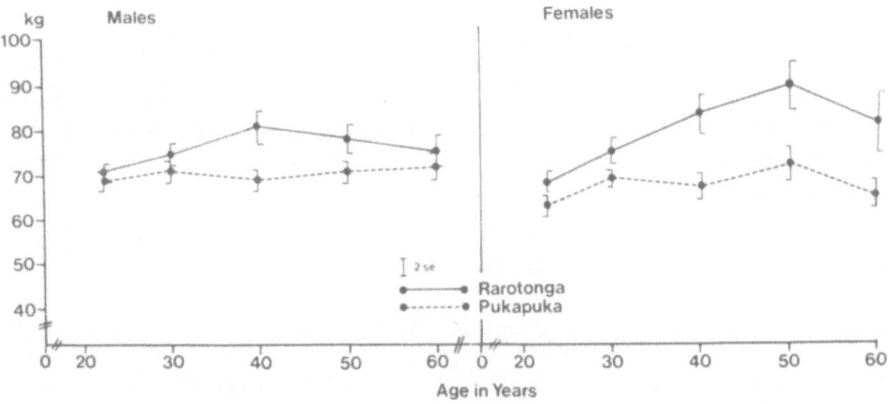

Figure 2. Mean weights (kg) in Rarotonga and Pukapuka by age and sex.

and age are shown for Rarotonga and Pukapuka in Table 1. The concentrations are higher in Rarotonga than Pukapuka in both men and women, and follow the same pattern shown in the 24-h urine outputs. No within-population correlations of 24-h urinary sodium output and systolic and diastolic blood pressures were shown in the Cook Island survey. The between-population differences in blood pressure and sodium output were highly significant, and only a small amount of the difference in blood pressure could be attributed to weight.

250

Table 1. Rarotonga and Pukapuka mean casual urinary sodiums (mmol/l) by age and sex.

Age (years)	Rarotonga			Pukapuka		
	n	Mean	SE	*n*	Mean	SE
MALE						
20–24	39	128.3	9.1	27	69.0	7.8
25–34	53	135.1	6.3	39	63.0	6.4
35–44	34	135.9	7.8	37	86.3	7.9
45–54	44	127.8	6.1	39	61.9	6.6
55–64	21	108.3	9.3	30	59.4	5.8
65–74	12	116.8	11.3	7	33.4	8.4
75–84	8	93.0	18.8	7	28.3	12.1
FEMALE						
20–24	39	122.0	7.5	23	80.4	8.8
25–34	42	126.3	7.9	50	68.0	6.5
35–44	34	118.2	8.4	29	77.0	8.9
45–54	29	114.5	8.4	25	65.9	7.1
55–64	24	90.5	7.4	31	59.4	6.1
65–74	9	109.1	12.8	11	64.0	15.3
75–84	7	104.6	6.2	4	43.0	18.3

3.2. Tokelau (1971) and Tokelauans in New Zealand (1972–74)

3.2.1. Cross-sectional studies: Blood pressure patterns. The systolic and diastolic pressures of the migrants to New Zealand are significantly higher than are the pressures of those who remained in Tokelau. The levels in Tokelau are higher than those found in Pukapuka, and the rate of increase with age is greater. Body weights show an increase in New Zealand. The weights in Tokelau are significantly higher than those in Pukapuka. The systolic and

Table 2. Tokelauan adults: mean systolic blood pressure (mmHg) by age group, sex and place.

Age group	Tokelau 1971						New Zealand 1972–74					
	Male			Female			Male			Female		
	n	Mean	SE	*n*	Mean	SE	*n*	Mean	SE	*n*	Mean	SE
15–19	71	113.5	1.3	84	113.5	1.2	88	115.8	1.2	77	107.7	1.2
20–24	28	119.1	2.1	58	115.6	1.6	94	124.2	1.2	79	113.0	1.3
25–34	52	120.3	1.7	66	115.9	1.7	155	130.8	1.1	116	118.4	1.2
35–44	63	120.5	1.5	88	120.9	1.7	87	133.6	1.6	60	130.7	2.9
45–54	64	124.6	2.2	61	137.8	2.3	61	135.3	2.2	45	140.5	3.7
55–64	39	134.5	4.1	43	142.9	4.3	39	143.0	4.0	34	155.8	4.6
65–74	36	142.8	4.4	57	150.4	3.9	18	156.8	6.4	20	164.4	6.2
75–84	13	161.3	7.8	17	159.3	6.2	6	150.2	12.6	4	150.2	5.0

Table 3. Tokelauan adults: mean diastolic (fourth phase) blood pressure (mmHg) by age group, sex and place.

Age group	Tokelau 1971						New Zealand 1972–74					
	Male			Female			Male			Female		
	n	Mean	SE	*n*	Mean	SE	*n*	Mean	SE	*n*	Mean	SE
15–19	71	65.8	0.8	84	66.8	1.0	88	68.8	1.0	77	67.6	1.2
20–24	28	65.0	2.2	58	67.5	1.2	94	72.0	1.0	79	69.0	0.9
25–34	52	68.2	1.4	66	69.6	1.4	155	81.1	0.9	116	75.1	1.0
35–44	63	70.1	1.1	88	72.6	1.1	87	84.3	1.0	60	81.2	1.8
45–54	64	71.3	1.4	61	81.7	1.4	61	82.4	1.4	45	83.3	2.2
55–64	39	75.8	2.4	43	78.6	2.4	39	84.8	2.1	34	87.8	2.8
65–74	36	74.8	1.8	57	78.7	2.0	18	85.7	3.3	20	88.7	3.0
75–84	13	80.1	3.8	17	83.4	3.5	6	79.6	5.7	4	80.5	8.5

Table 4. Tokelauan adults: mean body weight (kg) by age group, sex and place.

Age group	Tokelau 1971						New Zealand 1972–74					
	Male			Female			Male			Female		
	n	Mean	SE	*n*	Mean	SE	*n*	Mean	SE	*n*	Mean	SE
15–19	71	63.0	1.1	84	65.7	1.0	88	69.3	0.9	77	66.5	1.1
20–24	28	69.3	1.1	58	69.7	1.4	92	73.8	0.9	79	70.0	1.5
25–35	52	77.9	1.9	66	74.0	1.8	155	81.8	1.0	116	78.1	1.5
35–44	63	76.0	1.5	88	76.9	1.4	87	84.9	1.4	60	81.1	1.7
45–54	62	79.4	1.6	61	79.6	2.0	60	79.0	1.8	45	83.6	2.1
55–64	36	73.9	1.7	42	72.9	1.9	39	81.6	2.1	34	79.5	2.2
65–74	35	67.4	2.0	50	68.7	2.2	18	78.4	2.9	20	71.0	2.3
75–84	11	69.3	3.7	15	57.3	2.0	5	72.6	5.4	3	67.7	3.4

Table 5. Tokelauan adults in Tokelau: mean 24-h urinary sodium and potassium (mmol) excretion.

Age group	Sodium						Potassium					
	Male			Female			Male			Female		
	n	Mean	SE	*n*	Mean	SE	*n*	Mean	SE	*n*	Mean	SE
15–19	9	25.8	6.7	8	27.1	2.3	9	59.3	15.2	8	54.1	10.9
20–24	14	44.2	8.9	18	34.9	5.5	14	83.1	12.6	18	56.2	6.6
25–34	47	52.1	5.8	38	34.3	3.7	46	99.3	8.0	38	51.5	3.5
35–44	65	42.4	3.7	70	41.7	3.5	65	93.7	5.0	70	61.5	4.0
45–54	48	53.9	6.3	56	37.3	3.1	48	88.6	9.1	56	63.8	4.5
55–64	30	40.1	4.5	43	31.0	3.3	30	71.0	4.8	43	52.0	3.7
65–74	17	41.4	6.6	21	32.4	4.8	17	62.1	8.3	21	46.3	3.4
75–84	4	26.2	8.8	7	29.1	5.6	4	39.5	8.3	7	53.9	12.3

Table 6. Tokelauan adults in Tokelau: mean 24-h urinary creatinine and water excretion.

| Age group | Creatinine (mmol) | | | | | | Water (1) | | | | | |
| | Male | | | Female | | | Male | | | Female | | |
	n	Mean	SE	n	Mean	SE	n	Mean	SE	n	Mean	SE
15–19	5	8.1	1.9	8	4.9	1.0	9	0.69	0.09	9	0.62	0.09
20–24	7	10.3	1.7	10	5.9	0.7	14	0.91	0.09	19	0.62	0.08
25–34	34	11.0	0.7	29	6.4	0.4	47	0.98	0.06	38	0.71	0.05
35–44	47	10.3	0.6	53	6.7	0.4	65	1.06	0.05	70	0.85	0.05
45–54	38	10.7	0.8	42	6.1	0.3	48	1.05	0.07	56	0.81	0.05
55–64	22	8.7	0.8	35	5.4	0.4	29	0.87	0.05	43	0.75	0.05
65–74	14	6.9	0.8	18	5.6	0.4	17	0.98	0.11	21	0.82	0.08
75–84	4	6.1	0.5	5	3.7	0.6	4	1.12	0.36	7	0.86	0.24

Table 7. Tokelauan adults: mean early morning urinary sodium concentration (mmol/l) by age group, sex and place.

| Age group | Tokelau 1971 | | | | | | New Zealand 1972–74 | | | | | |
| | Male | | | Female | | | Male | | | Female | | |
	n	Mean	SE	n	Mean	SE	n	Mean	SE	n	Mean	SE
15–19	68	47.7	6.0	81	61.3	5.7	85	132.2	6.6	76	117.7	6.7
20–24	27	46.9	7.0	56	62.5	5.3	92	107.5	5.6	77	107.8	6.5
25–34	52	45.1	5.7	64	55.9	6.0	152	100.3	3.8	114	108.2	4.8
35–44	62	34.9	4.1	88	49.3	4.3	83	109.9	5.2	60	95.8	8.8
45–54	62	39.9	4.6	61	54.6	5.3	56	92.8	5.8	45	89.3	6.1
55–64	36	53.4	8.1	42	43.3	5.8	37	84.0	7.2	33	97.3	8.9
65–74	36	48.2	6.3	54	50.0	5.0	17	105.6	8.9	20	88.7	12.8
75–84	11	61.2	16.5	15	38.3	6.0	5	73.6	15.1	2	85.0	5.0

Table 8. Tokelauan adults: mean early morning urinary potassium concentration (mmol/l) by age group, sex and place.

| Age group | Tokelau 1971 | | | | | | New Zealand 1972–74 | | | | | |
| | Male | | | Female | | | Male | | | Female | | |
	n	Mean	SE	n	Mean	SE	n	Mean	SE	n	Mean	SE
15–19	67	110.0	8.4	81	113.3	9.0	85	64.0	3.9	76	63.6	3.3
20–24	27	106.9	10.1	56	112.7	9.2	92	57.0	3.5	77	58.6	3.4
25–34	52	109.0	8.0	65	85.9	7.4	152	62.1	2.5	114	63.6	2.8
35–44	62	89.2	6.4	88	90.2	7.9	83	56.9	3.0	60	55.4	3.5
45–54	62	82.9	7.1	61	80.5	6.8	56	55.4	3.5	45	53.4	3.8
55–64	36	90.1	8.4	42	77.7	7.3	37	54.0	5.0	33	52.0	4.8
65–74	36	74.0	6.4	54	91.1	7.4	17	47.8	5.2	20	53.6	7.6
75–84	11	98.5	17.1	15	76.4	20.6	5	34.8	6.0	2	52.0	24.0

diastolic fourth phase blood pressure (mmHg) and weights (kg) in the two environments are listed by age and sex in Tables 2–4.

The mean 24-h urine sodium and potassium outputs collected in Tokelau in 1968 and 1971 are listed by age and sex in Table 5. The 24-h urinary mean creatinine levels and urinary volumes by age and sex are shown in Table 6 for those seen in Tokelau. The early morning urinary sodium and potassium concentrations by age and sex for both Tokelau and New Zealand are listed in Tables 7 and 8. The notably high concentration of sodium in New Zealand and the lower concentration of potassium are clearly seen.

3.3. Correlation of blood pressures with urine constituents

The correlation of systolic and diastolic blood pressures with the 24-h urinary sodium, potassium, sodium–potassium ratio, creatinine and volume has been carried out on the 475 subjects from whom 24-h samples were collected in Tokelau. The correlations have been estimated with both the unadjusted and with age-adjusted blood pressures. The results of the correlation of the unadjusted systolic and diastolic pressures and 24-h urine sodium, potassium concentrations and sodium–potassium ratios, are shown in Table 9.

Table 9. Tokelauan adults: correlation of blood pressures with urinary sodium and potassium.

	Males		Females	
	Systolic	Diastolic fourth phase	Systolic	Diastolic fourth phase
24-Hour				
Sodium	(0.052)	(0.014)	(0.023)	(0.041)
Potassium	(−0.081)	(0.001)	(0.004)	(0.042)
Na/K ratio	0.192	(0.119)	(−0.003)	(0.006)
Early morning urine				
Sodium	0.122	0.186	−0.136	−0.074
Potassium	−0.092	−0.125	−0.105	−0.142
Na/K ratio	0.122	0.182	−0.062	(−0.020)

Coefficients in parentheses are non-significant ($P > 0.05$).

The only significant correlation is with Na/K ratio where the $R = 0.192$, and this became insignificant when age-adjusted pressures were used. The correlations of systolic and diastolic pressures with early morning sodium and potassium concentrations and sodium–potassium ratios have been examined in subjects from both Tokelau and New Zealand, and the results are also shown in Table 9. The significant correlations shown with early morning

Table 10. Tokelauan adults: regression of blood pressure with selected variables.

Variable	Unit	Regression coefficients				Standardised increments [a]			
		Systolic BP		Diastolic BP (4th)		Systolic BP		Diastolic BP (4th)	
		Males	Females	Males	Females	Males	Females	Males	Females
First examination	yes = 1, no = 0	(1.765)	2.176	2.644	2.709	0.826	1.052	1.238	1.310
Age	years	−0.403	−0.017	0.267	0.356	5.051 [b]	10.378	3.380	4.021
Age squared	years [b]	0.009	0.008	(−0.001)	(−0.002)				
Quetelet index	kg/m^2	1.580	1.527	1.046	0.861	6.174	7.975	4.088	4.48
Serum cholesterol	mmol/l	1.392	(0.098)	0.634	(0.274)	1.414	0.102	0.644	0.286
Serum uric acid	mmol/l	12.908	(13.748)	11.470	21.046	1.038	1.057	0.923	1.618
Haemoglobin	g/l	(0.038)	0.190	(0.013)	0.166	0.538	2.478	0.184	2.154
Time in New Zealand	years	0.373	(0.198)	0.382	(0.167)	1.232	0.565	1.263	0.477
Place of examination	NZ = 1, Tok = 0	(1.099)	−6.217	3.242	±3.232	0.542	−2.882	1.601	−1.498
Constant	mmHg	63.125	53.548	18.810	15.581				

[a] Change in pressure, in mmHg, associated with a one-standard-deviation increase in the selected variable.
[b] Change about the mean age, i.e. from 28.9 to 46.1 in males and from 29.2 to 47.6 in females.
Coefficients in parentheses are non-significant ($P > 0.05$).

concentrations also became insignificant when age-adjusted pressures were used.

3.4. Regression of blood pressure with selected variables

The regression coefficients of blood pressures with selected variables have been estimated in Tokelauan adults examined in Tokelau and in New Zealand, and are presented in Table 10. The standardised increments, which represent the change in systolic and diastolic pressures associated with a one-standard-deviation increase in the selected variable, are also shown in Table 10. This analysis confirms the greater effect of age on both systolic and diastolic pressures in females compared with males.

Body mass (Quetelet) changes make an important contribution to blood pressure increase in both sexes and influence change more than increases in cholesterol and uric acid levels. The decrease in systolic pressure in females in NZ compared with those in Tokelau in the regression analysis is anomalous and may be due to interaction of body mass and other changes related to time in New Zealand. The mean systolic pressures presented in Table 2 show those in Tokelau under age 24 were higher than those in NZ, while the converse is found in remaining age groups.

The body mass changes and age stand out as being most important factors contributing to blood pressure change in these studies.

3.5. Blood pressure and social interaction

The findings in this cross-sectional examination of blood pressure and social interaction show higher blood pressures and more subjects with significant hypertension in those who are interacting primarily with the NZ or non-Tokelau society than in those who are still involved in a more Tokelauan interaction family, work and community network. The amount of the variance that can be explained on the basis of social interaction is small, 2.1% in males and 1.4% in females, compared with that due to body weight and length of stay in New Zealand, which explained about five times as much of the total variance [14].

3.6. Tokelau children's study

The mean systolic blood pressures in children in Tokelau in 1976 and in New Zealand in 1975 are shown in Figures 3 and 4. In both boys and girls, the systolic and diastolic pressures are higher in New Zealand than in Tokelau. The weights and body mass are greater in the NZ children than in those in Tokelau, but weight differences account for only part of the blood pressure differences. The casual morning urinary sodium concentrations were lower in

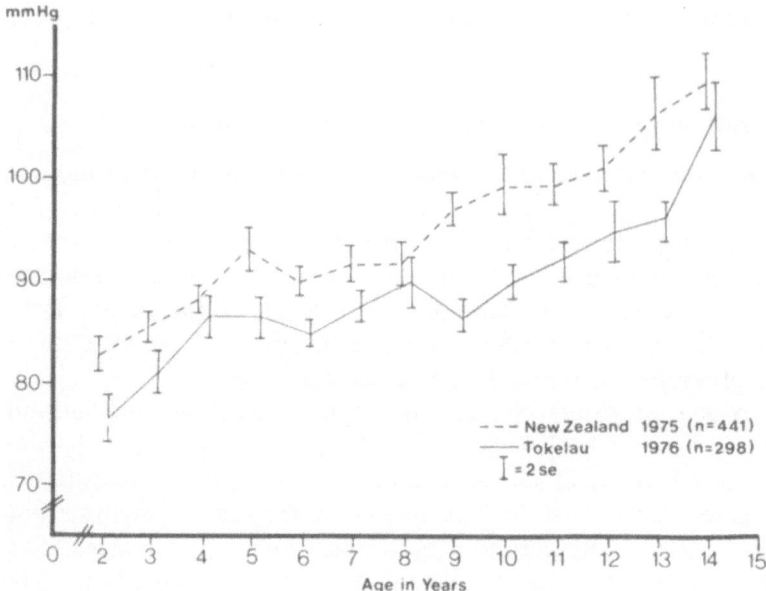

Figure 3. Mean systolic blood pressures* in Tokelau boys in Tokelau and New Zealand by age.

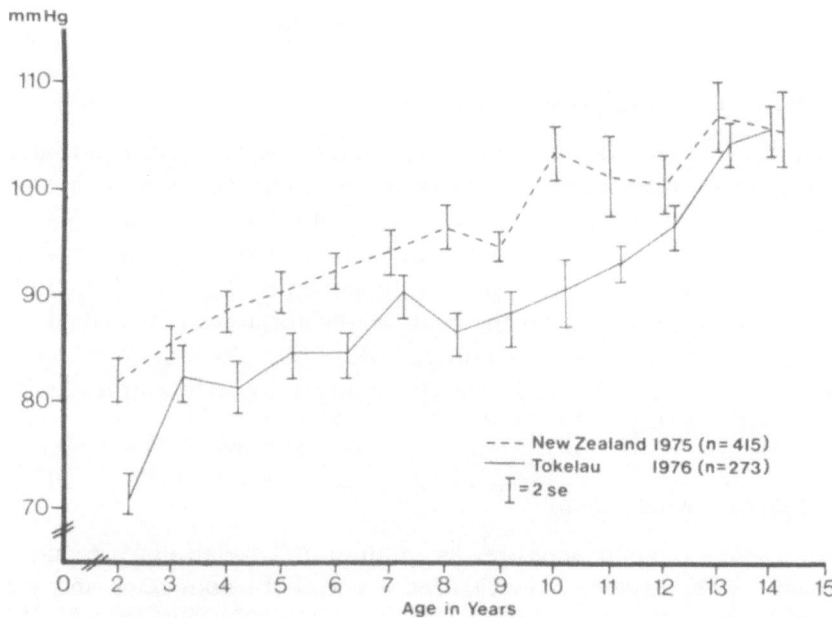

Figure 4. Mean systolic blood pressures* in Tokelau girls in Tokelau and New Zealand by age.

* Average of two readings adjusted for cuff size.

Tokelau than in New Zealand. A correlation of systolic blood pressure and urinary sodium was demonstrated, but this became insignificant when adjusted for age [15].

Longitudinal studies have shown a significantly greater increase in blood pressure and weight in younger migrant children in NZ than in non-migrants of the same age remaining in Tokelau. The differences in both blood pressure and weight were less marked in children who were aged 9–14 years at the time of migration to NZ [16].

4. DISCUSSION

The blood pressure patterns described in different Pacific populations have helped to confirm that an increase in blood pressure with age is not an inevitable characteristic of aging, and that the rate at which it occurs shows considerable variation.

Epstein and Eckoff [17], in their important review article on the epidemiology of blood pressure, pointed out that the level in young adults was also important in that some populations could have similar slopes of increase with age but still have higher or lower age-specific mean pressures.

Cassel [18, 19] drew attention to the way in which certain migrant studies could enable the testing of hypotheses during the dynamic process of change, providing certain conditions could be met. He confirmed that the majority, if not all, of those populations showing little or only minor increase of blood pressure with age came from isolated traditional societies where little in the way of urbanisation or modernisation had taken place, where traditional customs were respected, where subjects knew their place and the expected responses to different situations they faced as they grew up and took their place in the family and community. The concept of supportive or protective factors and stressful factors each playing a role and influencing the process of adaptation and the setting of blood pressure levels in individuals and groups was put forward.

Cassel suggested that a disjunction between the role a migrant found himself in in the new society and the extent of his preparedness for such, by virtue of his growth and development in a traditional, more-limited society, could be initiators of a series of neuro-endocrine and circulatory changes that contributed to blood pressure increase. This can be put forward as the psychosocial hypothesis while the alternate represents the physical hypothesis and attributes changes to environmental factors, including changes in diet, body weight, physical exercise and temperature.

Alteration in habitual salt intake, in sodium–potassium ratio in the diet, and increase in protein and overall calories are some of the specific dietary changes to be considered. It must be accepted that both hypotheses could contribute and that the balance could vary in different individuals and populations.

The Tokelau study provides valuable opportunities to examine the consequences of migration and urbanisation in a population of Polynesians who came from a traditional, small, isolated atoll society to the very different pattern of living in urban industrialised New Zealand [9].

Kempthorne [10] writing about genetic epidemiology and the opportunities and techniques it provides for examining the genetic versus environmental factors contributing to a variety of disorders, describes the limitations of observational population studies and stresses the need for an experimental research design if real progress is to be made.

The major complex pedigree files that have been developed from the anthropologists' genealogies, and the fact that the longitudinal Tokelau study includes those non-migrants remaining in Tokelau and those who have migrated to New Zealand, provides the basis of a quasi-experimental research design that has few counterparts in migrant studies.

The cross-sectional studies reported in this paper confirm that Tokelauans in Tokelau have blood pressure levels that are higher than those in Pukapuka, and show an increase with age in men and women which is greater in the women than in men. The Tokelau migrants in New Zealand have significantly higher pressures than those in Tokelau. The greater weight and body mass of those in New Zealand contributes in part to the blood pressure increase, but a considerable amount of the variance remains unexplained. The habitual sodium intake in Tokelau in the period 1968–71 has been defined by the 24-h urine outputs and is in the 40–50 meq Na/24 h range. Efforts were made to collect multiple samples in both 1968 and in 1971 in an effort to lessen the intra-individual differences: 53% collected two samples and smaller numbers collected three or more. The intake is not as low as in some groups, but is nevertheless less than that found in urban Rarotongans and most westernised groups.

The 24-h potassium outputs are high in Tokelau, and men have higher outputs than women. Quite clearly, the nature of the diet in Tokelau provides a balance of Na/K that is increasingly being recognised as having some protective role in relationship to the setting of individual and community blood pressure levels. Limited 24-h collections among Tokelauans in New Zealand have shown much higher Na and lower K output.

The early morning urinary Na, K and Na/K ratios were introduced as a further measure of Na and K use by individuals. The mean levels shown in Tokelau and in New Zealand support higher sodium use in Tokelauans in New Zealand with lower potassium, and indicate that this measure can be used to help characterise the overall Na/K use by a population subsample.

The introduction of timed overnight urine samples has been an important step, and the high correlation which urinary sodium and potassium output by this technique shows with 24-h output confirms the method as a valid technique for epidemiological studies[20].

The failure to show a significant correlation of 24-h urinary Na with systolic or diastolic pressures after adjusting for age in Tokelau may relate to the considerable intra-individual variability that can be present that is not properly defined unless multiple samples are collected. A similar lack of correlation was reported in the Cook Island study in 1964[2].

A correlation of Na and K in the early morning specimens and Na/K ratio to the systolic and diastolic pressure also became insignificant when pressures were adjusted for age.

The recent work by Guyton[7] and others, stressing the part which expansion of extracellular fluid in response to sodium intake may play in the initiation of hypertension, is gaining wider acceptance. The way in which the arterial wall sodium and calcium level may influence vascular reactivity and, in this way, contribute to peripheral resistance appears reasonable and needs further study.

The fact that there may be genetic factors controlling the cell membrane responsiveness to electrolytes, in particular to Na, Ca and K, that can thereby influence arteriolar tone could link in with the identification of subjects who, like Dahl's rats, may be salt sensitive or salt insensitive.

The availability of an indirect measure of the intramuscle cell sodium of the blood vessel wall by using red blood cells offers a new method for exploring these issues further.

Garay and Meyer[21] demonstrated differences in net Na^+ and K^+ fluxes in red cells of subjects with essential hypertension and in normotensive siblings of hypertensive and normotensive families. This seems to indicate genetic transmission and suggests that the method may help detect subjects liable to high blood pressure. The opportunity this method would give of examining for familial aggregation of cellular Na content in population subsamples, and of determining whether there are differences between close relatives in Tokelau and in New Zealand, raises some exciting possibilities in exploring the genetic versus environmental contribution to blood pressure level.

A preliminary examination of the genetic analyses comparing migrants in New Zealand, premigrants, prior to migration and non-migrants who have remained in Tokelau, suggests that genetic factors become more important, particularly in adult migrants in New Zealand, in influencing blood pressure levels. This is shown by much stronger familial aggregation of pressures in families in New Zealand where children are adult, compared with those where children are still under age 13 if female and 17 if male.

The combined genetic and socio-cultural factors account for around 58% of the variance in those in New Zealand with adult families, this compares with only 18% in those whose families are still juvenile [21].

The capacity to identify subjects who may be at risk and who are sensitive to Na and K intake could represent a most important advance and enable intervention in such subjects.

The results of the Tokelau children's blood pressure analyses show that factors are present in New Zealand which influence blood pressure levels from an early age leading to higher levels in New Zealand. Weight changes contribute partly to this, but there are clearly other unidentified factors. The casual urinary sodium concentrations were higher in New Zealand resident children, but in neither group was there a significant partial correlation controlling for age between casual urinary sodium concentrations and systolic blood pressure levels. Certainly, the fact that about one-half of the difference in systolic pressure in boys and one-third of the difference in girls under eight years of age can be attributed to the heavier weight of the New Zealand children is of potential significance from a preventive viewpoint.

The evidence that blood pressure levels in childhood may be predictive of adult pressures has been demonstrated in this and other studies [22]. Further evidence will be obtained from the longitudinal studies which will offer scope for identification of high-risk children.

The rapid changes associated with migration and urbanisation in many areas of the Pacific are contributing to increased risk of hypertension and coronary heart disease. However, much has yet to be learned of the factors contributing. Opportunities exist for exploration of new hypotheses and methods that could help identify the balance of genetic and environmental contributions. There is already sufficient data to confirm the part played by weight gain in migrants, both adult and child, and methods of effective intervention need to be developed.

Habitual salt intake stands out as important in contributing to between-population differences in blood pressure levels, but more work must be done to examine this hypothesis. There is a need for more detailed studies looking for within-population correlations between sodium and potassium intake and blood pressure, and for major intervention studies to test the effect of low-sodium high-potassium dietary regimes. If established, control of sodium and potassium intake could provide a public health and community approach of great value, particularly if linked with measures to control weight gain. Time, funding and more research will be needed to achieve these goals.

The Tokelau Island Migrant Study and its further development will help to contribute to these important areas of knowledge concerning the epidemiology of hypertension and its control and prevention.

5. SUMMARY

Epidemiological studies of blood pressure and cardiovascular risk have demonstrated wide gradients between different Pacific populations. Divergent patterns in Polynesians have suggested that ecological factors play an important role in the regulation of blood pressure and the development of increased cardiovascular risk status. Modernisation and moves towards western life styles with undue weight gain and a much greater habitual use of salt in the diet were shown in 1964 to be factors separating the low blood pressure and lower risk Pukapukans from the higher blood pressure and higher risk Rarotongans in the Cook Islands.

The Tokelau Island Migrant Study provides data on the effects of migration of atoll-dwelling Tokelauans from their traditional Polynesian society to the very different industrial New Zealand environment. This is being assisted by the development of a complex pedigree file linking all subjects in the two environments.

Higher blood pressures have been shown in migrants compared with non-migrants in both children and adults. Sodium intake in the migrants to New Zealand increases while potassium intake lessens, but a significant correlation with blood pressure has not yet been demonstrated in these studies. Weight changes in migrants are an important factor contributing to blood pressure change, while social interaction has a small but definite effect. Methods of effective intervention in these areas now require to be developed.

Acknowledgments. The authors wish to acknowledge the support of the Medical Research Council of New Zealand, the Cardiovascular Disease Unit of WHO, the Health Department of New Zealand, and the Wellington Hospital Board. The active participation of the Tokelau people in Tokelau and New Zealand has made the study possible and is gratefully acknowledged.

REFERENCES

1. Murphy W: Some observations on blood pressure in the humid tropics. NZ Med J 54:64-73, 1955.
2. Prior IAM, Evans JG, Harvey HPB, Davidson F, Lindsey M: Sodium intake and blood pressure in two Polynesian populations. N Engl J Med 279:515-520, 1968.
3. Page LB, Damon A, Moellering Jr RC: Antecedents of cardiovascular disease in six Solomon Island societies. Circulation 49:1132-1146, 1974.
4. Maddocks I: Possible absence of essential hypertension in two complete island populations. Lancet 2:396-399, 1961.
5. Sinnett PF, Whyte HM: Epidemiological studies in a total highland population. Tukisenta New Guinea. J Chronic Dis 16:265-290, 1973.

6. World Health Organisation: Report of WHO consultation on primordial prevention of cardiovascular diseases in developing countries. Geneva: WHO Cardiovascular Disease Unit, January 1979.
7. Guyton AC: A systems analysis approach to understanding long-range arterial blood pressure control and hypertension. Circ Res 35:159-176, 1974.
8. Dahl LK: Salt intake and hypertension. In: Genest J, Koiw E, Kuchel O (eds) Hypertension, physiopathology and treatment. Boston: McGraw-Hill, 1977, pp 548-559.
9. Prior IAM, Stanhope JM, Evans JG, Salmond CE: The Tokelau Island migrant study. Int J Epidemiol 3:225-232, 1974.
10. Kempthorne O: Logical, epistemological and statistical aspects of nature-nurture data interpretation. Biometrics 34:1-23, 1978.
11. Prior IAM, Harvey HPB, Neave MIE, Davidson F: The health of two groups of Cook Island Maoris. Spec Rep Ser 26. Wellington: Govt Printer, 1966.
12. Evans JG, Prior IAM: Experiences with the random zero sphygmomanometer. Br J Prev Soc Med 24:10-15, 1970.
13. Blackburn H, Rose FA: Cardiovascular survey methods. Geneva: WHO, 1968.
14. Beaglehole R, Salmond CE, Hooper A, Huntsman J, Stanhope JM, Cassel JC, Prior IAM: Blood pressure and social interaction in Tokelau migrants in New Zealand. J Chronic Dis 30:803-812, 1977.
15. Beaglehole R, Eyles E, Salmond C, Prior I: Blood pressure in Tokelauan children in two contrasting environments. Am J Epidemiol 108:283-288, 1978.
16. Beaglehole R, Eyles E, Prior I: Blood pressure and migration in children. Int J Epidemiol 8:5-10, 1979.
17. Epstein FH, Eckoff RD: The epidemiology of high blood pressure geographic distributions and ecological factors. In: Stamler J, Stamler R, Pullman TN (eds) The epidemiology of hypertension. New York: Grune and Stratton, 1967, pp 155-166.
18. Cassel JC: Hypertension and cardiovascular disease in migrants. Int J Epidemiol 3:204-206, 1974.
19. Cassel J: Studies of hypertension in migrants. In: Paul O (ed) Epidemiology and control of hypertension. New York: Symposia Specialists 1975, pp 41-61.
20. Liu K, Cooper R, McKeever I, et al.: Assessment of the association between habitual salt intake and high blood pressure: methodological problems. Am J Epidemiol 110:219-226, 1979.
21. Garay RP, Meyer P: A new test showing abnormal net Na^+ and K^+ fluxes in erythrocytes of essential hypertensive patients. Lancet 1:349-353, 1979.
22. Ward RH, Chinn PG, Prior IAM: The effect of migration on the familial aggregation of blood pressure hypertension. (in press) 1980.
23. Beaglehole R, Salmond CE, Eyles EF: A longitudinal study of blood pressure in Polynesian children. Am J Epidemiol 105:87-89, 1977.

PART SIX

DETERMINANTS OF BLOOD PRESSURE
IN HIGH BLOOD PRESSURE POPULATIONS

16. HOST AND ENVIRONMENTAL DETERMINANTS OF HYPERTENSION

Perspective from the Framingham Study

W.B. KANNEL

A large body of data has accumulated providing some insights into the way hypertension evolves in the general population and some clues to possible environmental determinants. A prominent genetic susceptibility has been repeatedly demonstrated, but in those so predisposed, environmental factors appear to exert a considerable influence. Together, these multiple environmental influences in genetically susceptible persons determine the level of blood pressure ultimately attained in adult life. Although it is now possible to control most of the hypertension encountered in the general population, its high prevalence makes primary prevention by avoidance or correction of predisposing factors the more desirable approach.

New underlying causes are discovered every decade, but the determinants of most hypertension in the general population remain elusive. However, vulnerable segments of the population and some correctable predisposing factors have been identified. The search for the causes of essential hypertension has thus far revealed no single major cause but rather a number of contributors. It is conceivable that, like fever, blood pressure elevation has no single or even major cause. However, the search must continue because of the great impact of hypertension on health and survival.

1. GENES VERSUS ENVIRONMENT

There seems little doubt that humans can inherit an increased susceptibility to hypertension [1–7]. More so than environmental factors, genetic predisposition has been accorded a major role as a determinant of essential hypertension [1, 2, 8]. It is not clear, however, whether either genetic predisposition or environmental factors can alone produce hypertension. The contribution of inheritance to hypertension may well be a permissive one allowing environmental influences to raise the blood pressure.

H. Kesteloot, J.V. Joossens (eds.), Epidemiology of Arterial Blood Pressure, 265–295.

Studies to detect a subgroup of essential hypertension in which genetic factors are chiefly responsible would seem more useful than those designed to evaluate the genetic components of all essential hypertension. The former, which appears to have greater utility, requires the identification of unique genetic markers, and progress in seeking these out has been slow.

It must be assumed that the rise in pressure in essential hypertension is a manifestation of some more basic disorder which has remained elusive. It is not even clear whether we are dealing with a deficiency of vasodilators or an excess of vasopressors or both. Serious impediments to the evaluation of a predominant genetic component are the high prevalence of hypertension and the lack of identified genetic markers.

Nevertheless, it seems likely that there is a substantial genetic component to most hypertension. This suspicion is based on observed racial differences, familial aggregation of blood pressure, twin studies, and animal experiments. Studies of blood pressures in twins, siblings, families with natural and adopted children, and spouses all support a powerful genetic influence. Offspring of hypertensive parents tend to have pressures at the higher end of the distribution, even at an early age, suggesting predestination [5–7]. The pressures of natural offspring have been found to correlate more closely than those of adopted children but many of these children were newly adopted. Twin studies have shown that monozygotic twins have a higher correlation of blood pressures than dizygotic twins, who in turn have higher correlations than ordinary sibs (Table 1). However, a major difficulty in most human genetic studies is that the closer persons are genetically, the more similar are their environments. A positive family history has been found in both mild and severe hypertension, but its predictive value is not established prospectively [4].

Genetically induced hypertension can be reliably produced in animals, and animals can be bred to be sensitive to salt intake so that they develop hypertension when fed salt early in life [2, 9, 10]. The hemodynamics, the

Table 1. Correlation of blood pressures among relatives.

	Systolic	Diastolic
MZ twins [a]	0.55	0.58
DZ twins [a]	0.25	0.27
Parent-offspring [b]	0.34	0.25
Siblings [b]	0.18	0.17
Spouses [b]	0.07	0.07

[a] NHLBI twin study.
[b] Framingham Study.

time lag, and permissive features of these animal experiments closely mimic the natural history of essential hypertension in humans.

However, the frequency distributions of arterial blood pressure have been shown to be unimodal both in the general population and in close relatives of patients with hypertension. This suggests that pressure differences are largely a matter of degree rather than kind, and that a polygenic inheritance much influenced by environmental factors must be involved. Hypertension, because it is very common, polygenic, and multifactorial, should lie more toward the environmental than the genetic end of the spectrum of causation. Yet Feinleib has estimated that the relative contribution of genetic factors is 60% [8]. It is likely that the genetic influence is permissive rather than absolutely determinative. Under this assumption the environmental influences must be widespread.

Although entire primitive societies exist in which blood pressure remains low throughout life, these people exhibit a rise in pressure when they migrate to or adopt the lifestyle of Western civilization. There are many indications of powerful environmental influences including socioeconomic gradients in hypertension, regional difference, secular trends, influences of acculturation, and salt intake.

Thus, genetic influences may be either enhanced or suppressed by environmental factors. Also, even if genetic endowment plays a major role, there is no reason for despair since it is likely that controllable environmental cofactors are involved and, whatever the cause, blood pressure can be controlled.

2. HOST FACTORS

A number of personal attributes have been examined in relation to blood pressure. Some have been found to be associated with blood pressure level and some have not. Among the factors studied are: age, sex, race, blood hemoglobin, heart rate, serum lipid, glucose tolerance, and weight.

2.1. Age and sex

In almost all population samples in which age can be accurately determined, there is a rise in pressure with age in both sexes. Such observations do not necessarily mean that blood pressures inevitably must rise with age or that those that do reflect a normal aging process. The magnitude of the rise observed with age is about 20 mmHg systolic and 10 mmHg diastolic from age 30 to 64. Age trends in blood pressure vary depending on whether based on cross-sectional data or longitudinal data.

Prevalence data clearly indicate that blood pressure increases with age in most population samples. In cross-sectional data, both systolic and diastolic pressures increase with age in adult life, with systolic pressures continuing to rise into the 80s in women and into the 70s in men (Fig. 1). Diastolic pressures tend to level off sooner and, in men, decline precipitously beyond age 56. The pressures start at a lower level in women and rise more steeply with age until they equal those of men at about age 50, and then progressively exceed those in men. This crossover in pressures in the sexes is observed for both the systolic and the diastolic component.

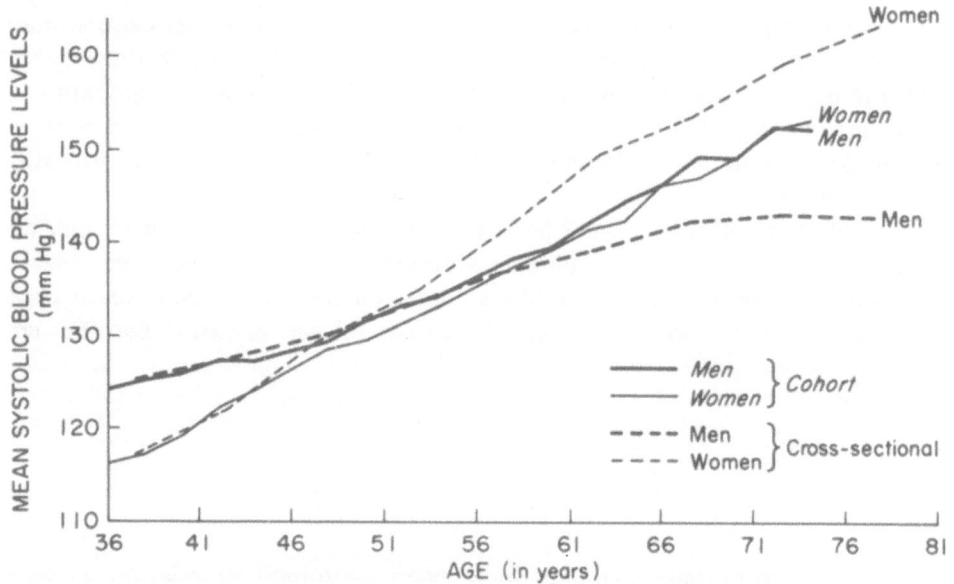

Figure 1. Average age trends in systolic blood pressure levels for cross-sectional and cohort data: Framingham Study, exams 3–10.

Longitudinal data, which are more apt to reflect pressures in the cohort as it actually ages, reveal diastolic pressures that are essentially parallel in the sexes, with women's pressures persistently lower than those of men (Fig. 2). Systolic pressures of women are initially lower than those of men, rise steeply to converge on those of men by age 60, but never exceed them. The data indicate a disproportionate rise in systolic pressure relative to diastolic pressure with advancing age, which is presumably due to a progressive loss of arterial elasticity. The reason for the difference in the picture of age trends

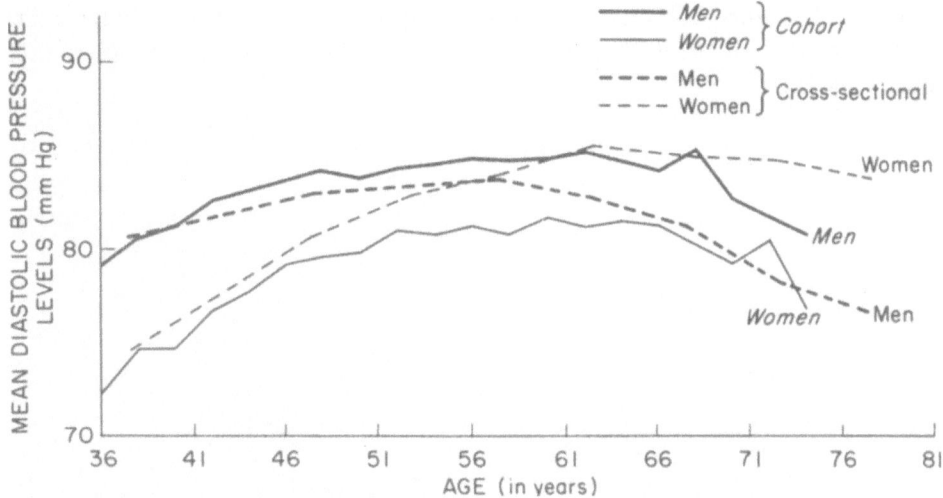

Figure 2. Average age trends in diastolic blood pressure levels. For cross-sectional and cohort data: Framingham Study, exams 3–10.

obtained cross-sectionally and longitudinally is not clear. It could reflect differential mortality in the two sexes or greater treatment of hypertension in women than men.

Epidemiologic studies have generally demonstrated that the blood pressure of females increases with age at a more rapid rate than that of males. Attempts to explain this phenomenon by such factors as pregnancy and urinary tract infection have not been convincing.

It is often assumed that the blood pressure rise with age is a consequence of the normal biologic aging process. However, there are examples of populations in which the blood pressure does not rise with age [11–14]. Even within populations where a rise in pressure with age is characteristic, not all subjects exhibit such a rise. Although there is no doubt that the mean blood pressure in Western populations rises with age, it is not certain that the pressure rises *because* of age. It might well be the time-dose product of environmental factors in susceptible persons.

2.2. Race

Blacks have been found to have higher pressures than whites in most Western cultures. How early in life this difference appears is unsettled because there is contradictory data as to whether the blood pressure in the black population is higher than that of the white in childhood and adolescence [15–19]. In adult blacks as in whites, there is a crossover in pressures in

270

the two sexes, with women's pressures rising to exceed those in men in later life. This crossover occurs at least ten years earlier in life in blacks than in whites (Fig. 3).

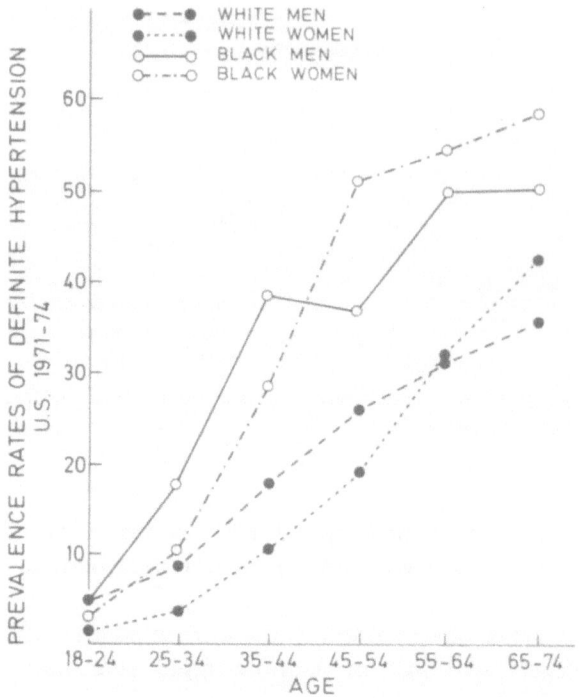

Figure 3. The prevalence of hypertension in the United States, defined as a systolic blood pressure of at least 160 mmHg or a diastolic blood pressure of at least 95 mmHg. Data from the Health and Nutrition Examination Survey 1971–1974. Source: Advance Data, Vital Health Statistics of the National Center of Health Statistics, no. 1, 18 October 1976.

The reason for this increased propensity to hypertension among blacks is uncertain. Attempts have been made to link this with social class, salt intake, psychologic stress, poor nutrition, infection, and secondary hypertension, but results have been inconsistent. While poverty and discrimination against blacks may play a role, at every income level blacks have been found to have higher pressures than whites. However, geographic variation in the prevalence of hypertension does seem to occur in blacks as in whites.

A major role of heredity has been suggested by Boyle, who noted a correlation between blood pressure and the degree of pigmentation in blacks [20]. This evidence is equivocal since socioeconomic status is also often

linked to the intensity of skin color in blacks. Nevertheless, genetic susceptibility is strongly suggested as the best explanation for the higher prevalence
of hypertension among blacks than whites. Blacks have been shown to
excrete sodium more slowly than whites, and to have lower renin values and
higher urinary sodium–potassium ratios [21–23]. The correlation between
blackness of skin and blood pressure is supported by data showing that blood
groups indicating African ancestry also correlate with blood pressure [24]. An
environmental influence, however, also seems likely since in the USA the
poor, uneducated and rural segments of the population have higher pressures,
and all these attributes are more common in blacks.

2.3. Host factors affecting trends in blood pressure

Aside from familial susceptibility, changes in a number of personal attributes
of subjects in the Framingham Study were found to be associated with
corresponding changes in pressure, and also with steeper trends in pressure
with age or over time. The strongest of these were changes in weight and
serum cholesterol, which tended to be mirrored by corresponding changes in
systolic pressure in both sexes (Table 2). A rising heart rate was associated
with an increase in blood pressure more prominently in men than women.

Table 2. Factors associated with trend in blood pressure.

	T-Values for significance [a]	
	Men	Women
Relative weight	5.91	9.60
Serum cholesterol	3.46	5.72
Heart rate	4.68	1.84
Blood glucose	2.76	0.01
Hematocrit	−0.49	2.49
Vital capacity	−1.89	1.65

[a] Significance of multivariate coefficients for regression of pressure on change in attribute
averaged over age groups.
Men and women aged 35–64; Framingham Study: 14-year follow-up.

Hemoglobin and hematocrit levels were found to be positively correlated
with blood pressure, with a twofold greater prevalence of hypertension in
those with high compared to low hematocrits (Table 3). There was no consistent evidence that the impact of blood pressure on the incidence of cardiovascular disease differed at different levels of hematocrit.

Using a multiple logistic function including these variables (blood pressure,
age, heart rate, cholesterol, glucose, relative weight, and hematocrit) Stamler

et al. were able to identify 20% of the population from which 55% of all expected hypertensives will emerge [25].

Table 3. Percent of persons hypertensive by level of hemoglobin or hematocrit. [a]

| Hct, Hb level | Prevalence of hypertension | | | | | |
| | 40–49 (years) | | 50–59 (years) | | 60–69 (years) | |
	Border. [b] HBP	Def. [c] HBP	Border. HBP	Def. HBP	Border. HBP	Def. HBP
MEN						
Low	22.6	11.6	28.4	14.2	30.1	18.8
Normal	29.6	13.0	31.0	19.9	35.2	22.4
High	34.0	20.2	34.3	27.2	38.2	30.8
WOMEN						
Low	17.2	6.7	25.0	14.8	41.1	25.6
Normal	21.4	9.3	32.5	18.3	40.0	29.7
High	31.1	17.0	33.4	31.3	34.9	43.5

[a] Classified by hematocrit at exams 1–3, and hemoglobin at exams 4–10.
[b] Borderline: 140–160/90–95.
[c] Def.: >160/95.

2.4. Menopause

It is tempting to attribute the steeper rise in systolic pressure with age in women than men to the menopause, but blood pressure rises with age before the menopause and does not abruptly rise thereafter. An examination of the blood pressure change in women who have undergone the menopause (whether natural or surgical), in comparison to women the same age who have not, reveals only trivial differences which are not statistically significant (Table 4).

Table 4. Systolic blood pressure according to menopausal status.

| Menopause | Natural menopause | | Bilateral oophorectomy | |
	Underwent menopause	Remained premenopausal [a]	Cases	Controls [a]
Exam prior	131	129	129	127
Exam of	132	130	131	129
Exam following	132	131	131	130

[a] Controls: women, matched by age, who remained premenopausal followed through same sequence of examinations.
Women aged 40–51; Framingham Study: 18-year follow-up.
None of the differences in pressure are statistically significant.

2.5. Diabetes

An association between diabetes and hypertension has been noted. Although renal involvement such as intercapillary glomerulosclerosis is associated with hypertension, the explanation for most hypertension in diabetics is obscure. In the Framingham cohort, a significant relationship of the deterioration in glucose tolerance under observation was associated with a rise in pressure only in men (Table 2). In neither sex was the base-line glucose value related to blood pressure.

2.6. Hyperresponsiveness

It has been proposed that an exaggerated pressor response is a hallmark of future hypertension. This assumption has never been properly tested. Hyperresponsiveness to cold has been implicated as a predictor of later hypertension [26]. However, such hyperresponsiveness has not been found to be characteristic of borderline hypertension [27, 28], and there is little correlation between blood pressure level and cold pressor response [29, 30]. Furthermore, prospective study of the cold pressor test has failed to predict future hypertension [30, 31].

Borderline hypertension leads to yet higher blood pressure, and most future hypertensives appear to come from the upper end of the normal distribution of blood pressure [32, 33]. However, there appears to be a positive relationship of the change in systolic pressure over time with the initial level, while for diastolic pressure the association is a negative one.

Blood pressure is a variable phenomenon and pressures have been shown to fluctuate over 100 mmHg systolic and 60 mmHg or more diastolic in a 24-h period. Since the variability of pressure increases as the mean level increases, the concept that normotension evolves into "fixed hypertension" by passing through a stage of labile hypertension would appear to be a myth which derives from the use of arbitrary thresholds for defining hypertension. The assertion that "fixed" hypertension usually arises from "labile" hypertension has not been established. The high pressures often considered "fixed hypertension" are actually more variable than those considered "labile" (Fig. 4). It is also not established that there is an identifiable subgroup of the population with characteristically labile pressures from one examination to the next. In fact the correlation (0.07) of lability of pressures from one examination to the next is trivial.

Nevertheless, it is possible that an exaggerated blood pressure response to a provocative test might identify future hypertensive persons. However, while it has been shown that tilting causes a "hypertensive response" in some patients with mild hypertension [34, 35], it is not clear that this type of

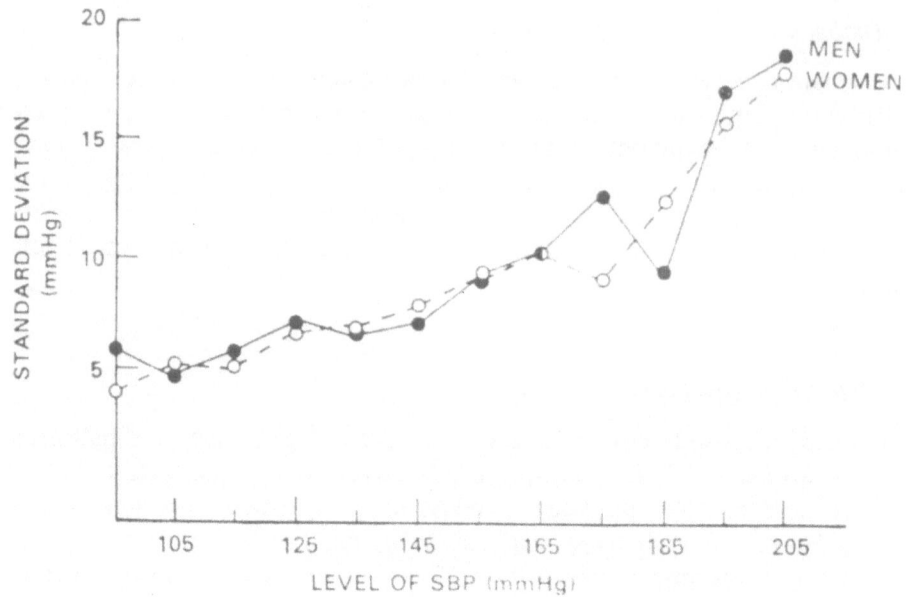

Figure 4. Average standard deviation of systolic blood pressure as function of level: Framingham Study, exam 3.

hyperreactivity predicts future hypertension in normotensive persons. Likewise, pressor responses to mental arithmetic, which are more pronounced in subjects with borderline hypertension and are associated with more catecholamine excretion [36], is not of established predictive value.

The heart rate has also been rather consistently noted to be associated with elevated pressures and to also predict future hypertension [25]. Framingham Study data have also shown a relationship of the heart rate to the increase in blood pressure over time, even taking the initial blood pressure into account (Table 2).

2.7. Possible physiologic predictors of hypertension

There are a number of correlates of borderline hypertension that deserve evaluation as possible precursors or predictors of future hypertension. Included among these are: the plasma volume, renin dependency, catecholamine levels, vagal vs sympathetic tachycardia, α-adrenergic dependency, peripheral vascular resistance, and the volume distribution in the capacity space [37]. Sodium loading may also be a useful procedure since borderline hypertensive subjects show an increased resistance in forearm flow rather than a decline [38]. It is possible that the prediction of hypertension can be improved by observing blood pressure, plasma volume, forearm flow, cardiac output, renin and kallikrein responses to sodium loading [37].

3. ENVIRONMENTAL DETERMINANTS

Although it seems clear that there are powerful genetic determinants of hypertension, there are some indications that environmental influences may be required for these inherited tendencies to become expressed as overt

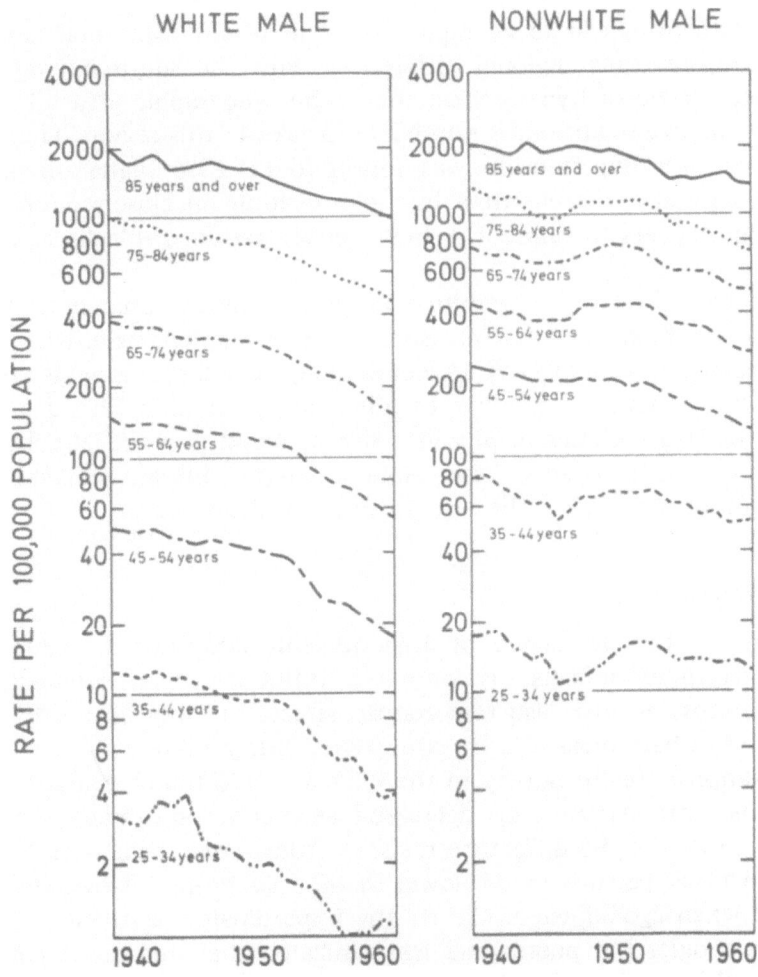

Figure 5. The mortality rates from hypertension in white and nonwhite males from 1940 to 1960. From Moriyama I, Kruger DE, Stamler J: Cardiovascular diseases in the United States (Cambridge: Harvard University Press, 1971).

hypertension. The downward trend in mortality attributed to hypertension (which preceded antihypertensive therapy), if not an artifact of reporting, would suggest a powerful environmental effect (Fig. 5). Social and regional differences in the prevalence of hypertension have been reported.

3.1. Regional differences

In the search for environmental determinants of hypertension, differences in blood pressure have been sought among populations in different geographic areas presumably exposed to varying environmental influences. In most instances, relatively modest differences have been found, but in many parts of the world there appear to be higher rates in urban than rural areas. In the USA there are some regional differences with the south having a slightly higher prevalence of hypertension than other geographic areas. This appears to reflect the disproportionate number of blacks in this region. The proportion of persons with hypertension was found to be 20% higher in populations living in central city areas than in those residing in closely adjoining areas. This again appears to reflect the high concentration of blacks in the central city.

A number of relatively primitive preindustrialized populations have been identified in which the blood pressure rise with age characteristic of Western society does not occur [39–49]. It seems likely that these findings are real and not simply a product of selective or other bias particularly, because migration to industrialized societies results in a rise in blood pressure [50]. These populations are usually small in size, isolated, highly inbred, and subsisting on foods without chemical additives, including sodium salts.

3.2. Socioeconomic status

Variation in the prevalence of hypertension according to education and income very likely reflects environmental influences. Once attained, the educational status, in turn, also importantly affects the way of life. In the USA, social class is best measured by educational attainment.

The National Health Survey in the USA in 1978 found that the proportion of persons with hypertension decreased as income and education increased (Table 5). Some of the difference resulted from a disproportionate number of older and black persons in the lower-income subgroups. However, the trend persisted when age-adjusted. Clearly the hypertensive population in the USA is not only older but poorer and less educated than the general population. Almost a third of hypertensive persons reported incomes below $5000 compared to 18% of the general population.

Data from the Framingham Study are quite consistent with the national

Table 5. Prevalence of hypertension according to family income and education, 1974: National health Survey.

	Prevalence of hypertension (per 100 POP)	
	Unadjusted	Age-adjusted
FAMILY INCOME		
Under $5000	26.7	22.9
$5000–9999	18.1	18.0
$10,000 or more	12.7	14.3
EDUCATION		
Under 9 years	28.6	20.0
9–11 years	17.6	18.9
12 years	14.0	16.1
13 years or more	11.1	13.6

Source: NHS. Characteristics of persons with hypertension. USA, 1974. DHEW Publ. no. (PHS) 74-1549, National Center for Health Statistics, December 1978.

data and, in addition, show a persistence of the trend when adjusted for degree of adiposity, which is also inversely related to educational status.

3.3. Work status

The work situation may influence blood pressure because of social stress, physical exertion, or exposure to noxious agents. While hard physical work can transiently raise the blood pressure, especially work involving the lifting of heavy objects, there is a paucity of evidence that this results in a sustained elevation of the resting blood pressure. Some believe that endurance exercise results in lower pressures, but adequately controlled trials to support this contention are lacking.

The Framingham Study cohort was classified into seven occupational categories (Table 6) and the systolic blood pressure was determined. This revealed

Table 6. Systolic blood pressure according to occupation: men and women aged 50–59.

Occupation	Men	Women
Professional	136	130
Executive	133	—
Supervisory	140	139
Technical	137	128
Laborer	139	140
Clerical	141	139
Sales	138	138
Housewife	—	140

278

no consistent pattern of blood pressure differences among the several categories of occupation. In men, the lowest pressures were recorded among executives, and in women among technical and professional workers. However,
none of the differences were striking or significant.

It did not appear that subjects who were self-employed had any different
pressures than those employed by others (Table 7). Also, those employed at
more than one job at the time of examination had blood pressure distributions which were almost identical to those of persons engaged in only one job.

Table 7. Systolic pressure according to employment status: Framingham Heart Study.

Age		Mean systolic pressure	
		Men	Women
TYPE OF EMPLOYMENT			
40–49	Self	131	128
	Others	132	130
50–59	Self	137	140
	Others	139	138
60–69	Self	140	154
	Others	142	151
NUMBER OF JOBS [a]			
40–49	One	132	129
	More	133	128
50–59	One	138	139
	More	137	139

[a] Jobs held at one time.

It is unlikely that these Framingham data adequately test the possible role
of the work situation in contributing to hypertension. For example, holding
down more than one job at a time may be stressful for some and stress-
relieving for others.

3.4. Psychosocial determinants

There is a common conception that hypertension may result from psychologic
stress. There is no doubt that psychologic stress will transiently elevate the
blood pressure, but it is not clear that this can result in sustained blood
pressure elevations.

Extensive research into possible psychosocial determinants of hypertension
span more than 30 years, but have not produced any conclusive
results [51–54]. No consistent hypertensive personality has been identified,

and most studies have been of questionable validity because of nonobjective methods, poor sampling, and inadequate controls [53].

However, associations with hypertension have been noted in demanding social situations where aspirations are blocked, human intercourse restricted, and where the outcome of important events is uncertain. Elevated pressures have been noted in emergency situations [55], prolonged combat duty [56], in air traffic controllers [57], with job termination [58], with stressful urban living, and in crowded prison situations [59].

A few psychosocial factors were examined in the Framingham cohort. Those who reported the use of tranquilizers may be presumed to have more emotional problems or perceive that they do. Framingham Study data indicate little difference in pressures of those taking tranquilizers compared to those the same age not using them (Table 8).

Table 8. Systolic blood pressure according to tranquilizer use (exams 9 + 10): Framingham Study.

	Mean systolic pressure tranquilizers		Mean change in systolic pressure tranquilizers				Population tranquilizers		Standard deviation	
	0	+	0/0	0/+	+/+	+/0	0	+	0	+
MEN										
Under 60	134.5	137.7	1.3	1.4	5.8	10.1	865	50	20.1	23.7
60 and over	142.2	143.7	−0.7	4.2	−0.9	3.6	666	43	21.6	26.2
WOMEN										
Under 60	131.8	134.6	0.6	0.2	2.2	3.3	1050	117	20.1	23.0
60 and over	151.6	151.8	0.1	−2.5	1.2	−2.7	911	69	25.0	23.7

Loss of a spouse is an emotionally and socially disturbing event. Comparison of blood pressures in married versus widowed persons in the Framingham cohort revealed higher pressures in the widowed in each sex, especially under age 60 (Table 9). However, the pressures of the widowed were found to be higher prior to the loss of their spouse.

Social factors which may well play a role are rapid cultural changes, migration to urban environments or to another culture, and adaptive strains from new roles in a different setting [53, 60–62]. Studies of personality and emotional stress are, however, too inconsistent and retrospective, so it is impossible to dissociate cause from effect. Even if the associations hold up prospectively, emotional stress may play either an initiating, predisposing, or sustaining role and may require a genetic predisposition. Also, it is not clear whether interventions to control the kinds of social and psychologic stress implicated are feasible.

Table 9. Systolic blood pressures in widowed vs married subjects (exam 9). Men and women aged 45–78; Framingham Study: 16-year follow-up.

	Mean systolic pressure		Standard deviation		Number	
	Married	Widowed	Married	Widowed	Married	Widowed
MEN						
Under 60	134.3	144.1	20.2	21.0	858	20
60 and over	142.3	146.5	21.8	23.2	637	50
WOMEN						
Under 60	131.5	136.0	20.4	23.4	912	85
60 and over	151.3	152.4	26.4	23.1	524	342

3.5. Diet

Various components of the diet have been incriminated as contributors to hypertension, including salt content, protein, and calories. Incrimination of protein appears to have been stimulated by the finding of proteinuria and renal disease in hypertensive patients. The rice fruit diet of Kempner was conceived because he believed that vegetable protein had a blood pressure lowering effect. Subsequently it was found that low sodium diets (<200 mg/day) were responsible for the reduction in blood pressure achieved. Dahl promoted the concept that dietary sodium was responsible for much of the

Table 10. Correlation of nutrient intake and blood pressure. Men aged 45–64 free of CHD Framingham, Puerto Rico and Honolulu.

Nutrient	Systolic blood pressure		
	Framingham	Puerto Rico	Honolulu
Number of men	859	8215	7272
Total calories	0.030	−0.009	−0.025 [a]
Total protein	0.009	−0.015	−0.034 [b]
Total fat	0.001	0.008	−0.040 [b]
SFA	−0.008	−0.021	−0.039 [b]
MFA	0.001	0.004	−0.039 [b]
PFA	0.015	0.060 [b]	−0.016
Total carbohydrate	0.004	−0.070 [b]	−0.046 [b]
Sugar	−0.009	−0.061 [b]	−0.048 [b]
Starch	−0.011	−0.054 [b]	−0.031 [b]
Other carbohydrate	0.040	−0.012	−0.013
Cholesterol	−0.023	0.007	−0.033 [b]
Alcohol	0.069 [a]	0.084 [b]	0.081 [b]

[a] Correlation coefficient differs from zero ($P<0.05$).
[b] Correlation coefficient differs from zero ($P<0.01$).

hypertension in the general population. The one aspect of diet which has been clearly substantiated is the role of excess calories leading to obesity.

Correlations between various nutrients and blood pressure, allowing for age, were determined in three epidemiologic studies supervised by the NHLBI (Table 10). Although many of the correlations observed were distinguishable from zero in both the Honolulu and Puerto Rico heart studies (because of large population samples), none were large enough to suggest a substantial impact of the major nutrients on blood pressure. Alcohol intake was the only consistent positive correlate of blood pressure in all three studies.

3.6. Alcohol, coffee, and cigarettes

The use of coffee and alcoholic beverages and cigarette smoking are common social practices which, because of the pharmacologic action of their chemical makeup, might be expected to raise the blood pressure. Epidemiologic evidence has incriminated only alcohol. A positive association between alcohol intake and blood pressure has been noted in a number of epidemiologic studies [63–66]. Blood pressures have been found to be higher in people who imbibe more than three drinks per day or more than 60 ounces of alcohol per month [63, 67].

An association between alcohol intake and blood pressure was noted in the Framingham Study cohort in all age groups under investigation (Fig. 6). It is interesting that in all age groups, those who drank modest amounts of alcohol

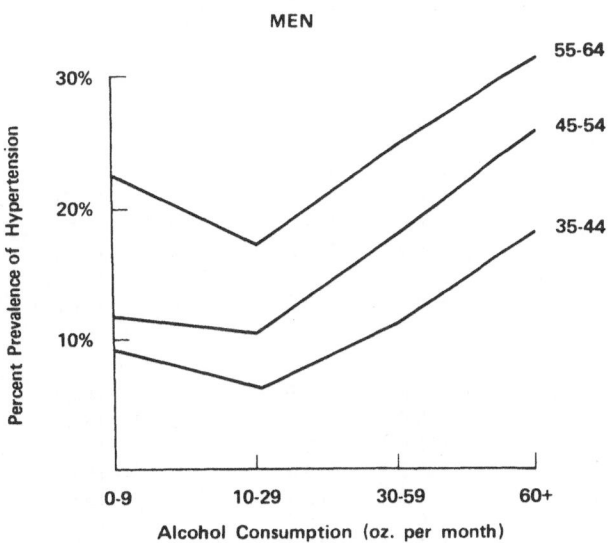

Figure 6. Percent prevalence of hypertension by alcohol consumption at exam 4: Framingham Study.

had a lower prevalence of hypertension than did those who abstained. This may be because among those who refused to admit any intake of alcohol there may have been some who were concealing excessive drinking. Among those who admitted alcohol intake there was a dose-related effect. There are correlations among alcohol, coffee, cigarettes, and adiposity which might account for the association. However, the association between alcohol and blood pressure has been shown to be independent of body weight in Framingham [67] and in the Kaiser Permanente Study, independent of age, sex, cigarette smoking, coffee use, schooling, and regular salt use as well [63]. It was also independent of past heavy drinking.

There is no support for the clinical adage that cirrhotics have low blood pressures, since alcoholics and patients dying of cirrhosis have been found to have more hypertension than expected [64].

Cigarette smoking has been shown to raise the systolic and diastolic pressures acutely as a result of local release of norepinephrine from adrenergic axon terminals [68, 69], but this does not appear to result in a sustained rise in blood pressure. Persons who smoked cigarettes in the Framingham Study actually had slightly lower blood pressures than those who did not, probably because they weighed less. Also, when smokers quit, they generally experience a slight rise in blood pressure probably reflecting weight gain [70, 71].

Table 11. Systolic blood pressure according to daily coffee intake: 6th biennial exam: men and women aged 35–65, Framingham Study.

Cups of coffee per day	Average systolic blood pressure					
Age:	35–39	40–44	45–49	50–54	55–59	60+
MEN						
0	131.2	131.1	132.9	126.2	134.4	141.8
1	124.8	124.8	129.7	137.7	134.1	151.5
2	125.0	127.7	132.2	134.1	134.3	141.9
3	125.4	127.3	133.0	135.5	139.2	137.0
4	124.7	131.7	130.7	129.3	141.0	137.5
5	125.9	127.6	135.9	129.6	136.3	136.6
6	134.8	131.4	132.4	133.0	146.6	129.2
7	134.7	129.8	129.4	131.6	140.5	130.1
WOMEN						
0	116.6	127.9	129.1	143.2	143.8	150.0
1	118.0	123.4	134.1	139.8	146.4	156.2
2	116.6	128.1	128.5	137.3	148.0	149.4
3	115.3	124.4	129.9	140.7	144.4	154.3
4	119.2	122.1	126.9	133.7	138.2	159.5
5	120.3	120.3	122.6	134.3	135.6	147.7
6	117.9	119.9	131.2	132.1	148.6	146.5
7	117.7	120.7	127.2	133.7	137.9	136.0

Because of the pharmacologic effect of caffeine, excessive coffee intake might be expected to influence blood pressure more than transiently. However, no association between coffee intake and blood pressure was noted in the Framingham cohort (Table 11). Evidently the slight rise in pressure and increased cardiac output associated with ingestion of 100–150 mg of caffeine with each cup of coffee or tea does not result in a sustained elevation of blood pressure.

3.7. Overweight

The connection between weight or obesity and blood pressure is quite firmly established by multiple clinical, metabolic, and epidemiologic studies [72–74]. Intervention studies have shown that weight reduction is accompanied by corresponding decreases in blood pressure [75, 76]. Also, subsequent regain of weight has been shown to be associated with a rise in blood pressure [73, 74]. By these criteria, a causal relationship seems likely.

Of the various factors examined for an association with trends in blood pressure in the Framingham cohort, change in relative weight is most prominent. Weight gain was found to be associated with a rise in pressure and weight loss with a corresponding reduction in pressure (Fig. 7). Regression

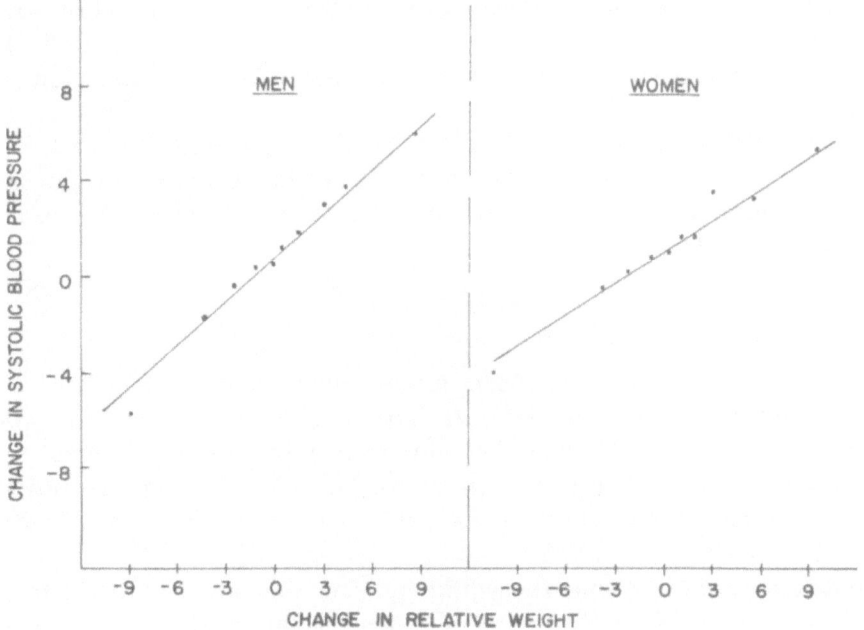

Figure 7. Change in systolic blood pressure according to change in relative weight between biennial exams.

analysis indicated a substantial relationship of weight *change* to changes in blood pressure, but no significant relationship to the basal weight [67]. Thus, taking into account the starting weight, change in weight was mirrored by corresponding changes in blood pressure. One standard deviation in weight change was associated with a 6.5-mmHg change in blood pressure in ten years.

Some have questioned the validity of elevated pressures in the obese as a fat arm artifact. However, the relationship of obesity to hypertension can be demonstrated using forearm blood pressures, and even intraarterial pressures correlate with adiposity [74].

Body fat rather than body mass or body volume seems to be the feature of overweight which is correlated with blood pressure. Blood pressure change has been shown to be related to changes in body weight, body mass index, skinfold thickness, and waist circumference. When weight is held constant, waist circumference is still correlated with blood pressure change [77].

Because there are many exceptions, it is clear that adiposity is not the chief determinant of hypertension, but the association has been demonstrated in multiple cultures, and in the young as well as adults. The well-documented association between overweight and hypertension requires a pathogenetic explanation. Discovery of causal mechanisms is handicapped by the common and variable occurrence of both conditions. Possible genetic, psychologic, social, and neurologic factors must all be considered. It is not clear whether those who respond with an increase in pressure exhibit an increased cardiac workload, or excessive plasma volume expansion for a given increment in weight.

The assertion of Dahl that it is attributable to increased salt intake is not supported by others who have found a relationship between weight change and blood pressure change, even when salt intake, determined by excretion, remains constant [76, 78].

3.8. Salt

Evolutionary arguments have been made which suggest that our sodium intake far exceeds our needs [79]. A large intake of sodium can produce hypertension in susceptible animals, and many forms of experimental hypertension are associated with sodium retention [83]. During man's evolution, he ate a low sodium, high potassium diet, which modern society has tended to reverse.

Population studies around the world indicate that areas with a very high salt intake have a high prevalence of hypertension, while areas with a low intake (i.e., less than 4 g of sodium chloride per day) have a low prevalence. In those low salt intake areas, blood pressures do not rise with age, and this is

Table 12. Population blood pressure characteristics according to salt intake.

Salt intake	Population blood pressure
<10 meq/day	Hypertension absent; no. increase in blood pressure with age.
10–70 meq/day	Low prevalence of hypertension.
70–350 meq/day	About 15% of adult population hypertensive; blood pressure increases with age.
>350 meq/day	About 30% of population hypertensive.

Freis, E. *Circulation* 53:589, 1976 [79].

all compatible with vigorous health. Freis has summarized this data (Table 12).

The most impressive epidemiologic support comes from studies of primitive societies subsisting on a very low sodium, high potassium intake. Hypertension apparently does not occur and the rise in pressure with age characteristic of affluent societies is not seen [38–50, 79]. Although other elements of their lifestyle may be responsible, salt intake seems the most likely explanation. This suspicion is supported by the fact that genetically similar natives who migrate to modern coastal cities develop the usual amount of hypertension [50].

The evidence relating sodium intake to the prevalence of hypertension within a given population sample is less persuasive [80–82], but some have shown a relationship [84]. Unfortunately most investigations attempting to correlate sodium intake or excretion with blood pressure have failed to show an association. This may be a consequence of failure to adequately take age, weight, and innate susceptibility to salt loading into account. It is also possible that the intraindividual variation in both blood pressure and sodium excretion is so great as to preclude demonstrating any correlation without large numbers of observations. However, Langford failed to show a relationship even after eight days of blood pressure determinations and six days of urine collections [81].

Another possible explanation is the failure to examine the relationship in subjects with a strong family history of hypertension. Other anions, such as calcium and potassium, may need to be considered. Although experimental data to provide a rationale are lacking, there is some evidence to suggest that calcium intake may modify the sodium effect. Also, potassium may suppress the sodium-induced rise in blood pressure. The sodium–potassium ratio has been found to correlate with blood pressure [81].

It is hypothesized that an increased salt intake leads to an increased extracellular volume which by circulatory and hormonal mechanisms leads to increased excretion of salt and water by the kidneys. Because in some persons the kidney's ability to excrete salt and water at a given pressure is limited to a greater extent, a higher pressure must be generated to augment filtration to maintain adequate excretion of salt and water.

3.9. Water minerals

Hardness of water or calcium and magnesium have been shown in various sets of data to be related to cardiovascular disease and hypertension [85, 86]. While some real relationship between cardiovascular mortality and the character of local water supplies seems likely, there is little agreement on what component of cardiovascular mortality is involved, on what substances that are present or absent are responsible, or whether the association is causal, From the evidence available, it seems unlikely that only one element is involved and more likely that an imbalance between substances is responsible. The issue is of some importance because water quality can be modified without causing any great change in lifestyle.

As tabulated by Masironi for the WHO, a majority of studies that have looked into the problem appear to show some relationship between water hardness and cardiovascular mortality [85]. Beginning with Kobayashi, various investigators around the world have examined the relationship of the character of drinking water to cardiovascular mortality [87–92]. The excess mortality, however, is not confined to cardiovascular causes [93–96]. In the USA, a strong negative correlation of water hardness with malignant neoplasm has been noted [97]. Canadian statistics show that more than half the excess mortality in soft water areas is actually certified to noncardiovascular causes of death [98].

Schroeder's theory that the soft water cardiovascular mortality is due to cadmium-induced hypertension is supported by animal experiments [99, 100]. The hypertensive effect of low doses of cadmium has been shown to be inhibited in rats when hard water is used to administer the metal [101, 102]. Increased cadmium and cadmium–zinc ratios have been found in the kidneys of persons dying with hypertension [101–103]. There is also some relation between the cadmium content of drinking water and the prevalence of hypertension [91].

Although at the point of use cadmium may be more abundant in soft water, its concentration does not correlate well with hardness and it is found in only a small percentage of municipal water supplies [91]. Also, more cadmium is absorbed from smoking than from water [104] and cigarette smokers have, if anything, lower pressures than nonsmokers.

Crawford postulated a protective effect of calcium against lead absorption in soft water areas [105, 106], and later implicated the ratio of magnesium plus calcium to sodium [91]. Joossens proposed sodium as the noxious element with calcium exerting a protective effect [107]. However, the sodium content of water in the USA and in Canada correlates *negatively* with mortality [91, 108, 109]. Langford and Watson also postulate that a low calcium intake may accentuate the hypertensive effect of sodium [110]. Blood and tap water lead concentrations have been noted to be higher in hypertensive persons in reports limited to England [113]. Also, at usual intake levels, a hypertensive effect has not been demonstrated either in animals or man [114, 115]. Furthermore, its concentration varies very little between hard and soft waters [91].

Thus, while potentially of great importance, the evidence relating the character of drinking water to the development of hypertension is too inconsistent and too incomplete to enable either firm conclusions to be drawn or recommendations to be made.

3.10. Oral contraceptives

Oral-contraceptive hypertension went unnoticed despite the use of this form of contraception for about a decade. Hypertension was then noted to occur in previously normotensive oral contraceptive users and to return to normal when the medication was discontinued [116, 117]. It has also been found to aggravate existing hypertension [116]. The pressor potential of oral contraceptives is a confirmed finding [118]. The hypertension, which may occur at any time after the institution of oral contraceptive use, is usually mild and reversible after 1–3 months without the medication. The risk of developing hypertension increases with the duration of oral contraceptive use, and in the fifth year the risk is five times that in the first year [118]. Also, older women are more susceptible than those below age 35.

In addition to occasionally promoting frank hypertension in some women and rarely malignant hypertension, oral contraceptives tend to raise the pressure slightly in practically all women [118]. In the Framingham Offspring Study, such a modest, and reversible increment in pressure was observed (Table 13). Both the estrogen and progestagen content have been implicated [118]. Induced renin and aldosterone abnormalities may require 2–3 months to disappear, and the accompanying hypertension may take as long as six months to subside.

Estrogen used in the postmenopausal female may also cause hypertension. The magnitude of the risk has not been established because hypertension is so prevalent in this stage of life.

Hormonal hypertension is now the commonest cause of secondary hypertension in the female. The atherogenic potential of decades of oral-contraceptive-induced hypertension, however mild, remains to be determined. It is also not established how reversible oral-contraceptive-induced hypertension will prove to be after prolonged use of the pill.

Table 13. Blood pressure and oral contraceptive use [a].

OC use		20–29		30–39
Av. systolic blood pressure				
None	(432)	111 ± 11	(589)	115 ± 13
Current	(168)	114 ± 12	(120)	117 ± 15
Ex.	(45)	111 ± 9	(54)	113 ± 11
Av. diastolic blood pressure				
None	(432)	72 ± 9	(589)	74 ± 9
Current	(168)	73 ± 9	(120)	75 ± 11
Ex.	(45)	71 ± 8	(54)	74 ± 9

[a] Framingham Offspring Study. Number of subjects in parentheses.

3.11. Urinary tract infection

Since pyelonephritis frequently occurs without symptoms, urinary tract infection has been considered as a possible cause of essential hypertension. Studies by Miall and co-workers in Jamaica appeared to show higher rates of asymptomatic bacteriuria in hypertensives than in nonhypertensives [119]. The prevalence of hypertension and bacteriuria both increase with age. However, studies in Framingham, where the prevalence of asymptomatic bacteriuria was quite low, failed to support the contention that either pyelonephritis or chronic bacteriuria is an important factor in the development of hypertension. No relationship between the bacterial colony counts and blood pressure was found, and the prevalence was too low to account for much of the high prevalence of hypertension in older women.

4. SUMMARY

Epidemiologic studies of the determinants of essential hypertension have revealed a number of host and environmental factors which appear to predispose. These factors, however, even combined do not appear to account for the high prevalence of hypertension in the general population. Efforts to clarify the epidemiology of hypertension have been only partially successful and many unresolved issues remain.

A number of facts have emerged which are worthy of consideration. While it seems apparent that genetic susceptibility plays a large role, this may only be permissive, requiring one or more environmental cofactors. There is an increasing conviction that the determinants of hypertension must be sought in childhood. Environmentally stressed susceptible persons after a latent period seem to develop into adult hypertensives.

With only a few exceptions, high blood pressure is a worldwide phenomenon reaching major proportions in the middle aged and elderly. It tends to run in families, and the rate of increase with age may be related to the level exhibited in youth. Blacks in the USA are distinctly more vulnerable, but this does not appear to be the case in Africa.

Genetic influences in combination with environmental factors appear to determine the level attained in later life. Weight gain has been consistently shown to raise the blood pressure, and this has been shown to be independent of salt intake. The contributions of salt and soft water have been the subject of considerable investigation and debate with more evidence favoring a role of salt in susceptible persons. Alcohol and high blood hematocrits have been noted to be associated with elevated pressures for reasons which are unclear. Urinary tract infection has not played a major role. Psychosocial factors appear to play a significant role, but the details are unclear. Menopause does not appear to play a role in the steeper climb of pressures with advancing age noted in women. Hyperresponsiveness of the pressure to various stimuli has not been demonstrated to predict future hypertension. Cigarettes and coffee intake do not play a role. Oral-contraceptive hypertension has emerged as the commonest form of secondary hypertension in women.

New underlying causes of hypertension are discovered every decade, but the determinants of most hypertension remain unclear. However, vulnerable segments of the population and some predisposing factors amenable to correction have been identified. Although it is now possible to control most of the hypertension encountered clinically, the very high prevalence of the condition makes this approach difficult. Primary prevention of hypertension by avoiding or correcting predisposing factors would be preferable.

REFERENCES

1. McKusick VA: Genetic factors in cardiovascular diseases. I. The four major types of C-V disease. Mod Concepts Cardiovasc Dis 28:535-542, 1959.
2. Dahl LK, Heine M, Tassinari L: Effects of chronic excess salt ingestion. Evidence that genetic factors play an important role in susceptible to experimental hypertension. J Exp Med 115:1173-1190, 1962.
3. Miall WE, Oldham PD: The hereditary factor in arterial blood pressure. Br Med J 5323:75-80, 1963.
4. Thomas CB, Ross DC, Higgenbottom CQ: Precursors of hypertension and coronary disease among healthy medical students. Discriminant function analysis. II. Using parental history as the criterion. Bull Johns Hopkins Hosp 115:245-264, 1964.

5. Zinner SH, Levy PS, Kass EH: Familial aggregation of blood pressure in childhood. N Engl J Med 284:401, 1971.
6. Klein BE, Hennekens CH, Jessee MJ, Gourley JE, Blumenthal S: Longitudinal studies of blood pressure in offspring of hypertensive mothers. In: Paul O (ed) Epidemiology and control of hypertension. Miami: Symposia Specialists, 1975.
7. Hennekens CH, Jessee MJ, Klein BE, Gourley JE, Blumenthal S: Aggregation of blood pressure in infants and their siblings. Am J Epidemiol 103:457-463, 1976.
8. Feinleib M, Garrison R, Borhani N, Rosenman R, Christian J: Studies of hypertension in twins. In: Paul O (ed) Epidemiology and control of hypertension. New York: Stratton Intercontinental Medical, 1975, pp 21-39.
9. Okamoto K, Poki K: Development of a strain of spontaneously hypertensive rats. Jpn Circ J 12:943-952, 1964.
10. Smirk FH, Hall WH: Inherited hypertension in rats. Nature 182:727-728, 1959.
11. Page LB, Sidd JJ: Medical management of primary hypertension. N Engl J Med 287:960-967, 1972.
12. Gordon T, Devine B: Vital Health Stat [Ser 11], no. 13, 1966.
13. Lóvell RRH: Race and blood pressure, with special reference to Oceanic. In: Stamler J, Stamler R, and Pullman TR (eds) The epidemiology of hypertension. New York: Grune and Stratton, 1967, pp 122-138.
14. Maddocks I: Possible absence of essential hypertension in two complete Pacific Island populations. Lancet 2:396-399, 1961.
15. Voors AW, Foster TA, Frerichs RR, Webber LS, Berenson GS: Studies of blood pressure in children aged 5–14 years in a total biracial community. The Bogalusa Heart Study. Circulation 54:319, 1976.
16. Kilcoyne MM, Richter RW, Alsup PA: Adolescent hypertension. I. Detection and prevalence. Circulation 50:758-764, 1974.
17. Kotchen JM, Kotchen TA, Schwurtman NC, Kuller LH: Blood pressure distribution of urban adolescents. Am J Epidemiol 99:315-324, 1974.
18. Johnson AL, Cornoni JC, Cassel JC, Tyroler HA, Heyden S, Hames CG: Influence of race, sex and weight on blood pressure behavior in young adults. Am J Cardiol 35:523-530, 1975.
19. Londe S, Gollub SW, Goldring D: Blood pressure in black and white children. J Pediatr 90:93, 1977.
20. Boyle Jr E: Biological patterns in hypertension by race, sex, body weight and skin color. JAMA 213:1637-1643, 1970.
21. Langford HG, Watson RL: Electrolytes and hypertension. In: Paul O (ed) Epidemiology and control of hypertension. New York: Stratton Intercontinental Medical 1974, pp 119-128.
22. Grimm CE, McDonough JR, Dahl LK: Dietary sodium potassium and blood pressure: racial differences in Evans County, Georgia. Circ Res [Suppl 3] 61, 62: 85, 1970.
23. Langford HG: Hypertension in blacks. In: Onesti G, Klimt CR (eds) Hypertension determinants, complications and intervention. Fifth Hahnemann International Symposium on Hypertension. New York: Grune and Stratton, 1979, pp 63-68.
24. Long WK: African genes and hypertension. N Engl J Med 284:708, 1970.
25. Stamler J, et al.: Relationship of multiple variables to blood pressure. Findings from four Chicago epidemiologic studies. In: Paul O (ed) Proceedings of the Second Symposium on the Epidemiology and Control of Hypertension. Miami: Symposia Specialists, 1976, pp 307-356.

26. Hines Jr EA: Vascular reactivity and hypertensive disease. Coll Pap Mayo Clin Found 42:317-325, 1950.
27. Thomas CB, Stanley JA, Kendrick MA: Observations on some possible precursors of essential hypertension and coronary artery disease. VII. The subjective reaction to the cold pressor test as expressed in the verbal response. J Chronic Dis 14:355-365, 1961.
28. Eich RH, Jacobsen EC: Vascular reactivity in medical students followed for 10 years. J Chronic Dis 20:583-592, 1967.
29. Armstrong HG, Rafferty JA: Cold pressor test follow-up study for 7 years on 166 officers. Am Heart J 39:454-490, 1950.
30. Harlan Jr WR, Osborne RK, Grabiel A: Prognostic value of the cold pressor test and the basal blood pressure: based on an 18 year follow-up study. Am J Cardiol 13:683-687, 1964.
31. Stamler J, Lindberg HA, Berksom DM, et al.: Epidemiological analysis of hypertension and hypertensive disease in the labor force of a Chicago utility company. Proc Counc High Blood Pressure Res 7:23-52, 1958.
32. Thomas CB: Developmental patterns in hypertensive cardiovascular disease: fact of fiction? Bull NY Acad Med 45:831-850, 1969.
33. Obermann A, Lane NE, Harlan WR, et al.: Trends in systolic blood pressure in the Thousand Aviator Cohort over a 24 year period. Circulation 36:812-822, 1967.
34. Esler MD, Nestel PJ: Sympathetic responsiveness to head up tilt in essential hypertension. Clin Sci 44:213-226, 1973.
35. Frohlich ED, Tarazi RC, Ulrych M et al.: Tilt test for investigating a neural component in hypertension. Circulation 36:387-393, 1967.
36. Nestel PJ: Blood pressure and catecholamine excretion after mental stress in labile hypertension. Lancet 1:692-694, 1969.
37. Julius S, Schork MA: Predictors of hypertension. In: Perry Jr HM and Smith WM (eds) Mild hypertension: to treat or not to treat. Ann NY Acad Sci 304:38-52, 1978.
38. Mark AL, Lawton WJ, Abbond FM, et al.: Effects of high and low sodium intake on arterial pressure and forearm vascular resistance in borderline hypertension. Circ Res [Suppl 1] 36-37: I-194-198, 1975.
39. Donnison CP: Blood pressure in the African native. Its bearing upon the actiology of hyperpiesia and arteriosclerosis. Lancet 1:6, 1929.
40. Burns-Cox CJ, Maclean JD: Splenomegaly and blood pressure in an Orang Asli community in West Malaysia. Am Heart J 80:718, 1970.
41. Kaminer B, Lutz WPW: Blood pressure in Bushmen of the Kalahari Desert. Circulation 22:289, 1960.
42. Kean BH: The blood pressure of the Cuna Indians. Am J Trop Med 24:341, 1944.
43. Maddocks I: Blood pressure in Milanesians. Med J Aust 1:1123, 1967.
44. Nye LJJ: Blood pressure in the Australian Aboriginal, with a consideration of possible artiological factors in hyperpiesia and its relation to civilization. Med J Aust 2:1000, 1937.
45. Oliver WJ, Cohen EL, Neel JV: Blood pressure, sodium intake and sodium related hormones in the Yanomamo Indians, a "no-salt" culture. Circulation 52:146, 1975.
46. Page LB, Danion A, Moellering Jr RC: Antecedents of cardiovascular disease in six Solomon Island societies. Circulation 49:1132, 1974.

47. Prior AM, Evans JG, Harvey HPB, Davidson F, Lindsey M: Sodium intake and blood pressure in two Polynesian populations. N Eng J Med 279:515, 1968.
48. Scotch N: A preliminary report on the relation of sociocultural factors to hypertension among the Zuhr. Ann NY Acad Sci 84:1000, 1960.
49. Shaper AG: Cardiovascular disease in the Tropics. III. Blood pressure and hypertension. Br Med J 3:805, 1972.
50. Creiz-Cohe R, Etcheverry R, Nagel R: Influence of migration on blood pressure of Easter Islanders. Lancet 1:967, 1964.
51. Glock CY, Lennard HL: Studies in hypertension. V. Psychologic factors in hypertension: an interpretive review. J Chronic Dis 5:174-185, 1957.
52. Howard J: Social, psychological and other selected factors associated with hypertension: a bibliography of articles indexed from 1962–1966. Chronic Dis Q Calif State Dep Public Health, no. 11, 1967.
53. Scotch NA, Geiger HJ: The epidemiology of essential hypertension: a review with special attention to psychologic and sociocultural factors in etiology. J Chronic Dis 16:1183-1213, 1963.
54. Stahl SM, Grim CE, Donald C, Neikirk HJ: A model for the social sciences and medicine. The case for hypertension. Soc Sci Med 9:31-38, 1975.
55. Ruskin A, Bear OW, Schaffer RL: Blast hypertension: elevated arterial pressure in victims of Texas City Disaster. Am J Med 4:228-236, 1948.
56. Graham JDP: High blood pressure after battle. Lancet 1:239-246, 1945.
57. Cobb S, Rose RM: Hypertension, peptic ulcer and diabetes in air traffic controllers. JAMA 224:489-492, 1973.
58. Kase SV, Cobb S: Blood pressure changes in men undergoing job loss: a preliminary report. Psychosom Med 32:19-38, 1970.
59. D'Atri DA, Ostfeld AM: Crowding: its effects on the elevation of blood pressure in a prison setting. Prev Med 4:550-566, 1975.
60. Christenson WN, Hinkle LE: Differences in illness and prognostic signs in two groups of young men. JAMA 177:247-253, 1961.
61. Stamler J, Berkson DM, Lindberg HA, et al.: Socio-economic factors in the epidemiology of hypertensive disease. In: Stamler J, Stamler R, Pullman TN (eds) The epidemiology of hypertension. New York: Grune and Stratton, 1967.
62. Syme Sl, Hyman MM, Enterline PE: Some social and cultural factors associated with the occurrence of coronary heart disease. J Chronic Dis 17:277, 1964.
63. Klatsky AL, Friedman GD, Siegabaub AB, Gerard MJ: Alcohol consumption and blood pressure. N Engl J Med 296:1194-1200, 1977.
64. Mathews JD: Alcohol usage as a possible explanation for socio-economic and occupational differentials in mortality from hypertension and coronary heart disease in England and Wales. Aust NZ J Med 6:393-397, 1976.
65. Gyntelberg F, Meier J: Relationship between blood pressure and physical fitness, smoking and alcohol consumption in Copenhagen males aged 40–59. Acta Med Scand 195:375, 1974.
66. Tibblin G: High blood pressure in men aged 50. A population study of men born in 1913. Acta Med Scand Suppl 470:1967.
67. Kannel WB, Sorlie P: Hypertension in Framingham. In: Paul O (ed) Epidemiology and control of hypertension. Miami: Symposia Specialists, 1975, p 553.
68. Aronow WS, Goldsmith JR, Kern JC, et al.: Effects of smoking cigarettes on cardiovascular hemodynamics. Arch Environ Health 28:330-332, 1974.
69. Cryer PE, Haymond MW, Santiago JV, et al.: Norepinephrine and epinephrine release and adrenergic mediation of smoking-associated hemodynamic and metabolic events. N Eng J Med 295:573-577, 1976.

70. Gordon T, Kannel WB, Dawber TR, et al.: Changes associated with quitting cigarette smoking: the Framingham Study. Am Heart J 90:322-328, 1975.
71. Seltzer CC: Effect of smoking on blood pressure. Am Heart J 87:558-564, 1974.
72. Kahn HA, Medalie JH, Neufeld HN, Riss E, Goldbourt U: The incidence of hypertension and associated factors. The Israel Ischemic Heart Disease Study. Am Heart J 84:171, 1972.
73. Chiang BN, Perlman LV, Epstein FH: Overweight and hypertension. A review. Circulation 39:403, 1969.
74. Kannel WB, Brand N, Skinner Jr JJ, Dawber TR, McNamara PM: The relation of adiposity to blood pressure and development of hypertension. The Framingham Study. Ann Intern Med 67:48, 1967.
75. Fletcher AP: The effect of weight reduction on the blood pressure of obese hypertensive women. Q J Med 23:331, 1954.
76. Reisen E, Abel R, Modan M, et al.: Effect of weight loss without salt restriction on the reduction of blood pressure in overweight hypertensive patients. N Engl J Med 298:106, 1978.
77. Svardsudd K: High blood pressure. A longitudinal study of men born in 1913. Goteborg, Sweden: Department of Medicine, Sahlgrenska Sjukhuset, 1978.
78. Dahl LK, Silver L, Christie RW: Role of salt in the fall in blood pressure accompanying reduction of obesity. N Engl J Med 258:1186-1192, 1958.
79. Freis ED: Salt, volume and the prevention of hypertension. Circulation 53:589, 1976.
80. Dawber TR, Kannel WB, Kagan A, Donabedian RK, McNamara PM, Pearson G: Environmental factors in hypertension. In: Stamler J, Stamler R, Pullman T (eds) The epidemiology of hypertension. New York: Grune and Stratton, 1967, pp 255-288.
81. Langford HG, Watson RL: Electrolytes and hypertension. In: Paul O (ed) Epidemiology and control of hypertension. New York: Stratton Intercontinental Medical Book Corp, 1975, pp 119-128.
82. Miall WE: Follow-up study of arterial pressure in the population of a Welsh mining valley. Br Med J 2:1204, 1959.
83. Meneely GR: The experimental epidemiology of sodium chloride toxicity in the rat. In: Stamler J, Stamler R, Pullman T (eds) The epidemiology of hypertension. New York: Grune and Stratton, 1967, p 240.
84. Joossens JV: Salt and hypertension: water hardness and cardiovascular death rate. Triangle 12:9-16, 1973.
85. Masironi R: Cardiovascular mortality in relation to radioactivity and hardness of local water supplies in the USA. Bull WHO 43:687-697, 1970.
86. Masironi R, Koirtyohann SR, Pierce JO, Schamschula RG: Calcium content of river water, trace element concentration in toenails and blood pressure in village populations in New Guinea. Sci Total Environ 6:41-53, 1976.
87. Kobayashi J: On geographical relationship between the chemical nature of river water and death rate from apoplexy. Ber Ohara Inst Landwirtsch Biol Okayama Univ 11:12-21, 1957.
88. Crawford MD: Hardness of drinking water and cardiovascular disease. Proc Nutr Soc 31:347-353, 1972.
89. Masironi R: Water quality, trace elements and cardiovascular disease. WHO Chron 27:534-538, 1973.
90. Punsar S: Cardiovascular mortality and quality of drinking water. An evaluation

of the literature from an epidemiological point of view. Work Environ Health 10:107-125, 1973.

91. Neri LC, Johanson HL: Water hardness and cardiovascular mortality. In: Perry M, Smith WM (eds) Mild hypertension: to treat or not to treat. Ann NY Acad Sci 304:203-219, 1978.

92. Sharrett AR, Feinleib M: Water constituents and trace elements in relation to cardiovascular disease. Prev Med 4:20-36, 1975.

93. Crawford MD, Gardner MJ, Morris JN: Mortality and hardness of local water supplies. Lancet 1:827-831, 1968.

94. Lowe CR, Roberts CJ, Lloyd S: Malformation of central nervous system and softness of local water supplies. Br Med J 2:357-361, 1971.

95. Crawford MD, Gardner MJ, Sedgwick PA: Infant mortality and hardness of local water supplies. Lancet 1:988-992, 1972.

96. Spiers PS, Wright SG, Siegel DG: Infant mortality and water hardness in the US. Pediatrics 54:317-319, 1974.

97. Sauer HI: Relationship between trace element content of the drinking water and chronic diseases, observed effects of trace metals in drinking water on human health. 16th Water Quality Conference, University of Illinois, 1974.

98. Neri LC, Mandel JS, Hewitt D: Relation between mortality and water hardness in Canada. Lancet 1:931-934, 1972.

99. Schroeder HA: Cadmium, chromium and cardiovascular disease. Circulation 35:570-582, 1967.

100. Schroeder HA, Vinton Jr HW: Hypertension induced in rats by small doses of cadmium. Am J Physiol 202:515-518, 1962.

101. Perry HM: Minerals in cardiovascular disease. J Am Diet Assoc 62:631-637, 1973.

102. Thind GS: Role of cadmium in human and experimental hypertension. J Air Pollut Control Assoc 22:267-270, 1972.

103. Schroeder HA: Cadmium as a factor in hypertension. J Chronic Dis 18:647-656, 1965.

104. Lewis GP, Jusko WJ, Coughlin LL, Hartz S: Cadmium accumulation in man: influence of smoking, occupation, alcohol habit and disease. J Chronic Dis 25:717-726, 1972.

105. Crawford MD, Crawford T: Lead content of bones in a soft and hard water area. Lancet 1:699-701, 1969.

106. Crawford MD, Clayton DG: Lead in bones and drinking water in towns with hard and soft water. Br Med J 2:21-23, 1973.

107. Joossens JV: Salt and hypertension: water hardness and cardiovascular death rate. Triangle 12:9-16, 1973.

108. Schroeder HA: Municipal drinking water and cardiovascular death rates. JAMA 195:81-85, 1966.

109. Sauer HI, Parke DW, Neill ML: Associations between drinking water and death rates. In: Hemphill DD (ed) Trace substances in environmental health IV. Columbia: University of Missouri Press, 1970, p 318.

110. Langford HG, Watson RL, Douglas BH: Factors affecting blood pressure in population groups. Trans Assoc Am Phys 81:135-146, 1968.

111. Foulger JH: Medical control of industrial exposure to toxic chemicals. Ind Med 12:214-225, 1943.

112. Einert C, Adams W, Crothers R, et al.: Exposures to mixtures of nitroglycerine and ethylene glycol dinitrate. Am Ind Hyg Assoc J 24:435-447, 1963.

113. Beevers DG, Erskine E, Robertson M, Beattie AD, Campbell BC, Goldberg A, Moore MR: Blood lead and hypertension. Lancet 2:103, 1976.
114. Stofen D: Environmental lead and the heart. J Mol Cell Cardiol 6:285-290, 1974.
115. Moore MR, Meredith PA, Goldberg A, Carr KE, Toner PG, Lawrie TDV: Cardiac effects of lead in drinking water of rats. Clin Sci Mol Med 49:337-341, 1975.
116. Woods JW: Oral contraceptives and hypertension. Lancet 2:653-654, 1967.
117. Laragh JH, Sealey JE, Ledingham JG, et al.: Oral contraceptives, renin, aldosterone and high blood pressure. JAMA 201:918-922, 1967.
118. Kaplan NM: Clinical complications of oral contraceptives. Adv Intern Med 20:197-214, 1975.
119. Miall WE, Kass EH, Ling J, Stuart KL: Factors influencing arterial pressure in the general population in Jamaica. Br Med J 2:497-506, 1962.

17. RELATIONSHIPS BETWEEN SODIUM AND POTASSIUM INTAKE AND BLOOD PRESSURE

W.G. WALKER

Kempner's demonstration of the effectiveness of a rice diet in reducing blood pressure in hypertensive individuals initiated a series of experiments that unequivocally established the therapeutic value of severe sodium restriction in lowering the blood pressure in hypertensive individuals [1, 2]. Subsequent studies by Murphy [3], Dahl et al. [4, 5], and others [6–8] provided documentation that this decrease in blood pressure was associated with a decrease in total body sodium as indicated by a negative sodium balance. The magnitude of the blood pressure drop could be quantitatively linked with the magnitude of sodium loss in these studies, thereby establishing a clear association between total body salt content and blood pressure. A number of population studies beginning with the observations of Dahl [9–11], and representing sampling from different geographic regions, have shown that those populations with a high sodium intake have a higher point prevalence of essential hypertension and populations with very low sodium intakes exhibit virtually no elevation of blood pressure.

Although studies of population samples from regions with very high sodium intakes reveal a high incidence of elevated blood pressure, this is not alone an adequate explanation for the blood pressure elevations observed in these individuals [12, 13]. Many individuals, despite extraordinarily high sodium intakes, have no difficulty with elevated blood pressure. Despite repeated efforts, nearly all attempts to identify a correlation between sodium intake and blood pressure within a segment of any given population have been unsuccessful [13]. Thus although large sodium intake clearly appears to be necessary for the development of high blood pressure, it alone is not sufficient. Some other factor or factors must be operative in order to produce progressive elevation of the blood pressure [14, 15].

Among factors that are possible candidates for this additional etiologic contribution to high blood pressure, heredity, other dietary influences, or possibly unique physiologic responses to the fluctuating salt intake require careful scrutiny.

As a means of providing some perspective on the current state of our knowledge relating salt intake to high blood pressure, pertinent data dealing with this and related associations, and possible inferences to be drawn from

H. Kesteloot, J.V. Joossens (eds.), Epidemiology of Arterial Blood Pressure, 297–309.

these data, will be reviewed here. In particular the question of the contribution of sodium, the possible physiologic responses to fluctuation in sodium intake that may exert a role on the blood pressure such as the concomitant behavior of the renin-angiotensin system, the possible modulating influences of other dietary factors, and the contributory influences of heredity will be examined.

In attempting to assess the importance of the contribution of each of these elements to the development of hypertension, the problem of defining high blood pressure is a confounding influence that presents artificial barriers. This difficulty is avoided by considering blood pressure the dependent variable and examining the association between this dependent variable and the candidate factors or influences that may possibly play a role in elevating blood pressure. Such data are of more value than those that arbitrarily group samples into normotensive and hypertensive groups and compare differences. Since it is generally agreed that the definition of hypertension is arbitrary [15], the sections that follow will attempt to place more weight upon those studies that examine the relationship between blood pressure and the dietary, environmental, and hereditary factors thought to exert some influence upon blood pressure, particularly those identifying factors that can be associated, at least statistically, with an increase in blood pressure.

1. ROLE OF SODIUM

The pathogenesis of high blood pressure was related to salt by Ambard and Beaujard [16], and articulated more clearly by Allen [17, 18], who proposed sodium restriction as an effective treatment, but it was Kempner's [1] demonstration of the effectiveness of the rice diet in lowering blood pressure that stimulated investigation of this relationship. The studies by Murphy and colleagues as well as those by Dahl and colleagues both established that the blood pressure lowering effect of the rice diet was attributable to the quantity of sodium lost by the individuals when they were subjected to the severe sodium restriction that the rice diet imposed [3, 4, 6]. These and subsequent studies made it abundantly clear that blood pressure in many instances could be effectively controlled by rigid sodium restriction alone; this was particularly true when dietary sodium reduction decreased intake to less than 15 meq/day [3, 6, 14].

Subsequent studies have followed two paths of investigation. Following Dahl's report that use of a questionnaire designed to provide a quantitative estimate of salt intake identified a relationship between sodium intake and blood pressure, subsequent studies by other investigators attempting to confirm this by demonstrating a relationship between blood pressure and urinary excretion within a single population sample have been uniformly unsuccessful [4, 9, 12, 13]. Population studies have, on the other hand, been more productive. Dahl first identified an association between the general level of sodium intake within a given population and the prevalence of elevated blood pressures in that population. He was able to show a linear relationship between the average salt intake of the population and the prevalence of elevated blood pressure in that population, based upon data obtained from Eskimos, at least two different regions of Japan, the United States, and the Marshall Islands. This observation has been repeatedly confirmed and documented in more elegant fashion by recent studies [9–13]. Page et al., in a series of experiments on small population isolates in the Solomon Islands, were able to demonstrate that those subjects who have quite low salt intakes have virtually no hypertension. Moreover, the population isolates with such low sodium intakes showed no tendency for the mean blood pressure to rise with age, the blood pressure for subjects in the 7th and 8th decades of life being indistinguishable from those obtained on subjects in the 2nd and 3rd decades. These observations indicate that increased sodium intake is responsible for the increase in blood pressure with age, a phenomenon previously regarded as a normal consequence of aging [10, 11, 19].

Meneely et al. demonstrated that the blood pressure in rats could be increased progressively by increasing the level of dietary sodium intake [20, 21]. Two important observations were made in this critical series of animal experiments: (a) blood pressure can be linearly related to sodium in the diet; (b) this influence of sodium can be modulated by potassium.

Despite convincing evidence relating the increase in prevalence of blood pressure elevation in a specific population to the general level of salt intake within that population, repeated efforts to identify an association between sodium intake and blood pressure within a single population sample have in general been unsuccessful [13, 22, 23]. Perhaps the nearest to a positive association was the demonstration by Sasaki that a positive correlation could be demonstrated between salt intake in a given region of Japan and the mortality rate within that region [12]. Moreover the principal cause of the fluctuations in mortality rate was a variation in the frequency of apoplexy. In the Akita prefecture, where the salt intake is well above 220 meq/day and may exceed 400 meq/day (measured excretions in this region have ranged from an average of 450 meq/day to a high of over 1000 meq/day), the prevalence of hypertension approaches 40% in the 5th decade of life and the frequency of fatal stroke is extremely high.

Despite these impressive associations, the case against salt is somewhat weakened by failure to demonstrate the intragroup (or intrapopulation) correlations between sodium and blood pressure. It is quite clear that some individuals take remarkably high levels of salt in their diets without any tendency to raise blood pressure. Since all available data from within single population groups indicate that not all of the subjects who take large quantities of salt develop high blood pressure, it is clear that some factor other than sodium must also be involved in this response. A plausible explanation for this failure to demonstrate such correlation may relate to the range of sodium intake where a relation between sodium and blood pressure may be demonstrated. Since studies in this country, Japan, and Europe [22–24] all indicate that sodium intake in these areas exceeds 200 meq/day, it may well be that the selection effect of increased sodium intake could be manifest well below this level. While this has not been tested directly, there is indirect evidence to suggest that this may be the case.

The data on the exact levels of sodium intake among the unacculturated populations that have been studied are relatively scant. Page has recently summarized the available evidence [25]. The sodium intake, as judged by measurement of urinary sodium excretion in these 'low blood pressure' populations, ranges from a level of 1.5 meq/24 h reported in the Yanomamo Indians in Brazil to a high of 85 meq/24 h in the Tarahumara Indians in Mexico. Since significant differences in the prevalence of hypertension have been noted among these low blood pressure populations with the highest prevalence of elevated blood pressures being seen in three Solomon Island groups (the Nasioi, Nagovisi, and Lau groups) with the highest levels of sodium intake [10, 11, 25], it seems evident that the selection of salt-sensitive individuals who respond by elevating blood pressure could be operating within this sodium range. If this is so, then it is not surprising that studies performed in populations whose sodium intake ranges between 170 and 250 meq/day fail to identify a significant correlation between dietary sodium intake and sodium excretion and elevations in blood pressure.

While there are no direct data to support this explanation of a failure to identify a clear correlation between sodium intake and blood pressure, there also is no evidence to contradict this inference. Perhaps the strongest indirectly supporting evidence comes from Shaper, dealing with Samburu men who were drafted into the Army in Kenya [26]. These individuals went from a sodium intake of 50 meq daily to an Army ration that contained approximately 275 meq. As a result, their blood pressure went up within the first two years of exposure to this diet and continued to rise through the sixth year. As further support for the existence of an important association between sodium intake and blood pressure elevations within populations, the question may be asked whether other evidence of interaction between sodium and blood pressure can be identified, as, for instance, changes in the renin-angiotensin-aldosterone system.

2. THE RENIN-ANGIOTENSIN-ALDOSTERONE SYSTEM AND BLOOD PRESSURE

We have recently reported [27] relevant blood pressure measurements, and plasma and urine data, on 574 ambulatory subjects with blood pressures ranging from 94/58 to 250/145 mmHg. No attempt was made to modify their sodium intake prior to study, and they were studied as ambulatory outpatients so that measurement of urinary electrolytes should reflect their usual intakes of sodium and potassium. Measurements were made on plasma renin activity, renin substrate, angiotensin II, and aldosterone in the plasma, plus urinary sodium and potassium and creatinine. Although we were unable to demonstrate any association between urinary sodium and measured blood pressure, the renin-angiotensin system appeared to change in the direction to be anticipated in the hypertensive subjects, and these changes correlated with the blood pressure (Table 1).

Table 1. Bivariate correlations in 574 subjects.

Variables tested for correlation	Correlation coefficient r	P value
Recumbent DBP vs PRS	+0.54	<0.000001
Recumbent DBP vs urinary K	−0.23	<0.00001
Recumbent DBP vs aldosterone	−0.20	<0.00001
Recumbent DBP vs PRA	−0.13	<0.005
Recumbent DBP vs urinary Na	−0.01	NS
Aldosterone vs urinary K	+0.24	<0.00001
Aldosterone vs urinary Na	−0.08	=0.06
PRA vs aldosterone	+0.14	<0.002
PRA vs urinary K	+0.14	<0.002
PRA vs urinary Na	−0.13	<0.005

DBP, diastolic blood pressure; K, potassium; PRA, plasma renin activity; Na, sodium; PRS, plasma renin substrate. From *Hypertension* 1:287, 1979 [27] (by permission of the American Heart Association, Inc.).

Plasma renin activity did exhibit a small but significant negative correlation with diastolic blood pressure, as did plasma aldosterone (Table 1). Both these negative correlations are in the direction to be expected if the renin-angiotensin system in those subjects with higher blood pressures has been suppressed by an increased salt intake. It is conceivable that such an explanation could also be extended to account for the positive correlation identified between renin substrate and diastolic blood pressure. Thus if the suppressed renin activity resulted in a decreased consumption of renin substrate without corresponding reduction in hepatic productions of renin substrate, the net result would be an increase in the mean levels of substrate among those subjects with elevated blood pressure, and a positive correlation between substrate and blood pressure. The demonstration of a significant negative correlation between plasma renin activity and urinary sodium can be construed as additional evidence in favor of a role for sodium in behavior of the blood pressure in this study.

The fact remains, however, that no differences in urinary sodium excretion were demonstrable when subjects with diastolic blood pressures of 90 mmHg or less were compared with those whose diastolic blood pressures exceeded 90 mmHg (Table 2). It thus seems necessary to postulate some additional

Table 2. Comparison of data on subjects grouped according to blood pressure.

Attribute	Diastolic BP ≤90 mmHg	Diastolic BP >90 mmHg	P value
Age (years)	31.3±0.4	32.1±0.4	NS
Height (inches)	69.1±0.2	67.5±0.2	<0.0001
Weight (lbs)	173.0±1.4	177.0±2.3	<0.0001
PRA	0.62±0.03	0.40±0.04	<0.0001
Aldosterone	14.5±0.61	11.1±0.61	<0.0001
Renin substrate*	1754±58.5	2076±54.5	<0.0001
Urinary potassium	66.6±1.74	53.9±1.74	<0.0001
Urinary sodium	129.0±2.91	128±3.16	NS
Urinary creatinine	165.0±5.03	164±4.74	NS
No. of subjects	274	300	

All labeled *P* represents probability that observed differences are chance variations due to sampling error.
BP, blood pressure; PRA, plasma renin activity; NS, not significant.
* For substrate $n = 187$ for normals and 108 for hypertensives.
From *Hypertension* 1:287, 1979 [27] (by permission of the American Heart Association, Inc.).

mechanisms. Some of the other findings in this study were so striking as to raise the question as to whether or not they may exert a stronger or more immediate influence upon blood pressure regulation, at least under the conditions of this study. For instance, in sharp contrast to the failure to identify a significant correlation between sodium and blood pressure, a highly significant correlation between potassium and blood pressure was identified in this group (Table 1).

3. RELATION BETWEEN POTASSIUM INTAKE AND BLOOD PRESSURE

The studies reported by us dealing with the patterns of electrolyte excretion and the state of the renin-angiotensin system in 574 ambulatory subjects revealed a surprisingly high correlation between urinary potassium and recumbent diastolic blood pressure. The correlation coefficient of −0.23 was significant at a *P* value of <0.00001. Moreover this urinary electrolyte was the only one to show any difference when the subjects with elevated blood pressure were compared with individuals whose diastolic blood pressure was

90 mmHg or less. Thus within these two groups (Table 2), urinary sodiums were virtually identical (129 ± 2.9 meq vs 128 ± 3.2 meq), as were measurements of urinary creatinine (165 ± 5.0 mg vs 164 ± 4.7 mg). None of these subjects had been previously treated for any blood pressure elevation, and there is no reasonable explanation for these urinary potassium differences except that they reflect differences in potassium intake.

An important and previously unrecognized association was also identified in this study series, namely a highly significant positive correlation between plasma aldosterone and urinary potassium. This correlation ($r = 0.24$; $P < 0.00001$) was virtually identical whether aldosterone was tested against the urinary concentration of potassium or excretion rates. It must be pointed out that this relatively strong association between urinary potassium and plasma aldosterone suggests that, in some fashion, plasma aldosterone is responsive to dietary potassium intake. We have described elsewhere that potassium appears to be the only stimulus for altering adrenal output of aldosterone once the kidneys are removed [28–31]. In the intact subject, it has not been possible, thus far, to establish the relative importance of the contribution of sodium versus potassium in regulating aldosterone output.

Potassium intake can clearly be demonstrated to influence aldosterone output in the intact subject [22, 32, 33], but how readily this can be overridden by changes in sodium intake is unclear.

In view of this highly significant association between aldosterone and urinary potassium and hence dietary potassium, the indirect argument associating sodium intake and high blood pressure via the renin-aldosterone system loses some of its force. The data much more strongly favor a major contribution of potassium to alterations in both the renin and blood pressure in hypertensives than they do for sodium. As we have pointed out elsewhere, the use of a more sophisticated statistical technique such as multiple linear regression identifies a significant contribution for potassium, but this technique also indicates that such a role for sodium cannot be demonstrated in these data [33–35].

These observations and the experimental studies of Meneely et al. (21, 27, 33] and other [36, 37] underscore the importance of a critical examination of the possible influence of potassium intake upon blood pressure within populations. The animal studies of Meneely and Dahl and their associates indicate clearly that increasing potassium intake in the rat effectively counters the adverse effect of increased sodium intake. As Meneely noted, when potassium intake in the diet of the salt-loaded animals was increased substantially, they actually survived longer than animals in the control group [21].

Whether a relative potassium deficit precedes the increase in blood pressure in human subjects or whether this is a secondary phenomenon occurring only in those patients who already have substantial elevations of blood pressure is unclear from our data. One point is clear, however; fluctuations in potassium intake and output do represent a confounding variable in studies that purport to show a relationship between sodium and blood pressure. This has usually not been taken into account in available studies [4, 5, 13, 22], and thus further caution must be exercised in interpreting the relationship between sodium and blood pressure as a direct one.

A potential association between potassium and the blood pressure was first noted more than 50 years ago. In 1928, Addison documented the beneficial effect exerted upon high blood pressure by potassium [38]. These studies, carried out in hypertensive individuals, demonstrated decreases in systolic blood pressure that in some instances exceeded 30 mmHg. Interestingly, this decrease in blood pressure could be completely counteracted by administration of sodium chloride. To be certain that potassium rather than chloride was responsible, he repeated the experiments using other salts of sodium and potassium with similar results; in fact, potassium citrate appeared to be more effective in lowering the blood pressure than did the potassium chloride. Addison noted further that administration of sodium chloride aggravated the hypertension with the result that the blood pressure exceeded pretreatment levels. These drops in blood pressure in response to potassium administration were accompanied by clinical improvement and a sense of well-being. Addison concluded as follows: 'One has forced on one the concept that the prevalence of arterial hypertension... is in large part due to a potash-poor diet, and an excessive use of salt (sodium chloride) as a condiment and as a preservative of meat.' It is of interest that Addison implied that this beneficial effect exerted by potassium in hypertension treatment was related to the natriuretic properties of potassium. Both Davies et al. [39] and Bunge [40] had previously shown that administration of potassium to normal subjects resulted in an increase in sodium excretion.

McQuarrie and associates [37] reported the same phenomenon in diabetic children approximately ten years later in studies designed to evaluate the influence of the administration of sodium and potassium upon glucosuria. They noted that the administration of large quantities of sodium chloride (30–40 g/day) produced significant increases in blood pressure with the systolic blood pressure rising from 115 to exceed 155 mmHg. Comparable but somewhat smaller increases in diastolic pressure were also observed. In contrast to the studies reported by Addison, McQuarrie and his associates administered potassium chloride while continuing the large sodium chloride intake. In this instance, the blood pressure returned to its base-line levels, i.e., those levels measured before the sodium chloride administration was begun. Upon withdrawal of the potassium chloride, the blood pressure again began to rise, returning promptly to levels reached prior to potassium administration. These studies were conducted over a three-week period. They suggested that 1 meq of potassium was capable of antagonizing the effects of at least 3 meq of sodium, a remarkable quantitative relationship, considering that their studies were based on data of only two or three patients. While the analogy between these acute studies and the situation created by an increased ingestion of salt in the diet can be questioned, they did conclude that 1–2 g of sodium chloride/kg of body weight increased the blood pressure between 30% and 50% above control levels in a period of 2–4 days. While these are admittedly very high levels, they are not much above the upper bounds of sodium intake that have been documented in some regions where the sodium intake is excessively high [12].

Sasaki [12], in his studies of the relationship between salt intake and high blood pressure in the Japanese, noted that in the Akita prefecture the dietary habits included frequent ingestion of a very salty soup as well as salt-laden soy sauce, and often yielded salt intakes in some provinces as high as 60 g daily. Furthermore, Sasaki noted that the high vegetable intake among the Japanese resulted in the consumption of a large amount of potassium, and comments that perhaps some of the differences in prevalence of hypertension may be related to potassium intake.

The evidence incriminating dietary potassium as a possible factor in the pathogenesis of hypertension is thus at least as compelling in studies within a given population as are the studies relating sodium intake and elevation of the blood pressure. Further studies are necessary to put the present observations in proper prospective, but it is evident that these factors acting alone are inadequate to account for the pathogenesis of hypertension. Some additional factor or factors must be evoked [12, 22]. Presently available data, both experimental and clinical, suggest that the most significant contributing factor is a genetic one [41, 42].

4. HEREDITARY INFLUENCES

The studies by Dahl et al. [41, 43, 44] and by Tobian et al. [45] clearly establish that there is a strong genetic component in the observed sensitivity of the blood pressure to sodium feeding at least in rats. Dahl and associates showed that it was a relatively simple matter to produce animals, as a result of selective inbreeding, that were exquisitely sensitive to increases in salt, responding by the development of severe hypertension. The same techniques also yielded animals that were quite resistant to increased salt intake, showing no tendency to elevate their blood pressures even with very high levels of sodium chloride. Tobian and associates have more recently shown at least a part of the susceptibility or resistance of these animals appears to be related to the kidneys facility for excreting increased quantities of sodium[45]. When kidneys were removed from such salt-sensitive animals and the relationship between arterial perfusion of the kidney and the rate of sodium excretion studied and compared with similar studies from kidneys of animals that were resistant to increased salt intake, the kidneys from the salt-sensitive rats required a higher pressure in order to excrete a given sodium load. If this is indeed the mechanism which these animals use to rid themselves of the increased sodium intake, the relationship between increased sodium intake and elevated blood pressure seems clear. These studies do not provide an explanation for the protective influence of potassium as demonstrated by Meneely et al.[20, 21]. Whether this potassium administration was related in any fashion to facilitation of the sodium excretion was a question addressed by these investigators in a later publication[46]. They demonstrated that administration of increased quantities of potassium chloride prevented the expansion of extracellular fluid seen otherwise with the increased sodium chloride ingestion in these animals.

No comparable direct data bearing on a genetic component to sodium excretion are available within humans. There is, however, a substantial body of evidence beginning with the studies of Pickering and his colleagues which clearly indicates that a significant genetic component can be demonstrated[15, 42]. These studies, which showed only that first-degree relatives of propositi with 'essential hypertension' had higher blood pressure than did comparable first-degree relatives of individuals who had no elevated blood pressure, constitute persuasive evidence that there is a substantial genetic component identifiable in instances of 'essential hypertension' in humans. They provide no evidence associating this genetic component with any unique susceptibility to salt. Such studies are yet to be done.

Acknowledgments. This worked has been supported in part by USPHS grants HL 03303, RR 35, RR 722, and grants from the Harris Foundation, The Irving Blum Memorial Fund, and the O'Neill Endowment Fund.

REFERENCES

1. Kempner W: Treatment of kidney disease and hypertensive vascular disease with rice diet. NC Med J 5:125, 1944.
2. Kempner W: Treatment of hypertensive vascular disease with rice diet. Am J Med 4:454, 1948.
3. Murphy RJF: The effect of 'rice diet' on plasma volume and extracellular fluid space in hypertensive subjects. J Clin Invest 29:912, 1950.
4. Dahl LK, Love RA: Evidence for relationship between sodium chloride intake and human essential hypertension. AMA Arch Intern Med 94:525, 1954.

5. Dahl LK, Love RA: Etiologic role of sodium chloride intake in essential hypertension in humans. JAMA 164:397, 1957.
6. Dole VP, Dahl LK, Cotzias GC, Eder HA, Krebs ME: Dietary treatment of hypertension: clinical and metabolic studies on patients on rice-fruit diet. J Clin Invest 29:1189, 1950.
7. Dustan HP, Cumming GR, Corcoran AC, Page IH: A mechanism of chlorothiazide enchanced effectiveness of antihypertensive ganglioplegic drugs. Circulation 19:360, 1959.
8. Wilson IN, Freis ED: Relationship between plasma and extracellular fluid volume depletion and the antihypertensive effect of chlorothiazide. Circulation 20:1028, 1959.
9. Dahl LK, Love RA: Evidence for relationship between sodium (chloride) intake and essential hypertension. AMA Arch Intern Med 94:525, 1954.
10. Page LB, Damon A, Moellering RC: Antecedents of cardiovascular disease in six Solomon Island Societies. Circulation 49:1132, 1974.
11. Page LB: Epidemiological evidence on the etiology of human hypertension and its possible prevention. Am Heart J 91:527, 1976.
12. Sasaki N: The relationship of salt intake to hypertension in the Japanese. Geriatrics 19:735, 1964.
13. Prior IAM, Evans JG, Harvey HPB, Davidson F, Lindsay M: Sodium intake and blood pressure in two Polynesian populations. N Engl J Med 279:515, 1968.
14. Dahl LK, Silver L, Christie RW and Genest J: Adrenocortical function after prolonged salt restriction in hypertension. Nature 185:110, 1960.
15. Hamilton M, Pickering GW, Roberts JAF, Sowry GSC: The aetiology of essential hypertension. Part 2: Scores for arterial blood pressure adjusted for differences in age and sex. Clin Sci 13:37, 1954. Part 4: Role of inheritance. Clin Sci 13:273, 1954.
16. Ambard L, Beaujard E: Causes de l'hypertension arterielle. Arch Gen Med 1:520, 1904.
17. Allen FM: Arterial hypertension. JAMA 74:652, 1920.
18. Allen FM: Treatment of arterial hypertension. Med Clin North Am 6:475, 1922.
19. Dahl LK: Medical progress. Salt intake and salt need. N Engl J Med 258:1152, 1205, 1958.
20. Meneely GR, Tucker RG, Darby WJ, Auerbach SH: Chronic sodium chloride toxicity in the albino rat. II. Occurrence of hypertension and a syndrome of edema and renal failure. J Exp Med 98:71, 1953.
21. Meneely GR, Ball COT: Experimental epidemiology of chronic sodium chloride toxicity and the protective effect of potassium chloride. Am J Med 25:713, 1958.
22. Freis EDP: Salt, volume and the prevention of hypertension. Circulation 53:589, 1976.
23. Dahl LK: Salt and hypertension. Am J Clin Nutr 25:231, 1972.
24. Padfield PL, Brown JJ, Lever AF, Scalekamp MAD, Beevers DG, Davies DL, Robertson JIS, Tree M: Is low renin hypertension a stage in the development of essential hypertension or a diagnostic entity? Lancet 1:548, 1975.
25. Page LB: Hypertension and atherosclerosis in primitive and acculturating societies. In: Hunt JC, Cooper T, Frohlich ED, Gifford RW, Kaplan NM, Laragh JH, Maxwell MH, Strong CG (eds) Hypertension update: mechanisms, epidemiology, evaluation, and management. Bloomfield NJ: Health Learning Systems, 1980.

26. Shaper AG: Cardiovascular disease in the tropics. III. Blood pressure and hypertension. Br Med J 3:805, 1972.
27. Walker WG, Whelton PK, Saito H, Russell RP, Hermann J: Relation between blood pressure and renin, renin substrate, angiotensin II, aldosterone and urinary sodium and potassium in 574 ambulatory subjects Hypertension 1:287, 1979.
28. Cooke CR, Ruiz-Maza F, Kowarski A, Migeon CJ, Walker WG: Regulation of plasma aldosterone concentration in anephric man and renal transplant recipients. Kidney Int 3:160, 1973.
29. Bayard F, Cooke CR, Tiller DJ, Beitins IZ, Kowarski A, Walker WG, Migeon CJ: The regulation of aldosterone secretion in anephric man. J Clin Invest 50:1585, 1971.
30. Cooke CR, Horvath JS, Moore MA, Walker WG: Modulation of plasma aldosterone concentration by plasma potassium in anephric man in absence of change in potassium balance. J Clin Invest 52:3028, 1973.
31. Walker WG, Cooke CR: Plasma aldosterone regulation in anephric man. Kidney Int 3:1, 1973.
32. Gann DS, Gill Jr JR, Thomas JP, Bartter FC: Control of aldosterone secretion by change of body potassium in hormonal man. Am J Physiol 207:104, 1964.
33. Walker WG, Saito H, Whelton PK, Russel RP, Hermann J: Blood pressure, renin, renin substrate, aldosterone and urinary electrolytes in ambulatory patients. In: Thurm RH (ed) Essential hypertension. Chicago: Year Book Medical, 1979, p 317.
34. Walker WG, Moore MA, Horvath JS, Whelton PK: Arterial and venous angiotensin II in normal subjects. Relation to plasma renin activity, plasma aldosterone concentration, and response to posture and volume changes. Circ Res 38:477, 1976.
35. Walker WG, Horvath JS, Moore MA, Whelton PK, Russell RP: Relation between plasma renin activity, angiotensin, and aldosterone and blood pressure in mild untreated hypertension. Circ Res 38:470, 1976.
36. Priddle WW: Observations on the management of hypertension. Can Med Assoc J 25:5, 1931.
37. McQuarrie I, Thompson WH, Anderson JA: Effects of excessive ingestion of sodium and potassium salts on carbohydrate metabolism and blood pressure in diabetic children. J Nutr 11:77, 1936.
38. Addison WLT: The use of sodium chloride, potassium chloride, sodium bromide and potassium bromide in cases of arterial hypertension which are amenable to potassium chloride. Can Med Assoc J 18:281, 1928.
39. Davies HW, Haldane JBS, Kennaway EL: Experiments on the regulation of blood alkalinity. J Physiol 54:32, 1920-21.
40. Bunge G: Über die Bedeutung des Kochsalzes und das Verhalten der kalisalze im menschlichen Organismus. Z Biol 9:104, 1873.
41. Dahl LK, Heine M, Thompson K: Genetic influence of the kidneys on blood pressure. Evidence from chronic renal homografts in rats with opposite predispositions to hypertension. Circ Res 40:94, 1974.
42. Hamilton M, Pickering GW, Roberts JA, Sowry GSC: Arterial pressures of relatives of patients with secondary and malignant hypertension. Clin Sci 24:91, 1963.
43. Dahl LK, Heine M, Tassinari L: Role of genetic factors in susceptibility to experimental hypertension due to chronic excess salt ingestion. Nature 194:480, 1962.

44. Dahl LK, Heine M, Tassinari L: Effect of chronic excess salt ingestion. Role of genetic factors in both DOCA-salt and renal hypertension. J Exp Med 118:605, 1963.
45. Tobian L, Lange J, Azar S, Iwai J, Koop D, Coffee K, Johnson MA: Reduction of natriuretic capacity and renin release in isolated blood-perfused kidneys by Dahl hypertension-prone rats. Circ Res 43:I-92, 1978.
46. Meneely GR, Ball COT, Youmans JB: Chronic sodium chloride toxicity: protective effect of added potassium chloride. Ann Intern Med 47:263, 1957.

18. DEVELOPMENT OF HIGH BLOOD PRESSURE AND ITS CONSEQUENCES FOR HEALTH

A Swedish population study

L.W. Wilhelmsen, K.S. Svärdsudd, and G.L. Berglund

In clinical medicine, biological traits are often described in qualitative terms such as healthy–ill, normal–abnormal, and normotensive–hypertensive. This dichotomy suggests that the contrasting groups are qualitatively different. Hypertension is not regarded as a defined disease, because it has been repeatedly shown that blood pressure is continuously distributed in the population, and hypertension most often represents only the upper end of the distribution. This is true for the majority of cases, namely those with primary (essential) hypertension. Another fact indicating that hypertension is a graded disorder is the gradually increasing risk with increasing blood pressure.

The increase of blood pressure with increasing age might depend on certain individual or environmental risk factors, which we studied in a representative population sample of men. First, review of these results will be given in this paper, followed by a discussion of the consequences of blood pressure elevation when other cardiovascular risk factors are also considered. A third important issue which will be considered is the concept 'population attributable risk.'

1. THE BLOOD PRESSURE CHANGE WITH TIME

There is little direct evidence about the time factor involved in the development of hypertension. Published blood pressure records which cover a long time period [1, 2] support the view that the blood pressure change over time for most people is a gradual process occurring over decades. Other indirect evidence includes the changes of the blood pressure distribution with age, and the stable blood pressure ranking. The blood pressure distribution at a young age is approximately normal (Gaussian). With increasing age, the upper end of the distribution extends toward higher values while the lower end is relatively unaffected [3–9]. Several studies have shown relatively stable blood pressure ranking, i.e. individuals in a certain blood pressure group tend to retain their relative positions in the blood pressure distribution on successive measurements [6, 7, 9–14]. An individual with high blood pressure at the first reading tends to remain at the upper end of the scale, an individual with

H. Kesteloot. J.V. Joossens (eds.), Epidemiology of Arterial Blood Pressure, 311–324.

moderate pressure remains in the middle of the scale, and so on. This stable ranking is observed in age groups from two years up to 70. The stability of the ranking decreases with increasing time interval between the measurements, but it is still observable after 30 years [11].

A model of the blood pressure change with time, and thus of the development of hypertension, which would satisfy this evidence is shown in Figure 1. According to this model, most people have about the same blood pressure at birth. With increasing age, the blood pressure of some people increases slowly, while that of others increases more rapidly. In the figure, the blood pressure change over time is assumed to be linear, even though it may be irregular in the short-term perspective.

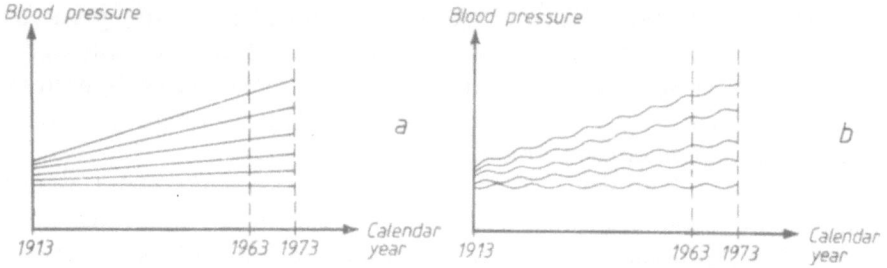

Figure 1. The presumed course of the blood pressure in the study population of men born in 1913 (a) under ideal calculatory conditions and (b) under more realistic conditions.

As a consequence of the model, a positive relationship should exist not only between the blood pressure increase and the blood pressure level attained, but also between the attained level and subsequent blood pressure change. This is called the horse-racing effect, in analogy with a horse race [15] where there is a close correlation between the speeds of the horses and their positions in the race. Such a relationship has been shown to exist [16] and is thus further indirect evidence supporting the model.

2. CAUSE AND EFFECT

The reason for constructing a model of the blood pressure change with time is to facilitate the search for factors causing a blood pressure increase, i.e., risk factors for the development of hypertension. If, as is assumed in Figure 1, the rate of blood pressure increase is a more or less personal characteristic, then the underlying cause should also be a rather stable personal characteristic or a stable environmental factor. Thus, the search for the underlying factors would be limited to a rather small group of factors. If, on the other hand, the development of hypertension is a sudden process, then any short-term or intermittently active factors could be responsible, and the search for the underlying cause could not be limited in the same way. In the following, we assume that the blood pressure increase is a gradual, long-term process.

Another consequence of the assumptions made relates to the interpretation of cause and effect. Suppose we make a survey of a group of individuals 50 years of age and that we follow these individuals up to the age of 60. We also assume that they have the blood pressure development shown in Figure 1. If a factor x, which causes a blood pressure increase, was active for a sufficiently long time before age 50, it would show a relationship not only with the blood pressure increase up to age 50, but also with the blood pressure level at age 50 since those who had the faster blood pressure increase would have attained the highest levels. Such a factor would also be related to the subsequent blood pressure change. But if factor x was a consequence of the raised blood pressure, for example hypertensive vascular lesions, a relationship would be expected only with the blood pressure level and not with the blood pressure change. If factor x and the blood pressure change had a common cause but were otherwise unrelated, the same pattern of relationships would be observed as if factor x were a cause of the pressure change. Since the blood pressure level and the blood pressure change are highly correlated, any analysis of a factor x against blood pressure change must be performed with the blood pressure level taken into account.

Thus, on the basis of a known causal relationship, a certain pattern of associations may be expected, In reality, however, the situation is the reverse. From the analysis, a pattern of relationships is obtained which is used for the interpretation of causality. The absence of a statistically significant association is no evidence that no true relationship exists. Therefore the results of the analysis must be interpreted with caution.

3. RISK FACTORS FOR BLOOD PRESSURE INCREASE

In the study of men born in 1913, an analysis of risk factors for blood pressure increase was performed. The study started in 1963 when a sample consisting of a random third of all 50-year-old males in Göteborg, Sweden, was selected. Of the 973 selected men, 855 participated in the base-line examination. These were reexamined in 1967 and 1973, i.e., at ages 54 and 60. On all three occasions, blood pressure and a number of suspected risk factors were measured. The model of the blood pressure change with time outlined in Figure 1 was employed in the study. The risk factors measured in 1963 were related to the blood pressure level in 1963 and to the blood pressure change from 1963 to 1973. In accordance with the cause and effect discussion above, only those factors which showed a correlation both with the

314

blood pressure level at start of the study and with the blood pressure change during follow-up were accepted as risk factors. To check the results, a similar analysis was performed using the 1967 data as base-line data against the blood pressure change from 1967 to 1973. The results were the same, and results from both follow-up periods are presented in the following presentation.

Body weight and body-mass index (a measure of relative weight) were both correlated with the blood pressure level in 1963 and 1967, and also with the subsequent blood pressure change. Skinfold thickness was positively correlated with both the initial pressure level and the change, even when body weight was taken into account, but body weight was not related to the initial pressure level or to the change when skinfold thickness was taken into account. In 1967, a number of body circumference measurements were used as indices of obesity. They were all correlated with the initial pressure level and with the pressure change, but only waist circumference was of importance when weight was kept constant. Uric acid, a history of maternal death from cardiovascular disease, total serum protein, and systolic and diastolic blood pressure during exercise and at rest 5 min after work were all positively correlated with the initial pressure level and the change of blood pressure.

Blood glucose, serum triglycerides and cholesterol, hematocrit, heart rate, eye-ground changes, heart volume, serum transaminases, urine albumin, and heart rate during work were all positively correlated with the initial pressure level, but not with the subsequent pressure change. Smoking was negatively correlated with the initial pressure level, but not with the pressure change.

Table 1. Regression analysis of suspected risk factors for blood pressure increase during 1963–73 and during 1967–73 taking the initial blood pressure level into account. The study of men born in 1913.

	Regression coefficient	$P \leqslant$
THE PERIOD 1963–73		
Subscapular skinfold thickness (mm)	0.46	0.001
Weight (kg)	−0.21	0.005
Mother died from cardiovascular disease	3.36	0.05
Income (Skr)	−0.0001	NS*
Uric acid (mg/100 ml)	0.79	NS*
THE PERIOD 1967–73		
Subscapular skinfold thickness (mm)	0.36	0.001
Systolic blood pressure at 600 kmp/min (mmHg)	0.10	0.01
Serum protein level (g/100 ml)	2.04	0.05

* NS, not significant.

A multivariate analysis was performed in which the variables related both to the initial pressure level and the pressure change were introduced. The result is shown in Table 1. Skinfold thickness, maternal death from cardiovascular disease, serum protein level, and systolic blood pressure during exercise were independently correlated with the blood pressure change when the initial blood pressure level was taken into consideration. However, the blood pressure increase that could be explained by these factors was rather small, as indicated by the regression coefficients. The effect of the strongest of them, subscapular skinfold thickness, is shown in Figure 2. The thicker the skinfold in 1967, the higher the blood pressure in 1973 regardless of the blood pressure level in 1967.

Body weight and skinfold thickness were both used in this study in an effort to differentiate the influence of obesity from that of body mass. The finding that skinfold thickness at a given weight was of importance for the pressure increase, but that body weight at a given skinfold was not, supports

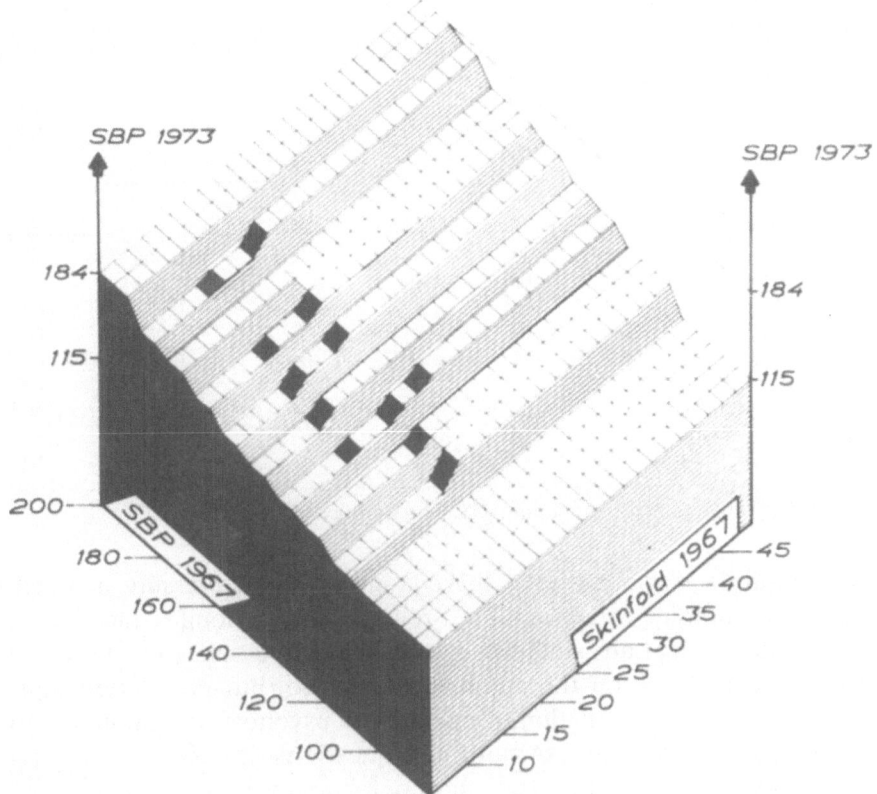

Figure 2. Systolic blood pressure in 1973 in relation to systolic blood pressure and skinfold thickness in 1967. From the study of men born in 1913.

the hypothesis that body fat or some factor closely associated with body fat is the variable related to the blood pressure. The findings were the same in another report from this study [17] using more sophisticated measurements of body fat and lean body mass.

The changes in a number of the variables used in this analysis were also analyzed in relation to the blood pressure change. The changes of body weight, body-mass index, skinfold thickness, waist circumference, heart rate, blood glucose, and serum triglycerides were all positively correlated with the blood pressure change, but the changes of serum cholesterol and hematocrit were not. When weight was kept constant, all the significant correlations were weaker, but still significant except for triglycerides (Table 2). When the change of skinfold thickness was kept constant, the change of weight was no longer significantly correlated with the blood pressure change. Thus, once again, body fat rather than body mass or body volume seems to be the variable strongest related to blood pressure.

Table 2. Correlations between the changes of anthropometric, physiological, and metabolic variables and the change of blood pressure during ten years except for change of waist circumference, which was over six years. The study of men born in 1913.

	Change		Correlation to systolic blood pressure change		Ditto given weight $P \leqslant$
	Mean	SD			
			Direction	$P \leqslant$	
Weight (kg)	1.7	5.3	+	0.005	—
Body-mass index (kg/cm^2)	0.6	1.7	+	0.001	—
Skinfold (mm)	1.3	4.4	+	0.01	0.01
Waist circumference (cm)	6.3	5.8	+	0.001	0.05
Heart rate (beats/min)	2.2	12.8	+	0.001	0.05
Blood glucose (mg/100 ml)	5.4	22.6	+	0.01	0.01
Triglycerides (mmol/l)	−0.02	0.7	+	0.05	NS
Cholesterol (mg/100 ml)	7.0	40.8		NS	NS
Hematocrit (%)	1.5	3.8		NS	NS

+ Denotes a positive (direct) correlation; NS, not significant.

In this study we also analyzed the change of blood pressure in relation to psychosocioeconomic variables. The relationship among education, social class, income, occupation, shift work, and subjective stress on the one hand, and the blood pressure on the other was analyzed, but no relationships were found. In the 1973 examination, a number of psychosocioeconomic variables were evaluated by interview. Among the questions answered, seven, relating to a worsened job situation, were chosen for analysis and a score was constructed. This score was negatively related to the pressure change, implying that men who reported the greatest deterioration in their work situation had the lowest blood pressure increase. A score based on self-rating in 15 questions relating to change in different aspects of the life situation was not related to pressure change. An affirmative answer to the questions 'Have you been unable to make full use of vacation periods during the last ten years?' and 'Have you had a divorce during the last ten years?' were positively related to the pressure change ($P<0.05$ and $P<0.01$, respectively). Other types of conflicts within the family, change of subjective stress, and receipt of sickness benefit or a disability pension were not related to the pressure change.

Using questionnaires, an attempt was also made to analyze the importance of alcohol consumption. No significant relationship could be found, but this does not exclude alcohol being of importance as there are several sources of bias when using this type of questionnaire.

Thus, high body weight and factors associated with body weight, heredity of cardiovascular disease, high blood pressure during exercise, and high serum protein level were the significant risk factors for blood pressure increase found in this study.

4. HIGH BLOOD PRESSURE AS A RISK FACTOR

In the previously mentioned 'Study of Men Born in 1913', morbidity data are available for 13.5 years of follow-up. The fact that only one age group—men aged 50 at entry to the study—are followed improves the possibility of eliminating the confounding factor age, which is important when dealing with such a strongly age-dependent variable as blood pressure. However, men with definite hypertension were treated with antihypertensive drugs, and the relationship between blood pressure level and subsequent disease is therefore underestimated in relation to what might be found in a less well-treated population.

In this study, as well as in several others, a strong association between the height of blood pressure and total mortality was found [18]. As regards specific diagnoses, death from myocardial infarction and cancer, and morbidity from myocardial infarction and stroke, were significantly related to the blood pressure level.

When considering risk for various diseases, it is not only important to analyze the relative risk at different blood pressure levels, but also to analyze the number of cases suffering the respective end points. In the present study, 37 died from coronary heart disease, but only four from stroke.

A Norwegian study by Holme and Waaler [19] followed 41,000 males of various ages during five years. They also found that coronary heart disease (CHD) was much more important as an end point at most blood pressure

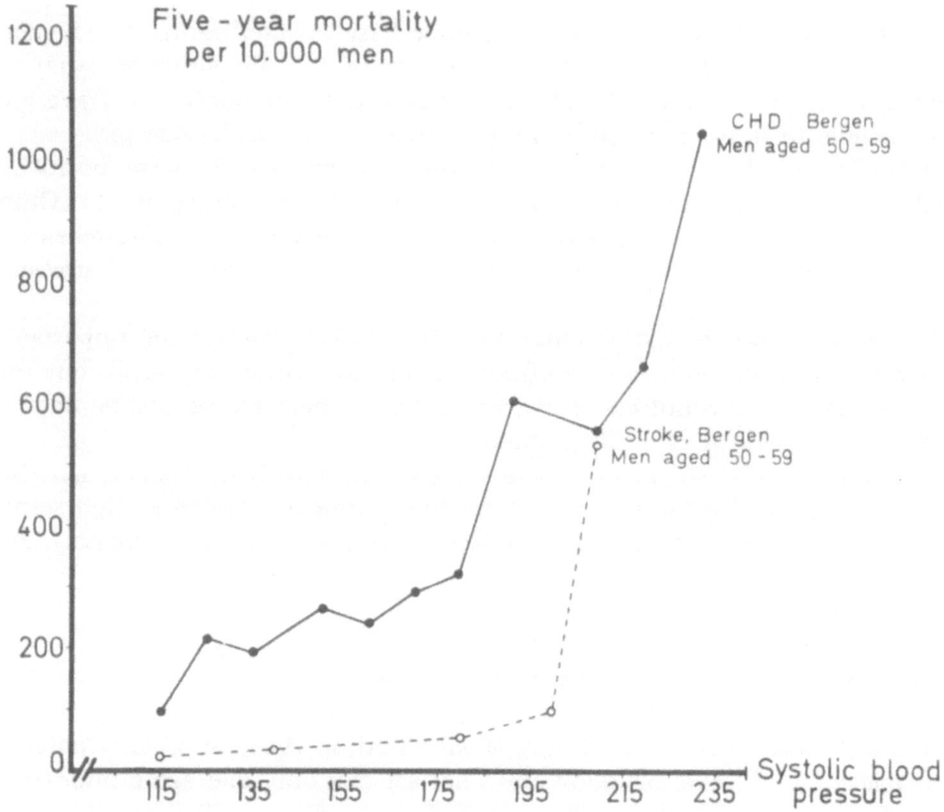

318

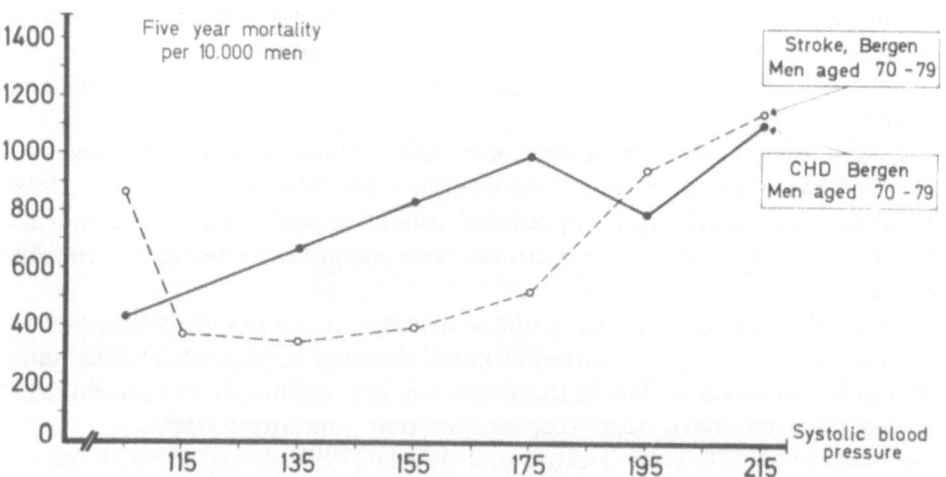

Figure 3. The relationship between five-year mortality and systolic blood pressure in the Bergen study [19]. Men aged 50–59 years. From *Clin. Sci.* 57:455s–458s, 1979.

Figure 4. The relationship between five-year mortality and systolic blood pressure in the Bergen study [19]. Men aged 70–79 years.

levels, excepting the highest among 50- to 59-year-old men (Fig. 3). The difference was less pronounced at ages 70–79 years and the increase with blood pressure was also less steep at the older ages (Fig. 4)[20].

However, CHD is more dependent on the two risk factors serum cholesterol and smoking than is stroke. Thus, in a country with a low prevalence of hypercholesterolemia and few smokers, stroke might be as important a cause of death as CHD, at least when the blood pressure is very high. There are relatively few studies available from countries with such low smoking and cholesterol levels, however. Recently, Ashcroft and Desai[21] reported results from a population study in rural Jamaica. The population had low mean serum cholesterol levels (4.7–5.0 mmol/l in men aged 35–64 years). The total

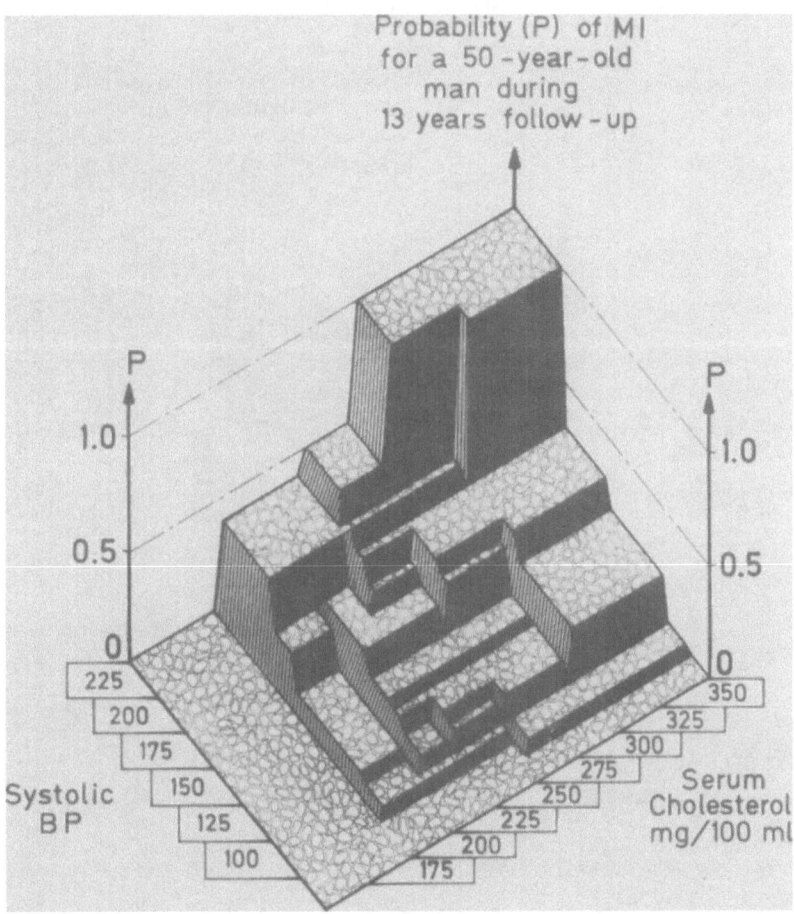

Figure 5. Probability (*P*) of nonfatal or fatal myocardial infarction (MI) or sudden coronary death for a 50-year-old man during 13 years of follow-up in relation to sytolic blood pressure and smoking habits. By permission ref. [20].

mortality during 13 years of follow-up was low and mortality was significantly increased only at blood pressure above 180 mmHg systolic or 110 mmHg diastolic.

This does not contradict the results from industrialized countries. Thus, in our study of men aged 50 at entry (followed for 13 years in this analysis), we found that coronary heart disease risk (nonfatal myocardial infarction, fatal myocardial infarction, and sudden coronary death) rose rather moderately with increasing blood pressure among nonsmokers and exsmokers (Fig. 5) or in men with low cholesterol values (Fig. 6). However, when the serum cholesterol was high or a person was a heavy smoker, the risk increased much more steeply. The data were analyzed with the aid of multivariate logistic analysis and isotonic regression [22, 23]. From these diagrams, it can easily be seen that the coronary heart disease risk for a certain blood pressure varies

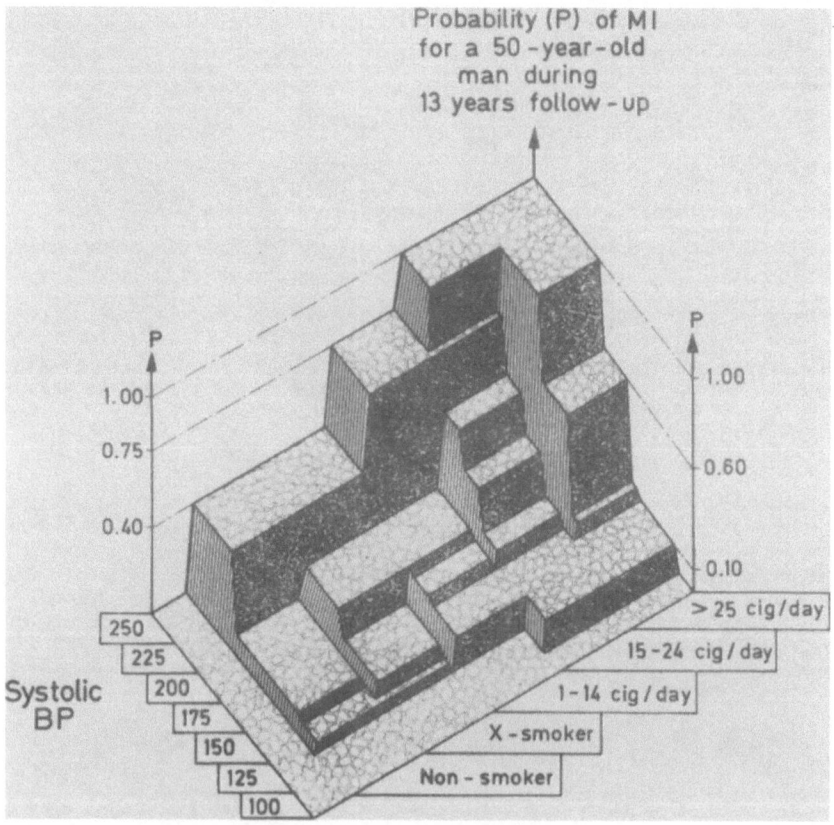

Figure 6. Probability (*P*) of nonfatal or fatal myocardial infarction (MI) or sudden coronary death for a 50-year-old men during 13 years of follow-up in relation to systolic blood pressure and serum cholesterol level. The study of men born in 1913. From *Clin. Sci.* 57:455s–458s, 1979.

between individuals—as well as between countries—according to the levels of the other risk factors. In women, who are at lower risk for coronary heart disease than men, there are less-marked incidence differences between coronary heart disease and stroke.

5. POPULATION ATTRIBUTABLE RISK

The probability (risk) for a coronary heart disease event was as high as 1.0 (100%) in those with high blood pressure and high cholesterol level, or in those who smoked heavily (Figs. 5 and 6). However, very few subjects have such high risk in the general population. Figure 7 shows the risk increase

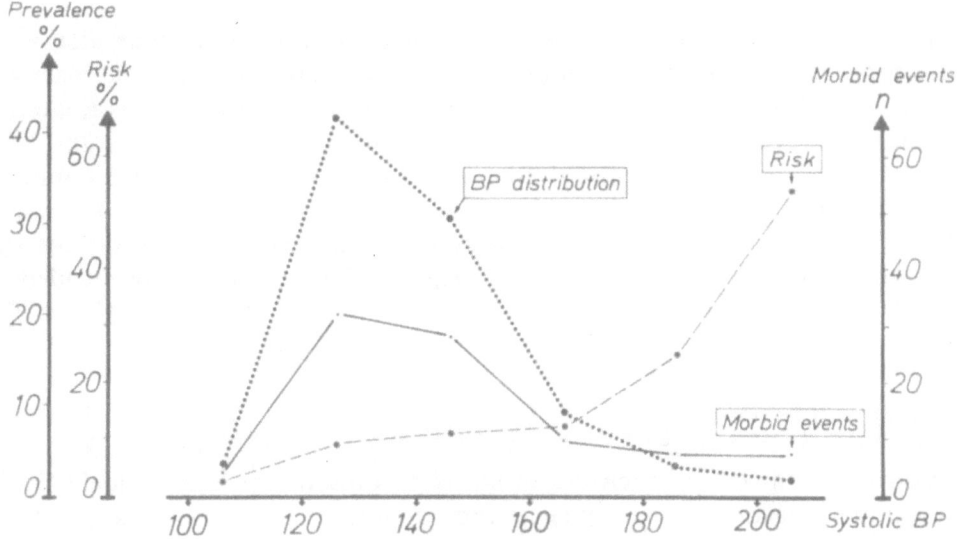

Figure 7. Blood pressure distribution, risk for coronary heart disease (CHD) or stroke, and number (*n*) of such morbid events in relation to blood pressure during 13.5 years of follow-up of 865 men aged 50 at entry to study. The study of men born in 1913. From *Clin. Sci.* 57:455s–458s, 1979.

with increasing blood pressure, the blood pressure distribution, and the number of fatal events in relation to blood pressure. As can be seen, it is important to not only consider the risk, but also the number of individuals exposed to the risk. Thus, the concept 'population attributable risk' denotes the product of risk and number of individuals exposed to the risk. The majority of events occurred among men with blood pressures commonly regarded as normal, or at least not considered in need of antihypertensive drug treatment.

Based upon theoretical calculations of the effect of intervention in this population sample, we obtained the following results.

If the 2% of the population with the highest blood pressures had been treated so intensively that their risk had been reduced to the same level as in the individuals with a systolic blood pressure of 140–155 mmHg, six of the seven cases in the group and 7% of the total infarction and stroke morbidity would have been avoided. If the highest 5% had been treated in the same way, 10 out of 14 events in the group and 11% of all events would have been avoided. The efficacy of measures taken declines rapidly, however, when lower blood pressure groups are being treated. In order to avoid 13% of all events, 14% of the population must be treated, and to reduce the number of events by 19%, 45% of the population would have to be treated. By treating virtually the entire population, the incidence of infarction and stroke would be reduced by about 65%.

Thus, it would seem impossible to eliminate the myocardial infarction and stroke problem from the community by drug treatment, Even a massive effort, with drug treatment at a low level in the blood pressure distribution, would not prevent more than 15%–20% of all cases in this age group. For comparison, it can be calculated that if a pressure reduction of 10 mmHg could be achieved for the whole blood pressure distribution except the lowest blood pressure group, the incidence of infarction and stroke would decline by 18%. If a pressure reduction of 20 mmHg could be achieved, the incidence would fall by 36% [24].

6. A POSSIBLE STRATEGY

Treatment with antihypertensive drugs is at present the most widely used preventive measure, but the main effort at present is to reduce the risk in individuals at high risk. To solve the problem of infarction, stroke and other sequelae *in the community*, case finding and drug treatment must be combined with other measures influencing the incidence in the low- and middle-risk intervals as well. Such measures should be simple, cheap, harmless, and applicable on a large scale in the entire population. They should also be self-generating, i.e., it must be possible to incorporate the measures into a normal life pattern in order to avoid expensive 'maintenance.' No such ideal instrument is available at present. Of the hitherto proposed nonpharmacological preventive measures, the effect of reduction of weight and of salt intake is fairly well documented [25–29]. Weight reduction is, however, neither a simple nor a cheap or self-generating measure. It might also be hard to apply on a large scale in the community.

If salt intake is as important for the blood pressure level as some studies indicate [30], reduction of the salt intake would be a natural preventive measure. A number of intervention studies have shown that a reduction of salt intake is followed by a reduction of blood pressure. However, most of the attention has been focused on treating hypertension with a reduced salt intake, often vigorously reduced. Little is known about the effect in lower blood pressure levels and of the effects of a slight to moderate salt intake reduction. By inference from the studies cited above, one would expect that a salt intake reduction large enough to produce a blood pressure fall of 5–10 mmHg on the average would be fully acceptable by the public. Such a small blood pressure reduction has earlier been regarded as insignificant from a clinical viewpoint, but it might be large enough to have a marked impact on the incidence of blood pressure related diseases, especially if combined with case finding and drug treatment of hypertensives.

These nonpharmacological preventive measures are still too little explored to be recommended for use on a large scale. More detailed information about the short-term and long-term effects of this type of intervention is needed. But if these measures can be applied in the majority of the population, it may be a further step toward the control of hypertension and its sequelae.

REFERENCES

1. Evelyn KA: The natural history and prognosis of hypertension. Proceedings of the 42nd Annual Meeting of the Medical Section, American Life Convention, 42:44–78, 1954.
2. Holmgren I: Studies of arterial tension on 4,864 patients from private practice. Acta Med Scand 151:237-257, 1955.
3. Bjerkedal T, Natvig H: Changes in blood pressure with age. A descriptive analysis based on a cross-sectional and a longitudinal study of Norwegian men, 15–70 years of age. Acta Med Scand 180:257-273, 1966.
4. Borhani NO, Hechter HH: A longitudinal study of blood pressure. Angiology 15:545-555, 1964.
5. Eilertsen E, Humerfelt S: The blood pressure in a representative population sample. Acta Med Scand 183:293-305, 1968.
6. Feinleib M, Halperin M, Garrison RJ: Relationship between blood pressure and age. Regression analysis of longitudinal data. Paper presented at the 97th Annual Meeting of the American Public Health Association, Philadelphia, 10–14 November, 1969.
7. Harlan WR, Osborne RK, Graybiel A: A longitudinal study of blood pressure. Circulation 26:530-543, 1962.
8. Miall WE, Chinn S: Blood pressure and ageing: results of a 15–17 year follow-up study in South Wales. Clin Sci Mol Med [Suppl] 45:23-33, 1973.
9. Zinner SH, Martin LF, Sacks F, Rosner B, Kass EH: A longitudinal study of blood pressure in childhood. Am J Epidemiol 100:437-442, 1975.
10. Diehl HS, Hesdorffer MB: Changes in blood pressure of young men over a seven year period. Arch Intern Med 52:948-953, 1933.

11. Harlan WR, Oberman A, Mitchell RW, Graybiel A: A thirty-year study of blood pressure in a white male cohort. Clin Res 19:319, 1971.
12. Hsu PH, Mathewson FAL, Rabkin SW: Blood pressure and body mass index patterns — a longitudinal study. J Chronic Dis 30:93-113, 1977.
13. Robinson SC, Brucer M: Range of normal blood pressure. A statistical and clinical study of 11,383 persons. Arch Intern Med 64:409-444, 1939.
14. Rosner B, Hennekens CH, Kass EH, Miall WE: Age-specific correlation analysis of longitudinal blood pressure data. Am J Epidemiol 106:306-313, 1977.
15. Fletcher C, Peto R, Tinker C, Speizer FE: The natural history of chronic bronchitis and emphysema. London: Oxford University Press, 1976.
16. Svärdsudd K, Tibblin G: A longitudinal blood pressure study. Change of blood pressure during ten years in relation to initial values. The study of men born in 1913. J Chronic Dis (to be published).
17. Larsson B: Obesity. A Population study of men born in 1913 with special reference to development and consequences for the health. PhD thesis, University of Göteborg, 1978.
18. Svärdsudd K, Tibblin G: Mortality and morbidity during 13.5 years' follow-up in relation to blood pressure. Acta Med Scand 205:483–492, 1979.
19. Holme I, Waaler HTH: Five-year mortality in the city of Bergen, Norway, according to age, sex and blood pressure. Acta Med Scand 200:229-239, 1976.
20. Wilhelmsen L, Berglund G, Wedel H: Benefits of blood pressure treatment in the general middle-aged male population. In: Gross F, Strasser T (eds) Mild hypertension — natural history and treatment. London: Pitman Medical, 1979, pp 47-55.
21. Ashcroft MT, Desai P: Blood pressure in a rural Jamaican community. Lancet 1:1167-1170, 1978.
22. Wilhelmsen L, Wedel H, Tibblin G: Multivariate analysis of risk for coronary heart disease. Circulation 48:950-958, 1973.
23. Wilhelmsen L, Bengtsson C, Elmfeldt D, Vedin A, Wilhelmsson C, Tibblin G, Wedel H: Multiple risk prediction of myocardial infarction in women as compared to men. Br Heart J 39:1179-1185, 1977.
24. Svärdsudd K: High blood pressure. A longitudinal population study of men born in 1913, with special reference to development and consequences for health. PhD thesis, University of Göteborg, 1978.
25. Chiang BN, Perlman LV, Epstein FH: Overweight and hypertension. A review. Circulation 39:403-421, 1969.
26. Reisin E, Abel R, Modan M, Silverberg DS, Eliahou HE, Modan B: Effect of weight loss without salt restriction on the reduction of blood pressure in overweight hypertensive patients. N Engl J Med 298:1-6, 1978.
27. Parijs J, Joossens JV, Linden L van der, Verstreken G, Amery AKPC: Moderate sodium restriction and diuretics in the treatment of hypertension. Am Heart J 85:22-34, 1973.
28. Carney S, Morgan T, Wilson M, Matthews G, Roberts R: Sodium restriction and thiazide diuretics in the treatment of hypertension. Med J Aust 1:803-807, 1975.
29. Morgan T, Cillies A, Morgan G, Adam W, Wilson M, Carney S: Hypertension treated by salt restriction. Lancet 1:227-230, 1978.
30. Freis ED: Salt, volume and the prevention of hypertension. Circulation 53:589-595, 1976.

19. EPIDEMIOLOGY AND CONTROL OF HYPERTENSION IN NORTH KARELIA, FINLAND

Observations from a five-year community control programme

J. TUOMILEHTO, A. NISSINEN, P. PUSKA, J. ELO, and T.E. KOTTKE

Arterial hypertension is a common problem in industrialized societies, and a major cause of disability and death in the adult populations. Although elevated blood pressure itself is not an incapacitating condition, a high proportion of severe cardiovascular disease (CVD) is due to hypertension. For these reasons, it has been called the epidemic of the modern world; it is a challenge to medical care and public health [1–6]. During the last 25 years, several potent and relatively harmless drugs for hypertension treatment have been introduced. Studies on long-term blood pressure reduction have made it clear that antihypertensive drug treatment is effective in preventing complications, morbidity, disability and premature death [7–12].

The evidence that drug therapy is beneficial in long-term hypertension management has caused a considerable increase in the number of treated hypertensive patients all over the world. Epidemiological studies conducted during the 1970's documented that in many populations, only a fraction of the total number of hypertensives is being treated at all, and a still smaller proportion receives systematic and effective treatment and follow-up. A community programme for hypertension control was started in 1972 in North Karelia, Finland. The pilot programme aim was to evaluate the effects carefully so that experiences could be used in other large-scale antihypertension programmes. To evaluate the change due to intervention, a reference population was also needed. The reference area had a similar age distribution, economic and social characteristics, and patterns of mortality and morbidity at the outset.

This report presents the findings in North Karelia between 1972 and 1977. It shows the changes in blood pressure and in antihypertensive treatment status resulting from the effort against hypertension in the entire population of North Karelia.

1. THE NORTH KARELIA PROJECT

Faced with an exceptionally large CVD problem in North Karelia [13–16], representatives of the local population in North Karelia signed a petition in

1971 asking for national assistance to reduce the high CVD mortality and prevalence rates. After the planning stage, the North Karelia Project was launched in 1972 to meet the local population's urgent need.

During the planning, it was decided to carry out a comprehensive CVD control programme within the service structure and social organization of the community. This intervention was to involve both primary and secondary prevention [17–19]. The main project objective was to reduce CVD morbidity and mortality among the population, with special reference to middle-aged men. Reduction of the levels of the known CVD risk factors (smoking, serum cholesterol, blood pressure) and promotion of early detection, treatment and rehabilitation of CVD was the strategy. The objective for national purposes was to test the feasibility and effect of this approach, and to provide tested methods for nationwide use in CVD control and related health programmes.

The subprogrammes were based on the steps in the natural history of coronary heart disease (smoking, diet, hypertension, coronary heart disease, acute myocardial infarction, rehabilitation) [20, 21]. The North Karelia Project was a five-year intensified community intervention and its evaluation from 1972 to 1977.

2. BRIEF DESCRIPTION OF THE HYPERTENSION PROGRAMME

The hypertension programme of the North Karelia Project included health service organization and intensification, health personnel training, health education for the public at large and patients in particular, and development of information services. A hypertension register was the major means of ensuring patient follow-up. It also served in the programme evaluation, together with the base-line and the terminal surveys [21, 22].

The North Karelia Project hypertension programme was a part of an international co-operative 'Community control of hypertension' study and followed the protocol prepared by the WHO expert group in Göteborg, Sweden, in 1971 [2].

2.1. Objectives of the hypertension programme. The main hypertension programme objective was reduction of high blood pressure among the whole population and especially among the middle-aged people in North Karelia. The special hypertension programme objectives were:

1) to identify hypertensives for treatment,
2) to control the blood pressure in these patients,

3) to unify the physicians' diagnostic and therapeutic procedures, and

4) to gather new information about the epidemiology of hypertension and the function of health services.

2.2. Implementation. The hypertension programme was implemented at three levels: at the national level by the National Medical Board (which took responsibility for the programme), at the county level by the North Karelia Province Department of Social and Health Affairs (which implemented the programme in the county), and at the local level by the health centre boards (which implemented the programme in the health centres).

The hypertension programme was integrated into the existing county health services and social organization. The majority of hypertensives were treated by the local health centre physicians. Special hypertension follow-up dispensaries were organized in each health centre. These dispensaries were run by public health nurses specially trained by the Project. The continuous hypertensive follow-up was thus dependent on these nurses. Physicians and public health nurses were advised to combine health education with treatment and follow-up. The aim was to reduce all CVD risk factor levels. The implementation has been described in detail elsewhere [23].

3. SUBJECTS AND METHODS OF THE EPIDEMIOLOGICAL SURVEYS

The base-line survey was carried out in spring 1972 in North Karelia and a reference area. A representative 6.6% sample was drawn from the national population register of the two counties. The sample included men and women born between 1913 and 1947 (aged 25–59 at the time of the survey). Exactly five years later, another cross-sectional survey, the terminal survey, was carried out in the two areas. The methods were strictly the same as those used in the base-line survey. The sample was an independent 6.6% random sample that included man and women born between 1913 and 1947 (aged 30–64 at the time of the survey).

Ten days before the examination, the subjects received a letter that contained an explanation of the study, an invitation to the examination, practical instructions and a questionnaire. The questionnaire was designed to evaluate multiple aspects of the programme, including hypertension epidemiology and control in the community. It contained questions on the following groups of items: general background, socioeconomic status, medical history (including present somatic and psychosomatic symptoms) and use of health services, health behaviour (smoking, diet, alcohol consumption, physical exercise) and attempts to change it, attitudes towards risk factors and health services, and social interaction and psychosocial stress levels. The subjects were asked to

328

complete the questionnaire at home and to bring it with them to the examination.

Casual blood pressure was measured at the examination. In the 1977 survey, the measurement was repeated if the first value exceeded 160 mmHg systolic and/or 95 mmHg diastolic. The measurement was done while the subject was in the sitting position, according to the standard technique [24]. The fifth phase of the Korotkoff sounds was recorded as the diastolic pressure. The questionnaire was checked at the examination when the subjects were also tested on their knowledge of other health aspects. Those with known hypertension were asked about their treatment. Additional questions were also asked about fat consumption.

The field work was carried out during February, March and April, mainly at local health centres, by six groups, each consisting of two specially trained nurses. Each group was aided by 2–4 local assistants, mostly public health nurses. The nurses took blood pressure and skinfold measurements and also checked the questionnaires. Subjects whose blood pressure was high at the examination were told so, and their blood pressures were checked afterwards by local health workers. Subjects were informed if their blood lipid concentrations were high. This was done in a letter that also contained instructions for visiting a doctor.

Table 1. Original and purified samples, participation and non-participation in the surveys.

| | 1972 | | 1977 | |
	Men	Women	Men	Women
Original sample	2576	2539	2355	2373
Purified sample	2407	2423	2317	2342
Participated	2228	2307	2002	2121
Also examination	2095	2196	2002	2121
Only questionnaire	133	111	—	—
Did not participate	179	116	315	221
Temporarily away	63	33	35	23
Unable to answer	17	14	30	14
Refused	8	3	23	19
Unknown reason	39	66	227	165
Participation rate (%)	92.6	95.2	86.4	90.6

Table 1 shows the sample sizes, participation rates, and reasons for non-participation, while Table 2 shows the subjects studied with stratification by age and sex. Because the same birth cohort was followed, the ages given in the tables refer always to the age of the subjects in 1972. Some subjects were excluded from the original sample because they had died or had moved permanently outside of the counties before the survey; thus they did not

Table 2. Responders of the surveys in North Karelia in 1972 and in 1977 by age and sex.

Age (years)	Men				Women			
	1972		1977		1972		1977	
	n	%	n	%	n	%	n	%
25–29	349	17.7	–	–	334	14.5	–	–
30–34	284	12.8	365	18.2	298	12.9	317	15.0
35–39	304	13.6	275	13.7	300	13.0	278	13.1
40–44	335	15.1	287	14.4	353	15.4	289	13.6
45–49	364	16.3	320	16.0	363	15.7	327	15.4
50–54	286	12.8	293	14.6	331	14.3	328	15.5
55–59	261	11.7	245	12.3	328	14.2	306	14.4
60–64	–	–	217	10.8	–	–	276	13.0
Total	2228	100.0	2002	100.0	2307	100.0	2121	100.0

really belong to the study population. The participation rates were high: 94% in the base-line survey (for about 6% of these subjects, only data from the questionnaire were available), and 89% in the terminal survey in North Karelia. The reasons for non-participation were mostly unknown: in most cases, addresses were not up to date and could not be corrected. People temporarily away from their homes comprised the second largest group of non-participants and the third largest group was comprised of people unable to answer (e.g. mentally retarded). Few people refused to participate. The data obtained in 1972 were compared with those obtained after five years of the intervention (1977).

4. RESULTS

Distribution of blood pressures are given in Figures 1 and 2 for men and women, respectively. Both systolic and diastolic blood pressures had non-normal distributions, skewed to the right. This skewness did not change from 1972 to 1977, but frequency distributions of both pressures shifted to the left despite the aging of the population during these five years.

Mean systolic blood pressure was associated with age in both sexes. This association was greater among women than men (Table 3). Men had significantly higher mean levels than women in age groups below 45 years. Lower age-specific mean systolic pressures were present in 1977 compared with those in 1972 for all age-sex groups. The association with age was also less marked in 1977 than in 1972. This was especially true among women; their mean systolic pressure values did not exceed those of men before 55 years of

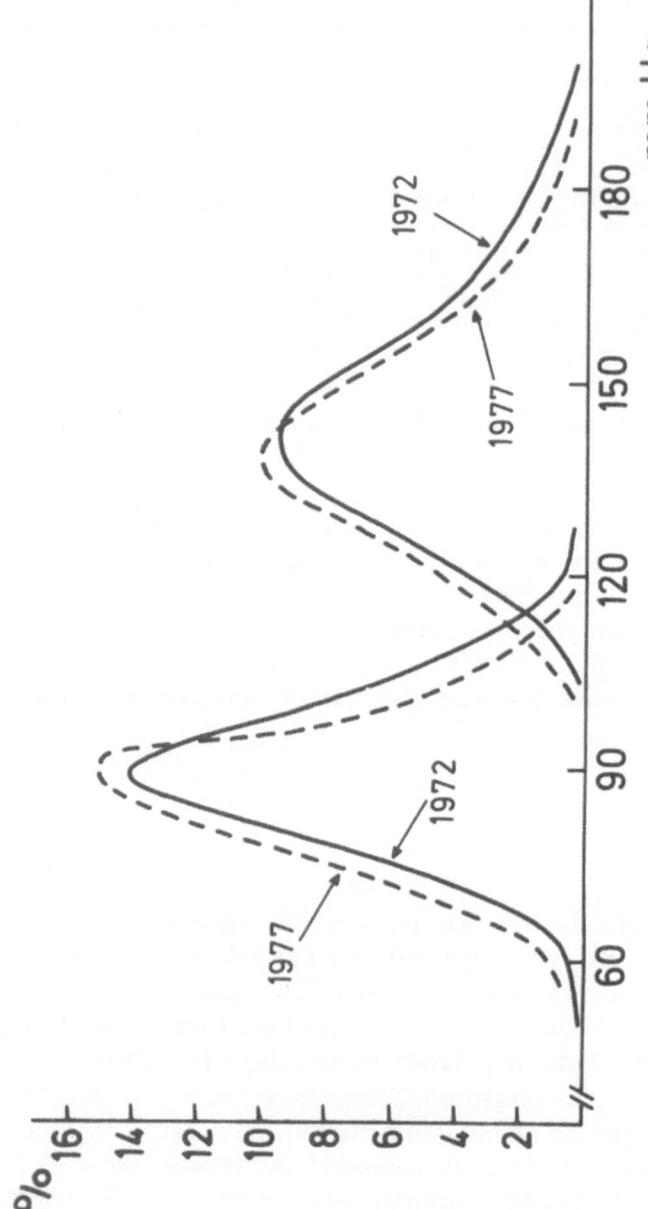

Figure 1. Smoothed distribution curves of blood pressures among men in 1972 and 1977.

331

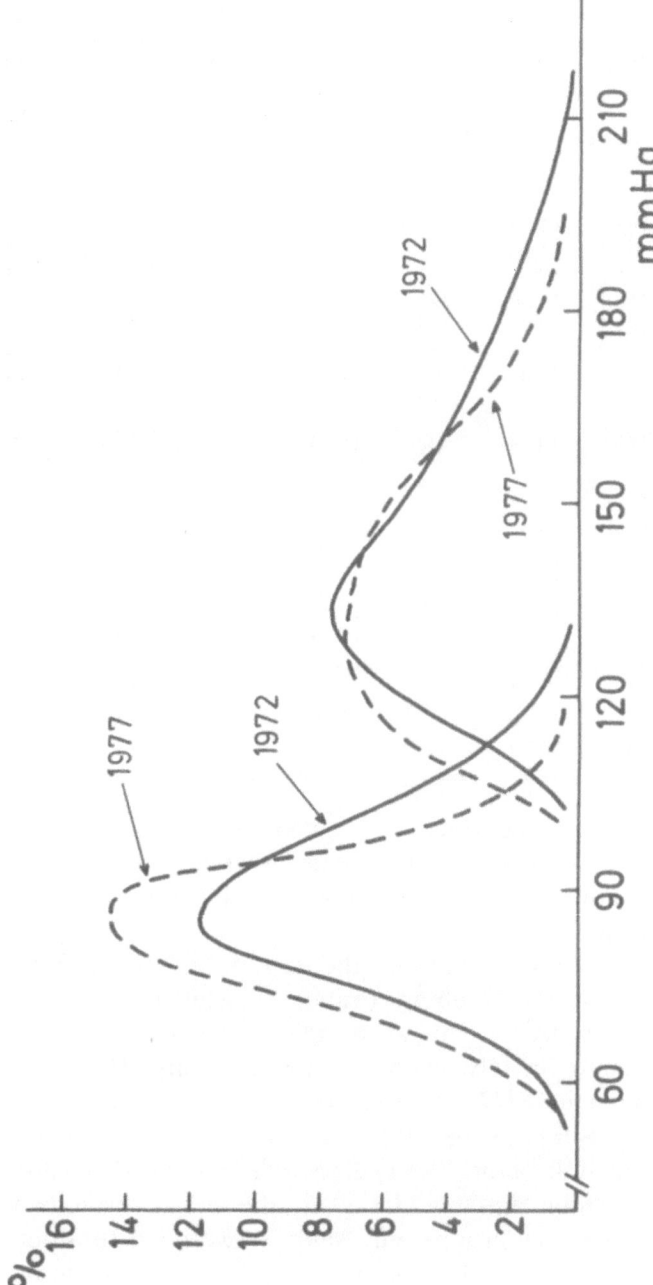

Figure 2. Smoothed distribution curves of blood pressures among women in 1972 and 1977.

Table 3. Means and standard deviations of systolic and diastolic blood pressure (mmHg) by age and sex.

Age (years)	Men				Women			
	1972		1977		1972		1977	
	Mean	± SD	Mean	± SD	Mean	± SD	Mean	± SD
SYSTOLIC PRESSURE								
25–29	141.1	15.93	—	—	129.9	14.54	—	—
30–34	142.1	15.60	139.0	14.87	136.0	16.38	127.7	15.33
35–39	145.2	18.63	141.2	17.07	140.2	19.44	132.5	16.36
40–44	146.1	18.30	140.2	17.82	147.5	21.33	137.2	18.04
45–49	147.9	19.92	145.5	17.63	155.6	25.37	144.7	19.78
50–54	154.3	23.17	144.9	18.00	163.0	25.32	147.6	20.78
55–59	157.4	25.81	148.1	19.56	181.4	27.38	156.0	21.40
60–64	—	—	152.1	23.05	—	—	159.2	21.25
Total	146.6	20.84	140.3	18.93	148.1	24.91	140.2	20.70
DIASTOLIC PRESSURE								
25–29	85.0	12.23	—	—	79.9	12.16	—	—
30–34	88.0	10.17	84.8	10.19	83.9	11.5	79.5	9.76
35–39	92.8	11.72	88.2	11.18	88.0	12.23	83.2	9.32
40–44	91.3	12.36	88.6	10.79	91.0	11.87	86.0	10.40
45–49	92.3	12.00	90.8	10.69	93.5	13.37	88.5	10.34
50–54	94.1	12.92	89.9	10.94	97.0	12.81	89.4	9.86
55–59	93.7	13.08	90.1	11.28	100.1	13.28	90.7	11.15
60–64	—	—	89.0	11.80	—	—	90.0	9.83
Total	89.9	12.65	85.7	12.06	89.8	13.76	84.8	11.71

age. Variation among individuals was greater with increasing age in both sexes at these two surveys, but this pattern was less marked in 1977 than in 1972. At both examinations, slightly more variability was seen among women than men with increasing age.

Diastolic blood pressure patterns did not differ much from the systolic pressure patterns described above (Table 3). The association of the mean value with age was found. Unlike systolic patterns, there was a plateauing among men at approximately age 50 both in 1972 and 1977. Among women, this was not found in 1972, but seen around age 60 in 1977. Higher mean diastolic blood pressures in men than in women were found until the age 45 years in 1972, but not before the age 55 in 1977—again a pattern similar to that found for systolic pressure. In 1977, the mean diastolic values of the women in the oldest age groups only slightly exceeded those of men so that the sex difference seen in the youngest age groups was more pronounced. Within-group variability of diastolic pressure was similar for all age-sex groups at each time, but was slightly smaller in 1977 than in 1972.

Table 4. Prevalence of elevated diastolic blood pressure in North Karelia in 1972 and in 1977 by age and sex.

	Age (years)	Men		Women	
		1972 %	1977 %	1972 %	1977 %
DIASTOLIC ⩾ 95 mmHg	25–29	15.6	—	10.1	—
	30–34	21.0	11.4	13.5	4.8
	35–39	34.8	20.7	23.0	9.0
	40–44	30.3	22.2	31.3	16.0
	45–49	35.2	30.7	40.6	22.8
	50–54	44.5	29.4	51.2	24.3
	55–59	41.6	29.2	60.0	27.5
	60–64	—	29.6	—	27.9
	Total	31.3	23.2	33.3	19.0
DIASTOLIC ⩾ 100 mmHg	25–29	11.0	—	8.1	—
	30–34	11.2	7.2	8.2	3.2
	35–39	26.3	16.7	17.5	4.3
	40–44	20.8	15.9	23.9	8.4
	45–49	27.6	19.9	31.7	13.2
	50–54	33.9	21.4	38.3	16.6
	55–59	34.4	21.3	50.7	19.3
	60–64	—	16.7	—	16.2
	Total	23.2	16.6	25.9	11.7
DIASTOLIC ⩾ 105 mmHg	25–29	4.9	—	3.3	—
	30–34	4.9	3.6	3.9	1.3
	35–39	14.3	8.4	9.3	1.4
	40–44	12.0	7.0	13.6	4.2
	45–49	15.5	8.2	19.1	4.3
	50–54	19.7	7.2	24.9	5.8
	55–59	22.0	9.2	35.5	9.8
	60–64	—	6.5	—	6.6
	Total	13.0	7.0	15.9	4.8

Table 4 gives the prevalence rates of elevated blood pressure in 1972 and in 1977 by age, sex and three different diastolic cut-off points. With a diastolic blood pressure of 95 mmHg as the cut-off, one-third of the men and women in 1972 had elevated blood pressure. The respective fraction was one-fifth in 1977. In 1972, women had slightly higher overall prevalence rates than men, but the situation was the reverse in 1977.

Prevalence of elevated blood pressure increased with age among women both in 1972 and in 1977, plateauing at approximately age 60. Among men, similar increases with age were seen in 1972, but the pattern was not so clear in 1977, when it levelled off at approximately age 50. Both among men and women, age-specific prevalence rates decreased during the five-year period. This decrease was greatest in the oldest age groups for both sexes.

Regression analysis was used to analyse factors associated with elevated systolic and diastolic blood pressures; 15 independent variables, which were chosen because of relationships found in other studies, were included in the analysis. In addition, the known risk indicators of coronary heart disease (cholesterol and smoking) were included.

Factors included in the analysis were: age, wrist width, systolic blood pressure, diastolic blood pressure, serum cholesterol, smoking, body-mass index [index = body weight (kg/height (m²)], triceps skinfold, height, serum triglycerides, fasting period, physical exercise at work, physical exercise at leisure time, coffee drinking, alcohol consumption, pork in diet, and stroke and/or myocardial infarction of mother and/or father under age 60.

The method was step-wise linear regression analysis which chose the variable that had the highest correlation with the dependent variable as the first independent variable. Selection was then made after each step, based on partial correlations. Body-mass index and age had the greatest numerical correlations with systolic pressure (0.44 and 0.40, respectively) and diastolic pressure (0.45 and 0.39, respectively). Only these two independent variables made a significant contribution (Table 5).

Table 5. Estimated coefficients of the two explaining variables in regression analysis on systolic and diastolic blood pressure.

Variable	b	se_b	t	P
SYSTOLIC BLOOD PRESSURE				
Body-mass index	1.73	0.077	22.6	<0.01
Age	0.67	0.031	21.9	<0.01
Constant	123.9			
Multiple $R^2 = 0.24$				
DIASTOLIC BLOOD PRESSURE				
Body-mass index	1.22	0.044	27.6	< 0.01
Age	0.28	0.018	15.8	< 0.01
Constant	67.5			
Multiple $R^2 = 0.24$				

The variables were ranked according to their t-values (b/se of b). Body-mass index and age were the most significant. These two variables explained 24% of the variance of both systolic and diastolic pressures. When those under antihypertensive drug treatment were excluded and men and women were treated separately, the explanatory power of the model did not increase. Age and body-mass index explained more of the variation in systolic and diastolic blood pressure among women than among men in the regression analysis.

The prevalence of hypertension in the community was estimated by using arbitrary criteria. Hypertension was defined as: blood pressure at least

175 mmHg systolic and/or 100 mmHg diastolic or under antihypertensive drug treatment. Prevalence of hypertension was associated with age among men and women both in 1972 and in 1977, but age-specific rates in 1977 were significantly lower than in 1972. There were dramatic differences between 1972 and 1977 among women.

Table 6 gives the prevalence rates and age-specific proportions of persons under antihypertensive drug treatment. Drug treatment increased four-fold among men and almost doubled among women during the five-year follow-up period. In 1972, antihypertensive drug treatment was more common among women in all age groups compared to men, despite the fact that men under the age of 40 had higher rates of hypertension. In 1977, only the men in the youngest age group had antihypertensive drug treatment more often than women. In general, the discrepancy between the prevalence of hypertension and antihypertensive drug treatment was greater among men. This was especially the situation in the youngest age groups.

Table 6. Prevalence of hypertension and antihypertensive drug treatment in North Karelia in 1972 and in 1977 by age and sex.

| Age (years) | Prevalence of hypertension[a] | | | | Currently on antihypertensive drug treatment | | | |
| | Men | | Women | | Men | | Women | |
	1972 %	1977 %	1972 %	1977 %	1972 %	1977 %	1972 %	1077 %
25–29	12.1	—	8.4	—	0.3	—	1.0	—
30–34	12.4	9.7	8.9	4.8	0.4	2.2	0.7	1.6
35–39	28.7	20.0	19.2	9.0	1.7	5.8	2.1	5.8
40–44	23.0	18.7	27.1	14.3	2.2	6.4	4.4	9.1
45–49	31.7	26.9	37.6	23.7	3.8	13.1	10.0	14.9
50–54	38.3	31.0	49.5	33.7	5.5	17.3	17.2	25.4
55–59	44.2	34.6	65.6	42.8	10.8	20.4	26.8	31.1
60–64	—	37.3	—	51.3	—	26.1	—	35.4
Total	26.6	24.3	31.6	25.6	3.3	12.1	9.1	17.5

[a] Blood pressure at least 175 and/or 100 mmHg diastolic or under antihypertensive drug treatment.

Table 7 presents four other indicators that are relevant to risk for severe CVD among hypertensives. The proportion of current smokers decreased significantly from 1972 to 1977. Also the mean level of serum cholesterol decreased. These changes were greater among men than among women. Coronary heart disease risk was estimated using logistic function model developed by Walker and Duncan [25], coefficients based on the follow-up of the base-line survey material of the North Karelia Project. The risk estimate

Table 7. Other CVD risk factors among hypertensives[a] in North Karelia in 1972 and in 1977 by sex.

	Men		Women	
	1972	1977	1972	1977
Current smokers[b] (%)	51	41		
Mean of serum cholesterol value, mg/dl ± SD	280	266	285	281
Mean of body-mass index[c]	27.5	27.9	29.2	29.4
Mean of CHD risk estimate[d]	6.3	4.5	—	—

[a] Blood pressure at least 175 and/or 100 mmHg or under antihypertensive drug treatment.
[b] Reported having been smoking regularly during the preceding six months.
[c] BMI = body weight (kg)/height (m^2).
[d] Logistic function model by Walker and Duncan [25].

decreased significantly also. Relative weight among hypertensives remained unchanged during the five-year period in both sexes.

Frequency and coverage of blood pressure measurements give some estimate of the case-finding activity in the population. In North Karelia in 1972, blood pressure measurements during the six months prior to the survey were more common among women than among men (Table 8). Among both sexes, the proportion of people with blood pressure measured increased with age. Only half of the hypertensive men and 70% of hypertensive women in 1972 had their blood pressure measured during the preceding six months. In 1977, 80% of the hypertensive men and 90% of the hypertensive women reported

Table 8. Percentage of persons whose blood pressure had been measured during the six months prior to the surveys in North Karelia in 1972 and in 1977 by age, sex and blood pressure status.

Age (years)	Men				Women			
	Total population		Hypertensives[a]		Total population		Hypertensives[a]	
	1972 %	1977 %	1972 %	1977 %	1972 %	1977 %	1972 %	1977 %
25–29	26.5	—	33.3	—	49.3	—	53.9	—
30–34	31.8	54.8	45.5	62.9	46.8	71.0	60.0	86.7
35–39	30.1	61.4	31.3	63.6	54.4	69.7	64.3	88.0
40–44	35.3	59.3	35.6	69.8	60.8	72.3	69.6	87.8
45–49	43.7	69.2	51.8	78.8	55.7	74.1	65.9	88.2
50–54	48.0	72.4	50.0	84.4	74.8	82.3	79.1	93.5
55–59	61.2	79.5	69.1	89.3	68.1	82.1	69.7	90.8
60–64	—	78.1	—	87.5	—	77.2	—	88.2
Total	38.8	66.8	47.9	79.3	58.8	75.7	69.7	89.8

[a] Blood pressure at least 175 and/or 100 mmHg or under antihypertensive drug treatment.

having their blood pressure measured within that time. Furthermore, the proportions were not so strongly related to age in 1977 as in 1972. In 1977, the majority of hypertensives had a satisfactory number of blood pressure control measurements. At the same time, blood pressure measurements among the old populations increased considerably, especially among young age groups.

Awareness of hypertension reflects also the case-finding activity. In 1972, 37% of hypertensive men and 67% of hypertensive women were aware of their high blood pressure. Among men, this proportion had no association with age; it was also weak among women. In 1977, the majority of men and women with hypertension were aware of it. This change in awareness between 1972 and 1977 was greatest in the youngest age groups in both sexes. Awareness was over 90% among young women in 1977 (Table 9).

Table 9. Awareness of hypertension in North Karelia in 1972 and in 1977 by age, sex and blood pressure status.

Age (years)	Hypertensive men[a]		Hypertensive women[a]	
	1972 %	1977 %	1972 %	1977 %
25–29	19.1	—	57.7	—
30–34	33.3	57.1	68.0	93.3
35–39	26.2	70.9	62.5	92.0
40–44	32.9	66.0	70.7	85.4
45–49	35.2	74.1	64.1	84.4
50–54	45.6	73.0	69.0	93.6
55–59	50.9	75.0	66.2	86.2
60–64	—	77.8	—	78.4
Total	37.3	72.2	66.5	85.8

[a] Blood pressure at least 175 and/or 100 mmHg or under antihypertensive drug treatment.

Tables 10 and 11 give the mean values and standard deviations of blood pressures according to age and sex in 1972 and in 1977 for normotensives and hypertensives. In 1972, the mean systolic pressure among normotensives rose slightly with age among men; this increase was greater among women. In 1977, the increase with age was similar. Among hypertensives, the increase with age was more progressive than among normotensives and more progressive in 1972 than in 1977; only a small increase with age was observed in 1977.

The mean diastolic blood pressure values did not vary much among normotensive men in 1972, but increased with age among normotensive women. In 1977, the diastolic level was lower among normotensive men and women

Table 10. Means and standard deviations of systolic and diastolic blood pressure (mmHg) among men by age and blood pressure status.

MEN Age (years)	Normotensive[a]		Hypertensive[b]		Normotensive[a]		Hypertensive[b]	
	1972	1977	1972	1977	1972	1977	1972	1977
	Mean of systolic blood pressure				Standard deviation of SBP			
25–29	138.2	—	162.1	—	17.5	—	13.3	—
30–34	139.0	136.8	163.2	159.7	16.6	15.5	12.8	13.0
35–39	138.2	136.8	162.5	158.9	18.8	17.9	13.3	13.7
40–44	139.8	135.3	167.2	161.8	17.2	16.9	13.2	13.9
45–49	139.6	139.5	166.0	161.9	18.2	18.2	14.4	13.0
50–54	142.6	138.2	173.2	159.7	21.8	16.2	14.8	14.4
55–59	142.3	140.8	176.4	162.3	23.6	19.5	15.4	15.1
60–64	—	141.8	—	169.4	—	22.5	—	16.3
Total	139.6	138.0	168.7	162.3	20.5	18.7	13.8	14.1
	Mean of diastolic blood pressure				Standard deviation of DBP			
25–29	82.4	—	103.6	—	10.6	—	6.8	—
30–34	85.8	82.9	103.7	102.8	8.4	8.5	7.3	6.6
35–39	87.4	84.2	106.0	104.2	7.8	7.7	9.0	8.2
40–44	86.4	85.0	107.7	103.8	7.9	7.9	10.3	8.0
45–49	86.4	86.5	105.1	102.5	7.6	7.9	9.5	8.4
50–54	86.9	85.2	105.6	100.4	8.9	8.0	9.6	9.2
55–59	86.0	85.0	103.4	100.0	8.6	8.3	11.1	9.7
60–64	—	83.8	—	97.9	—	9.6	—	9.9
Total	85.7	84.6	105.2	101.3	8.8	8.3	9.7	9.0

[a] Blood pressure under 175/100 mmHg and no antihypertensive drug treatment.
[b] Blood pressure at least 175 and/or 100 mmHg or under antihypertensive drug treatment.

compared with the figures of 1972. There was also an increase with age approximately up to age 50. Whereas the mean diastolic pressure among hypertensives was rather stable with age in 1972, there was a slight decrease with age in 1977 among both men and women. The diastolic blood pressure level among normotensives was much the same in 1972 as in 1977 among both sexes. It was significantly lower in 1977 among hypertensive men and women than in 1972.

In 1972, very few patients who were being treated for hypertension were under satisfactory blood pressure control. Only 29% of treated men and 18% of treated women had a blood pressure below 175/100 mmHg in 1972 (Table 12). The treatment effect was better among men than women and better in younger than older patients in both sexes. In 1977, when the proportion of treated persons was increased considerably, the proportion of those with satisfactory blood pressure control also increased significantly: it was 47% among men and 59% among women.

Table 11. Means and standard deviations of systolic and diastolic blood pressure (mmHg) among women by age and blood pressure status.

WOMEN Age (years)	Normotensive[a]		Hypertensive[b]		Normotensive[a]		Hypertensive[b]	
	1972	1977	1972	1977	1972	1977	1972	1977
	Mean of systolic blood pressure				Standard deviation of SBP			
25–29	127.5	—	155.6	—	11.9	—	16.3	—
30–34	133.2	126.0	164.8	163.5	12.9	12.6	20.4	20.6
35–39	134.7	129.8	163.3	159.2	14.7	13.8	20.0	15.6
40–44	138.5	133.3	171.6	160.7	14.1	13.9	18.6	22.1
45–49	142.2	138.2	177.9	165.4	15.4	14.7	22.9	20.0
50–54	146.4	140.9	180.6	160.9	14.4	15.5	22.4	23.4
60–64	—	147.0	—	171.0	—	14.5	—	20.1
Total	137.0	135.8	176.9	166.0	15.5	15.8	23.1	21.9
	Mean of diastolic blood pressure				Standard deviation of DBP			
25–29	77.6	—	105.5	—	9.5	—	7.0	—
30–34	81.8	78.4	105.3	101.9	9.0	8.1	8.2	12.6
35–39	83.8	81.7	105.7	97.9	8.8	8.2	8.1	7.4
40–44	85.6	83.5	105.5	100.5	7.7	8.4	8.3	9.6
45–49	85.8	84.8	106.5	100.4	8.4	8.1	9.6	7.6
50–54	88.4	85.6	106.0	97.0	7.2	7.2	11.2	10.1
55–59	88.3	85.5	106.4	97.6	7.9	7.2	11.1	11.7
60–64	—	85.4	—	94.4	—	7.6	—	9.8
Total	83.7	83.1	106.1	97.4	9.2	8.3	10.0	10.3

[a] Blood pressure under 175/100 mmHg and no antihypertensive drug treatment.
[b] Blood pressure at least 175 and/or 100 mmHg or under antihypertensive drug treatment.

Table 12. Proportion of treated hypertensives with blood pressures below the cut-off level for hypertension (175/100 mmHg).

Age (years)	Men		Women	
	1972 %	1977 %	1972 %	1977 %
30–39	50	43	38	76
40–49	20	37	14	54
50–59	31	46	19	57
60–64	—	58	—	63
Total	29	47	18	59

The summary of the data for hypertension control in the area in 1972 and 1977 are presented in Table 13. The proportion of undetected hypertension decreased significantly between 1972 and 1977 and, at the same time, the considerable sex difference in undetected hypertension decreased, too. Among

340

Table 13. Percentage of undetected, untreated and inadequately treated hypertensives in North Karelia in 1972 and in 1977 by sex.[a]

		Men		Women	
		1972 %	1977 %	1972 %	1977 %
Not previously aware, high BP at examination		63	28	34	14
Aware, never on treatment		15	19	21	11
Aware, sometimes treated, not on treatment at examination	37	12	6	66 · 20	8
Aware, on treatment, but high BP at examination		6	24	20	27
Aware, on treatment, normal BP at examination		4	23	5	40
Total hypertensives %		100	100	100	100
n		555	476	683	534

[a] Blood pressure at least 175 and/or 100 mmHg.

men, the proportion of hypertensives who were aware of their condition but never under treatment increased from 15% to 19% but the respective proportion among women decreased from 21% to 11%. The proportion of patients who had dropped out of treatment decreased significantly among men and women between 1972 and 1977.

While the proportion of treated patients among hypertensive men and women increased, the proportion of inadequately treated hypertensives increased, too. This was especially true among men. However, antihypertensive drug treatment among men was so uncommon in 1972 that, despite of the four-fold increase in the proportion of inadequately treated hypertensive men, this proportion did not exceed the respective proportion of hypertensive women. Approximately one-fourth of all hypertensives fell into this category. Finally, the aim of all hypertension control activities, normotension, was achieved in only a very small proportion of hypertensives in 1972, but increased six-fold among men and eight-fold among women between 1972 and 1977.

5. DISCUSSION

Epidemiological surveys carried out in North Karelia in 1972 and in 1977 were aimed at measuring cardiovascular risk factors among the middle-aged population of the county of North Karelia that had the highest cardiovascular disease rates in the world [13, 16, 21]. A large proportion of these diseases was related to elevated blood pressure. Examinations in 1972 and 1977 in North Karelia were based on exactly the same methods at those two time periods. Because the participation rate in the surveys was very high, the data can give a good estimate of changes during the five years when there was an intensified hypertension control programme at the local level in the area. Data on blood pressure changes are supplemented by data dealing with detection, treatment and follow-up of hypertensives in the community.

The base-line survey of the North Karelia project in 1972 confirmed that hypertension was a major health problem and indicated that a community approach should be developed to ensure adequate management of the problem. The main contributors to the prediction of hypertension in North Karelia were body mass and height as in many other studies [26–30]. The importance of high salt intake has also been suggested [31, 32]. It is known that the salt intake in North Karelia is high [33].

Among men in North Karelia, lack of awareness of hypertension was a significant problem and only a very few men were under treatment in 1972. Even fewer of those treated had normal blood pressure. The majority of women knew that they had high blood pressure, but achievement of normotension was still rare. Compared with some other surveys, the North Karelian population had higher blood pressure levels and hypertension prevalence in 1972. In the U.S.A., 8.4% of the population who participated in the survey of the hypertension detection and follow-up programme had a diastolic blood pressure above 100 mmHg. In North Karelia, 26.6% of the men and 31.6% of the women had a blood pressure of at least 175 mmHg systolic and/or 100 mmHg diastolic, or were under antihypertensive drug treatment. The mean diastolic blood pressure in the hypertensive population in North Karelia in 1972 was very similar to that in the mild hypertension category in the American group [34].

The intensive community programme carried out in North Karelia from 1972 to 1977 was aimed at changing this picture. By 1977, less than one-third of the men and less than 15% of the women were aware of their hypertension. Almost one-fourth of the men were controlled, as were 40% of the women. There was a 6-mmHg decline in systolic blood pressure among the men and an 8-mmHg decline among the women in the entire population, and a 4-mmHg and 5-mmHg decline, respectively, in diastolic pressure. These changes occurred even though the population had aged five years during the follow-up.

This age range was chosen in order to assess the changes in the same age cohort, although not in the same individuals. Using the same age cohorts increases the comparability of the base-line and terminal measurements, because if the sample at the end had had the same age range as at the outset, the comparability would have diminished due to possible and unknown differences in the age cohorts in the study and in the reference areas. This, however, means that the sample at the end is five years older, which is meaningful in terms of the absolute changes in the two areas (i.e. possible risk factor reductions could be counterbalanced by an increase due to aging), but not in terms of comparison with the development in the reference area or the net reduction in North Karelia.

The prevalence of the diastolic blood pressure of 95 mmHg or more in casual examination declined 30% among the men and almost 50% among the women. The proportion of those hypertensives who were under drug treatment increased from 12% to almost 50% among the men and to about two-thirds among the women. These data provide solid evidence on the favourable progress in the control of hypertension in North Karelia.

The observed changes in blood pressure were not as great as in the U.S. programme, where in the intervention ('stepped care group') 90% had a diastolic blood pressure of 95 mmHg or less at the end of the first year [34]. However, the change in North Karelia occurred in the total population of an entire community, and not only in a special group of persons under special treatment and follow-up. The fact that even the existing health care system can improve hypertension control in the community is encouraging. Stamler et al. [5] have reported similar trends in the United States after active treatment for hypertension was promoted in the beginning of the 1970s. The proportion of treated hypertensives with normalized blood pressures was the same in North Karelia in 1972 as in the Mayo three-community study (24%), and this proportion at the end of our study was also the same as that in the Mayo study [35].

It has been shown here that a community-based programme for treating hypertension can effectively increase the proportion of treated patients and decrease the proportion of uncontrolled hypertensives in the community, although not all hypertensives can be brought under complete control. Naturally, the figures obtained in epidemiological surveys based on casual blood pressure readings underestimate the proportion of persons with satisfactory blood pressure control through treatment. There is no question that attention must be given to further development of detection, treatment and follow-up of hypertensives in the community. At the same time, the results show that even more attention must be given to possibilities for the primary prevention of blood pressure elevation. This means that special hygienic efforts among young adults, mild hypertensives and in the whole community shift the entire blood pressure distribution. This has been discussed also in North Karelia, and a programme for reducing salt intake in the population was recently started with scientific evaluation concerning its feasibility and effects.

REFERENCES

1. Stamler J: Lectures on preventive cardiology. New York: Grune and Stratton, 1967.
2. World Health Organization: Ischaemic heart disease registers. Report of the fifth WHO working group. EURO 8201(5), Copenhagen 26-29.4, 1971.
3. Strasser T: Pilot programmes for the control of hypertension. WHO Chron 26:451, 1972.
4. National Conference on High Blood Pressure Education: Report of proceedings. DHEW Publ (NIH) 73-486. US Department of Health, Education, and Welfare. Public Health Service, National Institutes of Health, 1973.
5. Stamler J, Stamler R, Riedlinger W, Algera G, Roberts R: Hypertension screening of 1 million Americans. Community hypertension evaluation clinic (CHEC) program, 1973 through 1975. JAMA 235:2299, 1976.
6. World Health Organization: Arterial hypertension. Report of a WHO expert committee, Geneva, 1978.
7. Hamilton M, Thompson E, Wisniewski T: The role of blood pressure control in preventing complications of hypertension. Lancet 1:235, 1964.
8. Hood B, Aurell M, Falkheden T, Björk S: Analysis of mortality and survival in actively treated hypertensive disease. In: Gross F (ed) Antihypertensive therapy. Berlin: Springer, 1966, p 370.
9. Veterans Administration Study Group on Antihypertensive Agents: Effects of treatment on morbidity in hypertension. Results in patients with diastolic blood pressures averaging 115 through 129 mmHg. JAMA 202:116, 1967.
10. Veterans Administration Study Group on Antihypertensive Agents: Effects of treatment on morbidity in hypertension. II. Results in patients with diastolic blood pressures averaging 90 through 114 mmHg. JAMA 213:1143, 1970.
11. Berglund G, Wilhelmsen L, Sannerstedt R, Hansson L, Andersson O, Sivertsson R, Wedel H, Wickstrand J: Coronary heart disease after treatment of hypertension. Lancet 1:1, 1978.
12. Reader R: Initial results of Australian national blood pressure study (Abstr). In: Sixth scientific meeting of the international society of hypertension, Göteborg, 11–13 June 1979. Göteborg: International Society of hypertension, 1979.
13. Keys A: Coronary heart disease in seven countries. Am Heart Assoc Monogr 29, 1970.
14. Purola T, Nyman K, Kalimo E, Sievers K: Sairausvakuutus, sairastavuus ja lääkintäpalvelusten käyttö. Helsinki: Kansaneläkelaitoksen julkaisuja A:7, 1971.
15. Leppo K, Lindgren J, Ritamies M: Mortality trends in Finland in the 1960's. In: Yearbook of population research in Finland XII, 1971. Vammala, 1972.
16. Puska P: Sydän- ja verisuonisairauksien aiheuttaman kuolleisuuden erot. Suom Lääkärilehti 27:3071, 1972.
17. Puska P: The North Karelia Project: an attempt at community prevention of cardiovascular diseases. WHO Chron 27:55, 1973.
18. Puska P, Koskela K, Pakarinen P, Puumalainen P, Soininen V, Tuomilehto J: North Karelia Project: a programme for community control of cardiovascular diseases. Scand J Soc Med 4:57, 1976.
19. Puska P, Tuomilehto J, Mäki J, Salonen J: Principles and experiences of a community control programme for hypertension as part of the North Karelia Project. Acta Med Scand [Suppl] 626:22, 1979.

20. Puska P: North Karelia Project, a programme for community control of cardiovascular diseases. Publ Kuopio Community Health [A] 1, 1974.
21. Puska P, Mustaniemi H: Incidence of stroke in Finland. Duodecim 40:965, 1974.
22. Tuomilehto J, Nissinen A, Puska P: Principles and experiences with a programme for community control of hypertension as part of the North Karelia project. Acta Med Scand 602:40, 1976.
23. Nissinen A: An evaluation of the community based hypertension programme of the North Karelia Project with special reference to the awareness and treatment of elevated blood pressure and the blood pressure level in the population. Publ Univ Kuopio Community Health [Orig Rep] 2, 1979.
24. Rose G, Blackburn H: Cardiovascular survey methods. WHO Monogr Ser 56, 1968.
25. Walker S, Duncan D: Estimation of the probability of an event as a function of several independent variables. Biometrica 54:167, 1967.
26. Bøe J, Humerfelt S, Wedervang F: The blood pressure in a population. Acta Med Scand [Suppl] 321:78-79, 1957.
27. Miall W, Oldham P: Factors influencing arterial blood pressure in the general population. Clin Sci 17:409, 1958.
28. Miall W, Lovell H: Relation between change of blood pressure and age. Br Med J 2:660, 1967.
29. Sive P, Medalie J, Kahn H, et al.: Distribution and multiple regression analysis of blood pressure in 10,000 Israeli men. Am J Epidemiol 93:317, 1971.
30. Kesteloot H, Houte O van: An epidemiologic survey of arterial blood pressure in a large male population group. Am J Epidemiol 99:14, 1974.
31. Freis E: Salt, volume and prevention of hypertension. Circulation 53:589, 1976.
32. Meneely G, Battarbee H: High sodium–low potassium environment and hypertension. Am J Cardiol 38:768, 1976.
33. Karvonen M, Punsar S: Suomalaiset suolan käyttäjinä. Suom Lääkärilehti L, 33:572, 1978.
34. Hypertension Detection and Follow-up Cooperative Group: Mild hypertensives in the hypertension detection and follow-up program. Ann NY Acad Sci 304:254, 1978.
35. Labarthe D, Krishan I, Nobrega F, Brennan Jr L, Smoldt R, Mori H, Hunt J: The Mayo three-community hypertension control program. I. Design and initial screening results. Mayo Clin Proc 54:289, 1979.

20. RELATIONSHIP BETWEEN BLOOD PRESSURE AND SODIUM AND POTASSIUM INTAKE IN A BELGIAN MALE POPULATION GROUP

H. KESTELOOT, M. VUYLSTEKE, and A. COSTENOBLE

Although a causal relationship between sodium (Na) intake and blood pressure is generally admitted to exist, few data on the actual intake of Na in different populations are available. The purpose of our study has been to analyse the 24-h urine excretion of Na, K and creatinine in a large male population group, in which the blood pressure (BP) was also measured.

1. METHODS

The population group studied consists of army units localized all over Belgium. Participation was voluntary. The participation rate varied between 60% and 84% but, since the study is still not finished, the non-participants will get a second chance to participate.

The normal strength of an army unit at any time is about 80% of the total effective force. The participants belonged to five different units distributed over the country, and about 40% took their lunch in the military mess.

For each participant, a 12-lead electrocardiogram was recorded, blood pressure was measured and a blood sample was taken for the total cholesterol, HDL-cholesterol and γ-glutamyl transpeptidase determination. The 24-h urine was also collected for determination of volume, Na, K and creatinine content, and for the presence of glucose and albumine.

Cholesterol was measured by means of the enzymatic method (CHOD-PAP method, Boehringer Mannheim), HDL-cholesterol after manganese-heparine precipitation and creatinine by the method of Jaffé. The method employed for the creatinine determination yielded values which are comparable to the values found in the Belgian-Korean comparative study[1].

In order to avoid any conscious or unconscious change in diet during the study, the participants were unaware of the fact that Na and K would be measured in the urine. The urine collection started between 0900 and 1100 hours in the morning and lasted until the same time of the next day. The participants were instructed to void their bladder at the start and at the end of the 24-h period, retaining only the latter urine. Moreover, they were instructed to urinate before each defecation. The urine was collected in a plastic bottle with a maximum content of 2.7 l. If necessary, more than one container could be obtained.

Blood pressure was recorded at the start of the procedure, before the ECG and blood samples were taken, and measured at three intervals, at 0, 5 and 10 min, with the subjects in the supine position. Both phase 4 and 5 of diastolic BP were recorded, but only phase 5 (disappearance of sounds) was used in this study. The analysis was performed on the mean of the three BP and heart rate (HR) determinations.

BP was measured by six medical doctors specifically trained for this purpose. The examinations were performed locally in the army units during February and April, which are among the colder months of the year.

Each participant completed a questionnaire containing both medical and psychological questions. More than 6000 volunteers have participated in the study until now, but the results of only the first 2026 participants have been analyzed and will be reported here. To eliminate most cases with under- or overcollection of urine, only cases with a 24-h creatinine excretion of between 800 and 3200 mg were excluded from the analysis.

The results were submitted to univariate and multivariate analyses (MRA) using the BMDP2R program of stepwise multiple regression (stepdown method). To enable an evaluation of the relative weight of the different independent variables in MRA, standardized regression coefficients (SRC) are given (SRC = partial regression coefficient × SD predicting variable/SD dependent variable).

2. RESULTS

The values of the measured variables in the participating group are given in Tables 1–3. The Na/K ratio was 2.4. The ratio of mean SBP on mean DBP was 1.59, which points to the fact that the BP was recorded in a rather basal condition. This was confirmed by the fact that the mean heart rate was only 70.3 beats/min. The univariate correlation matrix between all measured variables is given in Table 4. The results of the multivariate analysis of SBP and DBP are listed in Tables 5 and 6. Age, height, weight and 24-h urinary sodium, up to their third powers, 24-h urinary K, creatinine and heart rate were included in the analysis.

From the results of the MRA, it appears that HR is an important determinant of SBP and DBP. No correlation was found by MRA between Na or K and SBP. An overall small but negative correlation was found between Na and DBP. The amount of the explained variation of SBP (14%) and DBP (21%) remains small.

Table 1. Characteristics of studied population: Anthropometric and lipid data.

n	Total group 2026	≤20 y 203	21–25 y 235	26–30 y 198	31–35 y 155	36–40 y 202	41–45 y 344	46–50 y 290	51–55 y 248	56–60 y 51
$\bar{m}$ Age (years)	37.6±11.6	18.0	21.9	27.6	32.6	37.9	42.8	47.5	52.2	57.0
$\bar{m}$ Height (cm)	173.6± 6.4	175.9	175.4	174.4	174.5	173.0	173.8	172.6	171.7	168.7
$\bar{m}$ Weight (kg)	75.9± 9.7	70.7	73.2	75.6	77.9	77.3	77.8	77.3	76.1	75.3
$\bar{m}$ Chol (mg %)	224.2±48.6	171.1	189.5	215.0	224.2	238.5	236.4	246.4	240.7	241.2
$\bar{m}$ HDL-Chol (mg %)	48.1±12.0	48.2	47.1	47.7	48.5	48.0	48.2	49.3	47.1	49.4
Non-HDL-Chol/HDL-Chol ratio	3.66	2.55	3.02	3.50	3.62	3.97	3.90	3.99	4.11	3.88

Table 2. Characteristics of studied population: Urinary excretion values.

	Total group 2026	≤20 y 203	21–25 y 235	26–30 y 198	31–35 y 155	36–40 y 202	41–45 y 344	46–50 y 290	51–55 y 248	56–60 y 51
$\bar{m}$ Na (mmol/24 h)	159.4±62.7	140.2	154.0	153.3	156.1	170.6	169.4	163.1	159.7	153.4
$\bar{m}$ K (mmol/24 h)	67.1±25.2	62.4	67.2	67.0	63.3	70.2	68.5	68.1	68.0	63.5
$\bar{m}$ Creat (mg/24 h)	1735.0±498.7	1565	1734	1754	1811	1810	1802	1728	1702	1581
$\bar{m}$ Urinary vol (1/24 h)	1.37±0.5	1.09	1.21	1.32	1.36	1.40	1.47	1.47	1.45	1.46
Na/K ratio	2.38	2.25	2.29	2.29	2.45	2.43	2.47	2.39	2.34	2.42
$\bar{m}$ Na (mmol/24 h) c [a]	.	158.6	157.2	154.7	152.6	166.8	166.4	167.1	166.1	171.7
$\bar{m}$ K (mmol/24 h) c [a]	.	70.5	68.6	67.7	62.3	68.6	67.4	69.9	71.0	71.0

[a] Values corrected to a 24-h creatinine excretion value of 1.770 mg (for reasons of standardization).

Table 3. Characteristics of studied population: Blood pressure and heart rate data.

	Total group 2026	≤20 y 203	21–25 y 235	26–30 y 198	31–35 y 155	36–40 y 202	41–45 y 344	46–50 y 290	51–55 y 248	56–60 y 51
$\bar{m}$ SBP (mmHg)	126.4	122.17	124.5	126.0	126.9	124.4	125.9	128.0	129.9	133.1
$\bar{m}$ DBP (mmHg)	79.3	71.1	74.0	77.6	78.8	79.4	81.1	82.9	83.0	85.7
$\bar{m}$ HR (beats/min)	70.3	76.6	70.3	71.2	69.9	70.1	69.5	71.2	71.5	74.2
SBP/DBP ratio	1.59	1.71	1.68	1.63	1.61	1.57	1.55	1.54	1.56	1.55

Table 4. Correlation matrix [a].

	A	W	H	Chol	HDL-Chol	Vol	Na	K	Creat	m̄ SBP	m̄ DBP	m̄ HR
A	1											
W	0.167	1										
H	-0.214	0.429	1									
Chol	0.469	0.208	-0.128	1								
HDL-Chol	—	-0.175	—	0.070	1							
Vol	0.236	0.078	—	0.163	0.062	1						
Na	0.094	0.180	0.059	—	0.058	0.315	1					
K	0.045	0.154	0.088	0.049	—	0.210	0.361	1				
Creat	—	0.287	0.128	0.059	—	—	0.314	0.373	1			
m̄ SBP	0.156	0.198	—	0.166	—	0.097	—	—	—	1		
m̄ DBP	0.382	0.211	—	0.271	0.061	0.149	—	—	—	0.637	1	
m̄ HR	0.067	0.028	-0.077	0.154	—	0.053	-0.052	—	—	0.298	0.212	1

[a] Limits of significance for r: 0.043, $P > 0.05$; 0.057, $P > 0.01$; 0.073, $P > 0.001$.

Table 5. Standardized regression coefficients and F value of independent variables [a] significantly correlated with SBP in MRA [b].

	Standard regr coeff	F value
Heart rate	0.281	184.7
Weight	0.199	82.01
Age^3	0.457	7.26
Creatinine	−0.052	5.89
Age^2	−0.341	4.03

[a] The following independent variables were included in the analysis: age, weight, height and sodium up to their third powers; and the linear terms of heart rate, creatinine and potassium.
[b] $R = 0.38$, $R^2 = 0.14$.

Table 6. Standardized regression coefficients and F values of independent variables [a] significantly correlated with DBP in MRA [b].

	Standard regr coeff	F value
Heart rate	0.181	83.2
Weight^3	0.154	56.11
Age	0.660	18.93
Age^2	−0.331	4.24
Sodium	−0.206	7.69
Sodium^2	0.158	4.57

[a] See Table 5.
[b] $R = 0.46$, $R^2 = 0.21$. Partial regression coefficient for Na is −0.034 and for Na^2 +0.0001 (Na in mmol).

The data show an SBP/DBP ratio of 1.71 in younger subjects, decreasing to 1.55 in older subjects. This is in accordance with our concept that this ratio reflects whether the BP is near basal (<1.5) or not. Both from the lower volume of 24-h urine and from the lower 24-h creatinine excretion, the conclusion may be drawn that in younger subjects the collection of 24-h urine was incomplete. For this reason, corrected values for a mean 24-h urine excretion of 1770 mg are included for the younger age groups in Table 1. The decrease in 24-h creatinine excretion in the older age groups is probably real, as the urine output is identical to that obtained in the age group 30–45 years.

Regarding the lipid data, the studied population behaves as a typical Western population, with a marked increase in serum cholesterol between the ages of 18 and 47 years, after which a plateau phase is reached. HDL-chol remains markedly stable while the non-HDL-chol/HDL-cholesterol ratio increases very rapidly between the ages of 18 and 38 years.

3. DISCUSSION

Only limited information is available on salt consumption in different populations, and this is due to the evident difficulty of assessing salt consumption. In regions with a temperate climate, the 24-h urinary excretion of sodium may be assumed to be a good measure of Na consumption. Even fewer data are available on K consumption, although the K consumption may play a role in compensating for the positive influence of Na on BP. The Na/K ratio, obtained by dividing mean Na by mean K excretion expressed in mmol, is 2.4 in this study, whereas the ratio was 2.3 in a Belgian study performed in 1973.

In Korea and Japan, however (see corresponding chapters in this book), the ratio was 5.5 and 5–7, respectively. Countries with a low BP appear to have lower Na/K ratios than countries with higher BP. A possible exception appears to be Finland, where cerebrovascular mortality is one of the highest in Europe and where the Na/K ratio is only 1.6 (see corresponding chapter in this book). In a nomad tribe in Southern Iran, the individual Na/K ratios averaged 3.64 for males [3].

In most studies, it has been impossible to obtain a significant correlation between Na consumption and BP, within one population, and this study is no exception. It has been shown in an earlier chapter that in Korea, a positive correlation was found between Na consumption and BP. In Belgium also, a positive correlation between BP and Na consumption was established in 1969 within some population groups [2].

Several hypotheses can be made to explain this lack of correlation in most studies, apart from the methodological problems of assessing BP and 24-h electrolyte consumption. Variability of Na consumption in Western populations is rather small (SD 61 mmol/24 h in Belgium, SD 133 mmol/24 h in Korea for Na excretion). If consumption is uniform, genetic factors probably dominate. The influence of Na could also be greater in the higher ranges of Na consumption and be counterbalanced by a high potassium intake.

Moreover, the population of Western countries and especially of Belgium, where several campaigns have been held in order to lower salt consumption, is generally informed about the possible harmful effects of Na in hypertension. This could lead to a decrease in Na consumption in hypertensives and even to an increase in subjects who know that their BP is normal. This could possibly explain the negative correlation between Na intake and DBP found by MRA in this study. Establishing a link between Na consumption and BP could thus become very difficult, if not impossible.

Longitudinal studies on Na and K intake in a population are virtually non-existent. If the Na hypothesis on the genesis of hypertension is true, the generally obtained decline in morbidity and mortality by cerebrovascular disease should be accompanied by a decrease in Na consumption. In a male Belgian population sample of 1121 subjects with a mean age of 39.7 years, 24-h sodium was 200 ± 67 mmol in 1967 [2], while it was 184 ± 45 mmol (mean of ten values in each individual) in a small sample of 133 male subjects with a mean age of 39 years in 1973; whereas in this study in a sample of 2026 male subjects with a mean age of 37.6 years, the mean Na consumption was 159 ± 65 mmol/24 h.

This is in accordance with the impression that, in recent years, Belgian Na consumption is decreasing. It is evident, however, that much more data on Na consumption and BP in different population groups are necessary and that longitudinal studies on sodium and potassium consumption in randomized population groups should receive the highest priority in order to understand the reasons for the decline in cerebrovascular mortality occurring in the Western world.

REFERENCES

1. Kesteloot H, Lee CS, Park BC, Brems-Heyns E, Claessens J, Joossens JV: A comparative study of blood pressure and sodium intake in Belgium and in Korea. In: Kesteloot H, Joossens JV (eds) The epidemiology of arterial blood pressure. The Hague: Martinus Nijhoff Medical Division, 1980.
2. Joossens JV, Willems J, Claessens J, Claes J, Lissens W: Sodium and hypertension. In: Morgnani (ed) Nutrition and cardiovascular diseases, Roma; pp 91-110, 1970.
3. Page LB, Vandervert D, Nadir K, Lubin N, Page JR: Blood pressure, diet and body form in traditional nomads of the Qash'qai tribe, southern Iran. Acta Cardiol (Brux) 33:102-103, 1978.

21. EPIDEMIOLOGICAL STUDIES ON HYPERTENSION IN NEWFOUNDLAND

J.G. FODOR and I.E. RUSTED

In the last few years, hypertension has been recognized as a major public health problem in North America. It is estimated that in the United States about 15% of white and 28% of black adults have high blood pressure, i.e. values of ≥ 160 mmHg systolic and/or ≥ 95 mmHg diastolic [1].

The estimates of prevalence of hypertension in Canada are similar to those of the white population in the United States [2].

Mortality data [3] suggesting an increased incidence of strokes in Newfoundland, and reports of practising physicians [4], indicate that hypertension may be more frequent in Newfoundland than in other parts of Canada.

Newfoundland, the most easterly province of Canada, consists of the island of Newfoundland and, on the mainland, of Labrador. Our study was carried out on the island of Newfoundland, which has more than 43,000 square miles of territory and more than 500,000 inhabitants. The population density is about 11 persons per square mile. Approximately half of the population is scattered in several hundred small communities, mostly along the coast of the island. Most Newfoundlanders are of English or Irish origin. For the past 400 years, the fishing industry has been the principal occupation of Newfoundlanders and still plays an important role in the island's economy. In this century, however, forestry, mining and logging have gained in importance. The climate of Newfoundland, influenced by the Labrador current, results in a short growing season that does not encourage agriculture. Thus, grain and grain products and most of the vegetables and fruits have to be imported. Traditionally, salted fish, beef and pork form a substantial part of the Newfoundlander's daily diet.

Newfoundland physicians have suspected for more than two decades that these environmental factors might be causally associated with the observed high incidence of hypertension in Newfoundland. In 1967, the newly formed Faculty of Medicine of Memorial University of Newfoundland initiated an epidemiological study of hypertension, with the intention of determining the prevalence of hypertension among the Newfoundland population and evaluating the extent to which the pattern of nutrition and other possible etiologic factors might be associated.

H. Kesteloot, J.V. Joossens (eds.), Epidemiology of Arterial Blood Pressure, 353–366.

354

1. METHODS

1.1. Determination of the blood pressure distribution

The population sample was drawn from four widely separated communities in Newfoundland (Fig. 1). Based on 1966 Census statistics [5], the total population for each of these four communities was: Ramea: 1160; Fogo: 1150; Bay de Verde: 838; Badger: 1192. The population of voting age (21 years and over) for each in 1966 was as follows: 513, 592, 483, and 522, respectively. Except for Badger, which was settled late in the 19th century, evidence exists that the origin of other towns was several centuries earlier, although permanent settlement probably did not occur until the 18th century. Fogo, Ramea, and Bay de Verde are fishing villages, and the majority of the employed men derive their income from the fishery. Ramea and Bay de Verde developed, only 15 years ago, fresh fish plants that employ a large number of men and women. For males in Badger, the principal occupations are mining and logging. It is close to an urban centre and the Trans-Canada Highway passes through the town. The population in each town is relatively stable, but there

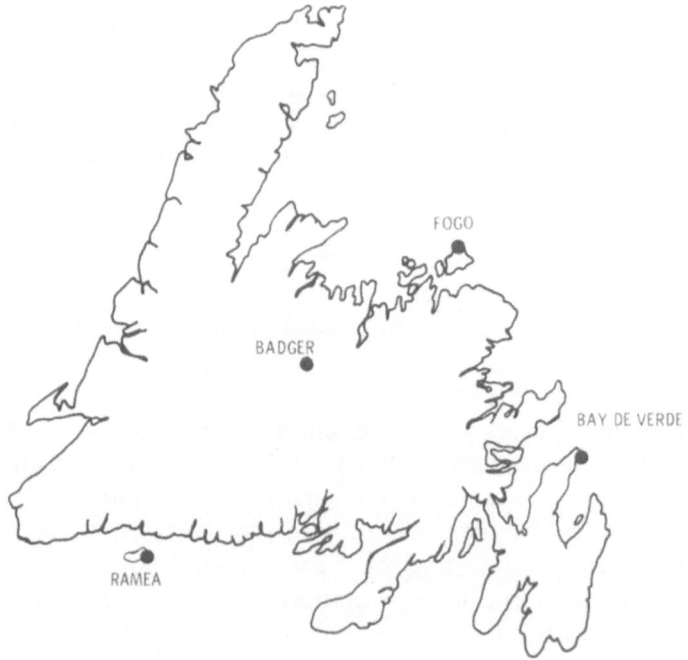

Figure 1. Four communities: Site of blood pressure survey in Newfoundland.

is some emigration, especially among the younger adults. Fogo and Ramea are situated on small islands off the coast and are accessible only by boat or plane.

'Blood pressure clinics' were held in each town within a one-month period during the autumn of 1967 to which each adult resident aged 19 and over was invited. A data card on each individual was completed prior to the examination, except for details pertaining to the individual's medical and family history. Height was recorded in inches without shoes, and weight was recorded in pounds in light clothing. All blood pressures were measured with the subject in the seated position after 3–5 min rest. During this period, further details of the personal and family history were recorded by the examiner.

Two examiners were involved in all blood pressure readings. To reduce observer bias and digit preference, all blood pressures were recorded on one of two sphygmomanometers of the London School of Hygiene and Tropical Medicine. Clip-on cuffs (14 × 40 cm size) were used with the above instruments.

The 15 subjects who were unable to attend the Clinic in Ramea were seen at home where their blood pressure was measured with a standard sphygmomanometer.

Phase I of the Korotkoff sounds was used as an indicator of the systolic blood pressure. Phase IV (change in tone prior to disappearance) and phase V (point of disappearance) were recorded as the diastolic pressure. In this report, the phase V diastolic blood pressure was considered for all further analysis.

1.2. Dietary survey

In the course of the above-described first part of the survey carried out in 1967–68, a sample of 60 individuals in each of the four towns was selected for inclusion in a dietary study. These groups consisted of residents who gave an assurance of co-operation with the study and adherence to the protocol. An attempt was made to have approximately equal numbers of each group (i.e. each decade) and a balanced composition of the sexes. Careful efforts were made not to reveal the purpose of this aspect of the study, and thus to avoid a modification of the diet on the part of respondents.

There were two survey periods, each lasting seven days. The first period was in the winter and the second in the summer. Of the 240 persons chosen, 210 completed the first survey; 127 respondents participated in the second survey.

The method of the dietary survey has been a so-called 'double portion' or 'phantom diet' system, during which the respondents (reimbursed financially) prepared twice the amount of food they had normally consumed. The additional daily 'phantom' diets were placed in individual one-gallon, polyethylene jars. Participants were asked to add equivalent amounts of liquid to all drinking water and other drinks consumed. Alcoholic beverages were excluded from the collection. Accurate collection of food samples was ensured by daily visits to each house by a dietician, who also reviewed the daily written record of all consumed foods and beverages. Each morning, all food and beverage collections from the previous day were weighed and homogenized in a Waring blender; 100-ml aliquots of the homogenate were removed and frozen.

Food aliquots were stored at $-17°C$ until thawed at room temperature. Duplicate 10-g aliquots were weighed into porcelain crucibles (Coors, 25-ml capacity) and dried initially at $80°C$ for 24 h, and then at $100°C$ for 48 h. The residues were ashed in covered crucibles at $450°-500°C$ for up to 16 h in muffle furnaces (Lindberg and Thermolyne) and, after cooling, dissolved in $2 N$ HCl (2 ml). The extracts were diluted to 25 ml with distilled water (final concentration $0.1 N$ HCl) and fine particulate material removed by filtration through Whitman no. 2 paper before storing in glass containers at $4°C$.

Sodium and potassium were measured by means of flame photometry (IL Flame Photometer) with lithium as the internal standard. The dietary zinc, calcium and magnesium contents were estimated for all samples by means of absorption spectrophotometry.

1.3. Five-year follow-up studies

Five years later (1974–75), an attempt was made to review the health status of respondents who participated in the original survey.

A total of 144 persons were revisited and a detailed examination was carried out, which included: (a) an interview concerning the medical history, (b) body height and weight measurements, (c) a 12-lead ECG, and (d) 12 blood pressure measurements after minimum half-hour rest periods (six measurements in supine and six in seated position). A total of 29 respondents were unavailable for follow-up examination, or had died since the first survey. However, they were included in the follow-up evaluation, as sufficient information was available from medical records and death certificates for determination of the blood pressure status. Ultimately, a complete set of information was collected on 125 'normotensives' and 48 'hypertensives', i.e. a total of 173 respondents.

Respondents were labelled as 'hypertensive' if, during the entire observation period, repeated measurements of blood pressure levels of at least 160 mmHg systolic and/or 95 mmHg diastolic were recorded, or if, following earlier diagnosis, they were receiving antihypertensive treatment.

2. RESULTS

A total of 1499 (810 women and 689 men) respondents over the age of 19 were seen during the initial study (Tables 1 and 2). Using the 1966 Census data, one estimates that from 60% to 90% of the population was covered by the survey. The response rate of women (82%) was better than that of men (60%). Some of the male residents were unavailable at the time of the survey because their occupation necessitated frequent periods away from home.

Figures 2 and 3 show the mean systolic and diastolic blood pressure values for six decades, for both sexes, in each of the four towns. Values for those persons 80 years and over were excluded because of small numbers in each of the four towns. An increase in mean systolic and diastolic pressure was noted with increasing age up to the age of 70–79, after which there was a tendency for blood pressure levels to stabilize.

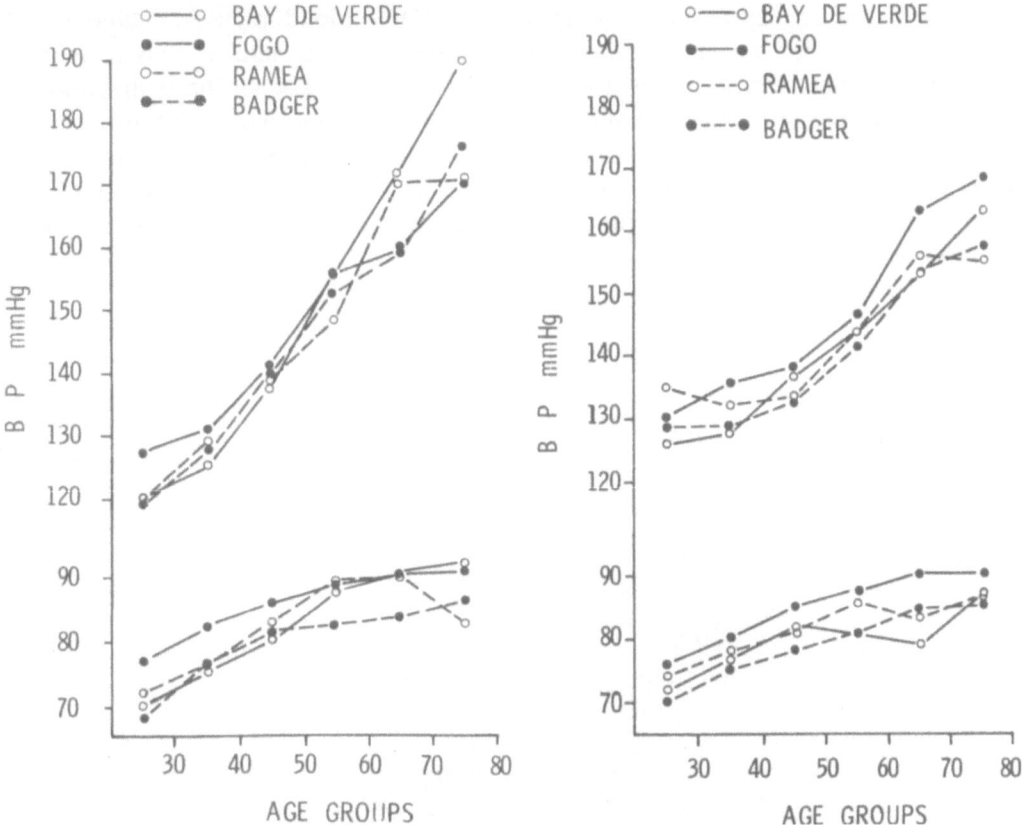

Figure 2. Mean values of the systolic blood pressure by age in four Newfoundland communities (Women *n* = 810).

Figure 3. Mean values of the systolic blood pressure by age in four Newfoundland communities (Men *n* = 689).

In each town, systolic pressures were higher in men than in women in the 30–40 age group. However, in the older age groups, the blood pressure levels of women exceeded those of men and, with the exception of Fogo, showed a steeper gradient, with the difference being maintained until the seventh decade.

Only minor differences were noted between the diastolic pressures in men and women with no constant trend to higher pressures in women. Systolic and diastolic blood pressure values of men from Bay de Verde and Ramea were between the highest levels in Fogo and the lowest in Badger. The same trend was discernible for female diastolic but not for systolic blood pressures. Curves for diastolic pressures tended to be parabolic, and the gradient was similar for the four towns and in both sexes.

As can be seen from Figures 2 and 3, the lowest blood pressure levels were recorded in the inland community of Badger, while the fishing village on Fogo Island had consistently the highest blood pressure values. Other calculations, using age and sex-adjusted scores of the blood pressure values [6], confirmed that the coastal fishing communities have generally higher blood pressure levels than the inland town studied. Figure 4 shows the distribution of the blood pressure levels in men in the two most-contrasting communities, Fogo and Badger. The distribution curves in both towns are normal, unimodal and skewed to the right. There is a distinct shift to the right in the distribution of the blood pressure values both in men and women of the Fogo population.

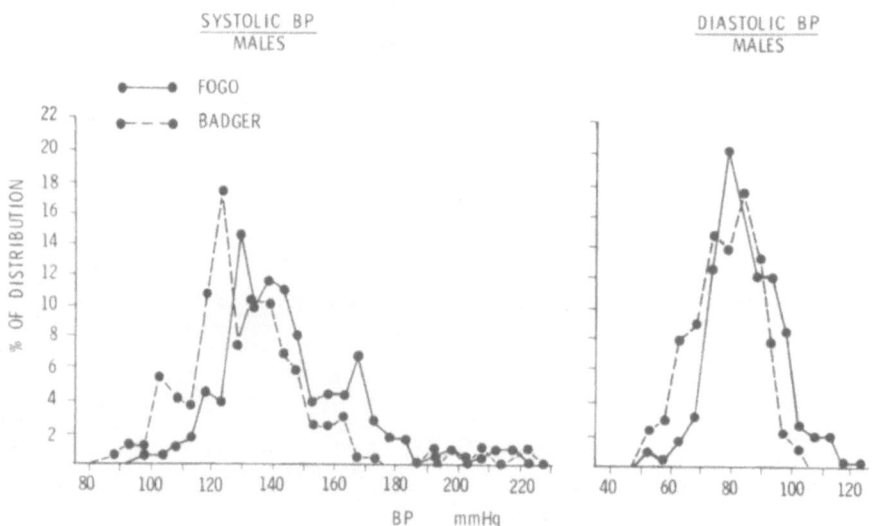

Figure 4. Distribution of the blood pressure levels of male respondents in two Newfoundland communities.

An analysis of our data by using quantitative criteria also indicates that the Newfoundland coastal fishing communities have a higher prevalence of high blood pressure than other parts of North America, with the exception of the south-eastern seaboard—the 'stroke belt' of the U.S.A.—which has a prevalence of hypertension similar to that of Newfoundland.

Table 1. Age-adjusted rates of high blood pressure [a] by community (rates per 100 population)[b].

Location	Men		Women	
	Rate	SE	Rate	SE
Badger (inland)	14.2	2.6	27.3	2.8
Bay de Verde[c]	20.4	3.0	28.6	2.9
Ramea[c]	23.9	2.9	30.3	2.6
Fogo[c]	26.5	3.0	26.3	2.7
U.S.[d] whites	13.0		15.1	
non-whites	27.8		29.7	

[a] High BP = systolic ≥ 160 mmHg or diastolic ≥ 95 mmHg.
[b] Number of respondents: 1499.
[c] Coastal fishing community.
[d] From U.S. National Health Survey [22].

Table 1 shows the age-adjusted prevalence rates for respondents with 'high blood pressure' in the adult population 19–79 years of age in the four surveyed communities. The cut-off point for the above-mentioned category was 160 mmHg systolic or 95 mmHg diastolic.

Prevalence rates for 'high blood pressure' were higher for women (27% – 30%) than for men (14% – 27%) in three towns. In Fogo, the rates were equal for men and women (26%), as compared with Badger where the rate for women was the same but only 14.2% in men.

2.1. Results of the dietary survey

2.1.1. Sodium intake. The day-to-day variation of the sodium intake can be substantial, as shown by two illustrative examples in Figure 5. The day-to-day variation of the sodium intake frequently exceeds 100 meq. Nevertheless, the mean values based on a seven-day observation show a remarkable stability and reproducibility for the same respondent a few months later.

Table 2 shows the mean values of the sodium intake in the four communities. The lowest intake was found in Badger, while the three fishing communities had a higher level of consumption, the highest being Fogo Island. The difference in sodium intake between Badger and Fogo is statistically significant at the 1% level.

360

DAILY SODIUM INTAKE

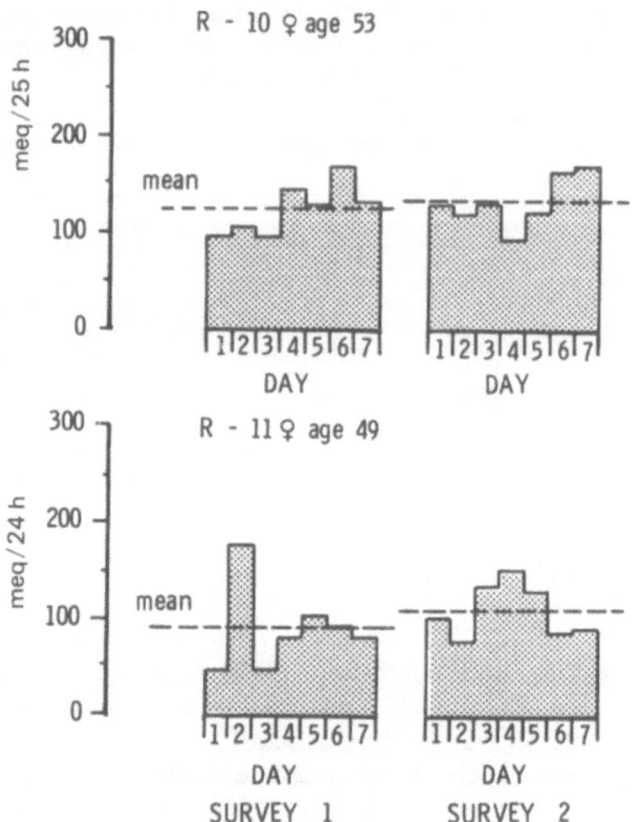

Figure 5. Variability of the dietary sodium intake: Survey 1: spring–summer; Survey 2: fall–winter.

Table 2. Dietary sodium content (mean of 7 days) meq/day.

Town	n	Sex	Survey I	Survey II
Fogo	29	M	177	168
	26	F	129	131
Badger	23	M	158	136
	31	F	104	116
Bay de Verde	19	M	177	183
	24	F	130	130
Ramea	20	M	160	145
	35	F	123	138

The sodium intake of the men is distinctly higher than that of the women (Table 2), but body mass did not seem to play a role in the magnitude of the sodium intake, as can be seen from Figure 6.

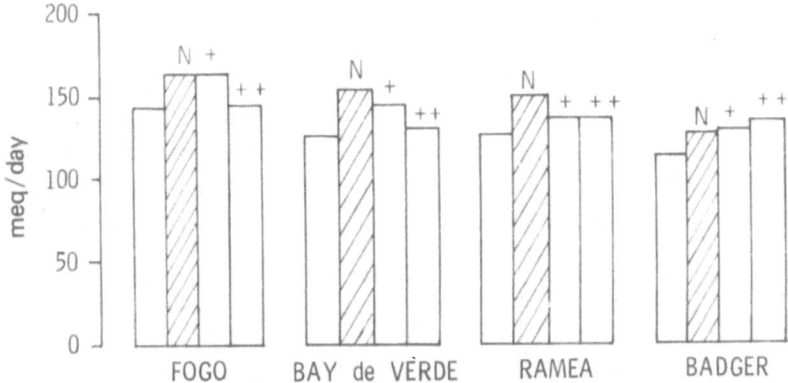

° Broca Index: Body weight in kg - (Body height in cm - 100)
    Deviations above and below are indicated by + or - values.
-   Underweight -6 or less
N   Normal weight -5 to +5
+   Overweight +6 to +15
++   Markedly overweight +16

Figure 6. Mean sodium intake of respondents by different body-mass categories expressed as Broca Index.

2.1.2. Potassium intake. The mean level of potassium intake in the coastal communities was 44 meq/day and in the inland town, Badger, 37 meq/day. The Na/K ratio was practically identical in coastal and inland communities, with a value between 3.2 and 3.4.

2.1.3. Calcium, magnesium and zinc intake. Table 3 shows the level of intake of Ca, Mg and Zn as determined in our survey. As could be seen from the

Table 3. Average concentration of elements in the daily diet of three coastal and one inland community (*n* = 210).

Community	Elements in daily diet (mg/day)		
	Ca	Mg	Zn
Coastal	506	170	6.0
Inland	473	150	5.1
Coefficient variation	0.32	0.28	0.38
Correlation of Na to	0.63	0.80	0.61

362

correlation coefficients between the sodium intake and these elements, only approximately 36% of variance in Ca and Zn intake can be explained by the variation in the sodium intake. The potassium and magnesium show a somewhat closer association with the sodium intake, with correlation coefficients of 0.73 and 0.80, respectively.

Finally, Table 4 shows the dietary intake of five measured electrolytes by 'normotensives' and 'hypertensives', classified into these two categories on the basis of long-term follow-up, as described above. The hypertensives had a lower intake of all electrolytes than the normotensives, with the exception of zinc. This difference was more pronounced in male hypertensives who consumed up to 1 g salt daily less than their normotensive counterparts.

Table 4. Measured intake of five electrolytes by diagnostic categories.

Electrolytes	Normotensives[a] mg/day	Hypertensives[b] mg/day	Coefficient variation
Na	3336 (~8.5 g NaCl)	3038 (~7.7 g NaCl)	0.30
K	1720	1525	0.30
Mg	173	155	0.28
Ca	555	492	0.32
Zn	5	6	0.38
Na/K ratio (mmol)	3.3	3.4	

[a] $n = 125$.
[b] $n = 48$.

3. DISCUSSION

The Newfoundland hypertension survey confirmed the earlier impression of practising physicians in the province that the prevalence of hypertension in this part of the world is substantially higher than in other parts of Canada, North America or Western Europe. Further confirmation of our findings can be seen in the fact that the mortality for stroke is higher in Newfoundland than in other parts of Canada [3].

We have now to examine how far we can explain, by environmental factors, this increased presence of hypertensive disease. The mean values of sodium intake are not exceedingly high—above 9 g in the coastal communities and above 7 g in the inland community. Nevertheless, this represents up to 18 times more than the calculated physiological need for sodium intake [7]. While this mean value may seem to be relatively moderate as compared to the estimate of the North American salt intake [8], we must stress that this is a mean value and that many of our respondents had a daily salt intake as high as 15–20 g/day.

In our population, we generally did not find evidence that an increased intake of sodium is associated with an increased blood pressure level within the groups studied, i.e. that the respondents who have high dietary salt consumption have higher blood pressure levels than those with lower dietary salt intake. This fact may be interpreted as evidence against the possible role of dietary sodium in the etiology and pathogenesis of essential hypertension.

On the other hand, one may speculate that once a sufficiently high 'threshold' level of salt intake has been reached in a given community, the 'dose-response' relationship disappears and every 'salt-sensitive' member of such a population will develop hypertension. In this situation, a continued high salt intake of the 'salt-resistant' individuals will obscure the inter-individual association of the salt consumption and blood pressure. In areas with high dietary salt intake, it would be more likely that even less susceptible individuals will develop hypertension. In our study, the lowest prevalence of hypertension was recorded among men in the inland settlement with the lowest level of salt consumption.

There is another possible explanation why, in our population, we were unable to replicate findings of other authors [7, 9, 10] who did find a positive association between salt intake and blood pressure in individuals within a studied population. The explanation may be found in the interaction of sodium with other dietary electrolytes like potassium, magnesium, calcium and zinc. The nutritional intake of these electrolytes can vary substantially. Thus, one of the most surprising findings of our dietary survey was the extremely low level of potassium intake among our respondents.

Generally, data on potassium are very scarce. Meneely and Battarbee [11] estimate that the ordinary North American diet supplies approximately 50–100 meq of potassium per day, corresponding approximately to 2–3 g of potassium salts. If this is true, then the sodium/potassium ratio in the daily diet in North America and Western Europe will be in most cases under 3. Priddle [12] observed a sodium/potassium ratio of 2.4 in his hypertensive patients. Langford and Watson [13] found in a group of high-school students that the 24-h urinary sodium/potassium ratio among whites was 2.98; only among blacks were the values of the sodium/potassium ratio above 4. The findings in Newfoundland population are approaching the levels of the dietary Na/K ratio of the black population in the United States.

It is of interest that the recently published 'Dietary Goals for the United States' [14] suggests as a desirable level of potassium consumption 2.5 g of potassium salts per day: far above the present dietary intake in Newfoundland.

Potassium is obviously antagonizing the hypertensiogenic effect of sodium [12], and thus the lack of this element in the diet may be a more important factor in eliciting hypertension in Newfoundland than the high level of salt intake itself.

364

Low calcium intake has also been implicated in the pathogenesis of hypertension. However, the available data in this respect are also scarce and ambiguous [15]. The magnesium and zinc intake is also very low. Both elements in Newfoundland are consumed substantially below the level of the recommended daily allowance. One may further hypothesize that the low dietary intake of zinc, which in biological organisms plays an antagonistic role toward cadmium [16], may also have an indirect effect on the blood pressure. Schroeder reported that higher than normal ratios of cadmium to zinc had been found in subjects dying of hypertensive complications [17].

A more-detailed study of the key electrolytes in human nutrition in relation to sodium is clearly needed.

Finally, we would like to comment on the fact that the male hypertensives in our survey consumed less salt than the normotensives. This finding is similar to those reported by Miall [18], Dawber et al. [19], and more recently by Berglund et al. [20]. As the hypertensives have a decreased ability to excrete salt compared to the normotensives, one wonders whether the repeatedly observed lower salt intake by hypertensives is a sort of 'feedback' mechanism.

In conclusion, the Newfoundland population, afflicted by a high prevalence of hypertension, has nutritional habits that result in a relatively high sodium and definitely low potassium intake. Fruits, green leaf vegetables, milk and milk products are very scarce in the Newfoundland diet. If this is considered as a type of nutrition associated with a low socio-economic class population, one wonders whether the inverse relationship that has been shown in the prevalence of hypertension with socio-economic class has not a basis in this type of food selection. The increased consumption of salt in low socio-economic classes has been demonstrated in Belgium by Joossens and Claessens [21]. It is possible that across the socio-economic structure, there is an inverse relationship between the social status and potassium consumption.

We feel that further studies are needed in this area, which would include a wider range of electrolytes than sodium only. Intervention studies, with corrective patterns of nutrition and with an analysis of its effect on hypertension may further clarify this problem area and could facilitate our effort in developing a programme of primary prevention of hypertensive disease.

4. SUMMARY

A survey of 1499 residents over the age of 19 in four rural Newfoundland communities ascertained that the prevalence of hypertension among the residents of the coastal areas is between 20% and 30%. The corresponding figures are somewhat lower in the surveyed inland town.

A total of 210 respondents participated in a dietary survey using a 'double portion' method of food collection. The dietary intakes of sodium, potassium, calcium, magnesium, and zinc was determined in homogenized aliquots of food and beverages for seven consecutive days in two survey periods. The mean sodium intake varies between 104 and 183 meq/day and the potassium intake between 37 and 44 meq/day.

The sodium intake was generally higher in the coastal fishing communities than in the inland town.

No relationship was found between the body-mass index and sodium intake. Males consumed more sodium than females. The hypertensive individuals among our respondents consumed less sodium than the normotensives. This phenomenon was more explicit among males.

We conclude that the interrelationship between electrolytes in the daily diet and the blood pressure level is a complex one. The most prominent feature in our population was the low level of intake of potassium. This factor may contribute significantly to the high frequency of hypertension in Newfoundland.

Acknowledgments. The authors would like to acknowledge and thank Dr. David Bryant of Memorial University of Newfoundland and Dr. Theodore Colton of Harvard Medical School for their help with the statistical analysis, and Dr. Siegfried Heyden of Duke University, North Carolina, for critical review and suggestions. We would also like to acknowledge the fine cooperation we received from the residents of the four communities involved in the study.

REFERENCES

1. National Center for Health Statistics: National health examination survey: blood pressure of adults by race and area, United States, 1960–62, Ser 11, no. 5. Washington DC: US Department of Health, Education and Welfare, 1964.
2. Hypertension: Report of the Ontario Council of Health, Toronto, 1977.
3. Hogan K: Stroke mortality in Newfoundland (unpublished results).
4. Ross J: A study of morbidity in family practice. Can Fam Phys 18:105-115, 1972.
5. Census of Canada population. 1, 1966.
6. Hamilton M, Pickering GW, Roberts JAF: The etiology of essential hypertension. Clin Sci 13:37, 1954.
7. Dahl IK, Lewis K: Salt and hypertension. Am J Clin Nutr 25:237-246, 1972.
8. Freis ED: Salt volume and the prevention of hypertension. Circulation 53:589-595, 1976.
9. Prior IAM, Evans JG: Sodium intake and blood pressure in Pacific populations. Isr Med Sci 5:608, 1969.
10. Shaper AG, et al.: Environmental effects on the body build, blood pressure and blood chemistry of nomadic warriors serving in the army in Kenya. East Afr Med J 46:282, 1969.
11. Meneely GR, Batarbee HD: High sodium–low potassium environment and hypertension. Am J Cardiol 38:768-785, 1976.

12. Priddle WW: Hypertension — sodium and potassium studies. Can Med Assoc J 86:1-9, 1962.
13. Langford HG, Watson RL: A study of the urinary sodium salt — taste threshold and blood pressure resemblance of siblings. Johns Hopkins Med J 131:143-146, 1972.
14. Dietary goals for the United States: supplemental views. Stock no. 052-070-042940, 49-51, 1977.
15. Langford HG, Watson RL: Electrolytes, environment and blood pressure. Clin Sci Mol Med 45:111-113, 1973.
16. Parizek J: The destructive effect of cadmium ion on testicular tissue and its prevention by zinc. J Endocrin 15:56-63, 1957.
17. Schroeder HA: Cadmium as a factor in hypertension. J Chronic Dis 18:647-656, 1965.
18. Miall WE: Follow-up study of arterial pressure in the population of a Welsh mining valley. Br Med J 1204-1210, 1959.
19. Dawber TR, Kannel WB, Kagan A: Environmental factors in hypertension. In: Stamler J, Stamler R, Pullman NT (eds) The epidemiology of hypertension, 1st ed. Grune & Stratton, 1967, pp 225-281.
20. Berglund G, Wallentin I, Wikstrand J, Wilhelmsen L: Sodium excretion and sympathetic activity in relation to severity of hypertensive disease. Lancet 1:324-327, 1976.
21. Joossens J, Claessens J: Epidemiologie de l'hypertension. Monographie Sandoz sur l'hypertension, Brussels, 1972.
22. National Center for Health Statistics: US national health survey: hypertension and hypertensive heart disease in adults, Ser 2, no. 1. US Gov Washington DC: US Government Printing Office, Public Health Service, 1966.

22. EPIDEMIOLOGICAL STUDIES ON HYPERTENSION IN NORTHEAST JAPAN

N. SASAKI

In the northeastern region of Japan, there is an expression, 'attata,' which literally means 'was being affected by.' This is an old expression and the exact meaning of the word is unclear, but it seems to be 'apoplexy,' which has been observed since the ancient Greek era. It occurs suddenly and the patient loses consciousness, resulting in motor paralysis. This is the so-called knocked-down condition that the people in the region call 'atari.' From its general symptoms, it can be differentiated from heart disease.

With regard to the diseases of the circulatory system in Japan, especially cerebrovascular disease, it is well known that the prevalence and the incidence differ in comparison with other countries. The mortality rate from cerebrovascular disease, particularly in Northeast Japan, is high, even in the young and in middle-aged subjects below the age of 60 years. The cause of death is mainly cerebral hemorrhage, and seasonal differences exist: it occurs more often in winter than in summer.

We started epidemiological studies in stroke and hypertension in Japan, especially in the inhabitants of the Northeast in 1954. Takahashi et al. [1] reported that the geographic distribution of cerebral apoplexy and hypertension in Japan could possibly be partly explained by the differences in atmospheric temperature. Cerebral apoplexy and hypertension were equally frequent in farm villages in which there was a surplus intake of rice and salt, and a lack of vegetables.

As an explanation of the nationwide regional difference in the mortality from cerebral apoplexy and in the blood pressure levels of the inhabitants, the author reported that the quantity of salt intake is the most influential factor from the standpoint of retrospective epidemiological studies [2].

1. BLOOD PRESSURE OF THE JAPANESE FROM A GLOBAL VIEWPOINT

Epidemiological studies on hypertension should be based on observations of blood pressure measurements in a specific population group. For this purpose, it should be known what level of blood pressure exists in different geographic regions in the world. There is still, however, a lack of coherent data in this

H. Kesteloot, J.V. Joossens (eds.), Epidemiology of Arterial Blood Pressure, 367–377.
Copyright © 1980 Martinus Nijhoff Publishers bv, The Hague/Boston/London. All rights reserved.

368

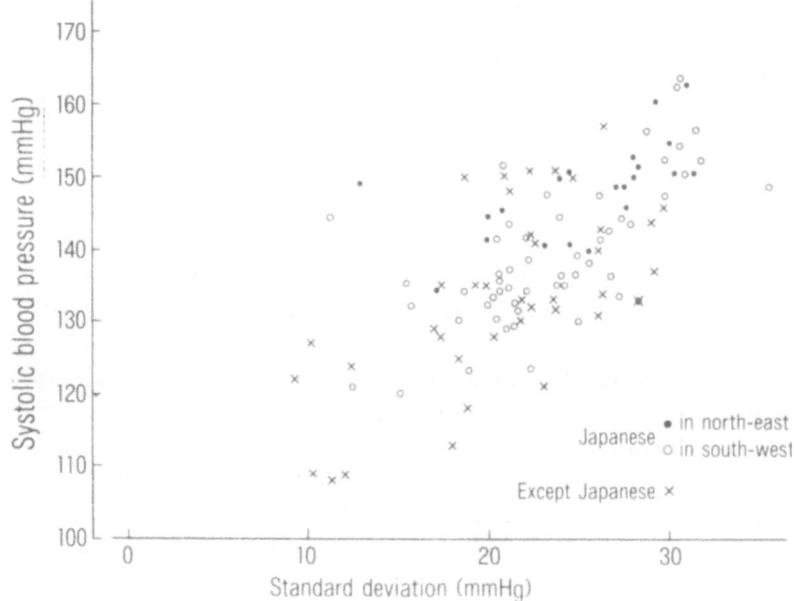

Figure 1. Mean and distribution of systolic blood pressure in various populations in the world (men aged 50 years).

field. Few international epidemiological studies on hypertension have focused on blood pressure, and not all methodological problems concerning blood pressure measurement are yet solved [3].

We could possibly get some clues from the data reported up to now. Figure 1 shows the correlation between the mean values and standard deviations of systolic blood pressure in 50-year-old men. These values were selected from various population groups reported from many countries in the world. The literature cited here consists of 211 papers dealing with the epidemiology of blood pressure of Japanese before 1970, and with 86 papers published in foreign countries before 1969 [4]. It appears from this figure that there seems to be a difference in blood pressure level and distribution between each population group, even if they are of the same age. Concerning the Japanese, especially the inhabitants of the Northeast, the measured blood pressure level seems to be high and has a wide range of distribution. In almost all Japanese groups, the blood pressure level increased with age; and in the group of young people with high blood pressure, the blood pressure level increased more rapidly at advanced age.

The author reported: 'For the investigation of blood pressure of a person, one must at first make mass surveys of levels and distributions of blood pressure of the population in which the person lives and compare it to the level of his own blood pressure' [5].

We have proceeded in our study mainly from the standpoint of cause analysis concerning the difference in blood pressure levels in various groups, and the differences in individual blood pressures. We have also examined the relationship of blood pressure and various living conditions. As working hypothesis for the differences in blood pressure in a population, the author proposed the relationship between the daily salt intake and the levels and distributions of blood pressure [6].

The blood pressure of humans varies from a low level with a narrow range of distribution, remaining so throughout life (e.g., natives of Brazil and New Guinea), to a high level with a wide distribution, beginning with childhood and progressing with age to a higher level and wider distribution (e.g., the inhabitants of Northeast Japan). Dahl reported the evidence that salt ingestion may be related to hypertension, and the results of the epidemiological findings in human hypertension, including the data from Japan, in an internation-

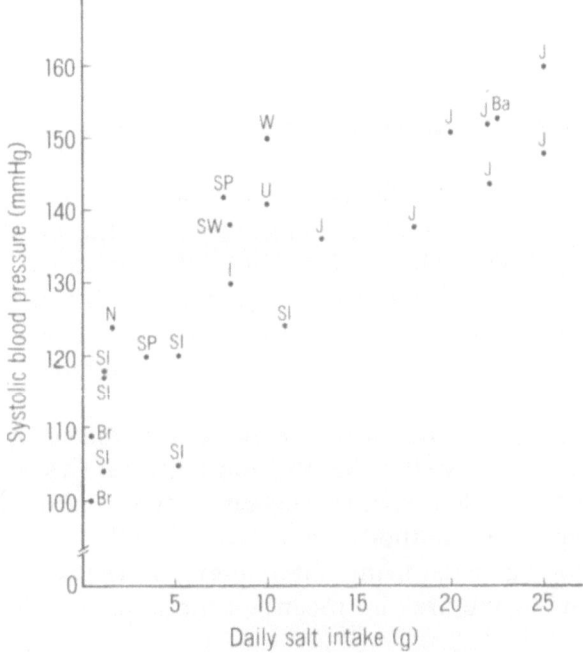

Figure 2. Mean systolic blood pressure of the populations aged 50 years, and average daily salt intake in various parts of the world (male). Ba, Bahamas; Br, Brazil; I, India; J, Japan; N, New Guinea; SI, Solomon Islands; SP, South Pacific; SW, South Wales; U, U.S.A.; W, West Indies. (Reproduced from the data of Sasaki N [10].)

al symposium on essential hypertension in 1960 [7]; he said that the frequency with which certain levels of blood pressure are found is more meaningful than the mean values of blood pressure by his subjective judgement [8].

In previous work, we have already shown the relationship between the mean levels of systolic blood pressure by age and sex in the various populations in which the salt intake of the subject population was actually measured [9, 10]. The correlation between blood pressure (both level and distribution) and daily salt intake is striking. The blood pressure level appears to be high already in a younger age group in areas with a salt intake of more than 10 g/day/person, with a subsequent increase of blood pressure with aging. In areas with a salt intake of less than 5 g, on the other hand, the blood pressure is low at a younger age and no increase is noted with advance in age.

Figure 2 shows the correlation between the mean systolic blood pressure of the population aged 50 years and the average daily salt intake in various parts of the world. The salt intake of the Japanese population is influenced by its traditional eating habits, and it is striking that, about 20 years ago, the Japanese population, especially the inhabitants of the Northeast, consumed 20–30 g of salt per day [2].

2. BLOOD PRESSURE OF THE JAPANESE POPULATION

It has been reported that the blood pressure of the applicants for life insurance and the blood pressure of the Japanese from the data of the National Survey in Japan are nearly the same as those of Americans. According to the summary of the WHO meeting held in Tokyo in 1974, high blood pressure is a prevalent condition in most parts of the world, and prevalence data presented from Japan did not appear to be essentially different from those from other areas.

However, there seem to be marked regional differences in the blood pressure of the Japanese, as well as in the mortality rate from apoplexy [1]. In order to determine the blood pressure levels of the inhabitants in the Northeast and to compare the author's own data with the results of other local studies, the author has made many observations on the arterial blood pressure of the populations in the area by means of local mass survey from 1954 to 1958 [11].

Blood pressure was measured by using a mercury sphygmomanometer with a 13-cm-wide cuff, while the subject was in the supine position. Blood pressure was measured several times, and the lowest level was recorded when different readings were obtained. The diastolic blood pressure was taken as the point at which the Korotkoff sounds disappeared (phase 5).

According to the results of mass observations on the blood pressure of the inhabitants of the Northeast, the blood pressure was higher among inhabitants of this region compared with other districts in all age groups. And the level and distribution of blood pressure actually differ between the communities. The blood pressure levels measured in the colder season (below a mean temperature of 10 °C) were higher than those measured in the warmer season (above 10 °C), even though the room temperature was around 20 °C in both seasons.

In the first mass survey on blood pressure of the inhabitants of the Northeast, the authors measured with precision the seasonal variation in the blood pressure of the same 831 subjects (274 male, 557 female) in winter and summer during five consecutive years [12]. The difference in blood pressure in winter and summer was always found to be significant, irrespective of sex, age group, or location, during each of the five years. The differences between winter and summer were around 10 mmHg for systolic blood pressure on average. Generally speaking, there was an obvious elevation in the blood pressure in winter among the inhabitants of the Northeast, so this elevation seems to be one of the causes of the seasonal variation in the number of deaths from cerebrovascular diseases in Japan.

The authors made observations on the blood pressure of middle-school pupils (aged 12–15 years) in the Akita prefecture twice a year, in winter and summer, from 1957 to 1962, and repeated the blood pressure measurement in the winter of 1967 [13]. According to the results (male $n = 20$, female $n = 26$), a statistically significant correlation was found between the systolic blood pressure level and the Probit value (an index representing the position of an individual in a population) of the blood pressure in middle-school age and in adulthood (aged 18–25 years).

In order to know whether there is a relation between the blood pressure of parents and their children, and between husband and wife, the authors calculated the correlation coefficients between the blood pressure by age and sex on the data obtained from the mass survey of blood pressure in the same farm village of Akita prefecture, the measurement being conducted twice a year from winter 1957 to summer 1961. The correlation coefficients between the blood pressures of parents and children by age and sex for systolic and diastolic blood pressures were almost significant, but the correlation coefficients between the blood pressure of husband and wife by age for systolic and diastolic blood pressures were not significant. From these results, we concluded that the blood pressure level at middle age or older might have been influenced partially by genetic and environmental factors at a certain stage of life, especially at an age earlier than marriage [14].

In the Aomori prefecture, the authors made observations on the blood pressure of schoolchildren: 357 primary-school pupils (aged 6–11 years) from

November to December 1971 [15], and 220 middle-school pupils (aged 12–14 years) from November to December 1973 [16], three times a day sequentially for three days by means of the auscultatory method with the subjects in the sitting position. Then, 28 subjects from a primary school and 36 subjects from a middle school were selected on the basis of a constant deviation from the average value, i.e., boys and girls who always had high blood pressure or who always had low blood pressure.

According to the results of blood pressure measurements that were carried out three times a day for 17 days for the primary-school pupils and 30 days for the middle-school pupils sequentially in the same subjects, it was found that the individual subjects distributed themselves in a mass according to their 'probit,' which was computed from their own and the average level and the standard deviation of blood pressure of the mass; in other words, some subjects always indicated somewhat high and some rather low levels of blood pressure from an early age onward.

As a result of the study on urinary potassium and sodium for five days [16, 17], no correlation was found between Na/K (mmol), NaCl/creatinine (g), and KCl/creatinine (g) in the casual morning urine and the blood pressure levels. The results are shown in Table 1.

The results of these epidemiological studies suggested that the interaction between genetic and environmental factors plays an important part in the causation of human hypertension.

Table 1. Casual morning urine electrolyte content in blood pressure subgroups.

	HPSP ↑	HPSP ↓	HMSB ↑	HMSB ↓	HMSG ↑	HMSG ↓
n	14	14	9	9	9	9
Na/K (mmol)	3.09 ± 1.53	4.03 ± 1.63	4.68 ± 1.63	5.60 ± 2.02	4.54 ± 1.67	4.13 ± 1.17
NaCl/creat (g)	13.6 ± 5.5	17.3 ± 5.97	10.8 ± 3.30	10.9 ± 2.86	12.2 ± 4.88	12.2 ± 3.74
KCl/creat (g)	3.16 ± 0.76	3.29 ± 0.71	1.87 ± 0.64	1.56 ± 0.77	2.10 ± 0.56	2.28 ± 0.82

HPSP ↑ : hypertensive primary-school pupils.
HPSP ↓ : hypotensive primary-school pupils.
HMSB ↑ : hypertensive middle-school boys.
HMSB ↓ : hypotensive middle-school boys.
HMSG ↑ : hypertensive middle-school girls.
HMSG ↓ : hypotensive middle-school girls.

3. LONG-TERM OBSERVATIONS ON BLOOD PRESSURE OF THE INHABITANTS OF THE NORTHEAST

The author has reported the results of our longitudinal epidemiological studies on hypertension in three farm villages in Northeast Japan [18]: Oinomori population, $n = 700$; Kanaya population, $n = 1400$, in the Aomori prefecture;

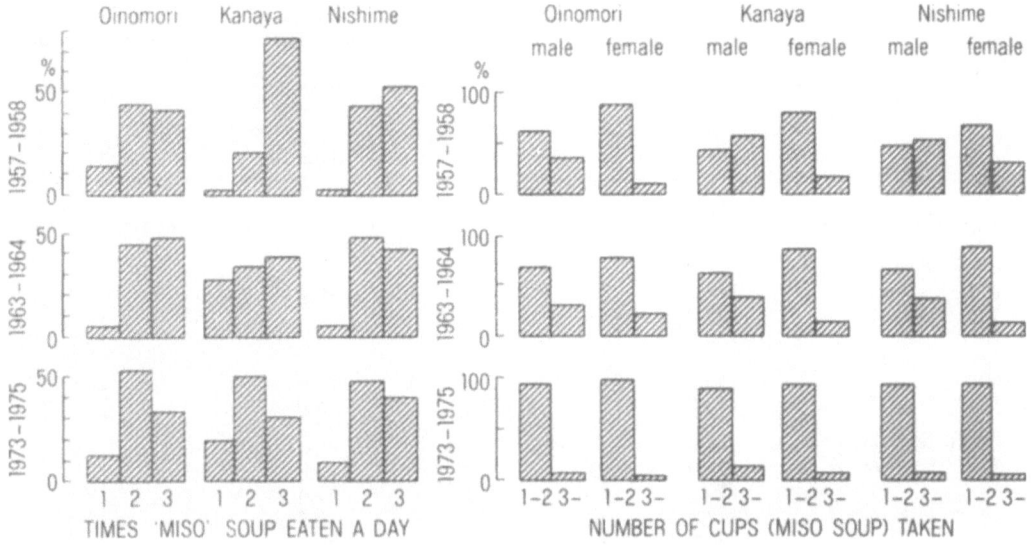

Figure 3. Changes in times 'miso' soup eaten and the number of cups (miso soup) taken per day by the middle-aged farmers of three farm villages.

and Nishime population, $n = 5000$, in the Akita prefecture. Blood pressure was determined once or twice a year by mass surveys in 1954, 1958, and 1957, respectively, up to 1975. The levels and distributions of blood pressure by age and sex in three villages were different at the beginning, as were the findings in the daily life of the inhabitants in the three villages. The differences in the blood pressure corresponded to the death rates fom cerebrovascular diseases in middle-aged subjects in the three areas.

Intervention studies on the hypertension control by reducing high salt intake have been carried out in Nishime village since 1957 and Kanaya village since 1958. The level of blood pressure of the inhabitants of these villages tends to become lower compared with the level at the beginning, in the late 1950s, not only in the middle-age group (Table 2) but also in a younger-age group, such as middle-school children [10]. We observed changes in dietary patterns such as how frequently, or how many, bowls of 'miso' soup were consumed per day (Fig. 3). The average salt content of 'miso' soup is 1.5%, and one bowl of Japanese 'miso' soup is usually 150–180 cubic centimeters. On the other hand, no changes occurred in the pattern of drinking 'sake' or in smoking. In the results obtained in field studies in December 1963, the urinary Na/K (mmol) ratios in the middle-aged farmers in Oinomori, Kanaya, and Nishime villages were 6.45 ± 3.28 ($n = 43$),

Table 2. Mean arterial blood pressure with standard deviation and frequency of persons with high blood pressure among the inhabitants of three farm villages in Northeast Japan by age and sex during 1954–1975.

Age (years)	Male	Systolic			Diastolic		
	n	m	σ	%	m	σ	%
Oinomori, Aug. 1954							
20–29	23	129.3	12.8	0	70.2	11.4	4.3
30–39	18	125.0	15.6	11.1	73.3	9.5	5.6
40–49	17	135.6	20.7	11.8	79.1	10.9	17.6
50–59	18	130.0	15.7	5.6	76.1	9.3	5.6
60–69	7	153.6	21.0	57.1	85.0	10.7	28.6
70–77	5	143.0	11.7	40.0	75.0	6.3	0
Oinomori. Sep. 1974							
30–39	10	127.0	9.8	0	75.0	6.3	0
40–49	11	120.5	14.4	9.1	71.4	9.8	9.1
50–59	14	127.1	10.1	0	76.4	11.2	14.3
60–69	15	146.3	26.0	46.7	86.3	9.6	33.3
70–79	9	129.4	16.4	11.1	73.9	7.4	0
80–89	3	135.0	8.2	0	75.0	8.2	0
Kanaya, Aug. 1958							
30–39	18	132.8	14.0	5.6	73.3	13.0	22.2
40–49	55	141.2	28.1	29.1	80.8	14.6	18.2
50–59	42	144.3	23.3	33.3	84.1	13.7	33.3
60–69	24	149.2	19.8	50.0	80.0	10.0	16.7
70–79	17	167.9	33.7	64.7	89.7	12.4	41.2
Kanaya, Sep. 1974							
40–49	20	122.5	16.7	10.0	73.5	12.4	10.0
50–59	24	131.3	21.9	20.8	80.0	12.2	25.0
60–69	25	133.8	23.4	24.0	77.0	11.7	16.0
70–79	13	146.5	20.7	53.8	78.8	8.4	7.7
80–89	4	150.0	32.8	25.0	82.5	8.3	25.0
Nishime, June 1958							
20–29	157	136.1	14.2	15.2	73.0	12.7	7.6
30–39	186	135.5	15.4	15.0	74.6	13.7	12.9
40–49	148	139.2	24.1	22.3	80.5	14.9	20.3
50–59	139	153.1	27.4	47.5	87.3	15.2	36.7
60–69	88	157.7	32.0	59.0	85.2	14.2	36.3
70–79	25	183.8	33.6	80.0	92.2	14.6	56.0
Nishime, Aug. 1975							
30–39	52	121.0	13.9	3.8	79.0	10.8	15.4
40–49	97	125.1	16.0	9.3	82.4	12.9	24.7
50–59	108	128.1	20.8	18.5	81.9	12.0	25.9
60–69	107	135.9	23.0	24.3	24.3	83.9	27.1
70–79	59	137.0	20.1	22.0	80.4	12.7	27.1
80–89	4	137.5	16.4	25.0	82.5	4.3	0

n, number.

m, mean blood pressure in mmHg.

σ, standard deviation in mmHg.

% incidence of persons in whom the blood pressure was 150 mmHg and above in systolic and 90 mmHg and above in diastolic.

Data of the blood pressure measurements which were made once or twice a year during above-mentioned periods in three villages were omitted from this table.

Female							
	Systolic				Diastolic		
n	m	σ	%		m	σ	%
31	123.7	13.4	3.2		70.5	11.0	3.2
29	122.6	11.0	0		73.3	7.4	0
25	121.0	16.0	8.0		75.8	7.9	4.0
16	135.6	24.6	25.0		78.1	10.4	18.8
9	143.9	22.8	33.3		80.6	9.6	22.2
6	158.3	11.1	83.3		83.3	9.0	33.3
21	116.9	6.6	0		70.7	9.0	4.8
18	120.0	8.3	0		71.7	7.5	0
17	130.3	20.9	17.6		75.6	10.6	11.8
20	130.0	20.1	15.0		74.5	12.0	15.0
9	148.3	22.6	33.3		86.1	14.5	44.4
3	148.3	34.0	33.3		78.3	9.4	0
21	130.2	12.6	9.5		73.1	11.8	9.5
68	135.1	24.4	19.1		80.7	13.7	22.1
38	145.5	24.8	39.5		83.4	12.6	21.1
38	155.5	31.0	55.3		84.7	16.4	34.2
15	191.0	30.5	93.3		93.0	13.3	66.7
28	117.5	15.0	7.1		72.1	9.9	7.1
34	121.8	17.4	5.9		73.8	9.6	2.9
20	132.5	20.5	15.0		76.5	9.6	15.0
18	137.2	16.9	16.7		73.9	8.1	0
4	135.0	10.0	0		72.5	4.3	0
300	129.7	15.2	9.0		71.2	12.8	6.3
314	129.2	17.7	10.2		73.1	11.9	5.4
253	135.7	23.6	19.0		78.5	13.8	17.4
193	149.5	28.7	41.4		84.0	13.8	28.0
126	162.1	29.3	65.9		87.3	13.8	38.1
36	182.2	27.7	86.1		90.3	12.6	38.9
112	111.9	11.9	0		70.8	10.2	5.4
186	113.5	14.2	2.7		73.2	9.8	3.8
217	120.0	19.5	8.9		77.0	11.4	10.6
169	128.4	21.9	15.4		77.1	11.1	11.2
91	133.4	19.3	19.8		75.0	11.9	12.1
7	153.6	21.7	57.1		76.4	9.9	14.3

7.01 ± 3.53 ($n = 223$), and 6.60 ± 3.12 ($n = 250$), respectively. And the urinary Na/K ratio of the 206 middle-aged farmers in Nishime villages was 5.47 ± 2.68, according to the results obtained in the field study in December 1970.

4. CONCLUSION

From the epidemiological viewpoint, the level and distribution pattern of the blood pressure of a population seems related to the daily salt intake, which is determined by dietary habits from childhood onward. Also, the results of epidemiological studies on the blood pressure of inhabitants in the Northeast suggested that interaction between genetic and environmental factors is important in the causation of human hypertension.

According to the results of intervention studies on hypertension, control by reducing salt intake changed both the level and the frequency distribution of blood pressure, as well as the way of life for the inhabitants of Northeast Japan.

REFERENCES

1. Takahashi E, Sasaki N, Takeda J, Ito H: The geographic distribution of cerebral hemorrhage and hypertension in Japan. Hum Biol 29:139-166, 1957.
2. Sasaki N: High blood pressure and the salt intake of the Japanese. Jpn Heart J 3:313-324, 1962.
3. Sasaki N, Hasunuma M: Objective recording of blood pressure for epidemiological study on hypertension (Abstr). 8th World Congress of Cardiology, Sept 1978, Tokyo, p 340.
4. Sasaki N: Blood pressure of Japanese from a global viewpoint. Hirosaki Med J 26:327-349, 1974.
5. Sasaki N: Studies on blood pressure. Hirosaki Med J 14:331-349, 1963.
6. Hatano S, Shigematsu I, Strasser T (eds): Hypertension and stroke control in the community. Geneva: WHO, 1976, pp 106-107.
7. Dahl LK: Possible role of salt intake in the development of essential hypertension. In: Bock KD, Cottier PT (eds) Essential hypertension. Berlin: Springer, 1960, pp 53-65.
8. Dahl LK: Evidence for minimal character of atherosclerosis in hypertensive Japanese farm laborers. At Bomb Casualty Commis Tech Rep 16:37-38, 1959.
9. Sasaki N: The salt factor in hypertension (Abstr). 6th World Congress of Cardiology, Sept 1970, London, p 24.
10. Sasaki N: The salt factor in apoplexy and hypertension — epidemiological studies in Japan. In: Yamori Y, et al. (eds) Proceedings of the international symposium on prophylactic approach to hypertensive diseases. New York: Raven, 1979, pp 467-474.

11. Sasaki N: Observations on the blood pressure of the inhabitants in North-East Japan. Jpn J Public Health 6:496-503, 1959.
12. Sasaki N, Takeda J, Fukushi S, Hasunuma M, Ichikawa H, Ichinohe M, Tanaka K, Sasaki I, Takei T, Sugita K, Takemori K, Yamada N: Seasonal variation in the blood pressure of the inhabitants in the northeastern parts of Japan. Hirosaki Med J 21:202-211, 1969.
13. Sasaki N, Takeda J, Fukushi S, Ichikawa H, Tanaka K, Ichinohe M, Takei T, Sugita K: Follow-up studies on blood pressure of the middle school pupils after 10 years in a farm village of the Akita prefecture (II report). Hirosaki Med J 20:400-408, 1968.
14. Ishiyama R: On the resemblance co-efficients between blood pressure of parents and child and husband and wife in a farm village of the Akita prefecture. Hirosaki Med J 17:607-615, 1966.
15. Sasaki N, Nakamura K, Ono E, Fukushi S: Observations on the blood pressure of primary school pupils in Aomori prefecture (I and II reports). Gakko-hoken kenkyu (Jpn J School Health) 16:174-179; 16:338-342, 1974.
16. Nakamura K: Observations on the blood pressure of middle school pupils in Aomori prefecture. Hirosaki Med J 30:603-630, 1978.
17. Sasaki N, Nakamura K, Takemori K: Observations on the blood pressure of primary school pupils in Aomori prefecture (III report). Gakko-hoken kenkyu (Jpn J School Health) 16:488-489, 1974.
18. Sasaki N: Epidemiological studies on hypertension in the northeastern parts of Japan. In: Proceedings of the first Asian-Pacific symposium on hypertension, Tokyo, 1976. Jpn Circ J 41:1139-1142, 1977.

23. REGIONAL DIFFERENCE OF BLOOD PRESSURE AND ITS NUTRITIONAL BACKGROUND IN SEVERAL JAPANESE POPULATIONS

Y. KOMACHI and T. SHIMAMOTO

Hypertension is the greatest risk factor for stroke, which is the primary cause of death for the Japanese people. Even though there is not much difference between the prevalence of hypertension in Japan and that in western countries, the incidence of stroke is higher in Japan whereas that of myocardial infarction is higher in the western countries. It might be logical to assume that hypertension in Japan tends to be causally related to stroke, but that hypertension in the western countries is apt to be associated with myocardial infarction. A clarification of this feature will make it possible to cast light on a qualitative difference between Japan and the western countries with respect to hypertension.

It is frequently emphasized that hypertension is closely related to obesity (overweight) in the western countries. There have been reports that when Polynesians and Africans came in contact with the western civilization and their life styles were westernized, the number of obese persons increased, thus raising their average blood pressure level [1, 2]. In Japan, however, it has been verified that there are signs of a higher prevalence of hypertension in the rural areas than in the urban areas, although the prevalence of obese persons is lower in rural areas [3, 4]. In other words, it is evident that the factors responsible for a rise in blood pressure level in Japan are different from those in Polynesia and Africa.

To clarify factors concerning the onset and evolution of hypertension, there is a need to sample groups with different environmental factors, elucidate the cause of differences in the mean blood pressure value and the prevalence of hypertension between groups, and check the differences against environmental factors.

From this aspect, seven groups with different environmental factors—i.e., residents in the Akita and Kochi prefectures, in a rural setting; and residents, manual workers, clerks, and company executives in the Osaka prefecture and physicians of the Osaka Medical Association—were sampled to carry out a cardiovascular survey, including blood pressure measurement, and an examination of dietary intake. Akita is a cold area in northeastern Japan, whereas Osaka and Kochi are warm areas in the center of Japan. Rice is the principal

H. Kesteloot, J.V. Joossens (eds.), Epidemiology of Arterial Blood Pressure, 379–394.

Table 1. Number of subjects and the characteristics of the study groups, men aged 40–69 years.

Group	Residents in two rural areas in Akita	Residents in a rural area in Kochi	Residents in a semiurban area in Osaka	Manual workers in several industrial companies in Osaka	Clerks in several offices in Osaka	Physicians in Osaka (Members of Osaka Medical Association, volunteers)	Executives in several industrial companies in Osaka
No. of subjects							
40–49	561	367	711	2258	1432	702	118
50–59	406	336	617	1130	673	351	137
60–69	311	310	389	291	123	204	97
Total	1278	1013	1717	3679	2228	1257	352
No. examined							
40–49	465	295	625	1896	1180	241	100
50–59	349	286	518	980	573	145	117
60–69	272	292	341	243	100	81	78
Total	1086	873	1484	3119	1853	467	295
Response rate (%)							
40–49	82.9	80.4	87.9	84.0	82.4	34.3	84.7
50–59	86.0	85.1	84.0	86.7	85.1	41.3	85.4
60–69	87.5	94.2	87.7	83.5	81.3	39.7	80.4
Total	85.0	86.2	86.4	84.8	83.2	37.2	83.8

farm product of Akita, while Kochi's farm products are of a wide variety, including vegetables in vinyl-greenhouse cultivation, and tangerines.

Age-adjusted death rate from stroke is highest in Akita, followed by Kochi and Osaka, respectively. In Osaka, four different vocational groups were sampled in addition to one group of residents, because it was conceivable that the living patterns differ, depending on the type of occupation in urban areas—i.e., general residents and manual workers stick to conventional life styles, whereas physicians and company executives maintain a more sophisticated life style.

The survey was carried out in 1965. The number of samples surveyed and the rate of participation are given in Table 1. The rate exceeded 80% for all groups except for the group of physicians, whose participation was voluntary. The survey method has been described previously in detail [4].

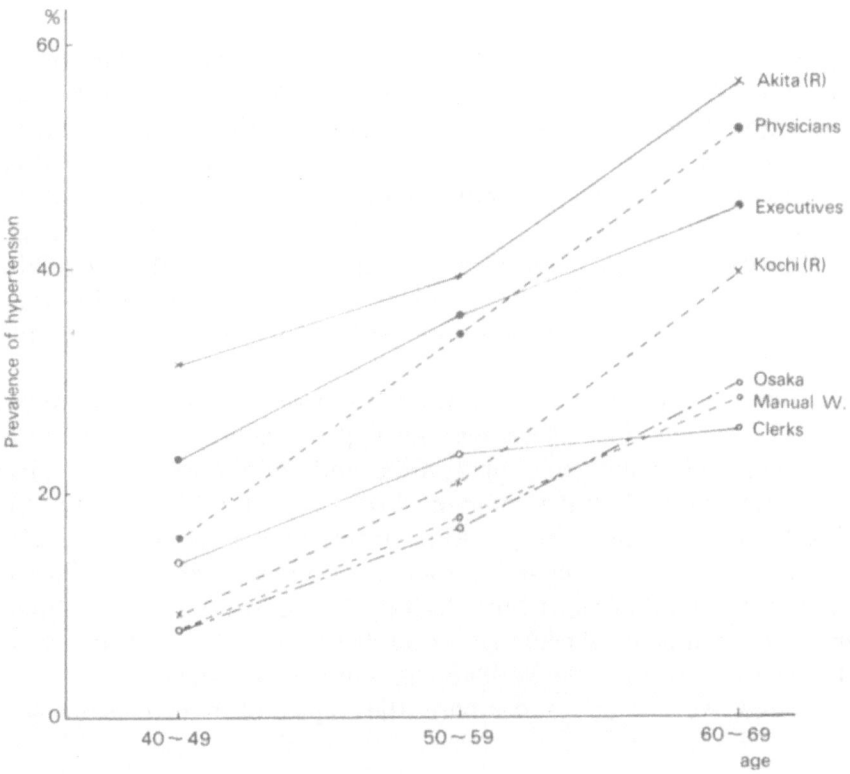

Figure 1. Prevalence rate of hypertension (160+ and/or 95+), men aged 40–69 years.

1. PREVALENCE OF HYPERTENSION IN RELATION TO AREA AND OCCUPATION

The prevalence of hypertension in each group by age is indicated in Figure 1. Hypertensives, as defined here, include those subjects whose blood pressure exceeded a systolic pressure of 160 mmHg and/or a diastolic pressure of 95 mmHg according to the WHO criteria [5], or those whose blood pressure did not exceed either the systolic or diastolic blood pressure level, but received medication for hypertension.

The prevalence of hypertension is highest in the Akita residents and in the Osaka company executives and physicians, followed respectively by the Kochi residents and the Osaka clerks. The prevalence is lowest in the group of Osaka residents and that of Osaka manual workers. In other words, the prevalence of hypertension is highest in two diametrically different groups—i.e., the group whose life style is highly westernized compared with the group that most vividly retains the remnants of the traditional practices.

2. MEAN SYSTOLIC AND DIASTOLIC BLOOD PRESSURE VALUES IN RELATION TO AREA AND OCCUPATION

The mean value and the standard deviation of systolic and diastolic blood pressures for each group are indicated in Table 2. With respect to the systolic blood pressure level, the mean value is highest for the groups of Akita residents, followed respectively by the groups of company executives in Osaka, physicians in Osaka, residents in Kochi, clerks in Osaka, residents in Osaka, and manual workers in Osaka. As for the diastolic blood pressure, the mean value is highest in the groups of Akita residents and Osaka company executives, followed respectively by those of physicians in Osaka, clerks in Osaka, residents in Kochi, residents in Osaka, and manual workers in Osaka.

When the relative position is compared between groups with respect to systolic and diastolic blood pressures, the highest values are registered in the group of Akita residents both for systolic and for diastolic blood pressure. Regarding the group of Osaka company executives, the highest values corresponding to those of the group of Akita residents are registered for diastolic blood pressure, but the values for systolic blood pressure are lower than in the Akita residents. In other words, the diastolic blood pressure value is higher in the group of company executives in Osaka than in the Akita residents, considering the way the systolic blood pressure value stands.

An attempt was made to compare the types of hypertension between residents in Akita and company executives in Osaka; the combination of blood pressure levels was classified into three categories: (a) a systolic level of more than 160 mmHg and a diastolic level of more than 95 mmHg, (b) a

Table 2. Means and standard deviations of systolic and diastolic blood pressures, men aged 40–69 years.

Group	Residents in Akita	Residents in Kochi	Residents in Osaka	Manual workers in Osaka	Clerks in Osaka	Physicians in Osaka	Executives in Osaka
No. examined							
40–49	465	295	625	1896	1180	241	100
50–59	349	286	518	980	573	145	117
60–69	272	292	341	243	100	81	78
Total	1086	873	1484	3119	1853	467	295
Systolic blood pressure (mmHg)							
40–49	142.9 ± 22.2	129.7 ± 14.6	127.6 ± 16.3	124.4 ± 17.6	128.9 ± 18.0	134.1 ± 20.3	142.1 ± 18.6
50–59	151.3 ± 26.6	137.3 ± 18.9	136.4 ± 20.2	132.2 ± 23.6	138.9 ± 20.4	143.0 ± 21.5	147.5 ± 20.2
60–69	162.1 ± 27.2	144.2 ± 22.1	146.7 ± 25.9	148.0 ± 23.8	146.3 ± 24.0	152.7 ± 24.5	152.8 ± 21.8
Total	150.4 ± 26.1	137.1 ± 19.7	135.0 ± 21.5	128.7 ± 21.3	132.9 ± 19.9	140.1 ± 22.6	147.1 ± 20.5
Diastolic blood pressure (mmHg)							
40–49	86.4 ± 14.1	78.0 ± 9.9	78.4 ± 11.2	76.8 ± 12.6	81.7 ± 12.6	83.3 ± 13.1	86.5 ± 11.5
50–59	90.4 ± 14.9	80.6 ± 10.6	82.3 ± 12.6	80.6 ± 14.1	86.1 ± 12.8	87.5 ± 13.1	89.7 ± 12.1
60–69	91.4 ± 15.3	80.9 ± 10.8	83.8 ± 14.8	85.4 ± 13.5	86.1 ± 12.5	89.1 ± 15.9	92.6 ± 12.8
Total	88.9 ± 14.8	79.8 ± 10.5	81.0 ± 12.8	78.7 ± 13.4	83.3 ± 12.6	85.6 ± 13.8	89.5 ± 12.3

384

systolic level of less than 160 mmHg and a diastolic level of more than 95 mmHg, and (c) a systolic level of more than 160 mmHg and a diastolic level of less than 95 mmHg; (a) accounted for 55%, (b) for 23%, and (c) for 23% of hypertensives in Akita; (a) amounted to 27%, (b) 48%, and (c) to 25% for company executives in Osaka. These percentages suggest that both systolic and diastolic blood pressure values are high for many Akita residents with hypertension, whereas the systolic blood pressure is not so high, but the diastolic blood pressure level is high, for Osaka company executives with hypertension.

A similar phenomenon can also be observed in blood pressure values when Akita residents and U.S. citizens are compared. The diastolic blood pressure levels of residents in Framingham [6], Tecumseh [7], and Evans County [8] in the United States are practically the same as, or slightly higher than, that of the Akita residents, but systolic blood pressure levels of these American residents are somewhat lower than that of residents in Akita [9]. It is interesting to note that the blood pressure pattern of company executives in Osaka, who enjoy a westernized life style in Japan, is similar to that of American citizens. It is also interesting to note that few hypertensives are observed among manual workers, clerks, and residents in Osaka, who do not stick adamantly to the traditional Japanese life style, but whose life styles are not westernized to a great extent. Not only on the basis of the afore-mentioned survey, but also on the basis of a joint epidemiological national survey [10] that included the groups sampled in our survey on cardiovascular diseases, the prevalence of hypertensives among the groups of residents, manual workers, and clerks in Osaka is the lowest.

3. HYPERTENSIVE CHANGES IN RELATION TO AREA AND OCCUPATION

The prevalence rate of those who had exceeded two grades of Scheie's classification [11] in fundus examination was compared among the groups. The prevalence is highest for Akita residents in all age brackets, but the prevalence of fundus changes is low, or practically the same, as that of other groups for company executives and physicians in Osaka, among whom the prevalence of hypertension is practically as high as that of residents in Akita. This suggests that even in groups with many hypertensives, hypertension tends to be accompanied by fundus changes when the traditional Japanese life style is maintained but that, particularly in groups enjoying a westernized life style, hypertension hardly tends to be accompanied by fundus changes.

Similarly, an attempt was made to compare the prevalence of ECG changes indicative of left-ventricular hypertrophy. Left high amplitude R plus ST depression and/or T-wave abnormalities were considered indicative of left-venticular hypertrophy. The prevalence is highest for Akita residents, followed respectively by Kochi residents, and Osaka physicians, company executives, and residents; whereas that of Osaka clerks and manual workers is somewhat lower.

Here, in order to clarify the difference in environmental factors that are responsible for the appearance of the traditional and western types of hypertension, the food intake was compared among the groups.

4. RELATIONSHIP OF HYPERTENSION AND HYPERCHOLESTEROLEMIA TO OBESITY

First, the total serum cholesterol value and the obesity (overweight) index were used as indices of food intake in order to examine their relationship to hypertension.

The prevalence of hypercholesterolemia for each group is shown in Figure 2. The modified Zak-Henly method [12] was used to measure the total serum cholesterol. For this study, a total serum cholesterol level of 220 mg/dl or higher was defined as hypercholesterolemia, and the values were classified for hypertensives and nonhypertensives in each group. No groups with a significant difference were observed: the more westernized the life style, the higher the prevalence of hypercholesterolemia; the more conspicuous the traditional life style, the lower the prevalence of hypercholesterolemia.

The correlation between total serum cholesterol and systolic and diastolic blood pressure levels was studied for each group, but no groups with a

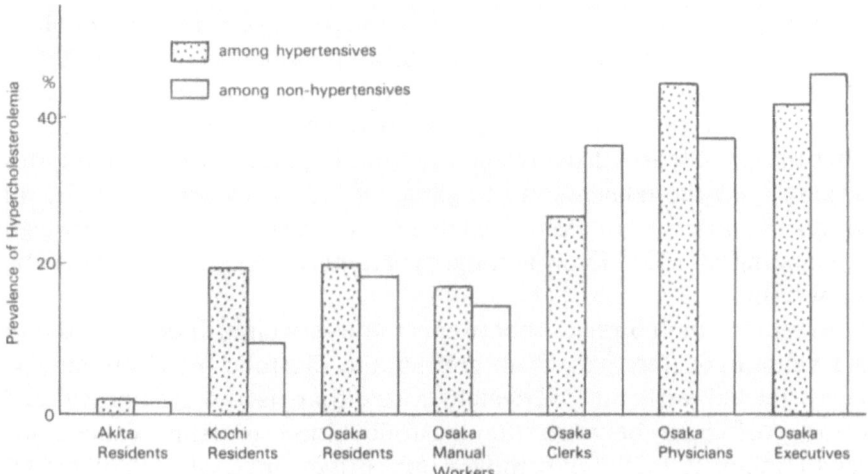

Figure 2. Prevalence rate of hypercholesterolemia (≥ 220 mg/dl), men aged 40–69 years.

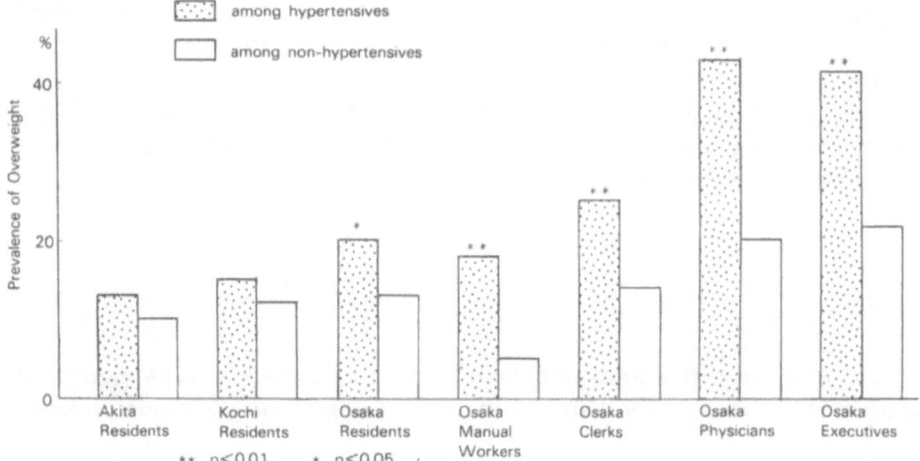

Figure 3. Prevalence rate of overweight ($\geq +20\%$), men aged 40–69 years.

significant correlation were observed. In other words, as demonstrated in many of the Western countries' studies, no significant correlation was observed between hypertension and hypercholesterolemia.

Next, a similar study was carried out with respect to overweight; the results are presented in Figure 3. Minowa's index[13] was computed on the basis of body height and weight, and an index standing at 20% and over was regarded as overweight. There were signs that the prevalence of overweight among hypertensives is higher than among nonhypertensives in each group. Particularly in the groups of physicians and company executives in Osaka, the difference between hypertensives and nonhypertensives is noticeable; the prevalence of overweight is high in both groups of physicians and executives, and about half of the hypertensives are overweight. In contrast, there are signs that the prevalence of overweight among hypertensives is slightly higher than among nonhypertensives in the group of Akita residents, but the difference is not significant. In Akita residents, the prevalence of overweight is lowest, standing at 12%. Even among hypertensive Akita residents, 85% are not overweight.

A close look at the correlation between the overweight index and the blood pressure value indicates that, in all groups, the diastolic blood pressure value is more correlated with the overweight index than is the systolic value. The correlation coefficient between the diastolic blood pressure value and the overweight index is 0.29 for company executives in Osaka, 0.29 for Osaka physicians, 0.11 for Osaka clerks, 0.10 for Osaka manual workers, 0.06 for Osaka residents, and 0.04 for Akita residents.

Table 3. Nutrient intake and salt intake (mean ±SD/day/person), men aged 40–69 years.

Group	Residents in Akita	Residents in Kochi	Residents in Osaka	Manual workers in Osaka	Clerks in Osaka	Physicians in Osaka
No. examined	12	15	11	10	9	13
Total calorie (cal)	3016 ± 881	2936 ± 708	2485 ± 464	2511 ± 141	2347 ± 240	2706 ± 269
Protein, total, g	104 ± 34	102 ± 24	74 ± 11	83 ± 9	81 ± 13	103 ± 17
(Animal protein)	(44 ± 23)	(44 ± 10)	(47 ± 6)	(41 ± 8)	(44 ± 10)	(56 ± 13)
Fat, total, g	41 ± 12	40 ± 10	45 ± 4	46 ± 7	58 ± 11	65 ± 23
(Animal fat)	(15 ± 2)	(15 ± 5)	(20 ± 4)	(18 ± 5)	(30 ± 10)	(37 ± 13)
Carbohydrates, g	502 ± 158	515 ± 153	407 ± 89	408 ± 35	356 ± 46	378 ± 72
Salt, g	20 ± 7	18 ± 5	13 ± 4	8 ± 3	13 ± 2	13 ± 4

Thus, the correlation between hypertension and overweight differs, depending on the group. In groups with highly westernized life styles, there are many overweight hypertensives, indicating that overweight is correlated with hypertension. In groups with noticeable traditional life styles, there are many hypertensives who are not overweight, suggesting that overweight is not correlated with hypertension.

5. DIETARY PATTERN IN RELATION TO AREA AND OCCUPATION

The dietary pattern of each group was examined, and the results are presented in Table 3. This survey was carried out from 1968 to 1971. About ten persons were sampled at random from each group, and registered dieticians measured the quantities of all drinks and food for three consecutive days. Company executives in Osaka were excluded from this survey because they would often eat their meals out, making it difficult for dieticians to make an accurate assessment.

The total calory intake is highest for residents in Akita, who are followed respectively by Osaka physicians, Kochi residents, Osaka manual workers, Osaka clerks, and Osaka residents. The protein intake is high for residents in Akita and Kochi, whereas the animal protein intake is high for physicians in Osaka. The fat intake (68 g/day) is highest for physicians in Osaka, and they are followed by clerks and manual workers in Osaka, whereas the intake is low for residents in Kochi, Osaka, and Akita. When animal fat intake alone is considered, the intake is highest for physicians in Osaka, but low for rural groups. The salt intake, as is elucidated in chapter 24 of this book, is highest (20 g/day) for residents in Akita, and they are followed by residents in Kochi (18 g/day) and the four groups in Osaka (8–14 g/day).

When the dietary patterns are compared between Akita residents and Osaka physicians, the intake of carbohydrates, primarily rice, and that of salt are high, but fat intake is low for Akita residents. In contrast, the intake of carbohydrates is relatively low for Osaka physicians. As relatively large quantities of meat are consumed, the fat and protein intake is high for Osaka physicians. The dietary pattern of Akita residents conspicuously retains features of the traditional Japanese diet. In contrast, the dietary pattern of physicians in Osaka is close to that of western countries.

6. INCIDENCE OF STROKE AND ISCHEMIC HEART DISEASE IN RELATION TO AREA AND OCCUPATION

The incidence of stroke and ischemic heart disease was surveyed in a follow-up study conducted on each group for 5–10 years. An attempt was also made to determine whether hypertension tended to develop into stroke or ischemic heart disease in groups with many hypertensives of the traditional type and with those of the relatively western type. The process evolving from a survey on stroke and ischemic heart disease to a diagnosis has been reported earlier. Millikan's criteria [14] were used for the diagnosis of stroke, whereas the WHO criteria [5] were used for that of ischemic heart disease. To ascertain the reliability of our diagnosis of stroke, the clinical diagnosis was checked against the post-mortem diagnosis in case of autopsy in Akita, which showed that the rate of coincidence was extremely high (97%) [15]. We also participated in WHO-sponsored joint studies, when the diagosis of stroke in Japan and western countries was compared. Regarding rhe diagnosis of stroke, the rate of coincidence was extremely high between Japan and western countries [16].

The age-adjusted incidence of stroke and ischemic heart disease in each group per year is shown in Figure 4. Myocardial infarction and angina pectoris were considered ischemic heart diseases. The incidence of stroke is highest for Akita residents, followed by Kochi residents. Although the prevalence of hypertension among Osaka company executives and physicians is as high as that of Akita residents, the incidence of stroke among Osaka company executives and physicians is only about 1/2.5 that of Akita residents and practically the same as that of Osaka residents. The incidence is lowest for Osaka clerks and manual workers.

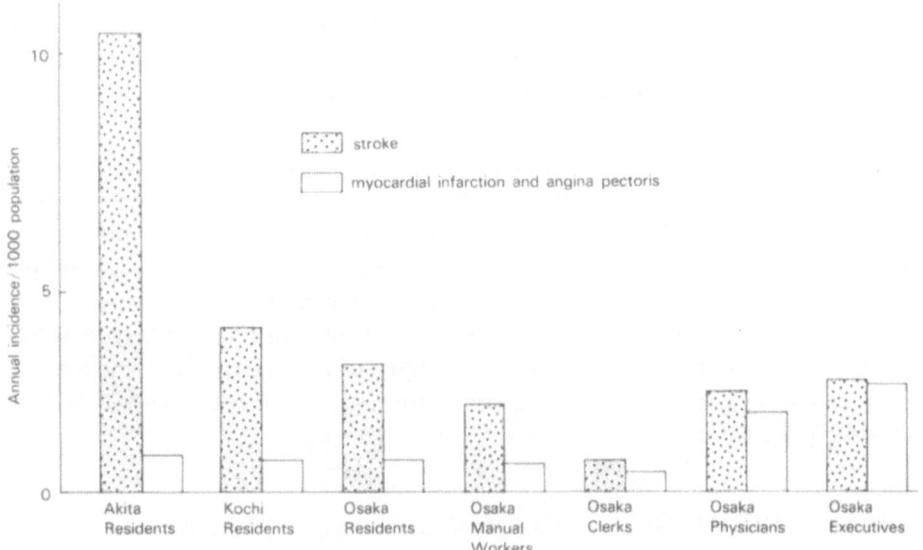

Figure 4. Age-adjusted incidence rate of cardiovascular diseases, men aged 40–69 years, follow-up 5-10 years.

As far as ischemic heart disease is concerned, the difference between groups is not as conspicuous as in the case of stroke, but the incidence is slightly higher for company executives and physicians, who enjoy westernized life styles to a greater extent than other groups.

In the Akita residents and Osaka company executives and physicians, among whom the prevalence of hypertensives is equally high, the incidence of stroke is particularly high for Akita residents but that of ischemic heart disease is low. For the Osaka company executives and physicians, the incidence of stroke is not as high as in the group of Akita residents, but that of ischemic heart disease is relatively higher than that in other groups. This coincides with the fact that stroke mortality is low, but mortality from ischemic heart disease is high in western countries, although it is argued that there is not much difference in the prevalence of hypertension between Japan and western countries.

Not only surveys on Akita residents, but also joint nationwide epidemiological surveys [10], have demonstrated that the incidence of stroke is high in rural groups with a high prevalence of hypertension. Among the Japanese people, apart from those in a westernized environment, joint epidemiological studies [10] have also demonstrated that the higher the prevalence of hypertension in a group, the higher the incidence of stroke.

It can be concluded thus far that there are at least two types of hypertension in Japan. One type makes its appearance and then develops, with no relation to overweight, against the background of hard farm work and a dietary pattern with a high salt and carbohydrate intake, but a low fat intake. This might be described as the traditional type of hypertension that is observed mostly in rural Japan. It is frequently accompanied by changes in fundus oculi and tends to develop into stroke with the systolic blood pressure standing at a relatively high level.

The other type, observed mostly in groups with westernized life styles, makes its appearance and develops with a close relation to overweight, as demonstrated in western surveys. It is relatively less likely to develop into stroke with a high diastolic pressure as opposed to a high systolic blood pressure, but the latter type may develop into ischemic heart disease. With the progressive westernization of the society, however, it is expected that the latter type will gradually increase, although it generally still is exceptional among Japanese people, insofar as the findings of our nationwide survey are concerned [17].

7. CHANGES IN LIFE STYLE AND CHANGES IN BLOOD PRESSURE

The change in the blood pressure value of each group over a ten-year period from 1965 or so, when the first survey was conducted, is shown in Figure 5.

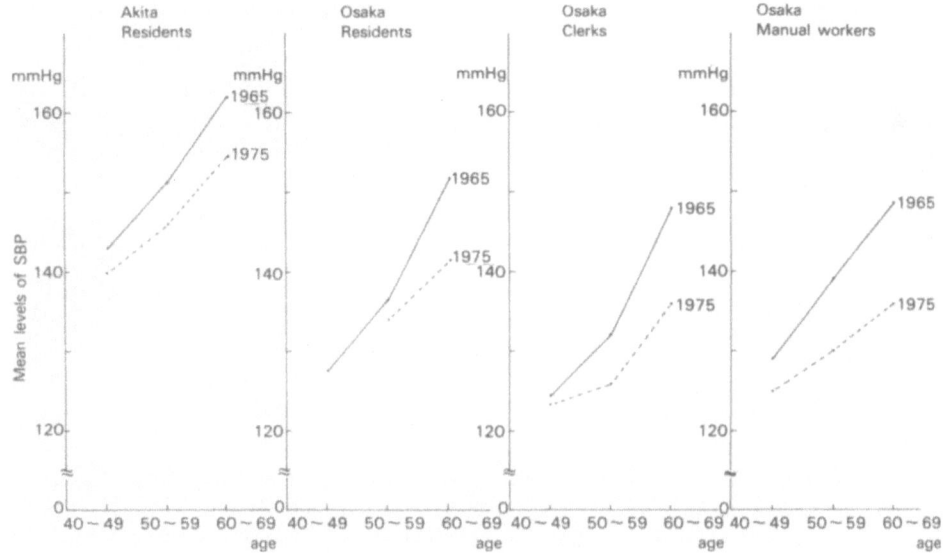

Figure 5. Mean levels of systolic blood pressure, 1965 and 1975, men.

When changes in the mean value of the systolic blood pressure are analyzed with respect to Akita residents, Osaka residents, Osaka clerks, and manual workers in Osaka—on whom survey findings are available—there are signs of a decrease in each age bracket for all groups. The mean value of the diastolic blood pressure does not feature equally conspicuous changes as the systolic blood pressure, and there are signs of a slight decrease in all groups.

In the groups of Akita residents and those in Osaka, the incidence of stroke has dropped by about 50% in the meantime. In the groups of Osaka clerks and manual workers—among whom the incidence of stroke used to be low— few fluctuations have occurred.

It is surmisable that these phenomena have been caused by western living practices being added to the traditional Japanese living pattern. As demonstrated in the Agriculture-Forestry Census, mechanization and motorization in the agricultural sector have reduced manual work. As observed in the National Nutrition Survey, the dietary pattern has changed, with a decrease in carbohydrate intake and an increase in fat intake. The use of heating equipment in winter has become widespread. Another significant factor is the widespread use of hypertension control—primarily, the use of antihypertensive drugs. There is no way of determining which is the greatest contributory factor, but, at least from the findings of joint nationwide surveys [17], the blood pressure level has noticeably decreased in areas where the level had been high. For this reason, it is surmisable that the difference in blood pressure value between urban and rural areas is diminishing.

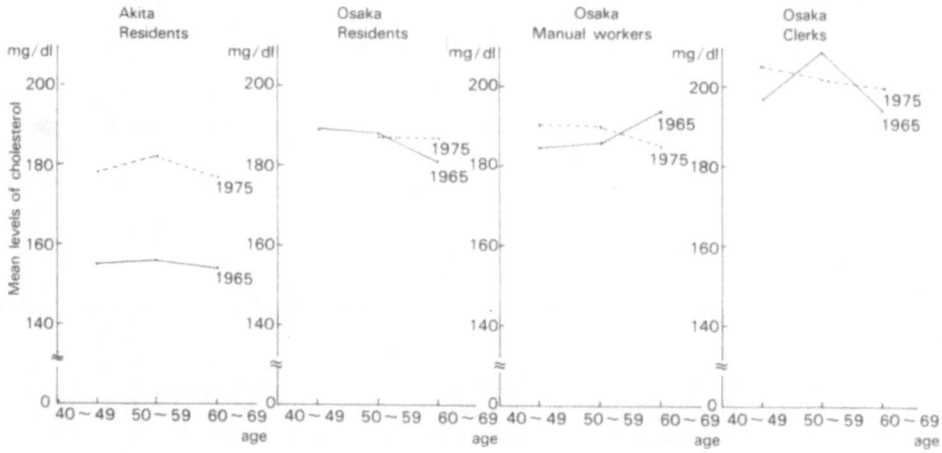

Figure 6. Mean levels of total serum cholesterol, 1965 and 1975, men.

To clarify the changes in the food intake in our survey areas during the last ten years, mean values of total serum cholesterol and the prevalence of overweight both in 1965 and 1975 are shown in Figures 6 and 7. As indicated in Figure 6, changes in the mean value of total serum cholesterol for the Akita residents, Osaka residents, Osaka manual workers, and clerks in Osaka are such that the mean value, which was low in the past, has steadily increased for Akita residents, but remains lower than that of Osaka residents. In the three Osaka groups, there has not been a significant change in the total serum cholesterol level.

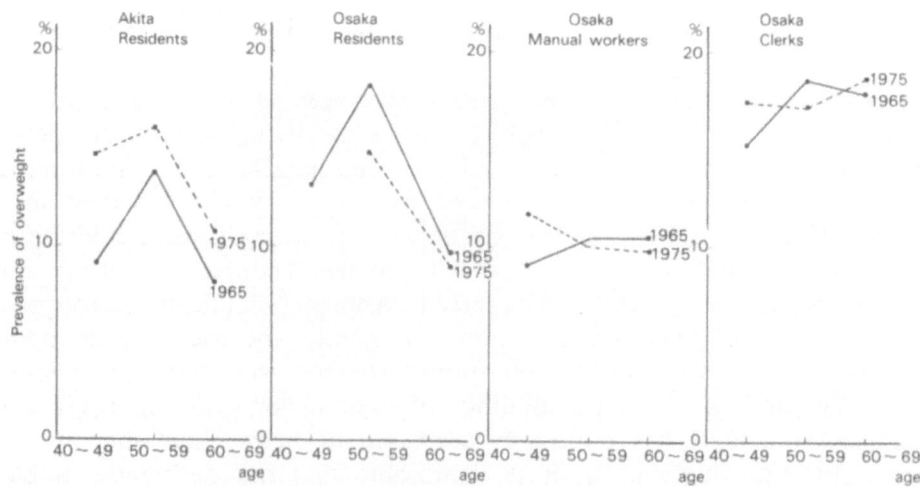

Figure 7. Prevalence rate of overweight ($\geq +20\%$), 1965 and 1975, men.

With respect to overweight, as schematized in Figure 7, there have been increases in the prevalence of overweight for Akita residents whose life style has noticeably changed because of an alleviation of manual work and changes in the food intake, but no conspicuous changes have been observed in the three Osaka groups.

Such changes in the total serum cholesterol level and in the prevalence of overweight have been observed not only in our surveys, but in joint nation-wide epidemiological studies as well [17]. The blood pressure level is gradually decreasing and the incidence of stroke is diminishing as western factors are being incorporated into the Japanese society in recent years.

8. SUMMARY

The authors have attempted to demonstrate that the factors responsible for the onset and evolution of hypertension are multiple and complex. It also is evident from this report that overweight and hypercholesterolemia, which are generally described as facilitating the onset of hypertension, have not contributed in the past to the onset of hypertension among the Japanese. However, it is a fact that, in recent years, the life style of the Japanese people has become astonishingly sophisticated, and the authors hope to elucidate in detail, on a separate occasion, how these changes affect hypertension.

REFERENCES

1. Kagan A: Epidemiology of hypertension and stroke in Oceania. In: Hatano S, Shigematsu I, Strasser T (eds) Hypertension and stroke control in the community. Geneva: WHO, 1976, pp 97-104.
2. Akinkugbe OO: Epidemiology of hypertension and stroke in Africa. In: Hatano S, Shigematsu I, Strasser T (eds) Hypertension and stroke control in the community. Geneva: WHO, 1976, pp 28-42.
3. Komachi Y, et al.: Epidemiological studies on Japanese hypertension and ischemic heart diseases. Jpn Circ J 31:563-580, 1969.
4. Komachi Y, et al.: Geographic and occupational comparisons of risk factors in cardiovascular diseases in Japan. Jpn Circ J 35:189-207, 1971.
5. WHO: Arterial hypertension and ischemic heart disease, preventive aspect. Tech Rep Ser 231, 1962.
6. Dawber TR, et al.: Coronary heart disease in the Framingham study. Am J Public Health 47:4-22, 1957.
7. Johnson BC, et al.: Distribution and familial studies of blood pressure and serum cholesterol levels in a total community, Tecumseh Michigan. J Chronic Dis 18:147-160, 1965.

8. McDonough JR, et al.: Blood pressure and hypertensive disease among negroes and whites, a study in Evans County, Georgia. Ann Intern Med 61:208-228, 1964.
9. Komachi Y, et al.: Epidemiology — characteristics of cerebral stroke in Japan (in Japanese). Saishin Igaku 25:1212-1219, 1970.
10. Shigiya R, Kimura N, Komachi Y, Isomura K, Kojima S, Watanabe T: Nutritional status of Japanese with special reference to epidemiology of cerebrovascular accident (CVA) and coronary heart disease (CHD). In: Asahina K, Shigiya R (eds) Physiological adaptability and nutritional status of the Japanese. Tokyo: University of Tokyo Press, 1975, pp 123-165.
11. Scheie HG: Evaluation of ophthalmoscopic changes of hypertension and arteriosclerosis. Arch Ophthamol 49:117-138, 1953.
12. Yoshikawa H, et al.: Quantitative analysis on serum cholesterol by the terric chloride method (in Japanese). Igaku no Ayumi 33:375-381, 1960.
13. Minowa S: Studies on the standard body weight of the adult in Japan (in Japanese). Jpn Med J 1988:24-28, 1962.
14. Millikan CH: A classification and outline of cerebrovascular diseases. Neurology 8:395-434, 1958.
15. Shimamoto T, et al.: Reliability of clinical diagnosis of stroke — comparison with autopsy diagnosis (in Japanese). In: Shigiya R, Komachi Y, Watanabe T (eds) Nutrition and cerebro-cardiovascular diseases in Japan. Tokyo: Hokendozin, 1976, pp 377-387.
16. Hatano S (ed): WHO collaborative study on the control of stroke in the community: observer variations in the diagnosis of stroke. Jpn Heart J 18:171-177, 1977.
17. Komachi Y, et al.: Cooperative epidemiological study on the prevention of hypertension and stroke (in Japanese). In:Agency of Science and Technology (ed) The prevention of hypertension and stroke. Tokyo: Ministry of Finance, 1979, pp 283-341.

24. SALT INTAKE AND ITS RELATIONSHIP TO BLOOD PRESSURE IN JAPAN

Present and past

Y. KOMACHI and T. SHIMAMOTO

Many epidemiological studies and animal experiments on the relationship between salt intake, on the one hand, and hypertension and stroke, on the other, have been documented in the past [1–4]. The death rate from stroke in Japan is high. For years, attention has been drawn to high salt intakes in the Tohoku region, where the prevalence of hypertension is high. There have been many epidemiological studies on the relationship between the excessive salt intake and hypertension, and also a number of studies on the dietary pattern that is responsible for such an excessive salt intake [2, 3].

Many of these studies on salt intake, however, reflected the situation in a limited time period, and it has been noted that there is a need to look into changes in the salt intake from the past to the present in order to study the effects of salt on hypertension, which develops over many years. To make an epidemiological study on the relationship between salt intake and the prevalence of hypertension or the blood pressure level, it is necessary—instead of being satisfied with only the survey data available from the Ministry of Agriculture, Forestry and Fisheries and the Ministry of Health and Welfare—to select a number of populations throughout the nation for a cardiovascular survey, including blood pressure, and also for a survey on their salt intake in order to clarify the relationship between blood pressure and salt consumption.

1. COMPARISON OF RECENT SALT INTAKE BETWEEN AKITA AND OSAKA

The prevalence of hypertension, the mean systolic blood pressure value, and the mean diastolic blood pressure value for residents in the Osaka and Akita areas are reported in chapter 23 of this book. With respect to these factors, the values are higher for residents in Akita than in Osaka. The prevalence of hypertensive changes in the examination of the ocular fundus and in the ECG examination is also higher for residents in Akita than in Osaka.

The salt intake in both areas was surveyed twice—that is, in 1965 and 1970 [5, 6]. The findings in 1965, as indicated in Table 1, suggest that the salt intake per person per day amounted to 23.2 g for Akita, as against 14.2 g for Osaka, i.e. the salt intake by residents in Akita was 1.63 times higher than in Osaka. In a 1970 survey, the salt intake per person per day was 20 g in Akita compared with 14 g in Osaka, suggesting that the values were close to those in 1965 for both areas and that there still remained a difference in the salt intake between residents of Osaka and Akita.

Table 1. Salt intake in Akita and Osaka in 1965 (g/person/day).

	Akita	Osaka
Salt	4.1	2.5
Salt from miso (bean paste)	5.9	0.9
Salt from soy sauce	7.5	5.8
Salt from pickles	2.6	1.9
Salt from other foods	3.2	3.1
Total salt	23.2	14.2

In the salt intake survey conducted in 1965, 30 families were selected, and the survey was continued for five days [5]. In a method of measurement on a family basis, the food intake was surveyed to compute the salt intake according to a food analysis table. At the same time, salt, 'miso' (soybean paste), soybean sauce, and other condiments were distributed to each family beforehand, and the quantity of each condiment was measured both at the beginning and at the end of the survey in order to measure the quantity used. The total salt intake was computed from the quantities of food and condiments consumed. The 1970 survey was carried out for three consecutive days on 10–15 males, 40–59 years old, sampled at random in both areas [6]. The survey was designed to measure each individual's intake of all food (including condiments).

2. COMPARISON OF SALT CONSUMPTION BETWEEN AKITA AND OSAKA IN THE PAST

The 1935–37 period, which was not affected by war or any other turbulence and in which the people's dietary life remained stable, was selected for a comparison [5]. For those years we were unable to secure reliable data on the salt intake, and the available data on the two areas have been used to compute the salt consumption, but not the salt intake. Therefore, whatever value was gained from these data could not be checked against the recent data.

The salt consumption in the 1935–37 period, as indicated in Table 2, was 34.0 g in Akita and 25.3 g in Osaka per person per day, suggesting that the salt consumption by residents in Akita was 1.4 times greater than in Osaka. One set of data used here was from the Ministry of Agriculture and Forestry, which surveyed tens of farm households in Akita and Osaka prefectures. Based on the housekeeping account books of the farm households, these data covered the quantities of rice, meat, fish, vegetables, miso, soybean sauce, and other necessities produced or purchased by these families in a year. The other set consists of data on farm families that have lived for generations in an area of Akita prefecture where epidemiological surveys are often conducted. This set includes elaborate data on what measures were prepared, how much money was spent for the food, what quantity of side foods was consumed, how much rice was produced by them, what quantities of rice and miso were purchased, etc., per year.

Table 2. Salt consumption in Akita and Osaka in 1935–37 (g/person/day).

	Akita	Osaka
Salt	32.8	18.1
Salt from miso (bean paste)	0.4	0.2
Salt from soy sauce	0.8	7.0
Total salt	34.0	25.3

On the basis of these two sets of data, an attempt was made to estimate the quantity of salt consumed per person per day in those years. By referring not only to the findings of surveys at present but also to variety of records and data in the past, it has been demonstrated that there is still as noticeable a difference in the salt intake between the Akita and Osaka prefectures, where there is an extremely big difference in the prevalence of hypertension, as in the past. In studying the relationship between chronic diseases, such as hypertension, and the dietary pattern, a survey on the prevailing dietary pattern alone would be of little significance now as distortions during a long span of time, such as 10, 20, and 30 years, are responsible for the onset of hypertension. This factor will of course be of increased importance for countries, such as Japan, where noticeable changes in the dietary pattern occur.

3. PREVALENCE OF HYPERTENSION AND SALT INTAKE IN RESPECT
   TO EIGHT GROUPS IN JAPAN

To further elaborate on the relationship between salt and hypertension, comparison was made on a nationwide scale [7]. On the basis of a joint epidem-

398

iological study on 10,112 males, 40–49 years old, in eight groups throughout Japan, including Akita and Osaka, an attempt will be made here to elaborate on the relationship between the prevalence of hypertension and salt intake in each group. The subject groups included five rural groups: Akita residents,

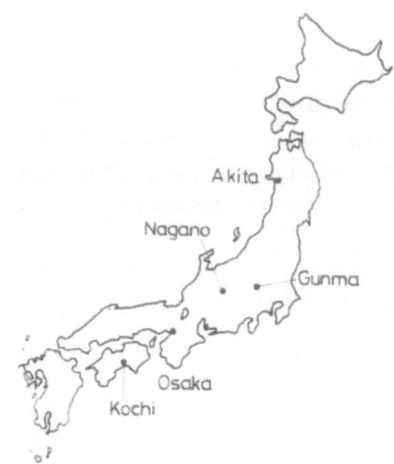

Figure 1. Study areas in the joint epidemiological survey.

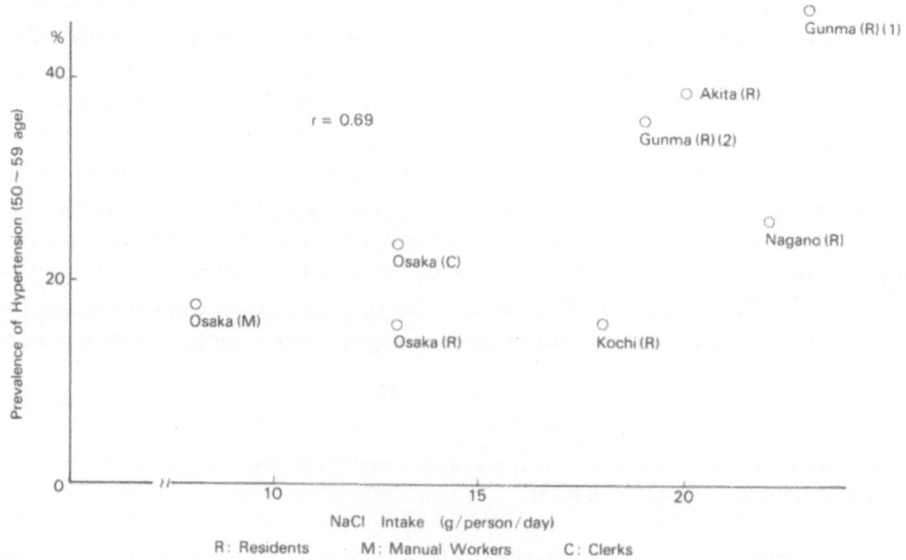

Figure 2. Prevalence rate of hypertension plotted against NaCl intake.

Nagano residents, two groups of Gunma residents[1, 2], and Kochi residents; and three urban groups: Osaka residents, Osaka clerks and company executives, and Osaka manual workers (Fig. 1).

The relationship between the prevalence of hypertension and the salt intake per person per day, as indicated in Figure 2, proves positive when all groups are compared with one another. With respect to salt intake, total salt intake was measured for three consecutive days in 10–15 males, 40–59 years old, sampled at random from each group. The close relationship between hypertension and salt, which will often be suggested as the result of a study on mortality statistics and existing data gained from surveys on dietary patterns in the past, has also been demonstrated as the result of an epidemiological survey on general residents.

As indicated in Figure 2, the salt intake is high and the prevalence of hypertension is also high among residents of Eastern Japan, such as Akita, Nagano, and Gunma prefectures, where Japan's traditional life styles persist.

Here, an attempt will be made to elaborate on the background of excessive salt intake in rural communities on the basis of surveys on the dietary practices of Akita residents for many years. In the rural communities in the past, salt was indispensable for the preservation of food in preparation for the coming winter season during which traffic would be disrupted. Also in the rural communities in the past, where farm mechanization was almost non-existent, housewives were quite busy with housekeeping and farm work. For this reason, 'miso' soups and pickles, the preparation of which did not require much time and which matched rice, the staple food, were excessively consumed. Given these factors, the excessive salt intake in the past might be described as an inevitable outcome.

In recent years, such environmental factors have been considerably eliminated as the distribution system, means of transport in the winter season, preservation of food, and economic standards of farm households have been improved in addition to enhanced farm mechanization. The traditional dietary practices, which have permeated Japanese society for many years, persist, presumably driving rural people to greater salt intakes than urban people.

Incidentally, it should be noted that the relationship thus far elaborated between salt and hypertension can be observed only between groups, but that no significant difference has been observed between individuals in a given group as the result of a study on the relationship between salt and hypertension. The inclination toward salty food spreads practically throughout this district. Between individuals in a group, there is a far more noticeable difference with respect to some competing factors other than salt, and we would think that salt intake in this situation does not appear to be a risk factor for the onset of hypertension.

REFERENCES

1. Dahl LK: Possible role of chronic excess salt consumption in the pathogenesis of essential hypertension. Am J Cardiol 8:571-575, 1961.
2. Kojima S: Distinctive features of cerebral apoplexy as seen around the Akita district (in Japanese). Jpn J Public Health 13:907-924, 1966.
3. Sasaki N: High blood pressure and the salt intake of the Japanese. Jpn Heart J 3:313-324, 1962.
4. Aoki K, et al.: Effects of high or low sodium intake in spontaneously hypertensive rats. Jpn Circ J 36:539-545, 1972.
5. Ozawa H: Geographic variation on mortality of cerebrovascular diseases and dietary life in the past (in Japanese). Jpn J Public Health 15:551-566, 1968.
6. Komachi Y, et al.: Geographic and occupational comparisons of risk factors in cardiovascular diseases in Japan. Jpn Circ J 35:189-207, 1971.
7. Shigiya R, Kimura N, Komachi Y, Isomura K, Kojima S, Watanabe T: Nutritional status of Japanese with special reference to epidemiology of cerebrovascular accident (CVA) and coronary heart disease (CHD). In: Asahina K, Shigiya R (eds) Physiological adaptability and nutritional status of the Japanese. Tokyo: University of Tokyo Press, 1975, pp 123-165.

25. BLOOD PRESSURE OF QASH'QAI PASTORAL NOMADS IN IRAN IN RELATION TO CULTURE, DIET, AND BODY FORM

L.B. PAGE, D. VANDEVERT, K. NADER, N. LUBIN, and J.R. PAGE

Population studies have disclosed a general tendency for blood pressure to rise with age in many parts of the world. The prevalence of hypertension varies among different racial and ethnic groups, but no race has been found to be genetically resistant to its development. Contrary to the general trend, over 20 isolated populations have been described that are virtually free of hypertension and show no age-related upward trend in blood pressure. These 'low blood pressure populations' represent many different races, climates, diets, habitats, and modes of life [1, 2]. Despite wide diversity, they share several common features: all adhere to traditional modes of life different from those of the dominant Western culture, and all are physically active peoples who show little or no tendency to gain weight as they age. When low blood pressure populations become acculturated or modernized by adopting the ways of Western civilization, they promptly develop an age-related upward trend in blood pressure [1, 3], thus demonstrating that they are not genetically protected from hypertension.

Several environmental influences have been suspected of playing an important role in bringing about rising blood pressure and other biologic changes in acculturating populations. Among them are dietary changes, especially in intake of sodium and potassium [2, 4, 5], the psychosocial stresses imposed by modern industrial life [6, 7], and the effects of acculturation on body weight, activity, and biologic fitness [2, 7, 8].

The relative importance of these and other potential determinants of blood pressure may be assessed by cross-comparing traditional cultures that remain relatively uninfluenced by the forces of Western civilization, but differ in habitual diets, habitats, and modes of life. The study reported here examined a population sample of traditional Nomadic herdsmen of the Qash'qai tribe in Southern Iran.

1. ETHNOLOGIC DESCRIPTION OF POPULATION

The Qash'qai are a large tribal confederation located in the province of Fars in Southern Iran (see map, Fig. 1). Of Turkish origin, they have been in this area

H. Kesteloot, J.V. Joossens (eds.), Epidemiology of Arterial Blood Pressure, 401–420.

402

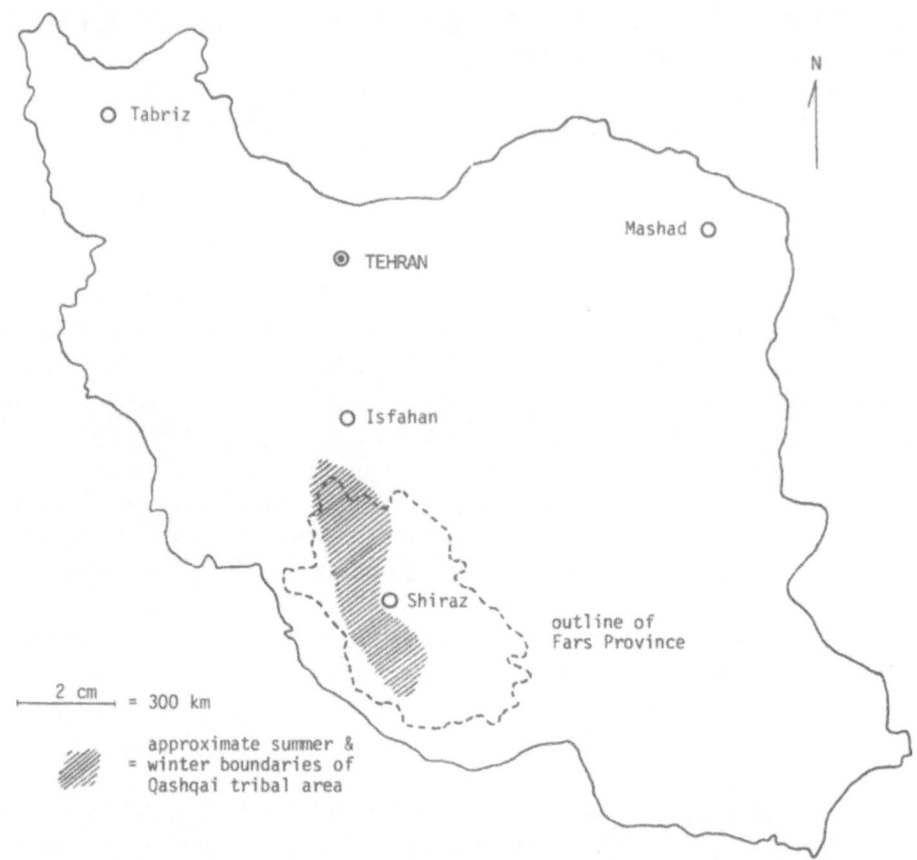

Figure 1. Outline map of Iran and of Fars Province. Shaded area shows approximate area traditionally occupied by the Qash'qai tribe of Normardic herdsmen.

for approximately 400 years. Estimates of population size vary considerably, ranging from 100,000 to 400,000 [9]; the latter figure is probably closest to being the most accurate. Many are now settled in villages and urban areas, but a large portion of the tribe continue to practice pastoral nomadism, herding goats and sheep over the arid and semiarid mountain ranges and plateaus of Southern Iran. Although other ethnically distinct tribes such as the Khamseh confederacy of Arabs, Lurs, mountain tribes (*Kohi*), and Bohri Ahmad bound the area, the Qash'qai were traditionally, economically and politically, a controlling force in major portions of the province.

Like other pastoral nomads of the Iranian plateau, the Qash'qai migrate semiannually to summer (*sarhad*) and winter (*garmsir*) areas, primarily as a response to the needs of their animals for pasture and water, and as a physiological adaptation of their animals to a relatively limited range of temperatures. Lengths of migrations vary considerably, from 40 or 50 km to

600 km [10]. Their social organization is based on patrilineal descent groups, with major lineages (*tiefeh*) being further divided into hundreds of clans (*tiereh*). The *tiefeh* is generally an endogamous group, although formerly alliances were often established by marriages between children of *khans* and tribal elites of differing *tiefehs*.

2. POPULATION SAMPLE

During October and November of 1976, six fall/winter campsites were surveyed and chosen on the basis of an adequate number of households within a

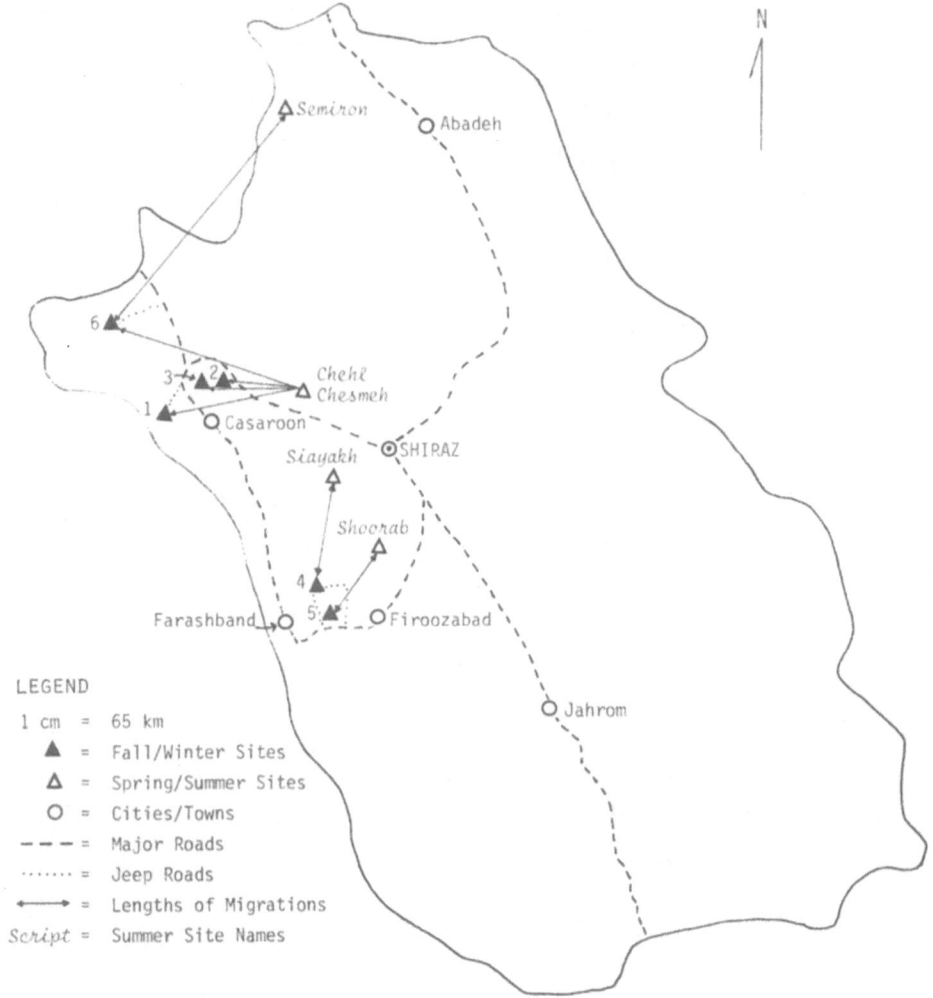

Figure 2. Outline map of Fars Province showing sites of winter campsites studied (1–6). Location of summer campsites from which migration had recently been completed are indicated (see text).

Table 1. Qash'qai: subjects and study sites (winter campsites).

Site	No. males	No. females	Total	Permanent bldgs	Health center	School	Seasonal wage labor	Markets accessible	Summer campsite
1	23	19	42	+	+	+	+		Chehl Chesmeh
2	9	14	23			+			Semiron
3	20	17	37				+		Chehl Chesmeh
4	8	10	18					+	Siayakh
5	50	44	94			+			Shoorab
6	22	28	50	+	+	+		+	Semiron Chehl Chesmeh
Totals	132	132	264	2	2	4	2	2	

2–4 km² area for the 2- to 4-day survey of each site. In each tent household were 1–4 adults over the age of 14. While most agreed to participate in the survey, a few of the older women refused. Free medical checks and distribution of drugs were offered to all camp residents, which enhanced cooperation with the medical survey team. Figure 2 shows locations of the spring/summer and fall/winter camp areas for the six sites. Table 1 shows numbers of subjects in each of the survey sites, presence or absence of factors tending to enhance 'acculturation' or external culture contact (discussed below), and the summer campsites from which they had recently migrated.

3. METHODS AND PROCEDURES

An interview was conducted with each subject in the local (Turkic) dialect. Information obtained included demographic data, 24-h diet recall, and length and circumstances of any exposure to nonpastoral living. A portion of the interview dealing with the time placement of important life events and data from other family members were used to verify biologic age. Age distribution for the 264 subjects is shown in Figure 3.

Interviews were separately conducted with women concerning cooking practices. Cooks were asked to prepare proportionate samples of ingredients for preparation of bread and rice, and these ingredients were retained and weighed.

All subjects were instructed in the collection of overnight urine samples. These were collected and measured, and 20-ml aliquots were preserved in the field by addition of 5 drops of pure formaldehyde. The samples were subsequently frozen until analysis several weeks later.

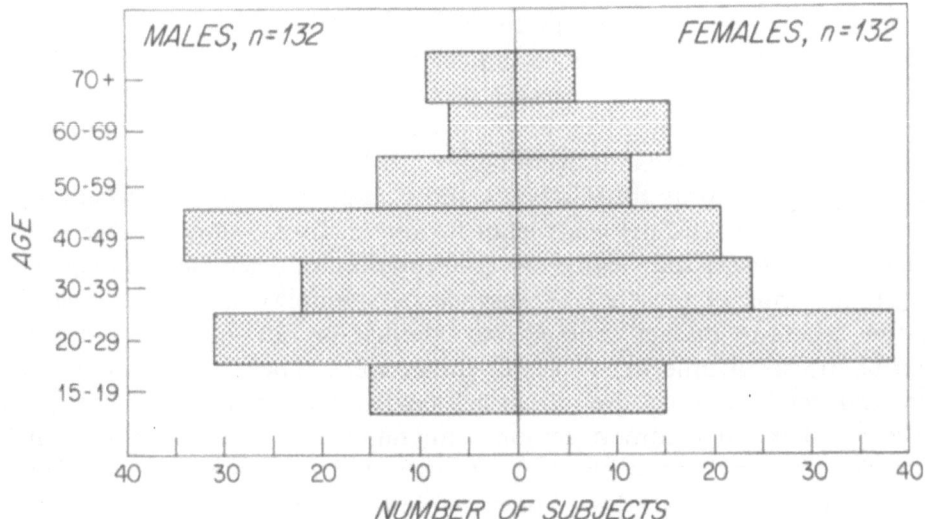

Figure 3. Age and sex distribution of population sample by deciles of age.

Height, weight, and triceps skinfolds were determined. In males, weights were obtained with subjects lightly clothed. Women were weighed fully clothed. Since traditional Qash'qai women wear from two to nine skirts one over the other, it was necessary to correct for this. An average weight for skirts was determined and a correction factor based on number of skirts was subtracted.

Two independent determinations of blood pressure and pulse were recorded by a single observer, using a mercury manometer, with the subject seated comfortably in a chair.

4. ACCULTURATING FACTORS

Contrary to popular beliefs, pastoral nomads throughout history have never been cultural isolates. There have most likely been important pastoral-sedentary interrelationships, especially in the exchange of goods and services since their coevolution [11–14]. These interrelationships have been characterized by various authors as 'symbiotic'[15], 'polar opposites'[16], 'polar complementaries'[17], 'reciprocally dependent'[18], and 'encapsulated'[19] to various degrees. Gellner[15] notes that 'The history of the Islamic Middle East can, from its very beginnings, be written to a large extent in terms of the interaction between the nomads and the sedentary and urban populations'. Nomads have depended either directly or indirectly upon the products of agriculturalists (especially grains) and upon urban dwellers for such items as cloth, jewelry, tea, sugar, and other materials and services; while agriculturalists and urban dwellers have been dependent upon nomads as a major source of their meat supply, milk, and wool products [20–22].

In 1976, with the processes of industrialization extending to and reaching many rural residents of Iran, varying degrees of modernization were occurring throughout the country. The primary changes affecting the nomads were access to public vehicular transportation and improved access roads, certain public services such as tribal schools and occasional rural health clinics, and the availability of seasonal wage labor for males. In addition to these external sources of change, the degree of acculturation of each site surveyed was judged in terms of presence or absence of stationary fall/winter dwellings, relative access to market centers, and whether or not individuals had more than briefly spent time in villages or urban areas. These factors of acculturation and modernization are discussed below. However, all of the groups surveyed share in common seasonal migrations, a total or at least major dependency upon their flocks of goats and sheep for economic subsistance, and a basic nomadic 'ideology,' or belief and committment to the advantages of pastoral life.

4.1. Employment. Traditionally, wage labor was seldom pursued as a source of income. Only those tribesmen whose herd size fell below a certain minimum for household subsistance chose this demeaning alternative [23]. Of the six groups surveyed, two had males who were engaged in outside wage labor: At site 1, a majority of the males worked on construction of the Cazaroon-Bushire road, or on a water pipeline being built from the area southward. A few were also involved in local agricultural work. At site 3, a few men were employed in nearby agriculture, or in small industries in the town of Cazaroon. At the other sites, there were no nearby sources of outside labor, seasonal or otherwise, with the exception of the tribal teachers.

4.2. Permanent dwellings. At site 1, small one-room adobe houses were either built or in the process of being built by each household. Generally, the black tent adjoined the house; the latter was used primarily for storage and comfort during times of excess winter cold and rain. At site 6, approximately one-half of the households had permanent dwellings, and at site 2, a few permanent houses were being constructed. At the other sites, no form of permanent dwellings were present, and short movements of camp location occur periodically during the fall and winter months.

4.3. Public services. Tribal schools were present at all sites except 3 and 4. The teachers are Qash'qai, often from the same camping group to whom they teach, and they migrate along with the tribes. Classes through the fifth grade are offered. Upon completion, the students could continue their education in urban schools or in the Tribal Teacher-Training school in Shiraz. Only at sites 1 and 6 were there rural health clinics, staffed by often-absent Health Corps physicians.

4.4. Relative isolation. Only at sites 4 and 6 was access to markets, towns, and urban areas difficult, and diets reflected this isolation. For example, at these two sites, almost 50% of the tribesmen ate bread alone for at least one meal; and consumption of only bread for the remaining two or three meals occurred more than at the other sites. At the other sites, trips into local towns could easily be made in a day's journey. A tribesman making the journey usually brought back with him goods for several households, including vegetables, fruits, and miscellaneous items such as batteries for radios and tape recorders, kerosene for lamps, and occasional heaters.

4.5. Experiences of nonnomadic living. Of the total sample, 16 males had lived in cities or towns for periods ranging from six months to five years. The majoritiy of these residences were for military service, in such cities as Tehran, Kermanshah, Isfahan, and Shiraz. Four of five females who had experienced urban living stayed in Shiraz from three months to one year, primarily because of pregnancy complications. One female had lived in Shahreza for three years. Six males had spent from six months to three years in villages, and three females, one, two, and seven years.

The villages resided in are traditional, without electricity or any 'modern' conveniences. All are within the Qash'qai tribal area, inhabited by both Iranian peasants and other settled tribesmen. Cities and towns, of course, are generally quite modernized with most modern facilities available. The presence or absence of various acculturating influences discussed here are indicated in Table 1 for the six study sites.

5. DIET

5.1. 24-Hour diet recall. Diet among the pastoral nomads probably varies seasonally to some degree. The survey was conducted in the fall, soon after migration to winter campsites had been completed. Milk production by the herds diminishes during migration and remains low for a period afterward. This limits the variety, and to some degree, the quantity of foodstuffs available. Milk products, in particular, are limited at this time of year. Thus the

Table 2. Number and percent consuming certain classes of foods* in each of six campsites based on 24-h recall.

Food	Site No.						Totals 264
	1 $n = 42$	2 $n = 23$	3 $n = 37$	4 $n = 18$	5 $n = 94$	6 $n = 50$	
Bread	42 (100%)	23 (100%)	37 (100%)	18 (100%)	94 (100%)	50 (100%)	264 (100%)
Rice	25 (59.5%)	15 (65.2%)	18 (48.6%)	9 (50%)	54 (55.1%)	19 (38%)	140 (52.2%)
Meat	11 (26.2%)	3 (13%)	8 (21.6%)	3 (16.7%)	33 (33.7%)	18 (36%)	76 (28.3%)
Milk and milk products	10 (23.8%)	4 (17.4%)	5 (13.5%)	1 (5.6%)	9 (9.2%)	19 (38%)	48 (17.9%)
Fruit	14 (33.3%)	1 (4.3%)	11 (29.7%)	2 (11.1%)	3 (3.1%)	—	31 (11.6%)
Eggs	9 (21.4%)	5 (21.7%)	9 (24.3%)	4 (22.2%)	15 (15.3%)	5 (10%)	47 (17.5%)
Vegetables	16 (38.1%)	10 (43.5%)	23 (62.2%)	7 (38.9%)	36 (36.7%)	8 (16%)	100 (37.3%)

* Very sweet tea is consumed at every meal and often alone. Also miscellaneous foods *occasionally* are consumed (e.g., nuts, jams, honey, wild greens), but have not been included here.

data obtained during the survey cannot be confidently accepted as representative for all periods of the year. The 24-h diet recall shows a correlation between access to markets and agricultural areas and the variety of foods reported in the interview (Table 2). Sites 4 and 6 were the most isolated from sources of fruits and vegetables, and this is reflected in the results of the survey.

For all groups, the most important dietary staple is the very thin flat bread (*tannook* in Persian *cherak* in Turkish) baked daily and consumed at every meal. Fourteen samples of the usual quantity of salt added to a certain quantity of flour were obtained. The results indicated that an average of 2.01% salt by weight is added to the flour, with a range of 0.84% to 3.28%. This bread is most likely the major source of salt in the diet. Rice is also of importance in the Nomads' diet, being eaten at one meal 2–4 times per week, depending on the relative wealth of the household. It is likely the second largest source of salt intake of their diet. Nine samples of the usual quantity of salt added to the water of a certain amount of cooking rice were collected. The samples ranged from 1.25% to 3.58% by weight, with a mean of 2.3%. However, the actual amount consumed via the cooked rice is difficult to determine by the interview technique, as a small portion of the salted water is emptied off during the process of cooking.

Table 3. Number and percent consuming certain classes of food: 24-h recall in total population sample (*n* = 264).

Food	No.	%
Bread	264	100
Rice	140	52.2
Vegetables	100	37.3
Meat	76	28.3
Milk and milk products	48	17.9
Eggs	47	17.5
Fruit	31	11.6

Table 4. 24-Hour recall of bread, rice, and meat consumption for three meals.

	Total No.	Percent
Bread*	264	100.0
Rice*	140	52.2
Meat*	76	28.3
Bread only		
1 meal	127	47.4
2 meals	57	21.3
3 meals	18	6.7

* Consumed during at least one meal of the recall period.

Bread was eaten at every meal by all persons surveyed. It was supplemented in varying degrees by other foods (Table 3). Bread alone often comprises the entire diet for one, two, or even three meals (Table 4).

5.2. Nutrient analysis of food samples. Analysis of four samples of bread and two samples of cooked rice (performed by H.V. Shuster Co., Inc., Boston, Massachusetts) are recorded in Table 5. Values for the various constituents vary so widely that no generalizations can be made. Variations in concentration of constituents appear primarily to reflect variation in moisture content, although correction for this variable still leaves a large sample to sample variation in several constituents.

Table 5. Food analysis of prepared bread and rice.

Sample No:	Bread				Rice	
	1	2	3	4	5	6
Moisture, % by weight	75.13	68.84	25.04	29.96	63.62	63.87
Fat, % by weight	0.90	1.29	2.74	2.52	3.68	2.99
Protein, % by weight	2.39	3.34	7.26	7.54	3.38	3.88
Ash, % by weight	1.06	1.41	8.32	2.78	2.79	0.55
Crude fiber, % by weight	0.8	1.1	2.1	1.9	0.3	0.7
Carbohydrate, % by weight	19.72	24.02	54.54	55.30	26.23	28.01
Calories/100 g	97	121	272	274	152	154
Calcium, mg/100 g	47.4	58.4	143	97.9	13.5	10.5
Sodium, mg/100 g	176	299	2570	632	329	217
Potassium, mg/100 g	115	118	317	231	17.2	27.5

A high content of phylate in bread samples from rural Iran has been found by Haghshenass et al. [24]. Binding of dietary iron by phylate may result in a high prevalence of iron deficiency anemia in this population.

5.3. Sodium and potassium content of staple foods. Ten samples of bread from several different study sites were ashed, and sodium and potassium content determined by atomic absorption spectrophotometry (H.V. Shuster, inc., Boston). Results of these analyses are shown in Table 6. The variability in electrolyte content is too wide to allow generalization, but parallel variability of moisture content is apparent in these samples, and a high sodium–potassium ratio is usually present. For comparison, sodium content of commercial breads in the United States averages approximately 550 mg/100 g and potassium 115 mg/100 g [36].

Salt is used liberally by the nomads, both in cooking and at the table. It is readily available to them from commercial sources, and also from natural

Table 6. Sodium and potassium content of bread samples.

No.	Site	Sodium		Potassium		Water	
		mg/100 g	meq/100 g	mg/100 g	meq/100 g	Na/K	Content %
1	6	176	7.65	115	2.88	2.66	75.1
2	1	299	13.0	118	2.95	4.41	68.8
3	3	2570	111.7	317	7.9	14.1	25.0
4	3	632	27.5	231	5.8	4.74	30.0
5	3	258	11.2	139	3.5	3.2	—
6	3	399	17.3	221	5.5	3.2	—
7	6	944	41.0	365	9.1	4.5	—
8	6	492	21.4	306	7.7	2.8	—
9	6	821	35.7	264	6.6	5.4	—
10	3	96	4.2	358	8.95	0.47	—
Means		669	29.1	243	6.1	4.55	49.7

deposits that occur throughout the tribal area. Salt is added in the preparation of cheese, and dried milk cake (*Kashk*). It is used liberally in cooking of meats. At the table, additional salt is often added to most foods, including bread. While drinking-water supplies are usually low in sodium, salty-water supplies are recognized by the people and are sometimes used for drinking during periods of travel. Two of these were sampled, and contained 50 and 80 meq/l of sodium.

6. URINARY EXCRETION OF SODIUM AND POTASSIUM

A total of 248 timed overnight urine samples were obtained and analyzed for sodium, potassium, and creatinine. The ratio of creatinine excretion to body weight was calculated and samples were rejected if this was more than 3 SD from the mean for sex. Samples were also rejected if urine volume was less than 16 ml/h.

Mean 24-h excretion of sodium and potassium was extrapolated for men and women from the 228 samples that met the criteria for inclusion. Results are given in Table 7. Several recent studies have shown that overnight urine

Table 7. 24-Hour sodium and potassium excretion extrapolated from timed overnight urine samples.

	n	Na	K	Na/K	Creatinine (mg)/24 h
					Body Wt (kg)
Males	118	186.46 ± 105.9	56.36 ± 32.51	3.62 ± 1.7	32.6 ± 14.1
Females	110	141.28 ± 73.0	49.54 ± 26.05	3.24 ± 1.5	28.3 ± 11.7

412

sodium excretion correlates well with 24-hour excretion [25–27]. The overnight and 24-h electrolyte excretion are not linearly related, since the overnight samples tend to somewhat underestimate 24-h excretion [25]. The extrapolated values used here may therefore be somewhat below the true value for 24-h excretion. The difference in excretion rate for sodium between men and women (ratio 1.32) is highly significant ($P < 0.001$). A higher sodium excretion in males than in females has been found in other populations [35]. In the Qash'qai no correlation was found between sodium excretion and measures of body size. The magnitude of this difference is unexplained and is presumed to be culturally determined. Urinary Na/K ratios are moderately high for both sexes in comparison with other populations [37].

7. BLOOD PRESSURE

Unlike traditional populations in several parts of the world, systolic, diastolic, and mean blood pressure increase significantly with age both in males and in

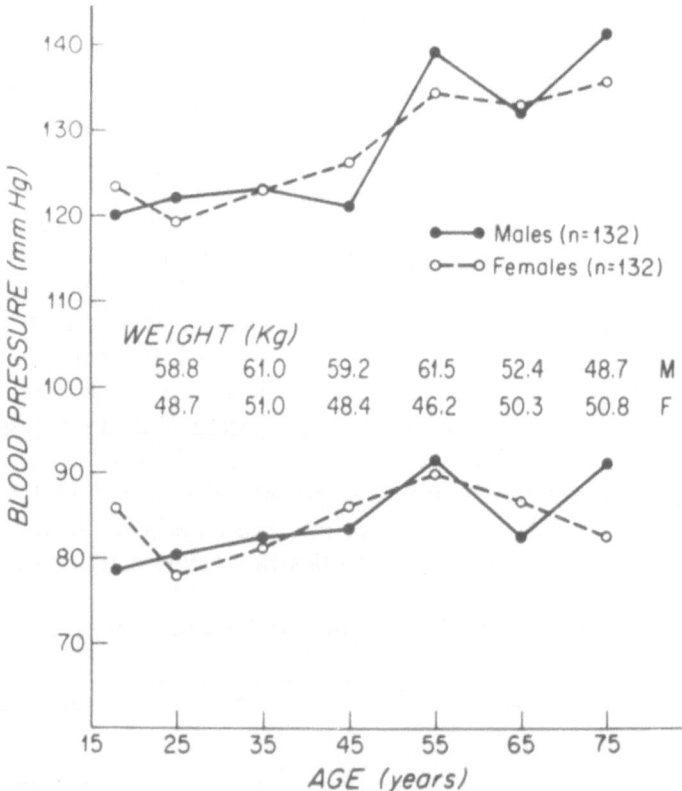

Figure 4. Mean values for systolic and diastolic blood pressure and body weight by deciles of age.

Table 8. Qash'qai subjects exceeding certain levels of blood pressure.

Subjects	n	Systolic ≥ 140		Systolic ≥ 160		Diastolic ≥ 90		Diastolic ≥ 95		BP ≥ 140/90		BP ≥ 160/95	
		n	%	n	%	n	%	n	%	n	%	n	%
Subjects aged 15 years and over													
Males	132	24	18	6	4.5	23	17	12	9.1	13	10	6	4.5
Females	132	23	17	6	4.5	30	23	19	14.3	15	11	6	4.5
Subjects aged 30 years and over													
Males	86	19	22	6	7.0	17	20	9	10.5	10	12	6	7.0
Females	79	19	24	6	8.0	23	29	16	20.3	14	18	6	8.0

Table 9. Qash'qai nomads: mean blood pressure by deciles of age.

Age (years)	Males		Females	
	n	Mean and SD	*n*	Mean and SD
15–19	15	92.5 ± 10.3	15	98.3 ± 9.0
20–29	31	94.4 ± 9.3	38	91.8 ± 7.8
30–39	22	96.1 ± 8.1	24	95.0 ± 12.9
40–49	14	107.1 ± 15.0	12	104.6 ± 15.0
60–69	7	98.8 ± 17.7	16	102.1 ± 19.0
70 +	9	107.6 ± 21.6	6	100.4 ± 17.9
Totals	132	97.3 ± 12.1	132	97.1 ± 12.9

females in the Qash'qai. The frequency of hypertension in this population, using various cutoff points, is shown in Table 8. Calculated average values for mean blood pressure are given in Table 9. Regression coefficients of blood pressure on weight, ponderal index, and electrolyte excretion are given in Table 10. Age-related changes in systolic and diastolic blood pressure and body weight are shown in Figure 4 by deciles of age. Although blood pressure is correlated with body weight in males in this population, there is no

Table 10. Coefficients of correlation for blood pressure, body form, and electrolyte excretion, all adults, aged 15 years and over ($n = 264$) (M = 132; F = 132).

	Males	Females
Age and weight	−0.07	0.11
Age and ponderal index	0.06	−0.07
Age and systolic pressure	0.31[b]	0.31[b]
Age and diastolic pressure	0.29[b]	0.21[a]
Age and mean blood pressure	0.32[b]	0.26[b]
Weight and systolic pressure	0.22[b]	0.10
Weight and diastolic pressure	0.13	0.06
Weight and mean blood pressure	0.19[a]	0.08
Ponderal index and systolic pressure	−0.31[b]	−0.03
Ponderal index and diastolic pressure	−0.18[a]	−0.02
Ponderal index and mean blood pressure	−0.26[b]	−0.03
Partial correlation coefficients controlling for age and ponderal index		
Systolic pressure and Na excretion	0.27[b]	0.08
Diastolic pressure and Na excretion	0.15	0.09
Mean blood pressure and Na excretion	0.22[a]	0.09
Systolic blood pressure and Na/K ratio	0.17	0.24[a]
Diastolic blood pressure and Na/K ratio	0.02	0.16
Mean blood pressure and Na/K ratio	0.10	0.21[a]
Mean blood pressure and age (controlling for weight)	0.34[b]	0.26[b]
Mean blood pressure and weight (controlling for age)	0.22[a]	0.06

[a] $P < 0.05$.
[b] $P < 0.01$.

tendency for body weight to increase with age. Furthermore, ponderal index is correlated negatively with blood pressure in males and shows no significant correlation in females. The increase of blood pressure with age therefore cannot be attributed to associated changes in body mass.

Partial correlations (Table 10) show a direct relationship of systolic and mean blood pressure with sodium excretion in males, and with Na/K ratio in females. These relationships suggest that the high sodium intake and/or Na/K ratio may be important determinants of rising blood pressure in this population.

8. DISCUSSION

Among ethnological studies of Middle Eastern nomadic herdsmen, there are few recent references to the Qash'qai Tribe. Biomedical observations, in particular, are very scanty for the Qash'qai and culturally similar societies. More extensive and prolonged observations would be required to determine the extent to which cultural change in Iran has caused new stresses in this nomadic tribal society, or has altered the traditional life patterns of its members in recent years.

In this study, an effort was made to focus observations on some segments of the tribe who appear to be adhering to traditional life values and activities. The tribal schools introduced 20 years ago are now widespread and generally accepted, but their impact on the daily life and attitudes of persons in this population sample is probably not great, since the teachers are themselves Qash'qai, and the schools have become adapted to nomadic life.

Occasional residence in villages and urban areas is not a recent phenomenon, although the cities have become more Westernized in the past few decades, and a larger percentage of both men and women have lived in them, or at least visited them periodically. Despite these temporary experiences, subjects in the study population had returned to nomadic life in the tents, bringing with them very few of the goods and habits of the cities. They frequently expressed a strong ideational preference for the nomadic life. They volunteered a strong preference for the tent and the open spaces, over the walled-in dwellings of the city. There was widespread preference for the traditional goat milk products, and use of animal fats over Westernized foods and vegetable oils. The work and activity patterns of males and females were those described as traditional in these nomadic societies [23].

A secular trend toward increasing adult height is usually seen in societies undergoing acculturation [28, 29]. No such trend was present either in males or females in the Qash'qai population.

We conclude, within the limitations of our observations, that the popula-

416

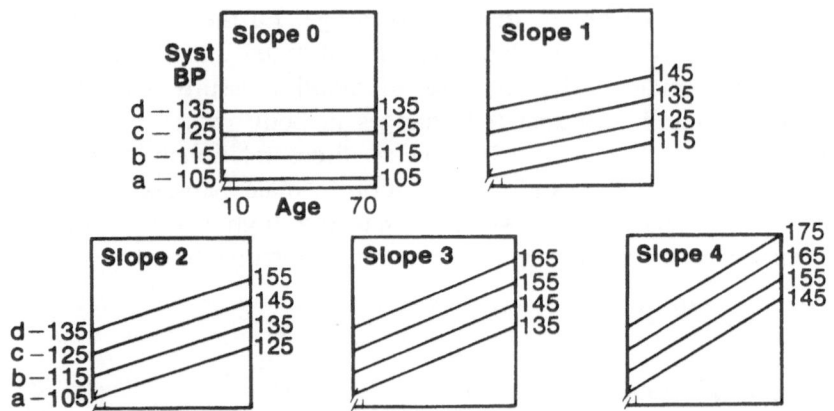

Figure 5. System for classifying age-related systolic blood pressure trends in populations by level and slope (after Epstein and Eckoff [3]).

tion sample was at a low level of acculturation, and undergoing cultural change at only a very slow pace.

In this nomadic population, systolic, diastolic, and mean blood pressures are clearly rising with age. Epstein and Eckoff have proposed a system for classifying level and slope of age-related systolic pressure change in order to compare different populations [3] (Fig. 5). By this classification, both males and females in the Qash'qai rank at slope 2 and level b. This is higher and steeper than most traditional populations, although less high and steep than many acculturated and industrial populations.

Like most traditional societies, these Qash'qai nomads are generally lean and active, showing no tendency for weight to increase with age (Fig. 4 and Table 10). Indeed, ponderal index is negatively correlated with systolic, diastolic, and mean pressure, at least in males. The relationships of blood pressure to body form in this population clearly cannot account for the age-related upward trends in blood pressure.

Based on the data obtained in this survey, these traditional Qash'qai nomads consume a large amount of salt. Urinary sodium excretion, based on overnight samples, is equal to or greater than in most European and U.S. population samples. Our data also suggest that Qash'qai men consume substantially more sodium than women. In males of this population sample, a strong correlation is seen between urinary sodium excretion and both systolic and mean blood pressure. In females, systolic pressure is correlated with Na/K ratio. These relationships, found in a 'low acculturation–high salt population' support the hypothesis that dietary intake of electrolyte, especially sodium, is a powerful determinant of blood pressure trends.

The relationship of electrolyte intake to hypertension has been, and remains, controversial. When comparisons are made *between* different populations, blood pressure trends often appear to be related to average daily sodium excretion [2, 4, 5]. On the other hand, studies *within* populations have often failed to find a significant relationship between these variables [1, 30, 31]. The absence of a clear relationship between blood pressure and electrolyte excretion among individuals has been cited as evidence against a role of sodium as an important determinant of blood pressure. On the other hand, most intrapopulation studies have been done in highly acculturated or industrial populations. Failure to find such a relationship in these populations may be due to several factors that tend to obscure the relationship. While day-to-day intake of electrolyte varies widely in modern societies, most studies have based conclusions on a single timed urine sample. Recent studies suggest that, for United States populations, as many as six [25, 32] or even 14 [26] samples are necessary to adequately assess sodium excretion. Although day-to-day variation has not been rigorously examined in traditional societies, observations suggest that diet in such societies varies very little from day to day, and processed 'snack' foods are unavailable. Thus it is likely that their urinary electrolyte excretion varies much less than in industrialized populations.

It has also been suggested that the relationship of dietary electrolyte to blood pressure in modern populations may be obscured by excessive 'noise' due to effects of other variables known to influence blood pressure [2]. These include genetic variability [33], variation in body weight and fatness [34], alcohol intake, and possibly psychosocial stress factors [6, 7].

Observations in free-living traditional societies that are largely free of these confounding variables may help to resolve this controversy. The high sodium intake of the Qash'qai, occurring in the absence of a general change in diet, age-related weight gain, or rapid acculturation, may account for rising blood pressure and hypertension in genetically susceptible members of this population. Data on this relatively small sample of pastoral nomads thus lends support to the hypothesis that electrolyte intake is an important determinant of blood pressure in free-living populations.

9. SUMMARY

A study of blood pressure, diet, urinary electrolyte excretion, and body form was conducted on 264 traditional nomadic herdsmen of the Qash'qai tribe, Fars Province, Southern Iran. The population sample included most male and female members over 14 years of age of tent households at six winter campsites. Interviews established biologic age, any experience of nonnomadic living, and 24-h dietary recall. Selected interviews recorded cooking practices. Height, weight, triceps skinfolds, and blood pressures were measured. Over-

418

night urine samples were aliquoted and analyzed for sodium, potassium, and creatinine content. Samples of dietary staples were collected and analyzed for nutrient and electrolyte content.

The main dietary staple was bread. Use of rice, meat, fruit, vegetables, and milk products varied at the different campsites. Urinary sodium excretion averaged 186 meq/24 h in males, and 141 meq/24 h in females. Urinary Na/K ratios were 3.64 and 3.24 in males and females, respectively.

Systolic, diastolic, and mean blood pressure in both males and females increased significantly with age. Blood pressure $\geqslant 140/90$ mmHg was found in 12% of males and 18% of females aged 30 years or over. Body weight showed no tendency to increase with age in either sex. Ponderal index, in males, was negatively correlated with blood pressure. Systolic and mean blood pressure correlated with urinary sodium excretion in males and with urinary Na/K ratio in females. From cultural observations, the population sample was considered traditional in orientation and at a low level of acculturation.

The data suggest that blood pressure trends in this population are related to habitual dietary intake of electrolyte intake. They support the hypothesis that sodium intake is an important determinant of blood pressure trends in free-living populations.

Acknowledgments. The authors gratefully acknowledge the encouragement and assistance of Dr. Hossain Ronaghy, former Chairman, Department of Community Medicine, Pahlavi University Medical School, and Mrs. M. Mohalati of the Department of Pathology for analysis of the urine samples.

REFERENCES

1. Page LB: Epidemiological evidence on the etiology of human hypertension and its possible prevention. Am Heart J 91:527-534, 1976.
2. Page LB: Hypertension and atherosclerosis in primitive and acculturating societies. In: Hunt JC (ed) Dialogues in hypertension. Vol 1: Hypertension update. Bloomfield NJ: Health Learning Systems, 1979.
3. Epstein FH, Eckoff RD: The epidemiology of high blood pressure — geographic distribution and etiologic factors. In: Stamler J, Stamler R, Pullman TM (eds) Epidemiology of hypertension. New York: Grune and Stratton, 1967, pp 155-1611.
4. Page LB: Salt and hypertension: epidemiology and mechanisms. In: Onesti G, Klimt C (eds) Hypertension: determinants, complications and intervention. New York: Grune and Stratton, 1979, pp 3-11.
5. Tobian L: Salt and hypertension. Ann NY Acad Med 304:178-197, 1978.
6. Henry JP, Cassel JC: Psychosocial factors in essential hypertension. Am J Epidemiol 90:171, 1969.
7. Beaglehole R, Salmond CE, Hooper A, et al.: Blood pressure and social interaction in Tokelauan migrants in New Zealand. J Chronic Dis 30:803-811, 1977.

8. Baker PT: Migration and human adaptation. In: Seminar on migration and health, Wellington, NZ, 1979 (in press).
9. Oberling P: The Qash'qai nomads of Fars. The Hague: Mouton, 1974.
10. Monteil V: Les Tribus de Fars. Paris: Mouton, 1966.
11. Spooner B: The status of nomadism as a cultural phenomenon in the Middle East. In: Irons WG, Dyson-Hudson N (eds) Perspectives on nomadism. International studies in sociology and social anthropology, Vol 12. Leiden: Brill, 1972.
12. English P: Urbanites, peasants, and nomads: the Middle Eastern ecological triology. J Geogr 66:54-59, 1967.
13. Bates D: The role of the State in peasant-nomad mutualism. Anthropol Q 44:109-131, 1971.
14. Pastner S: Ideological aspects of nomad-sedentary contact: a case from southern Baluchistan. Anthropol Q 44:172-184, 1971.
15. Gellner E. Introduction: approaches to nomadism. In: Nelson C (ed) The desert and the sown: nomads in the wider society. Inst Int Stud Univ Calif Berkeley Res Ser 21:1-9, 1973.
16. Lewis I: Nomadism: an anthropological view. FAO Conference Paper, Cairo, 1971.
17. Mohammed A: The nomadic and the sedentary: polar complementaries — not polar opposites. In: Nelson C (ed) The desert and the sown: nomads in the wider society. Inst Int Stud Univ Calif Berkeley Res Ser 21:97-112, 1973.
18. Gulick G: The Middle East: an anthropological perspective. Pacific Palisades: Goodyear, 1976.
19. Fazel G: The encapsulation of nomadic societies in Iran. In: Nelson C. Ref 15, 129-142.
20. Spooner B: The cultural ecology of pastoral nomads. Addison-Wesley, pp 129-142.
21. Swidler W: Adaptive processes regulating nomad-sedentary interaction in the Middle East. In: Nelson C (ed) The desert and the sown: nomads in the wider society. Inst Int Stud Univ Calif Berkeley Res Ser 21, 1973.
22. Stouffer T: The economics of nomadism in Iran. Middle East J 19:284-302, 1965.
23. Barth F: Nomads of South Persia. Boston: Little, Brown and Co, 1961.
24. Haghshenass M, Mahloudji M, Reinhold JG, Mohammadi N: Iron deficiency anemia in an Iranian population associated with high intakes of iron. Am J Clin Nutr 25:1143-1146, 1972.
25. Watson RL, Langford HG: Usefulness of overnight urines in population groups. Am J Clin Nutr 23:290-304, 1970.
26. Liu K, Dyer AR, Cooper RS, Stamler R, Stamler J: Can overnight urines replace 24-hour urine collection to assess salt intake? Hypertension 1:529-536, 1979.
27. Pietinen PE, Wong O, Altshul AM: Electrolyte output, blood pressure, and family history of hypertension. Am J Clin Nutr 32:997-1005, 1979.
28. Tobias PV: On the increasing stature of the Bushman. Anthropos 57:801, 1962.
29. Page LB, Damon A, Moellering Jr RC: Antecedents of cardiovascular disease in six Solomon Islands societies. Circulation 43:1132-1146, 1974.
30. Dawber TR, Kannel WB, Kagan A, Donabedian RK, McNamara PM, Pearson G: Environmental factors in hypertension. In: Stamler J, Stamler R, Pullman TN (eds) The epidemiology of hypertension. New York: Grune and Stratton, 1967, p 255.

31. Swaye PS, Gifford Jr RW, Berritoni JN: Dietary salt and essential hypertension. Am J Cardiol 29:53, 1972.
32. Liu K, Cooper P, Soltero I, Stamler J: Variability in 24-hour urine in children. Hypertension 1:631-636, 1980.
33. Feinlieb M: Genetics and familial aggregation of blood pressure. In: Onesti G, Klimt CR (eds) Hypertension: determinants, complications, and intervention. New York: Grune and Stratton, 1979, pp 35-48.
34. Chiang BN, Perlman LV, Epstein FH: Overweight and hypertension — a review. Circulation 30:403-421, 1969.
35. Kesteloot H, Song CS, Park BC, Brems-Heyns E, Joossens JV: An epidemiological survey of arterial blood pressure in a Korean population using home reading. In: Rorive G, Van Cauwenberge H (eds) The Arterial hypertensive disease. New York: Mossen, 1976, pp 141-148.
36. Agriculture Handbook 456: Nutritive value of American foods. Washington DC: US Department of Agriculture, US Government Printing Office, 1975.
37. Langford HG, Watson RL: Electrolytes and hypertension. In: Paul O (ed) Epidemiology and control of hypertension. New York: Stratton Intercontinental Medical, 1975, pp 119-130.

PART SEVEN

INTERNATIONAL COMPARATIVE STUDIES

26. THE NI-HON-SAN STUDY OF CARDIOVASCULAR DISEASE EPIDEMIOLOGY

Population characteristics and epidemiology of stroke

A. KAGAN, M.G. MARMOT, and H. KATO

International data show marked geographic variability in mortality from coronary heart disease (CHD)[1]. Mortality in the United States is among the highest and that in Japan is among the lowest reported. The determination of reasons for these marked differences is made difficult by confounding genetic, environmental, and cultural variation and by the differences in diagnostic techniques and reporting practices used in various countries. One of the methods that has been found useful in overcoming some of these difficulties is the study of migrant populations[2]. Large numbers of Japanese migrated to Hawaii and California late in the 19th century and early in the 20th century. Gordon reported a gradient of CHD mortality with men of Japanese ancestry living in the United States experiencing risks that were intermediate between the low levels in Japan and the high levels among Caucasian Americans[3, 4]. Gordon also demonstrated a gradient of increasing CHD mortality among Japanese men in Japan, Hawaii, and California. The gradient of mortality from cerebrovascular disease was the reverse.

Ni-Hon-San is an acronym for Nippon-Honolulu-San Francisco (in Japanese, Ni-Hon-San may be freely translated as 'the Japanese three').

The Ni-Hon-San study was established to document the status of the three populations with regard to a variety of factors including demographic characteristics, diet, exercise habit, cigarette smoking, physical findings, serum biochemical variables and the like, to confirm the reported mortality statistics, to attempt to validate these mortality gradients by prevalence and incidence determinations, and to eliminate insofar as possible those methodological problems that made interpretation of published mortality data difficult. This was to be accomplished by using standardized methods for collecting the data in ethnically similar cohorts living in diverse environmental and cultural conditions[5].

1. STUDY POPULATIONS

In Japan, the study cohort was selected from the group under observation by the Atomic Bomb Casualty Commission (now renamed the Radiation Effects

H. Kesteloot, J.V. Joossens (eds.), Epidemiology of Arterial Blood Pressure, 423–436.

Research Foundation) located in Hiroshima and Nagasaki. This is a free-living population made up of exposed and nonexposed subjects. Observations have not revealed an effect of atomic radiation on cardiovascular disease [6]. The data are based on an examination of the men in the Adult Health Study population who have been receiving general biennial examinations since 1958 [7]. Special forms designed for the Ni-Hon-San Study have been included in cycles of these periodic examinations since 1965 for the men aged 40–69 years at that examination. For the purposes of Ni-Hon-San comparisons, the cohort was limited to men aged 45–69 years at the time of examination.

The study cohort in Honolulu consisted of all men of Japanese ancestry born in the years 1900–1919 and resident on Oahu in 1964. They were identified through World War II Selective Service records and located through searches of telephone, business, and state agency records [8].

The target population in California was all the male Issei (born in Japan) and male Nisei (born of Issei parents in the United States), aged 40–69 years and residing in eight San Francisco Bay counties. For purposes of the Ni-Hon-San comparisons, the cohort was limited to those men aged 45–69 years at the time of examination. Details of the identification procedures and sampling techniques for California have been documented [5].

2. METHODS

Self-administered questionnaires were filled out by each subject to provide basic demographic, socio-economic, health, and dietary information at the time of examination. Family, social, and past medical histories were obtained in California by self-administered questionnaires filled out under supervision, and in Japan and Honolulu from a structured interview carried out by a nurse. Height and weight were measured while the subjects were without shoes; skinfold thickness was measured over the left triceps and left subscapular areas by means of constant-tension skin calipers. Blood pressure was measured by a nurse using a mercury manometer attached to a standard-sized cuff applied to the left arm of the seated subject. Diastolic blood pressure was recorded at the 5th Korotkoff phase (disappearance of sound). Standard 12-lead electrocardiograms were recorded by using Sanborn Electrocardiographs at a paper speed of 25 mm/s.

Each man's diet was evaluated by a dietitian using the 24-h recall method on all the men in Japan and Hawaii and on a sample of the men in California. Food models, photographs, and serving utensils were used to determine portion size. A common food grouping system was used to estimate nutrient composition, and standard food composition tables were used.

Venous blood specimens were collected 1 h following a 50-g oral glucose load, except in California, where glucose was not administered to men with known diabetes mellitus. Hematocrit and blood-group determinations were performed in each local laboratory. Serum was separated from the sample and frozen at $-20\,°C$ in preparation for transfer to the laboratory for analysis. Details of the laboratory procedure have been published [9]. In summary, the method of determination of glucose was the Auto-Analyzer N-2B modification of Hoffman's method. Cholesterol was determined by the Auto-Analyzer N-24A method, and the uric acid determination was performed using the Auto-Analyzer N-13B method.

Disease incidence was detected by means of biennial examinations in Japan, supplemented by death certificate surveillance. In Honolulu, repeat examinations were conducted two and six years after the first examination. Hospital discharges and death certificate records were also monitored. In California, only one examination was performed. Surveillance by mail was conducted two and four years after the examination, supplemented by hospital follow-up and by death certificate surveillance.

The prevalence of stroke was assessed using two criteria: first, by the response to the question 'Have you ever had a stroke?'; second, after an evaluation by a consultant neurologist at each study site. Referral to the neurologist in California was based on a questionnaire supplemented by a screening examination by nurses and paramedical personnel; in Japan and Hawaii, the screening examinations were performed by physicians. Stroke diagnoses were made on the basis of all available pertinent records. In the majority of cases, records were supplemented by a thorough examination by a neurologist.

3. DEFINITIONS OF DISEASE

Hypertension was classified on the basis of World Health Organization criteria: hypertension represented systolic blood pressure $\geqslant 160$ mmHg and/or diastolic blood pressure $\geqslant 95$ mmHg; normotension implied both systolic blood pressure less than 140 mmHg and diastolic pressure less than 90 mmHg; borderline hypertension represented the residual category in which systolic blood pressure was less than 160 mmHg and diastolic blood pressure was less than 95 mmHg, but pressures were not simultaneously both below 140 mm systolic and 90 mm diastolic.

Left-ventricular hypertrophy was defined by ECG criteria alone, and was diagnosed in the presence of high-voltage QRS complex and ST-T-wave abnormalities (Minnesota Codes 3-1 plus 4-1, 4-2, or 4-3 plus 5-1, 5-2, or

5-3)[10]. Hypertensive heart disease was diagnosed on the basis of the presence of hypertension plus ECG evidence of left-ventricular hypertrophy.

The diagnosis of definite stroke[11] required a relatively sudden onset of brain deficit lasting at least two weeks (or until death) or the presence of blood in the cerebrospinal fluid. Strokelike episodes attributable to other disease processes were excluded. Definite strokes could usually be classified as thromboembolic or hemorrhagic on the basis of the clinical picture, surgery, or autopsy findings (computerized axial tomography was not available during the time of this study). Focal deficits usually without prolonged unconciousness, nuchal rigidity, fever, or pronounced leukocytosis, and in the absence of known bloody spinal fluid, were considered to indicate a thromboembolic event. Cases of intracranial hemorrhage were diagnosed on the basis of bloody spinal fluid obtained from a nontraumatic lumbar puncture or on the basis of surgical findings. Intracerebral hematoma was distinguished from subarachnoid hemorrhage by the presence of lateralizing signs or occasionally by the evidence of a space-occupying lesion from radiologic or ultrasonic studies in patients in deep coma.

Possible stroke was diagnosed when a brain deficit of relatively sudden onset lasted at least 24 h, but the exact duration of the impairment was shorter than two weeks or of unknown duration and there were no permanent residuals. Some patients with headaches and meningismus consistent with subarachnoid hemorrhage, but with possibly traumatic or absent lumbar puncture, were also included in this group. A number of cases had inadequate or conflicting documentation in the hospital records. A few fatal cases without autopsy also fell into this group. 'Possible stroke' cases were categorized using the same criteria as for definite cases. A large proportion of the 'possible stroke' group could not be classified. This subset was considered to be possible stroke, unknown type.

To avoid noncomparability of clinical judgments among the three study areas, standardized procedures were used to assess CHD prevalence. A history of angina pectoris and the pain of possible myocardial infarction were assessed by means of the London School of Hygiene Cardiovascular Questionnaire[10]. Angina pectoris was diagnosed by the report of substernal chest pain while walking uphill or hurrying, if the pain went away in 10 min or less when the subject stopped or slowed down. Possible myocardial infarction was diagnosed if the subject had experienced a severe pain across the front of the chest which lasted for half an hour or more.

Myocardial infarction (MI) was diagnosed by abnormal Q and QS patterns on the electrocardiogram. Minnesota Codes 1-1-1 to 1-1-7 constituted definite MI, and 1-2-1 to 1-3-6 constituted possible MI[10].

Men without ECG evidence of infarction at the initial examination were followed-up for incidence. Biennial follow-up examinations including electrocardiograms were performed in Japan and Hawaii, but not in California. However, surveillance procedures performed in California were comparable to those performed in Hawaii. It was therefore possible to make separate comparisons of incidence between Japan and Hawaii, and between Hawaii and California [12].

In the Japan-Hawaii comparison, incidence of coronary heart disease was based exclusively on the diagnosis of myocardial infarction as indicated by ECG changes between two successive examinations, or by the occurrence of death from coronary heart disease. Rigid criteria were specified for ECG changes and for the clinical findings required for diagnosis of myocardial infarction or death due to coronary heart disease.

In the Hawaii-California comparison, hospital and death certificate surveillance carried out in all of the hospitals on the island of Oahu was used for determination of cases in Hawaii. In California, a questionnaire was mailed to each cohort participant two and then four years after the initial examination to report health problems in general, and specifically, the occurrence of CHD. Medical records including electrocardiograms were obtained for all persons in whom occurrence of CHD was suspected. The records of suspect California cases were sent to Hawaii for review, identical to the case review employed for the Hawaii records. The specific criteria utilized in these comparative studies have been published [12].

4. COHORT CHARACTERISTICS

The characteristics presented are based on the examination of 2183 men in Japan, 8006 men in Hawaii, and 2296 men in California, aged 45–69 years, at the time of their initial examinations for the Ni-Hon-San Study [13]. The age distributions of the three cohorts were dissimilar: the Japan cohort was slightly older and the California cohort was slightly younger than the Hawaiian cohort (Table 1).

Nearly 70% of the immigrants to Hawaii came from some four adjacent prefectures: Hiroshima, Yamaguchi, Kumamoto, and Fukuoka. An additional 14% came from Okinawa. In total, 12% were Issei or first-generation immigrants, while 88% were Nisei or second generation.

The majority of immigrants to California, also, came from the first four mentioned prefectures, and an additional 12% migrated from Wakayama in the southern part of Honshu Island. In the California cohort, the Issei comprised 14%, the Nisei 86%.

Age-specific mean values for selected variables are shown in Table 1. The California and Honolulu cohorts were similar in height, and both were slightly taller than their counterparts in Hiroshima.

Table 1. Mean values of cohort characteristics by site and age.

Characteristic	Site [a]	Age (years)				
		45–49	50–54	55–59	60–64	65–69
Number of men	N	322	436	454	519	452
	H	1832	2792	1593	1338	451
	S	901	663	346	206	180
Height (cm)	N	162.1	161.6	161.0	159.6	158.9
	H	164.3	163.6	162.6	160.5	159.8
	S	165.4	163.7	162.4	161.1	159.3
Weight (kg)	N	55.3	56.1	55.5	53.7	51.7
	H	65.9	64.3	62.8	60.3	59.3
	S	67.8	66.4	64.6	61.8	60.4
Sum of skinfolds[b] (mm)	N	17.6	18.5	19.1	18.6	16.8
	H	25.4	24.7	24.3	23.3	23.0
	S	25.7	25.2	24.6	23.4	23.2
Systolic blood pressure (mmHg)	N	125.7	129.9	136.2	140.1	144.4
	H	128.6	132.0	134.3	138.6	142.2
	S	133.5	137.3	141.7	144.2	150.4
Diastolic blood pressure (mmHg)	N	80.4	82.0	84.7	83.0	83.5
	H	81.8	82.2	82.6	82.1	81.1
	S	87.3	88.6	89.2	88.9	89.0
Hematocrit (%)	N	43.6	43.1	42.7	41.8	41.9
	H	45.1	44.8	44.6	44.2	44.0
	S	45.2	44.8	44.6	44.1	44.4
Cholesterol (mg/dl)	N	176.3	176.4	174.9	178.1	176.6
	H	219.4	219.4	218.7	216.7	211.1
	S	223.4	228.2	226.8	223.6	224.0
Glucose (mg/dl)	N	137.4	147.8	139.9	146.8	152.7
	H	150.3	158.8	164.1	173.4	182.1
	S	155.3	154.6	162.7	158.7	171.3
Uric acid (mg/dl)	N	5.3	5.4	5.3	5.3	5.5
	H	6.1	6.0	5.9	5.9	6.0
	S	5.9	6.0	6.0	5.8	5.8

[a] N Nippon; H Honolulu; S San Francisco.
[b] Triceps + subscapular.

California men were slightly heavier than those in Honolulu who, in turn, were heavier than the men in Japan by an average of 8 kg. Skinfold thickness was measured over the left triceps and subscapular areas; the ratios of body weight in the three cohorts were similar to the ratios for the sum of skinfolds.

Blood pressure values were similar in Hawaii and Japan except that the men in Japan showed a slight increase in the older age groups, particularly in the diastolic pressure. In all age groups, both systolic and diastolic pressures

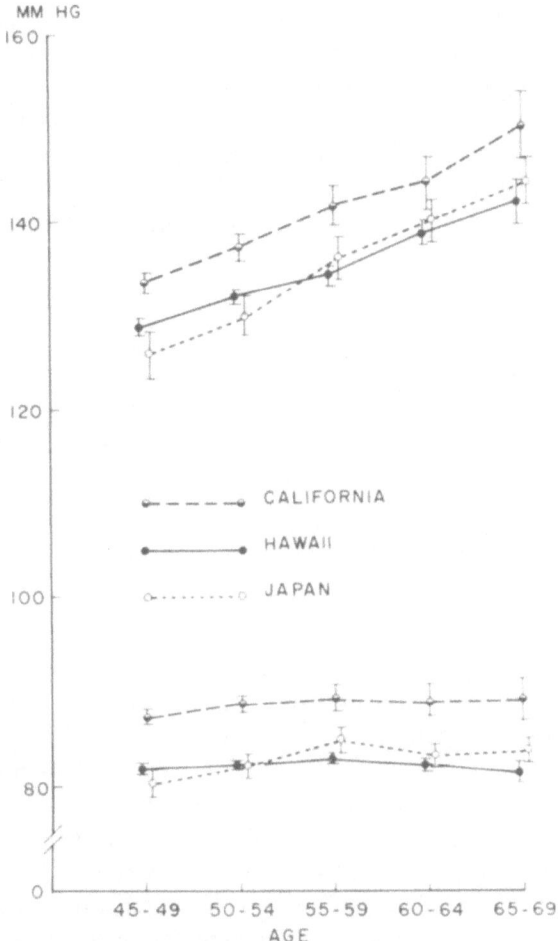

Figure 1. Mean levels of systolic and diastolic blood
pressure by age (years), Ni-Hon-San Study; error bars
indicate two standard errors of the mean.

were higher in the California cohort (Fig. 1). Blood pressure levels correlated
with body weight; and when the blood pressures were adjusted for relative
weight, the differences among the cohorts became smaller and, for some age
groups, disappeared [14].

The hematocrit values were similar in California and Hawaii; the values
were somewhat higher than those found in Japan. There was a slight difference between California and Hawaii men in serum cholesterol values. Men in
California had only slightly higher levels, and both American cohorts had
markedly higher values than those found in the Japanese cohort.

Serum glucose values in Hawaii were greater than those in Japan; the California data were similar to the Hawaii data except in the oldest age groups. To some extent, this difference may be accounted for by the fact that California diabetics were not given a glucose load, whereas diabetics were given a glucose load in the other two cohorts.

Mean uric acid levels were similar in the Hawaii and California cohorts, and they were significantly higher than the values in the Japan cohort.

Table 2. Mean values of nutrients.

Nutrient	Nippon	Honolulu	San Francisco
Calories	2132	2274	2268
Animal protein (g)	40	71	66
Vegetable protein (g)	37	24	23
Saturated fat (g)	16	59	66
Unsaturated fat (g)	21	26	29
Simple carbohydrate (g)	61	92	96
Complex carbohydrate (g)	278	169	155
Alcohol (g)	28	13	9
Cholesterol (mg)	457	545	536

Analysis of dietary data indicated that the mean value for total calories was only slightly lower in Japan than in Hawaii, but the differences in composition were substantial (Table 2). Subjects in Japan ate less protein and fat and more carbohydrates than did the American subjects. Alcohol intake was higher in Japan while dietary cholesterol was lower. Furthermore, the larger intake of protein in Honolulu and California was derived from excess animal protein. The mean value of vegetable protein was higher in Japan than in the American cohorts. The proportion of dietary fat in Hawaii was substantially greater than that in Japan, and the amount of fat consumed in California was the greatest. The proportion of calories derived from fat was 15.1%, 33.2%, and 37.6% of calories consumed in Japan, Hawaii, and California, respectively. Much of the excess fat was accounted for by the greater intake of predominantly saturated animal fat in both Honolulu and California. The excess of total carbohydrate in Japan was derived from a great excess of complex carbohydrate, primarily rice, while the intake of simple cabohydrate was substantially greater in both Honolulu and California than in Japan. Sodium intake was higher in Japan than in the American cohorts.

Cigarette-smoking patterns differed in the three areas. A larger proportion of men in Japan were smokers, but they fell predominantly in the mild to moderate category (20 cigarettes or less per day). The proportion of heavy smokers (more than a pack a day) was similar in Japan and California. The Hawaiian cohort had the largest number of heavy smokers.

When the ratio of total caloric intake to body weight was used as an indirect index of physical activity, the ratio was higher in Japan than in Hawaii, suggesting greater physical activity in Japan.

5. STROKE PREVALENCE

Stroke mortality in Japan, as a whole, has declined since 1970 [15], and stroke mortality in Hiroshima and Nagasaki prefectures, as well as stroke incidence and mortality in the cities of Hiroshima and Nagasaki, have also declined during that time [16]. The mortality from stroke of men of Japanese ancestry living in Hawaii and California has fallen sharply from the experience in Japan to approximately the experience in whites in Hawaii, which in turn is close to that of whites in the United States as a whole [17]. In a comparison of stroke mortality in the Ni-Hon-San Study, the experience in these comparable cohorts showed that stroke mortality in Japan was three times that of the American Japanese cohorts [18].

Table 3. Age-adjusted [a] prevalence rates/1000 of stroke by site and by method of diagnosis.

Method of diagnosis	Nippon	Honolulu	San Francisco
Simple history	43.9	17.3	13.0
Evaluation by neurologist (definite only)	35.4	10.7	10.4
Definite + possible	42.5	15.0	13.0

[a] Age-adjusted by the direct method to the age structure of the Honolulu cohort.

The prevalence of stroke tabulated according to a simple history is shown in Table 3; the age-adjusted rates in Japan, Hawaii, and California were 43.9, 17.3, and 13.0 per thousand, respectively. Age adjustment was done by the direct method and related to the age structure of the Hawaii cohort. Using this criterion the stroke prevalence was $2\frac{1}{2}$ times higher in Japan than in Hawaii and more than three times higher in Japan than in California. The differences between Hawaii and California were not statistically significant.

The prevalence of stroke in the three sites according to the diagnosis of the consulting neurologist (Table 3) indicated relationships similar to those determined by history alone. The age-adjusted prevalence rates of definite stroke were 35.4, 10.7, and 10.4 in Japan, Hawaii, and California, respectively. In the instance of definite and possible cases, the rates were 42.5, 15.0, and 13.0, respectively.

No attempt was made in the California cohort to distinguish specific types of stroke. In both the Hawaii and the Japan cohorts, the great majority of stroke prevalence cases were due to cerebral infarction [11]. Of course, caution is necessary in the interpretation of prevalence data for a disease with such a high mortality as stroke, particularly since mortality from specific types of stroke differs.

These findings of differences in stroke prevalence and mortality have been supported by an autopsy study that showed a greater frequency of cerebro-vascular disease, both as an incidental finding and as a cause of death, in Hiroshima decedents than in Honolulu decedents. Cerebral infarction was found more frequently in Hiroshima than in Honolulu in a ratio of 2:1 [19].

6. STROKE INCIDENCE

No repeat examination was conducted in the California study. The comparable incidence data based on repeat examinations from the study in Japan have not yet been completely analyzed, so the following data on stroke incidence are limited to findings in the Honolulu study. In six years of follow-up based on examinations and on surveillance, 133 new cases of definite stroke were diagnosed with an additional 49 diagnosed as possible stroke. A division of definite cases showed 94 (71%) thromboembolic, 14% due to intracerebral hemorrhage, 11% due to subarachnoid hemorrhage, and 4% of unknown type. Stroke incidence increased with age. After age adjustment, the variables related to the incidence of thromboembolic stroke included blood pressure, number of cigarettes smoked daily, hematocrit, and serum glucose after a 50-g glucose load. In the univariate analysis, the prevalence of coronary heart disease and the ECG finding of left-ventricular hypertrophy or strain (LVH/LVS), or nonspecific ST-T abnormalities were also related to thromboembolic stroke.

In multivariate analysis, using the Walker-Duncan method [20], those risk factors retaining significant association with the development of thromboem-

Table 4. Cerebral infarction: multivariate logistic function.

Variable	Standardized coefficient	t [a]
Age	0.357	3.51
Glucose	0.247	3.21
Systolic blood pressure	0.450	5.20
LVH/LVS	0.155	3.15

[a] $t = \dfrac{\text{standard coefficient}}{\text{standard error}}$

A value of 2 or greater indicates statistical significance at $P < 0.05$.

bolic stroke were systolic blood pressure, age, serum glucose, and the ECG finding of LVH/LVS (Table 4). In the case of intracranial hemorrhage, the univariate analysis showed risk attributed to age, elevated blood pressure, alcohol consumption and ECG evidence of LVH/LVS. Serum cholesterol was inversely related to the occurrence of intracranial hemorrhage. In the multivariate analysis, significant risk factors for intracranial hemorrhage were systolic blood pressure, alcohol consumption, LVH/LVS on the ECG, and, inversely, serum cholesterol level (Table 5).

Table 5. Intracranial hemorrhage: multivariate logistic function.

Variable	Standardized coefficient	t [a]
Age	0.144	0.81
Glucose	−0.355	−1.66
Systolic blood pressure	0.537	3.70
LVH/LVS	0.218	2.80
Alcohol	0.263	2.63
Cholesterol	−0.380	−2.03

[a] Cf. footnote to Table 4.

As in the case of coronary disease, the presence of multiple factors magnified the risk. In this form of analysis, as is indicated by standardized coefficients and t values in the multivariate logistic function, the presence of elevated blood pressure was the preponderant risk factor for both cerebral infarction and intracranial hemorrhage.

7. DISCUSSION

The Ni-Hon-San Study was organized to take advantage of the natural experiment occasioned by the migration from Japan to Hawaii and California to elucidate the epidemiology of hypertension, coronary heart disease, and stroke.

The initial examination of the men revealed that these ethnically similar cohorts of indigenous and migrant Japanese males were similar in characteristics largely genetically determined, such as stature and skeletal size. They differed in those characteristics largely influenced by environment and sociocultural forces, factors such as diet and smoking habit. They differed also in features influenced by a mixture of genetic and sociocultural factors, variables such as weight, glucose tolerance, and levels of serum lipids and uric acid.

The differences noted in height in the three cohorts are of questionable biological significance; they may reflect nutritional differences. The differences in weight between the American and Japan cohorts were substantial. They clearly reflect significant differences in energy balance, and the similarity of the curves for weight and for skinfold measurements suggests that the weight differences are due to differences in adiposity. The differences in serum cholesterol determinations were large and not to due to differences in laboratory methodology. The lower glucose and uric acid values in the Japan cohort are of interest. The differences may be attributable in part to the differences in body weight [21].

Despite the progressive alteration of the diet in Japan since World War II [22], at the time of these examinations the differences were still great, particularly in terms of the proportion of animal and vegetable proteins and fats and in simple and complex carbohydrates.

The findings with regard to blood pressure distributions were unexpected. Independent studies in Hiroshima [6, 23] and Honolulu [17] have shown a strong relation between blood pressure and stroke incidence; and the prevalence of and mortality from stroke were highest in the Japan cohort, intermediate in the Hawaii cohort, and lowest in the California cohort [11] despite the findings of higher blood pressures in the California cohort. One possible explanation may lie in the relation between blood pressure, weight, and disease in these cohorts, the evidence suggesting only minor differences in blood pressure among the three cohorts after adjusting for differences in relative weight [14].

The finding that the Japanese migrants to the United States and their offspring have lower prevalence and mortality from stroke than ethnically similar residents in Japan suggests some factor in the environment or in the life style of Japanese-Americans that acts protectively against stroke. One possibility that comes to mind is the significant difference in dietary intake as well as in the serum cholesterol levels between the indigenous and migrant Japanese populations. Kimura [24] has suggested a deficiency in protein, Komachi et al. [25] a relative lack of animal fat, and Sasaki et al. [26] an excess of salt in the diet as being related to the susceptibility to stroke of the people in Japan. Studies on rats (SHRSP strain) have provided experimental support for all three of these hypotheses [27].

Our finding with regard to the preponderance of cerebral infarction is quite similar to reports about Caucasian populations. At the Hisayama Study [28] in Kyushu, cerebral infarction was also the predominant type of stroke. Vital statistics from Japan [14] show both an absolute and a relative decline in mortality from cerebral hemorrhage. It is uncertain to what extent this reported fall is attributable to changes in diagnostic practice and coding rules, and to what extent it is due to a change in the susceptibility of the population.

REFERENCES

1. Report of Inter-Society Commission for Heart Disease Resources: Primary prevention of the atherosclerotic diseases. Circulation 42:A55-A95, 1970.
2. Reid DD: The future of migrant studies. Isr J Med Sci 7:1592-1596, 1971.
3. Gordon T: Mortality experience among the Japanese in the United States, Hawaii and Japan. Public Health Rep 72:543-553, 1957.
4. Gordon T: Further mortality experience among Japanese Americans. Public Health Rep 82:973-984, 1967.
5. Belsky JL, Kagan A, Syme SL: Epidemiologic studies of coronary heart disease and stroke in Japanese men living in Japan, Hawaii and California. Research Plan, Atomic Bomb Casualty Commission Technical Report 12-71, 1971. (Microfiched and stored at: Bay Microfilm, Inc, 737 Loma Verde Avenue, Palo Alto, CA.)
6. Robertson TL, Shimizu Y, et al.: Incidence of stroke and coronary heart disease in atomic bomb survivors living in Hiroshima and Nagasaki, 1958–74: The Adult Health Study of the Radiation Effects Research Foundation. RERF TR 12-79, 1979.
7. Belsky JL, Tachikawa K, Jablon S: ABCC-JNIH Adult Health Study, Report 5. Results of the first five cycles of examinations, Hiroshima-Nagasaki 1958–68. Atomic Bomb Casualty Commission Technical Report 9-71, 1971.
8. Worth RM, Kagan A: Ascertainment of men of Japanese ancestry in Hawaii through World War II Selective Service registration. J Chronic Dis 23:389-397, 1970.
9. Nichaman MZ, Hamilton HB, Kagan A, Grier T, Sacks ST, Syme SL: Epidemiologic studies of coronary heart disease and stroke in Japanese men living in Japan, Hawaii and California: distribution of biochemical risk factors. Am J Epidemiol 102:491-501, 1975.
10. Rose GA, Blackburn H: Cardiovascular survey methods. Geneva: WHO, 1968.
11. Kagan A, Popper J, Rhoads GG, Takeya Y, Kato H, Browne Goode G, Marmot M: Epidemiologic studies of coronary heart disease and stroke in Japanese men living in Japan, Hawaii and California: prevalence of stroke. In: Scheinberg P (ed) Cerebrovascular diseases, 10th Princeton Conference. New York: Raven Press, 1976, pp 267-277.
12. Robertson TL, Kato H, Rhoads GG, Kagan A, Marmot MG, Syme SL, Gordon T, Worth RM, Belsky JL, Dock DS, Miyanishi M, Kawamoto S: Epidemiologic studies of coronary heart disease and stroke in Japanese men living in Japan, Hawaii and California: incidence of myocardial infarction and death from coronary heart disease. Am J Cardiol 39:239-243, 1977.
13. Kagan A, Harris BR, Winkelstein Jr W, Johnson KG, Kato H, Syme SL, Rhoads GG, Gay ML, Nichaman MZ, Hamilton HB, Tillotson JL: Epidemiologic studies of coronary heart disease and stroke in Japanese men living in Japan, Hawaii and California: demographic, physical, dietary and biochemical characteristics. J Chronic Dis 27:345-364, 1974.
14. Winkelstein Jr W, Kagan A, Kato H, Sacks ST: Epidemiologic studies of coronary heart disease and stroke in Japanese men living in Japan, Hawaii and California: blood pressure distributions. Am J Epidemiol 102:502-513, 1975.
15. Health and Welfare Statistics Association: Trends in nation's health, 1978 (in Japanese). Kosei-no-shihyo 25:380, 1978.
16. Lin CH, Shimizu Y, Kato H, Robertson TL, Furonaka H, Fukunaga Y: Cerebrovascular disease in a fixed population of Hiroshima and Nagasaki, with special

reference to relationship between type and risk factors. RERF Technical Report (in preparation).

17. Kagan A, Popper JS, Rhoads GG: Factors related to stroke incidence in Hawaii Japanese men: the Honolulu Heart Study. Stroke (in press) 1980.

18. Worth RM, Kato H, Rhoads GG, Kagan A, Syme SL: Epidemiologic studies of coronary heart disease and stroke in Japanese men living in Japan, Hawaii and California: mortality. Am J Epidemiol 102:481-490, 1975.

19. Mitsuyama Y, Thompson LR, Hayashi Y, Lee KK, Keehn RJ, Steer A: An autopsy study of cerebrovascular disease in Japanese men who lived in Hiroshima, Japan and Honolulu, Hawaii. Stroke (in press) 1980.

20. Walker SH, Duncan DB: Estimation of the probability of an event as a function of several independent variables. Biometrika 54:167-179, 1967.

21. Yano K, Rhoads GG, Kagan A: Epidemiology of serum uric acid among 8000 Japanese-American men in Hawaii. J Chronic Dis 30:171-184, 1977.

22. Insull W, Oiso T, Tsuchiya K: Diet und nutritional status of Japanese. Am J Clin Nutr 21:753-777.

23. Johnson KG, Yano K, Kato H: Cerebral vascular disease in Hiroshima, Japan. J Chronic Dis 20:545-559, 1967.

24. Kimura N: Epidemiology of hypertension and stroke in Asia. In: Hatano S, Shigematsu I, Strasser T (eds) Hypertension and stroke control in the community. Geneva: WHO, 1976, pp 55-59.

25. Komachi Y, Iida M, Ozawa H, Shimamoto T, Konishi M, Ueshima H, Goda N, Furukawa M: Interrelationship of food and stroke in Japan. Ann Rep Cent Adult Dis Osaka 15:82-93, 1975.

26. Sasaki N, et al.: High blood pressure and the salt intake of the Japanese. Jpn Heart J 3:313-324, 1962.

27. Yamori Y, Ooshima A: Nutritional prevention of hypertensive diseases. In: Inoue G, Yoshimura H (eds) Effects of alterations of dietary patterns and food habits on health. Osaka, US-Japan Cooperative Medical Sciences Program, 1978, pp 200-209.

28. Omae T, Takeshita M, Hirota Y: The Hisayama study and joint study on cerebrovascular disease in Japan. In: Scheinberg P (ed) Cerebrovascular diseases, 10th Princeton Conference. New York: Raven Press, 1976, pp 255-265.

27. HYPERTENSION AND HEART DISEASE IN THE NI-HON-SAN STUDY

M.G. MARMOT, A. KAGAN, and H. KATO

Blood pressure is a powerful predictor of the occurrence of coronary heart disease (CHD). Within a population, the measurement of an individual's blood pressure is perhaps the single most accurate guide to that individual's risk of subsequently developing CHD. This 'within-population' accuracy of prediction does not extend to comparisons between populations. In the United States, for example, blacks have higher mean blood pressures than whites, but not higher rates of CHD[1]. In the West Indies, average blood pressure levels are high, but not the rate of occurrence of CHD[2]. Similarly, blood pressure levels in Japan are comparable to those in western countries[3, 4], but the rate of occurrence of CHD in Japan is much lower than in western countries[5, 6].

In other words, knowledge of the distribution of blood pressure in a population is *by itself* an unreliable guide to that population's CHD risk, relative to other populations. In a multifactorial disease such as CHD, one must consider the interrelationship of blood pressure and other risk factors. The case of the Japanese is particularly interesting. In broad terms, Japan is a high blood pressure/high stroke area and the USA is a high blood pressure/high CHD area. Japanese living in the USA show a decreased mortality from stroke and increased mortality from heart disease relative to the rates in Japan[5].

The Ni-Hon-San study of men of Japanese ancestry living in Japan, Hawaii, and California, described in the previous chapter, has measured risk factors and assessed disease frequency in three groups of men aged 45–69 years. It offers the potential for a better understanding of the interrelationship of blood pressure and other risk factors in the aetiology of heart disease and stroke. The previous paper showed blood pressure to be a risk factor for stroke in Japan and among Japanese-Americans in Hawaii. However, the difference in stroke rates between Japanese in Japan and Japanese-Americans was greater than could have been predicted from differences in blood pressure. It seems likely that factors other than blood pressure account for the high rates of stroke in Japan.

In this paper, we shall consider (a) the levels of blood pressure and other coronary risk factors in Japan, Hawaii, and California; (b) the relationship

H. Kesteloot, J.V. Joossens (eds.), Epidemiology of Arterial Blood Pressure, 437–452.

438

between blood pressure and hypertensive heart disease in the three groups of men; (c) whether, despite the low CHD rates in Japan, blood pressure is associated with the occurrence of CHD in Japan as well as in Hawaii and California; and (d) what factors other than blood pressure might account for the higher CHD rate amongst Japanese-Americans.

1. HYPERTENSION AND OTHER RISK FACTORS IN JAPAN, HAWAII, AND CALIFORNIA

The age-specific means of coronary risk factors are shown in the previous chapter. The distributions have been published [4, 7]. For ease of summarization, Table 1 shows the age-adjusted means and prevalence of hypertension (WHO criteria), hypercholesterolaemia (serum cholesterol ≥ 260 mg%), and proportion of cigarette smokers. The California-Japanese have a higher prevalence of hypertension and higher mean blood pressure than the Japanese in Japan, who have a higher prevalence of hypertension than the Hawaii-Japanese.

Table 1. Blood pressure, serum cholesterol, and smoking in Japan, Hawaii, and California (figures are age-adjusted).

Characteristic	Japan (n = 2127)	Hawaii (n = 7998)	California (n = 1795)
Hypertensives [a]/100	22.4	19.4	31.6
Mean systolic BP (mmHg)	133.1	133.4	138.6
Mean diastolic BP (mmHg)	82.6	82.1	88.6
Serum cholesterol ≥ 260 mg% (/100)	3.2	12.4	16.3
Mean serum cholesterol (mg%)	181.5	218.1	225.7
Smokers/100	74	44	35

[a] Hypertension = systolic BP ≥ 160 mmHg or diastolic BP ≥ 95 mmHg.

As shown in the previous paper [8], the Japanese in America have greater average skinfold thickness than Japanese in Japan. Consistent with this, the Japanese-Americans are also heavier for their height. Adjusting for these relative weight differences reduces the magnitude of the blood pressure differences, but the ranking is preserved: Hawaii—low, Japan—intermediate, California—high [4]. Thus, part of the explanation for the higher blood pressures in California is the greater average body mass of the California-Japanese, but part of the difference remains unexplained. We have no accurate information on salt intake in the three groups. The high salt content of the Japanese diet has been well documented. We have no reason to believe that the shift to a more western diet by the Japanese-Americans involves a *higher* salt consumption.

Whenever blood pressures are measured in different places, the possibility must be considered that the observed differences are due to differences in measurement technique rather than to biological factors. Despite the adoption of similar methods of measurement in the three study areas, this doubt must be borne in mind when evaluating the comparison of the groups.

The figures for serum cholesterol show the expected low mean levels in Japan and the much higher levels among the Japanese-Americans. Only 3.2% of Japanese in Japan have a serum cholesterol ⩾ 260 mg%, compared with 12.4% in Hawaii and 16.3% in California.

Smoking is more prevalent in Japan than among Japanese-Americans. The strikingly high figure—74% of Japanese men report that they smoke cigarettes—hides the fact that fewer of the smokers in Japan were 'heavy smokers' (⩾ 20/day) as compared with men in Hawaii and California [9].

2. HYPERTENSIVE HEART DISEASE

As shown in Table 2, left-ventricular hypertrophy (LVH) is common among the Japanese in Japan. It is more frequent there than among the other two groups. When comparison is made of the prevalence of hypertensive heart disease, defined as LVH *plus* hypertension, the Hawaii-California-Japan gradient of increasing prevalence is still in evidence. This higher prevalence of LVH in Japan occurs despite lower levels of blood pressure than in California.

Table 2. Prevalence of left-ventricular hypertrophy and hypertensive heart disease among Japanese men by geographical location.

Diagnosis	Age-adjusted prevalence/1000		
	Japan (n = 2127)	Hawaii (n = 7998)	California (n = 1795)
Left-ventricular hypertrophy [a]	16.4	5.7	6.1
Hypertensive heart disease [b]	9.3	1.4	4.6

[a] Left-ventricular hypertrophy = Minnesota Codes 3–1 plus 4–1, 4–2 or 4–3 plus 5–1, 5–2 or 5–3.
[b] Definite hypertension (systolic ⩾ 160 mmHg or diastolic ⩾ 95 mmHg) plus left-ventricular hypertrophy.

One possible explanation for this discrepancy is that the methods of measuring blood pressure differed between Japan and California, so that the Japanese levels of blood pressure are artificially low, or the California figures artificially high.

It has also been suggested that the higher voltages recorded on the ECG in Japan may be a function more of thin chest wall than of increased myocardial

440

bulk [10]. However, the finding of ECG-determined LVH cannot be ignored, as Japanese in whom LVH is found have an increased risk of subsequent CHD mortality [11]. It does seem, therefore, that at a given level of blood pressure, hypertensive heart disease is more common in Japan than among Japanese-Americans.

3. PREVALENCE OF CHD IN JAPAN, HAWAII, AND CALIFORNIA

In the three groups, objective criteria were used to measure CHD prevalence: electrocardiograms were coded centrally according to the Minnesota codes and, in addition, the London School of Hygiene Cardiovascular Questionnaire was used to assess the prevalence of angina pectoris or possible myocardial infarction [12]. The age-adjusted prevalence of CHD is shown in Table 3. When CHD is defined by the presence of Q/QS abnormalities on the ECG (Minnesota codes 1-1, 1-2, or 1-3) a clear Japan-Hawaii-California trend of increasing CHD prevalence is seen. When the definition is confined to only major Q/QS abnormalities (Minnesota Code 1-1), the higher prevalence in California is still observed [13].

Table 3. Prevalence of coronary heart disease among Japanese men by geographical location.

	Age-adjusted prevalence/1000		
Diagnosis	Japan (n = 2141)	Hawaii (n = 8003)	California (n = 1834)
ELECTROCARDIOGRAM			
CHD — definite Q/QS [a]	5.3	5.2	10.8
CHD — definite plus possible Q/QS [b]	25.4	34.7	44.6
LSH and TM questionnaire			
Angina pectoris	11.2	14.3	25.3
Possible infarction	7.3	13.2	31.4

[a] Major Q/QS abnormalities: Minnesota Code 1-1.
[b] Major and minor Q/QS abnormalities: Minnesota Codes 1-1, 1-2 or 1-3.

The London School of Hygiene Cardiovascular Questionnaire was administered in Japanese in Japan, and in Japanese and English in Hawaii and California. It has been shown that the cultural background of the respondents and the mode of administration of the questionnaire can affect prevalence estimates [14]. It is, therefore, interesting to note that prevalence of angina pectoris and, to an even greater degree, prevalence of possible myocardial infarction show the same Japan-Hawaii-California gradient as the prevalence of Q/QS abnormalities on the ECG.

3.1. Blood pressure and CHD prevalence

The differences in blood pressure between Japan, Hawaii, and California do not show the same pattern as the CHD differences. For CHD prevalence, the trend (from low to high) is Japan-Hawaii-California. By contrast, the trend for prevalence of hypertension is Hawaii-Japan-California.

Despite this inconsistency in the *between*-population comparison, blood pressure is associated with prevalence of CHD *within* populations, as shown in Figure 1; particularly in Japan, the higher the blood pressure, the higher the prevalence of CHD. The lack of a clear dose-response relationship between blood pressure and CHD in California may be due to problems of cross-sectional studies. For example, it is possible that men with hypertension who developed CHD have a higher case-fatality ratio than normotensive men who develop CHD; in which case, in a cross-sectional study, men with hypertension and CHD would be missed to a disproportionate extent, thus blurring the apparent relation between blood pressure and CHD.

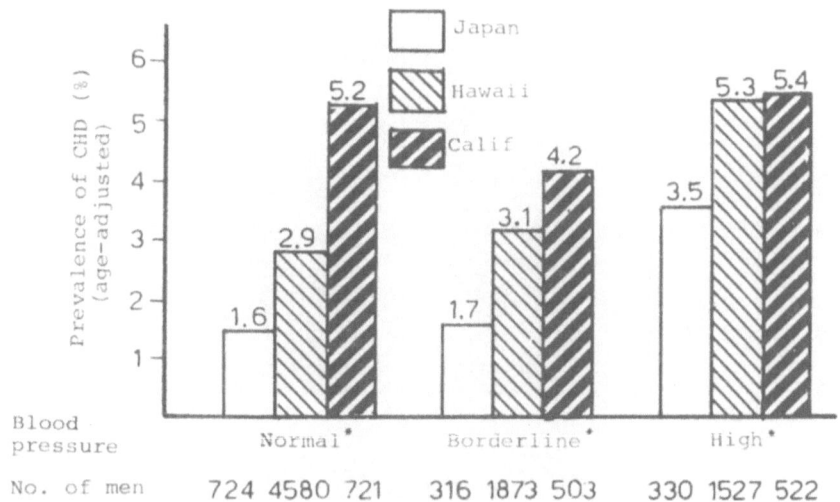

Figure 1. Prevalence of CHD in Japan, Hawaii, and California, controlling for blood pressure (age-adjusted). CHD = Minnesota Codes 1-1, 1-2 or 7-1 *or* angina pectoris from cardiovascular questionnaire; * = WHO criteria. By permission of ref. [24].

It is interesting to note, in Figure 1, that in each blood pressure category there is a Japan-Hawaii-California gradient in CHD prevalence. Although blood pressure is associated with CHD in individuals, these data suggest that factors other than blood pressure are responsible for the higher CHD rates among the men of Japanese ancestry living in America.

442

3.2. Serum cholesterol and CHD prevalence

An obvious candidate for the 'missing' factor is diet. The Japanese in Japan consume less total fat in their diet and less saturated fat (average = 16 g/day) than the Japanese in Hawaii and California (average = 59 g/day and 66 g/ day, respectively). The differences in serum cholesterol between the three groups (Table 1) is consistent with the possible importance of differences in the dietary intake of fat in the explanation of the Japan-Hawaii-California gradient in CHD. As shown in Figure 2, there is a clear association between CHD prevalence and level of serum cholesterol. It may also be noted from the 'denominators' in Figure 2 how few men in Japan have a serum choles- terol greater than 260 mg%. If indeed the low levels of serum cholesterol in Japan are related to the low per cent of dietary calories derived from fat, then these data do suggest that the Japanese-Americans are at higher risk of CHD because of their higher fat consumption.

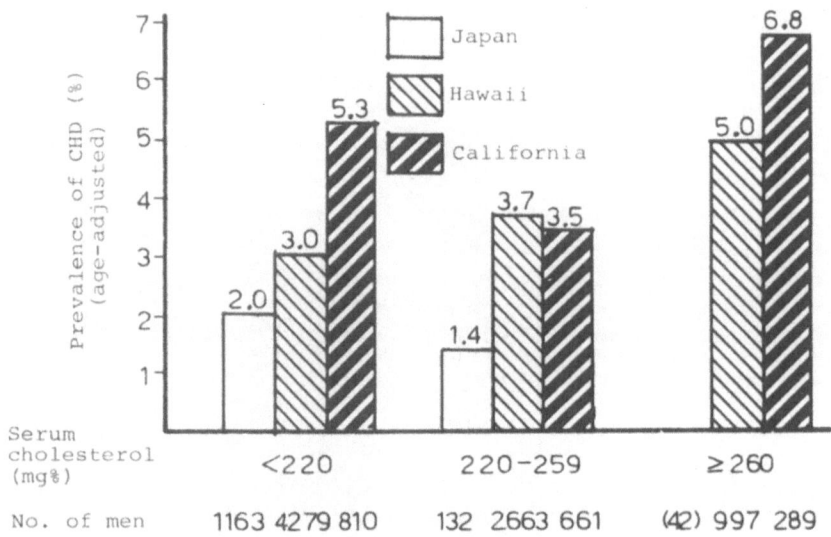

Figure 2. Prevalence of CHD in Japan, Hawaii, and California, controlling for serum cholesterol (age-adjusted). CHD = Minnesota Codes 1-1, 1-2 or 7-1 *or* angina pectoris from cardiovascular questionnaire. By permission of ref. [24].

This is unlikely to be the complete explanation, however. In Figure 2, there is the clear suggestion that the Japan-Hawaii-California CHD gradient exists among these men regardless of the serum cholesterol category into which they fall. For example, among men with serum cholesterol in the range 220 mg%, the age-adjusted CHD prevalence ranges from 2.0% in Japan to 5.3% in California.

To assess the combined effects of blood pressure and serum cholesterol on CHD prevalence, the three populations were subdivided according to blood pressure, serum cholesterol, and age. The data were then combined by using the Mantel-Haenszel procedure. Controlling for these three variables and taking the prevalence in Japan as 1, the relative risk in Hawaii is 1.6, and in California is 2.1. In other words, the combined influences on CHD prevalence of blood pressure and serum cholesterol are insufficient to account for the Japan-Hawaii-California gradient.

A similar analysis has been performed for smoking[13]. As described above, smoking is more common in Japan than among the Japanese-Americans, and there is little association between smoking and CHD prevalence in Japan. Hence the difference in smoking rates per se is not a likely explanation of the higher CHD prevalence in America.

4. CHD INCIDENCE IN JAPAN, HAWAII, AND CALIFORNIA

The data in the previous sections come from cross-sectional studies of the three populations in the Ni-Hon-San study. Such cross-sectional data have limitations when analysing aetiological relationships. In particular, fatal cases are missed and the variables under study may change consequently upon the development of the disease. For example, the prevalence figures from Hawaii show the prevalence of CHD to be higher among ex-smokers than among

Table 4. Incidence of myocardial infarction and CHD death in Japan, Hawaii, and California.

| Age (years) | CHD incidence/1000 person years at risk (Person years at risk) | | | |
	Japan	Hawaii Examination[a]	Surveillance[a]	California
45–49	— (1622)	1.7 (3756)	1.7 (3568)	3.0 (2660)
50–54	1.3 (2250)	2.6 (5390)	2.4 (5412)	2.8 (2148)
55–59	2.6 (2352)	3.9 (3082)	3.9 (3088)	3.2 (1254)
60–64	2.0 (2496)	4.4 (2526)	4.0 (2542)	10.7 (652)
65–68	1.7 (1188)	4.8 (836)	3.6 (838)	4.4 (458)
Total (age-adjusted)	1.4 (9908)	3.1 (15,410)	2.9 (15,448)	4.3 (7172)

[a] See text for explanation.

current smokers[13]. A likely explanation is that many men may have given up smoking *after* developing clinical CHD.

The three cohorts in the Ni-Hon-San study have been followed for 4–6 years, and data on incidence of CHD in the three cohorts have recently become available[15, 16]. It is interesting to note that the incidence figures largely confirm the conclusions from the analysis of prevalence. The incidence rates for CHD (CHD death and non-fatal myocardial infarction) are shown in Table 4. Two sets of figures are presented for Hawaii. The Japan-Hawaii comparison is based on physical examinations—at two, four, and six years of follow-up in Japan and at two years in Hawaii. The California sample was not re-examined. Hence the Hawaii-California comparison is based on surveillance of morbidity and mortality over two years in Hawaii and four years in California. The incidence figures obtained in Hawaii by the two different methods agree very closely[17]. As seen in the age-specific rates, and as summarised in the age-adjusted rates, there is a confirmation of the Japan-Hawaii-California gradient in the occurrence of CHD.

4.1. Blood pressure and CHD incidence in Japan and Hawaii

The relation of blood pressure levels to CHD incidence (fatal and non-fatal) is shown in Figure 3. It confirms that blood pressure is related to the occurrence of CHD amongst Japanese in Japan, but that factors other than blood pressure must be responsible for the higher CHD incidence in Hawaii[16]. Preliminary analyses of the Hawaii-California incidence figures show similarly that the California excess in CHD incidence cannot be explained by the higher blood pressure in California.

4.2. Other risk factors

Table 5 summarises the relation of other risk factors to CHD incidence in Japan and Hawaii, by comparing the mean values at base-line examination for those who subsequently developed CHD and those who remained free of CHD during the follow-up period. As already shown, blood pressure is related to CHD. Significant associations were also observed for serum cholesterol in both Japan and Hawaii. The small number of cases in Japan ($n = 22$) makes the appraisal of the other associations difficult. As shown by the lack of statistical significance, some of the differences between cases and non-cases in Japan may be due to chance.

In passing, it is of interest to note the lower calorie consumption at base line of the men who subsequently developed CHD compared with those who remained free of the disease. This has been reported from other studies[18]

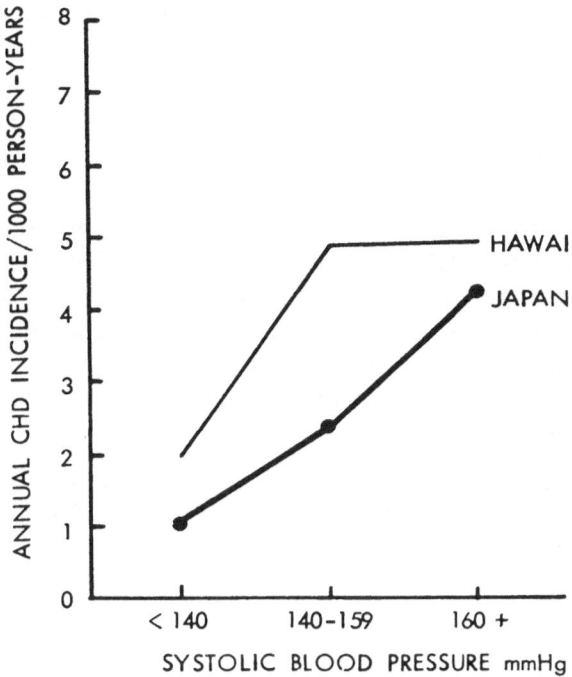

Figure 3. CHD incidence (fatal and non-fatal) according to blood pressure in Japan and Hawaii. By permission of ref. [16].

Table 5. Mean values of selected attributes of men, aged 45–68 years at first examination, in Japan and Hawaii with and without subsequent coronary heart disease (myocardial infarction or coronary heart disease death). By permission of ref. [16].

	Japan			Hawaii		
	CHD cases	Others	Significance test	CHD cases	Others	Significance test
Weight (kg)	56.2	55.1	NS	67.9	63.3	$P<0.01$
Relative weight (%)	105.0	101.9	NS	121.4	113.9	$P<0.01$
Subscapular skinfold (mm)	11.6	10.2	NS	19.2	16.4	$P<0.01$
Serum cholesterol (mg/dl)	209.5	181.0	$P<0.01$	232.9	218.0	$P<0.01$
Serum triglyceride (mg/dl)	170.9	134.3	NS	305.9	229.3	$P<0.01$
Serum uric acid (mg/dl)	5.7	5.4	NS	6.7	6.0	$P<0.01$
One-hour serum glucose (mg/dl)	172.1	146.4	NS	177.4	160.9	NS
Systolic blood pressure (mmHg)	153.3	133.0	$P<0.01$	145.2	132.7	$P<0.01$
Diastolic blood pressure (mmHg)	92.6	83.1	$P<0.01$	89.0	81.9	$P<0.01$
Pulse pressure (mmHg)	60.4	49.2	$P<0.01$	56.2	50.8	$P<0.05$
Hematocrit (%)	41.9	43.1	NS	46.2	45.0	NS
Total calories/24 h	2159	2180	NS	2030	2289	$P<0.05$

Values based on 47 cases in 7705 men observed for two years in Hawaii and 22 cases in 1963 men observed for approximately five years in Japan. Significance test results by Student's *t*-test; CHD, coronary heart disease; NS, not significant.

and could be explained by a lower level of physical activity amongst the future cases, i.e. by a protective effect of physical activity.

To assess the independent effects on CHD incidence of blood pressure, serum cholesterol, relative weight (measured as a per cent of ideal weight for height), and cigarette smoking, a multivariate analysis was performed using the multiple logistic function. The standardised coefficients are shown in Table 6. Blood pressure and serum cholesterol are significantly and independently associated with CHD in Japan and Hawaii. The lack of association between smoking and CHD in Japan is in clear contrast to the strong association in Hawaii. This lack of association with smoking has been found in other populations where the overall rate of CHD is low [19, 20]. It suggests that smoking may be important in the aetiology of CHD only when other risk factors are present.

Table 6. Standardised multivariate logistic function coefficients [a] for risk of coronary heart disease in Japan and in Hawaii: men aged 45–64 years. By permission of ref. [16].

Risk factors	Standardised coefficients [b]		Test for difference between cohorts [c]
	Japan	Hawaii	
Age (years)	0.547*	0.340**	NS
Systolic blood pressure (mmHg)	0.465*	0.432**	NS
Serum cholesterol (mg/dl)	0.410*	0.318**	NS
Relative weight (%)	0.270	0.109*	NS
Cigarette smoking	0.009	0.626**	Sug

[a] Calculated by maximum likelihood (Walker-Duncan) method [16].
[b] Coefficient times standard deviation of independent variable; Tests of significance are one-sided.
[c] Two-sided test for significance of difference in absolute coefficients between cohorts.
NS, not significant; Sug, suggestive $= 0.1 < P < 0.05$; *$0.01 < P < 0.05$; **$P < 0.01$.

Finally, the question of whether all these risk factors, particularly the higher levels of serum cholesterol in Hawaii, explain the higher CHD incidence in Hawaii is difficult to answer. Because of the small number of cases in Japan, conclusions must await a longer period of follow-up. Nevertheless, when the multiple logistic function summarising the relation of risk factors to disease in Japan is applied to the Hawaii population, the number of incident cases predicted in Hawaii agrees fairly closely with the number actually observed [16].

The cautious interpretation of these analyses is that (a) serum cholesterol is related to CHD in both Japan and Hawaii, and the higher levels in Hawaii are part of the explanation for the higher CHD rates; (b) in the presence of raised serum cholesterol, or other factors operating in Hawaii, the effect on CHD occurrence of smoking is enhanced; and (c) the *absolute* risk of CHD attributable to blood pressure is increased in the presence of raised levels of other risk factors such as serum cholesterol; but (d) there is little evidence for a difference between Japan and Hawaii in the *relative* risk of CHD associated with raised blood pressure.

Whether the crucial 'missing factor' in Japan is lack of dietary fat remains uncertain. The higher levels of serum cholesterol among the Hawaii-Japanese are likely to be related to their higher level of saturated fat consumption. Within the Hawaii population, however, there is little association between fat intake and serum cholesterol[21] or CHD incidence[22].

4.3. CHD incidence in Hawaii and Framingham

Although the Japanese-Americans have higher rates of CHD than Japanese in Japan, the rate for all Americans is even higher[5]. Japanese-Americans appear to be only partly exposed to the factors that are responsible for the high CHD rate in the USA; or alternatively, Japanese-Americans have only partly lost the protection enjoyed by the Japanese in Japan. To explore further the reasons for the difference in CHD rates, Gordon et al. compared data on CHD incidence in the Hawaii-Japanese in the Ni-Hon-San study with data from the Framingham study in Massachussets[20]. Such comparisons contained fewer of the usual dangers of comparisons between studies, because the two studies were carried out by the same institute using similar methods. Figure 4 plots the probability of developing CHD in two years in Framing-

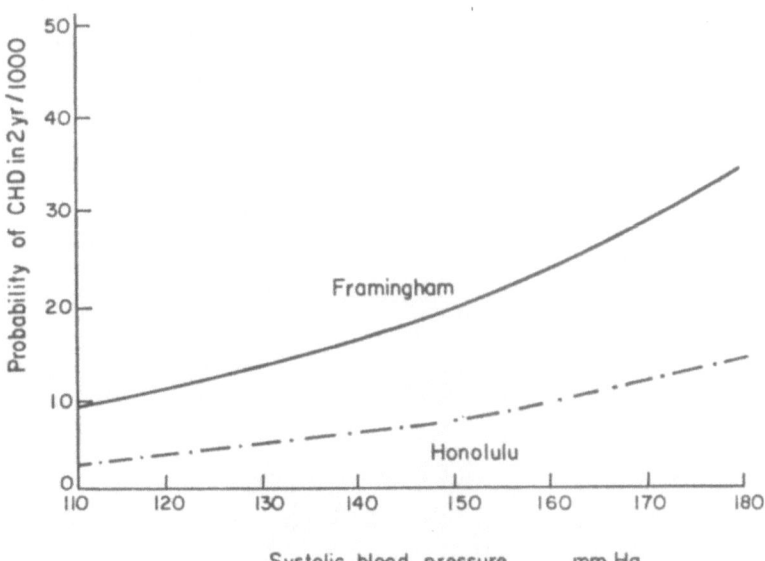

Figure 4. Probability at age 55 of CHD (fatal and non-fatal) occurring in two years in Hawaii, Japanese and Framingham men according to systolic blood pressure. By permission of ref. [20].

ham and Honolulu according to systolic blood pressure. These probabilities are taken from a logistic function. At a given level of blood pressure, the CHD incidence rate in Framingham is more than twice the rate among the Hawaii-Japanese. Similarly when serum cholesterol, cigarette smoking, and age are included with systolic blood pressure in a multiple logistic function, the rate in Framingham is more than twice the Hawaii rate for a given level of risk factors. Clearly the excess CHD rate in Framingham is not simply a matter of higher levels of blood pressure or other known risk factors.

5. CULTURAL DIFFERENCES IN CHD

Among the other factors considered that might account for the higher coronary rates among Japanese-Americans were cultural factors, other than patterns of diet or physical activity. It had been suggested that the Japanese were protected from CHD because the Japanese culture has devices for dealing with stress[23]. In particular, the tightly knit social groupings in Japan are thought to provide emotional and social support that make easier the handling of stressful situations. In addition, competitiveness in Japan tends to be between groups rather than between individuals. To test the hypothesis that the higher rate of CHD among Japanese-Americans is related to loss of the protective effects of Japanese culture, attempts were made to classify the Japanese of California according to their degree of 'Japaneseness' of culture. One such index of acculturation was labelled 'culture of upbringing.' It reflects the degree to which an individual grew up in a Japanese environment. Figure 5 shows that among the California Japanese, those who were brought

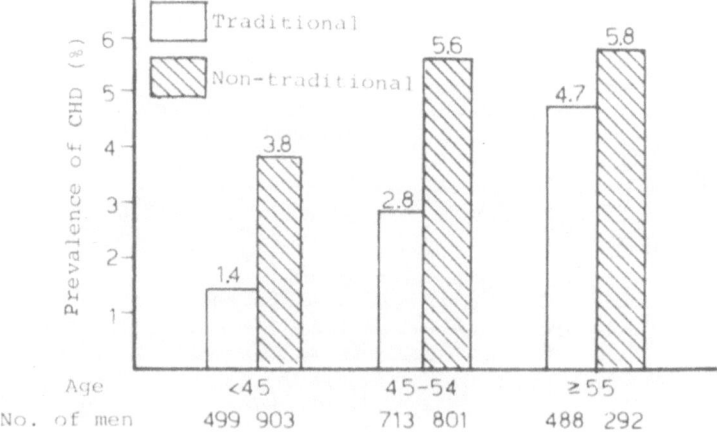

Figure 5. Prevalence of CHD according to culture of upbringing in California Japanese men. By permission of ref. [24].

up in a more traditional pattern have less than half the CHD prevalence of the more non-traditional men[24]. This association between cultural pattern and CHD is independent of differences in blood pressure, serum cholesterol, smoking, relative weight, or serum triglyceride. Using a somewhat different measure, in Hawaii the culture of upbringing has also been shown to be related to incidence of CHD[25].

6. DISCUSSION AND CONCLUSIONS

These studies of men of Japanese ancestry living in different environments have confirmed that blood pressure is a risk factor for the development of CHD in Japan, as well as in the USA. The *relative* risk of CHD associated with blood pressure was similar in Japan and in Japanese-Americans. By contrast, the *absolute* risk associated with a given level of blood pressure depends on the levels of other risk factors. This implies that blood pressure is playing a similar aetiological role in the development of CHD in Japan as in western countries. The relative rarity of heart disease as a complication of elevated blood pressure in Japan is related to the low levels of other risk factors and the low overall rate of CHD occurrence in Japan.

There appears to be a factor (or factors) operating in Japan that puts a hypertensive individual at risk of stroke; and a different set of factors in the USA that puts a hypertensive individual at risk of heart disease. The balance of evidence points to the importance of elevations of serum cholesterol. Serum cholesterol level is related to CHD risk in Japanese men in Japan and in the USA, and the average level of serum cholesterol is 30–40 mg% higher among the Japanese-Americans than among Japanese in Japan. Hence it would be expected, on the basis of serum cholesterol distributions, that the CHD rate would be higher among the Japanese in America. Levels of serum cholesterol do not appear to provide the whole explanation however. The differences in CHD between California and Hawaii (higher in California) are greater than would be expected from the small differences between them in level of serum cholesterol. In addition, the comparison between Hawaii Japanese and Framingham showed differences in levels of serum cholesterol and other risk factors to be inadequate explanations of the lower incidence of CHD in Hawaii[20].

Of course, in the search for causes, the statement that higher levels of serum cholesterol are part of the 'explanation' of the higher CHD rate in the USA is incomplete. One wishes to know the reasons for the higher levels. The findings of the Ni-Hon-San studies on dietary fat are similar to those from other studies (e.g. Keys[19]). Comparing whole populations, those with higher levels of saturated fat intake (California and Hawaii) have higher levels of serum cholesterol, and higher rates of heart disease than those with low levels of fat intake (Japan). Within population groups, however, little association has been found between an individual's level of fat intake and his or her level of serum cholesterol or his or her risk of CHD. In the present study, the one exception to this was the finding in Japan of a correlation between grams of saturated fat in the diet and level of serum cholesterol. Apart from this exception, the failure to find the expected associations with dietary fat have been ascribed to the difficulties of accurately characterizing individual diets [26]. It seems unlikely that this could be the sole reason for the negative findings on diet within populations. More likely is that differences between populations in the level of fat intake are indeed causally related to differences between them in the risk of CHD. *Within* populations, however, factors other than dietary fat intake appear to be responsible for interindividual differences in risk.

Within the California population and separately in Hawaii, it was possible to test the hypothesis that there are features of Japanese culture which are protective against the type of stresses that lead to CHD [23]. Evidence was found that Japanese-Americans who were more traditional in their culture had a lower frequency of CHD than those who were more Americanized. There was, however, little association between the cultural features studied and levels of blood pressure.

Putting these various findings together, we are left with a complex web of causation: (a) smoking is related to CHD only when the overall rate of occurrence of CHD is high; (b) blood pressure is significantly related to CHD risk in all three Japanese populations studied, but the absolute level of CHD risk is dependent on the level of other factors; (c) these other factors appear to include both level of serum cholesterol and dietary fat intake, but also other features of a traditional Japanese way of life that may be related to ways of handling stress.

REFERENCES

1. Stamler J: Lectures on preventive cardiology. New York: Grune and Stratton, 1967.
2. Miall WE, Campo ED, Fodor J, Rhode JRN, Ruiz L, Standard KL, Swan AV: Longitudinal study of heart disease in a Jamaican rural population. 2. Factors influencing mortality. Bull WHO 46:685-694, 1972.
3. Komachi Y, et al.: Geographic and occupational comparisons of risk factors in cardiovascular disease in Japan. Jpn Circ J 35:189, 1971.
4. Winkelstein W, Kagan A, Kato H, Sacks S: Epidemiologic studies of coronary heart disease and stroke in Japanese men living in Japan, Hawaii and California: blood pressure distribution. Am J Epidemiol 102:502-513, 1975.

5. Gordon T: Further mortality experience among Japanese Americans. Public Health Rep 82:973-984, 1967.

6. Worth RM, Rhoads G, Kagan A, Kato H, Syme SL: Epidemiologic studies of coronary heart disease and stroke in Japanese men living in Japan, Hawaii and California: mortality. Am J Epidemiol 102:481-490, 1975.

7. Nichaman MZ, Hamilton HB, Kagan A, Grier T, Sacks ST, Syme SL: Epidemiologic studies of coronary heart disease and stroke in Japanese men living in Japan, Hawaii and California: distribution of biochemical risk factors. Am J Epidemiol 102:491-501, 1975.

8. Kagan A, Marmot MG, Kato H: The Ni-Hon-San study of cardiovascular disease epidemiology: population characteristics and epidemiology of stroke. (This volume, chapter 26.)

9. Kagan A, Harris BR, Winkelstein W, et al.: Epidemiologic studies of coronary heart disease and stroke in Japanese men living in Japan, Hawaii and California — demographic, physical, dietary, and biochemical characteristics. J Chronic Dis 27:345-364, 1974.

10. Takahashi N, Kato K, Suzuki K, Watanabe H, Furumi C, Kuroda M, Koyama S: Epidemiologic studies on hypertension and coronary heart disease in a Japanese rural population. III. Electrocardiographic findings in Chiyoda. Jpn Heart J 5:37-48, 1964.

11. Johnson KG, Yano K, Kato H: Coronary heart disease in Hiroshima. Report of a six-year period of surveillance, 1958–1964. Am J Public Health 58:1355-1367, 1968.

12. Rose GA, Blackburn H: Cardiovascular survey methods. WHO Monogr Ser 56, 1968.

13. Marmot MG, Syme SL, Kagan A, Kato H, Cohen JB, Belsky J: Epidemiologic studies of coronary heart disease and stroke in Japanese men living in Japan, Hawaii and California: prevalence of coronary and hypertensive heart disease and associated risk factors. Am J Epidemiol 102:514-525, 1975.

14. Marmot MG, Syme SL, Kagan A, Kato H: The use of a standard questionnaire to diagnose angina pectoris in international studies. Presented at the sixth annual meeting of the Society for Epidemiologic Research, Winnipeg, Canada, 21–23 June 1973.

15. Robertson TL, Kato H, Rhoads GG, et al.: Epidemiologic studies of coronary heart disease and stroke in Japanese men living in Japan, Hawaii and California: incidence of myocardial infarction and death from coronary heart disease. Am J Cardiol 39:239-243, 1977.

16. Robertson TL, Kato H, Gordon T, et al.: Epidemiologic studies of coronary heart disease and stroke in Japanese men living in Japan, Hawaii and California: coronary heart disease risk factors in Japan and Hawaii. Am J Cardiol 39:244-249, 1977.

17. Rhoads GG, Kagan A, Yano K: Usefulness of community surveillance for the ascertainment of coronary heart disease and stroke. Int J Epidemiol 4:265-279, 1975.

18. Morris JN, Marr JW, Clayton DG: Diet and heart: a postscript. Br Med J 2:1307-1314, 1977.

19. Keys A (ed): Coronary heart disease in seven countries. Circulation [Suppl 1] 41:1–211, 1970.

20. Gordon T, Garcia-Palmieri MR, Kagan A, Kannel WB, Schiffman J: Differences

in coronary heart disease in Framingham, Honolulu and Puerto Rico. J Chronic Dis 27:329-344, 1974.

21. Kato H, Tillotson J, Nichaman MZ, Rhoads GG, Hamilton HB: Epidemiologic studies of coronary heart disease and stroke in Japanese men living in Japan, Hawaii and California: serum lipids and diet. Am J Epidemiol 97:372-385, 1973.

22. Yano K, Rhoads GG, Kagan A, Tillotson J: Dietary intake and the risk of coronary heart disease in Japanese men living in Hawaii. Am J Clin Nutr 31:1270-1279, 1978.

23. Matsumoto YS: Social stress and coronary heart disease in Japan: a hypothesis. Milbank Mem Fund Q 48:9-36, 1970.

24. Marmot MG, Syme SL: Acculturation and coronary heart disease in Japanese Americans. Am J Epidemiol 104:225-247, 1976.

25. Yano K, Blackwelder WC, Kagan A, Rhoads GG, Cohen JB, Marmot MG: Childhood cultural experience and the incidence of coronary heart disease in Hawaii Japanese men. Am J Epidemiol 109:440-450, 1979.

26. Epstein FH: Nutrition, atherosclerosis and coronary heart disease: evidence from epidemiological observations. Atherosclerosis Rev 5:149-182, 1979.

28. A COMPARATIVE STUDY OF BLOOD PRESSURE AND SODIUM INTAKE IN BELGIUM AND IN KOREA

H. Kesteloot, B.C. Park, C.S. Lee, E. Brems-Heyns, and J.V. Joossens

Although the value of international studies in the field of epidemiology and especially concerning the distribution and causation of cardiovascular diseases is now widely recognized[1], few standardized international comparative studies on blood pressure have been performed. This is the more astonishing since hypertensive disease, in contrast to ischemic disease, is an almost universal problem. Much remains to be learned about the exact geographical distribution of blood pressure and of the factors that are associated with blood pressure in different populations. The purpose of our study was to demonstrate the practical value of using home reading and to perform a comparative cross-sectional survey of the relationship between urinary 24-h sodium and potassium excretion, as a measure of intake, and arterial blood pressure in two different populations.

1. METHODOLOGY

The procedure used to measure arterial blood pressure (ABP) was as follows. Both in Belgium and in Korea, blood pressure was measured by the participants themselves[2]. The same type of blood pressure recorder was used in both countries (model auto-test SK, Presso-Stabil). In order to obtain precise BP data, it was necessary to have the BP meters periodically checked, which was done by direct comparison with a mercury manometer.

The more-detailed procedure has been published[3, 4]. In brief, the participants recorded their blood pressures (BP) while in the standing and lying position, both when rising in the morning and when retiring in the evening. Both systolic blood pressure (SBP) and diastolic blood pressure (DBP), phase 5, were recorded to the nearest even number. Blood pressure was measured during three consecutive days in Korea and during ten consecutive days in Belgium. During the period of blood pressure measurement, 24-h urine was collected, and samples were taken for analysis of electrolyte and creatinine content. Aliquots of the 24-h Korean urine were sent to Belgium where all urinary determinations were performed.

H. Kesteloot, J.V. Joossens (eds.), Epidemiology of Arterial Blood Pressure, 453–470.

The Korean population group discussed in this article differs from the group on which the BP data have been published previously [4] and for which no urinary electrolyte excretion data are available. The group studied consists of two subgroups, one living in the city of Seoul in a densely populated area, and the other living in the countryside in a farming area about 200 miles southeast of Seoul. A third group living in Seoul has also been examined, but this group was more heterogeneous and has not been analyzed separately. Those data, however, have been included in the final analysis.

The measurements in Korea were carried out from mid-September to mid-December. At that time, the climate is relatively temporate, thus minimizing the loss of electrolytes through sweat. Traditionally, salt (i.e., sodium chloride) consumption in Korea is very high and three gradients are recognized: a higher salt consumption is present in the farming area compared with the city, in the south compared with the north, and in lower compared with higher social classes.

In Belgium and in Korea, participation was voluntary, since a strict randomization was impossible. No subjects taking drugs that could influence BP were included in the investigation. In Korea most participants were relatives or neighbors of medical students or nurses, who introduced to them the method of ABP home reading.

The participants of the Belgian population group studied from 1970 to 1974 [2] belong to a community living in or near the city of Leuven. The participants are mostly from the middle social class, many of them affiliated with the University of Leuven and in all probability somewhat more health-conscious than the population at large. They participated on a voluntary basis.

Statistical data processing of the study was performed by means of multiple regression analysis (MRA). Thus, the independent contribution of each factor to the dependent variable can be determined, taking into account all factors included in the analysis. The MRA has been performed in a stepdown fashion, eliminating at each step the least significant variable until all remaining independent variables are significant at the $P < 0.05$ level.

The 24-h urinary creatinine value has also been included in order to compensate for possible variations in the completeness of the 24-h urinary collection. The mean value of all variables, both dependent and independent, obtained in each subject during three days in Korea and ten days in Belgium, has been used in the analysis.

Covariance analysis of the data was also performed with the introduction, depending on the data analyzed, of group (Korea or Belgium) and/or sex. In order to simplify the analysis, only the linear terms of age, height/weight^2 (Quetelet index) and sodium, potassium, and creatinine were included in the analysis as independent variables. The covariance analysis was performed by means of multiple regression analysis, using a stepdown procedure until all residual variables were significant at the $P < 0.05$ level.

As dependent variables SBP and DBP were used, and as independent variables the measured variables mentioned above together with dummy variables for group, sex and group, and group $\times$ sex, and the interaction of the dummy variables with the measured independent variables.

In Korea heart rate was also measured at the time of each BP measurement, and the data were analyzed separately (Table 1).

Table 1. Multivariate analysis of blood pressure: men and women/Belgium and Korea (N = 758).

Factors included in the analysis				
Age (years)	G (BE + 1, KO − 1)	$G \times A$	$S \times A$	$G \times S \times A$
W/H^2 (W: kg; H: cm)	S (M + 1, F − 1)	$G \times W/H^2$	$S \times W/H^2$	$G \times S \times W/H^2$
Na (mmol)	GS	$G \times Na$	$S \times Na$	$G \times S \times Na$
K (mmol)		$G \times K$	$S \times K$	$G \times S \times K$
Creat (mg)		$G \times Creat$	$S \times Creat$	$G \times S \times Creat$

M, males; F, females; G, group; S, sex; GS, interaction between group and sex. The interactions with G, S, and G $\times$ S were used on within data from Korea (KO) and Belgium (BE) (1968), from both sexes (S) or on the total data (G $\times$ S).

Finally, the data from Korea and Belgium were also analyzed separately, but not the combined data, including as independent variables higher powers (up to the third power) of age, weight, height, and sodium together with the linear terms for potassium and creatinine. The independent t-values for sodium and potassium were determined from this analysis.

In all subgroups, the value of the multiple correlation coefficient increased whenever higher powers of age, height, weight, and sodium were included. The multiple regression equations obtained in Belgium are presented in Table 1.

2. RESULTS

2.1. Anthropometric data, urinary electrolyte excretion, and BP

Table 2 shows that the anthropometric characteristics and the urinary electrolyte excretion and blood pressure are somewhat higher in the farming area than in the city area. The mean potassium and calcium excretion values are also higher in the farming area. Tables 3–5 present the data obtained in Korea and in Belgium, as well as the combined data.

Table 2. Anthropometric data, urinary electrolyte excretion, and blood pressure; mean values ±standard deviation: men and women/Korea.

	Seoul			Farming area		
	M (N=43)	F (N=51)	M+F (N=94)	M (N=44)	F (N=61)	M+F (N=105)
m̄ Age (years)	41.1±11.8	40.6±11.6	41±11.7	39.9±14.5	41.8±14.7	41±14.6
m̄ W (kg)	59.6±7.8	50.6±8	54.7±9	58.1±7.1	47.6±5.9	51.9±8.2
m̄ H (cm)	165.8±7.5	153±6.1	158.8±9.3	164.9±5.8	154.2±4.7	158.6±7.4
m̄ Na (mmol/24 h)	261±125	276±99	269±112	321±125	282±95	298±110
m̄ K (mmol/24 h)	39±20	40±16	40±18	58±29	62±32	60±31
m̄ Ca (mmol/24 h)	4.8±2.9	4.9±2.6	4.8±2.7	7.3±4.8	5±3.6	6±4.3
m̄ Creat (g/24 h)	1.1±0.45	0.9±0.27	0.98±0.38	1.2±0.48	0.94±0.42	1.05±0.46
m̄ SBP (mmHg)	132.2±8.6	128.5±16.4	129.8±14.8	132.2±13.2	130.4±22	131.2±18.8
m̄ DBP (mmHg)	88.1±8.6	84.9±10.8	86.3±10	87.7±10.2	86.2±13.2	86.8±12

M, males; F, females; W, weight; H, height.

Table 3. Anthropometric data, urinary electrolyte excretion, and blood pressure; mean values ±standard deviation: men and women/Korea.

	M (N = 200)	F (N = 258)	M + F (N = 458)
$\bar{m}$ Age (years)	37.5 ± 14.3	39.7 ± 13.7	38.8 ± 14
$\bar{m}$ H (cm)	166.6 ± 6.6	155.4 ± 5.2	160.3 ± 8
$\bar{m}$ W (kg)	60.2 ± 8.2	50.4 ± 7.3	54.7 ± 9.1
$\bar{m}$ W/H² (×100)	0.22 ± 0.024	0.21 ± 0.029	0.21 ± 0.027
$\bar{m}$ Na (mmol/24 h)	294.2 ± 133.4	266.5 ± 107.6	278.6 ± 120.2
$\bar{m}$ K (mmol/24 h)	57.1 ± 43.8	54.7 ± 27.5	55.8 ± 35.6
$\bar{m}$ SBP (mmHg)	125.2 ± 14.2	120.5 ± 18.6	122.6 ± 16.9
$\bar{m}$ DBP (mmHg)	81.2 ± 10.6	77.9 ± 12.0	79.4 ± 11.5

M, males; F, females; H, height; W, weight.

Table 4. Anthropometric data, urinary electrolyte excretion, and blood pressure; mean values ±standard deviation: men and women/Belgium.

	M (N = 133)	F (N = 167)	M + F (N = 300)
$\bar{m}$ Age (years)	39.3 ± 11.0	40.0 ± 12.2	39.7 ± 11.7
$\bar{m}$ H (cm)	174.0 ± 6.4	161.3 ± 6.4	166.9 ± 9.0
$\bar{m}$ W (kg)	75.4 ± 10.8	60.7 ± 8.2	67.2 ± 11.9
$\bar{m}$ W/H² (×100)	0.25 ± 0.033	0.23 ± 0.031	0.24 ± 0.033
$\bar{m}$ Na (mmol/24 h)	183.9 ± 44.6	152.6 ± 43.8	166.5 ± 46.8
$\bar{m}$ K/(mmol/24 h)	76.7 ± 15.4	65.3 ± 12.5	70.4 ± 15.0
$\bar{m}$ SBP (mmHg)	121.4 ± 12.6	114.6 ± 13.9	117.6 ± 13.7
$\bar{m}$ DBP (mmHg)	78.5 ± 8.6	73.0 ± 8.4	75.4 ± 8.9

M, males; F, females; H, height; W, weight.

Table 5. Anthropometric data, urinary excretion of electrolytes, and blood pressure; mean values ±standard deviation: men and women/Korea and Belgium.

	M (N = 333)	F (N = 425)	M + F (N = 758)
$\bar{m}$ Age (years)	38.2 ± 13.0	39.8 ± 13.1	39.1 ± 13.1
$\bar{m}$ W (kg)	169.6 ± 7.5	157.7 ± 6.4	59.7 ± 12.0
$\bar{m}$ H (cm)	66.3 ± 11.9	54.5 ± 9.2	162.9 ± 9.0
$\bar{m}$ W/H² (×100)	0.23 ± 0.032	0.22 ± 0.032	0.22 ± 0.032
$\bar{m}$ Na (mmol/24 h)	250.2 ± 119.9	221.7 ± 104.3	234.2 ± 112.2
$\bar{m}$ K (mmol/24 h)	64.9 ± 36.3	58.9 ± 23.4	61.6 ± 30.1
$\bar{m}$ SBP (mmHg)	123.7 ± 13.7	118.2 ± 17.1	120.6 ± 15.9
$\bar{m}$ DBP (mmHg)	80.1 ± 9.9	76.0 ± 11.0	77.8 ± 10.4

M, males; F, females; W, weight; H, height.

The data from Korea include all the data obtained, most of them from Seoul city. It is apparent that at about the same mean age, important differences in height and weight exist between the Belgian and Korean populations. From the height/weight ratio, it clearly appears that the Belgian population is more obese. Important differences also exist in the mean daily urinary electrolyte excretion, with a markedly higher excretion in Korea. This difference is even more clear when the existing differences in body weight are taken into account.

Table 6. Blood pressure and urinary excretion of electrolytes on different days; mean values ± standard deviation: men and women/Korea.

	SBP (mmHg)	DBP (mmHg)	Na (mmol/24 h)	K (mmol/24 h)	Creat (mg/24 h)
MEN[a]					
Day 1	126.0 ± 14.6	81.5 ± 10.7	390 ± 146	57 ± 45	1160 ± 707
Day 2	124.7 ± 14.3	81.0 ± 11.0	291 ± 150	55 ± 45	1133 ± 682
Day 3	124.9 ± 14.6	81.0 ± 10.8	302 ± 154	59 ± 49	1180 ± 776
WOMEN[b]					
Day 1	121.7 ± 19.8	78.4 ± 12.9	264 ± 123	53 ± 29	870 ± 384
Day 2	119.7 ± 18.5	77.7 ± 12.0	265 ± 120	55 ± 33	892 ± 515
Day 3	120.2 ± 18.8	77.4 ± 12.4	270 ± 124	56 ± 34	912 ± 594

[a] N = 200, $\bar{m}$ age = 38 years, $\bar{m}$ height = 167 cm, $\bar{m}$ weight = 60 kg.
[b] N = 258, $\bar{m}$ age = 39.7 years, $\bar{m}$ height = 165 cm, $\bar{m}$ weight = 50 kg.

Table 7. Blood pressure and urinary excretion of electrolytes on different days; mean values ± standard deviation: men and women/Belgium.

	SBP (mmHg)	DBP (mmHg)	Na (mmol/24 h)	K (mmol/24 h)	Creat (mg/24 h)
MEN[a]					
Day 1	121.9 ± 13.9	79.0 ± 9.3	193 ± 70	79 ± 23	1835 ± 370
Day 2	121.2 ± 13.5	78.8 ± 9.0	189 ± 73	77 ± 20	1820 ± 350
Day 3	121.7 ± 12.5	78.8 ± 8.8	186 ± 82	79 ± 26	1849 ± 390
WOMEN[b]					
Day 1	115.8 ± 14.8	73.5 ± 9.4	153 ± 57	66 ± 23	1269 ± 319
Day 2	114.8 ± 14.9	73.4 ± 9.1	156 ± 62	65 ± 22	1298 ± 262
Day 3	114.9 ± 14.4	73.1 ± 9.0	149 ± 59	66 ± 20	1307 ± 344

[a] N = 133, $\bar{m}$ age = 39 years, $\bar{m}$ height = 174 cm, $\bar{m}$ weight = 75 kg.
[b] N = 167, $\bar{m}$ age = 40 years, $\bar{m}$ height = 161 cm, $\bar{m}$ weight = 61 kg.

As expected, sodium excretion is higher in the farming area than in Seoul, but the potassium excretion is markedly lower in Korea and especially in Seoul than in Belgium. For a higher body weight, the creatinine excretion is somewhat lower in Seoul than in the farming area. This possibly points to a slightly incomplete urine collection in Seoul.

The mean blood pressure, i.e., the mean of all recorded blood pressure measurements for the three participating groups and for both sexes, is markedly higher in Korea than in Belgium, and slightly higher in the farming area than in Seoul, except for diastolic pressure in male subjects. Both SBP and DBP are higher in men than in women, this difference being more marked in Belgium than in Korea. The validity of the approach using home reading for the measurement of BP is confirmed by the small difference in mean BP found between the different days (Tables 6 and 7).

2.2. Multiple regression and covariance analysis

The mean systolic and diastolic blood pressure, i.e., the mean value of all systolic and diastolic blood pressures obtained in one day, has been correlated with different independent variables. The results are presented separately for the different population groups. For Korea, heart rate has been included in some of the analyses. This heart rate was measured at the time of each blood pressure measurement, and the mean heart rate of all values obtained each day was used. Heart rate was not determined in Belgium, and therefore this factor has been omitted from the overall analysis. All factors included in the multivariate analysis are listed in Table 1. As can be seen from the MRA, sodium is positively correlated with SBP and DBP in several subgroups in Korea and in Belgium, and in the combined data from Belgium and Korea.

In some subgroups, the potassium is negatively correlated with BP. As expected, age and the Quetelet index (weight/height^2) are also correlated with BP in nearly all subgroups. The independent contribution of sodium to BP is small. For every increase in urinary sodium excretion of 100 mmol/24 h, SBP and DBP increase about 1–3 mmHg, depending on the sex. Whenever potassium is significantly correlated with BP, its negative influence per mmol is about three times greater than that of sodium (Tables 8–16). The independent t-values for Na and K both for SBP and DBP, together with the multiple correlation coefficients when all significant factors are included, are listed in Table 17. From this table, it appears that the multiple correlation coefficient obtained in Belgium is always higher than the value obtained from the Korean data. It also demonstrates that the inclusion of heart rate in the Korean data significantly improves the multiple correlation coefficient obtained.

In order to further clarify the problem, we have submitted the BP data to

Table 8. Multivariate analysis of blood pressure: men/Korea (N = 200).

	BP		t-value		BP		t-value
$\bar{m}$ SBP = (mmHg)	107.6			$\bar{m}$ DBP = (mmHg)	67.84		
	+0.219	A	3.1		+0.2361	A	4.6
	+0.00609	Creat	3.1		+0.003848	Creat	3.4
	+0.0271	Na	3.0				
	-0.0980	K	-3.1				

$R = 0.37$, $R^2 = 0.14$, SEy $= 13.3$ mmHg $R = 0.34$, $R^2 = 0.12$, SEy $= 10.0$ mmHg

In this table and in Tables 9–16: A, age (years); H, height (cm); W, weight (kg); Na, sodium (mmol/24 h); K, potassium (mmol/24 h); Creat, creatinine (mg/24 h); R, multiple regression coefficient.

Table 9. Multivariate analysis of blood pressure: women/Korea (N = 258).

	BP		t-value		BP		t-value
$\bar{m}$ SDP = (mmHg)	87.25			$\bar{m}$ DBP = (mmHg)	64.45		
	+0.4213	A	5.2		+0.2451	A	4.6
	+7916.96	W/H^2	2.0		+0.01414	Na	2.1

$R = 0.32$, $R^2 = 0.10$, SEy $= 17.7$ mmHg $R = 0.28$, $R^2 = 0.08$, SEy $= 11.6$ mmHg

Table 10. Multivariate analysis of blood pressure: men and women/Korea (N = 458).

$\bar{m}$ SBP = (mmHg)	BP		*t*-value	$\bar{m}$ DBP = (mmHg)	BP		*t*-value
	90.5				66.62		
	+0.3292	A	5.9		+0.2386	A	6.4
	+5808.49	W/H^2	2.0		+1.38	M: +1; F: −1	3.7
	+0.0212	Na	2.8		+0.00362	Creat	2.6
	−0.06408	K	−2.2				
	+0.0047	Creat	2.6				
	+6.15	M: +1; F: −1	2.8				
	−0.1167	S×A	−2.1				

$R = 0.37$, $R^2 = 0.14$, SEy = 15.9 mmHg

$R = 0.33$, $R^2 = 0.11$, SEy = 10.9 mmHg

M, male; F, female; S, sex.

Table 11. Multivariate analysis of blood pressure: men/Belgium (N = 133).

SBP = (mmHg)	BP =		*t*-value	DBP = (mmHg)	BP		*t*-value
	83.50				50.55		
	+0.487	A	5.5		±0.329	A	5.5
	+7531.47	W/H^2	2.6		+6016.77	W/H^2	3.0

$R = 0.51$, $R^2 = 0.26$, SEy = 10.9 mmHg

$R = 0.53$, $R^2 = 0.28$, SEy = 7.31 mmHg

Table 12. Multivariate analysis of blood pressure: women/Belgium (N = 167).

SBP = (mmHg)	BP		*t*-value	DBP = (mmHg)	BP		*t*-value
	75.87				53.63		
	+0.5181	A	6.5		+0.3863	A	9.0
	+7690.31	W/H^2	2.5		+0.0254	Na	2.1

$R = 0.55$, $R^2 = 0.30$, SEy = 11.7 mmHg

$R = 0.59$, $R^2 = 0.35$, SEy = 6.80 mmHg

Table 13. Multivariate analysis of blood pressure: men and women/Belgium (N = 300).

	BP		t-value		BP		t-value
SBP = (mmHg)	79.5			DBP = (mmHg)	51.2		
	+0.506	A	8.6		±0.351	A	9.5
	+7634.85	W/H^4	3.5		+4377.91	W/H^2	3.3
	+1.926	S×Creat	4.4		+1060.69	S×W/H^2	6.1

$R = 0.57$, $R^2 = 0.33$, SEy = 11.3 mmHg $R = 0.61$, $R^2 = 0.38$, SEy = 7.0 mmHg

S, sex.

Table 14. Multivariate analysis of blood pressure: men/Korea and Belgium (N = 333).

	BP		t-value		BP		t-value
$\bar{m}$ SBP = (mmHg)	87.07			$\bar{m}$ DBP = (mmHg)	59.59		
	+0.368	A	6.0		+0.245	A	6.5
	+5933.3	W/H^2	2.3		+5104.3	W/H^2	2.8
	+0.0218	Na	2.9		−0.0041	G×Creat	−4.5
	−0.0743	K	−2.7		+1762.15	G×W/H^2	2.8
	+0.00548	Creat	3.2				
	−8.82	BE: +1; KO: −1	−3.5				
	+0.1564	G×A	2.6				

$R = 0.44$, $R^2 = 0.20$, SEy = 12.4 mmHg $R = 0.42$, $R^2 = 0.18$, SEy = 9.0 mmHg

BE, Belgium; KO, Korea; G, group.

Table 15. Multivariate analysis of blood pressure: women/Belgium and Korea (N = 425).

BP		t-value	BP		t-value
$\bar{m}$ SBP =	81.9		$\bar{m}$ DBP =	52.6	
(mmHg)	+0.442 A	7.6	(mmHg)	+0.297 A	7.9
	+8265.9 W/H²	3.2		+4172.5 W/H²	2.5
	-3.78 BE: +1; KO: -1	-4.5		+0.0116 Na	1.9
				-0.002 G×Creat	-3.4

$R = 0.41$, $R^2 = 0.17$, SEy = 15.6 mmHg

$R = 0.42$, $R^2 = 0.19$, SEy = 10.0 mmHg

BE, Belgium; KO, Korea; G, group.

Table 16. Multivariate analysis of blood pressure: men and women/Belgium and Korea (N = 758).

BP		t-value	BP		t-value
$\bar{m}$ SBP =	82.52		$\bar{m}$ DBP =	55.78	
(mmHg)	+0.3845 A	9.18	(mmHg)	+0.2985 A	10.42
	+7214.06 W/H²	3.94		+4107.89 W/H²	3.31
	+0.01908 Na	3.02		+0.0082 Na	2.13
	-0.04758 K	-1.99		+0.04273 G×A	2.14
	+0.004184 Creat	2.79		+465.27 G×S×W/H²	2.78
	-3.08 G	-3.75		-0.002776 Creat	-4.53
	+4.99 S	2.97		+2.186 S	5.91
	-0.0836 S×A	-2.05			

$R = 0.45$, $R^2 = 0.20$, SEy = 14.32 mmHg

$R = 0.47$, $R^2 = 0.22$, SEy = 9.75 mmHg

G, group; S, sex.

Table 17. Independent *t*-values Na and K.

		N	SBP		DBP		R [a]	
			Na	K	Na	K	SBP	DBP
Belgium	M	133	—	—	—	—	0.51	0.53
	F	167	—	—	+ 2.01*	—	0.55	0.59
	M + F	300	—	—	—	—	0.57	0.61
Korea	M	200	+ 3.0**	− 3.1**	—	—	0.37	0.34
	F	258	—	—	+ 2.1*	—	0.32	0.28
	M + F	458	+ 2.8**	− 2.2 +	—	—	0.37	0.33
Korea (+ HR)	M	200	+ 3.4***	− 2.6**	—	—	0.46	0.46
	F	258	+ 2.4**	—	+ 2.9**	—	0.41	0.44
	M + F	458	+ 4.1***	—	+ 2.6**	—	0.45	0.47
BE + KO	M	333	+ 2.9**	− 2.7**	—	—	0.44	0.42
	F	425	—	—	+ 2.0 +	—	0.41	0.42
	M + F	758	+ 3.0**	− 2.0*	+ 2.1*	—	0.45	0.47

[a] R = value obtained with all significant factors included.
*$P < 0.05$; **$P < 0.01$; ***$P < 0.001$.
M, Males; F, Females.

MRA with the inclusion of higher powers of age, height, and weight and also of sodium. This was done because previous work had shown the relationship of age, height, and weight with BP to be nonlinear [5, 6].

It was also postulated that since the effect of sodium on BP could be pharmacological, a nonlinear effect could also be expected. The multiple

Table 20. BP vs A, A^2, A^3, W, W^2, W^3, H, H^2, H^3, Na, Na^2, Na^3, K, Creat (sex; sex × independent variable) [a]: men (N = 199); women (N = 257)/Korea (N = 458).

t-value [b]		Na	Na^2	Na^3	K	R
M	SBP	2.9	− 2.2	—	− 2.9	0.45
	DBP	—	—	—	—	0.37
F	SBP	—	—	—	—	0.37
	DBP	2.2	—	—	—	0.31
M + F	SBP	2.9	− 2.0	—	− 2.3	0.42
	DBP	—	—	—	—	0.35
M + HR	SBP	3.2	− 2.4	—	—	0.52
	DBP	—	—	—	—	0.47
F + HR	SBP	2.7	− 2.1	—	—	0.48
	DBP	3.2	—	—	—	0.47
M + F + HR	SBP	3.8	− 2.8	—	—	0.50
	DBP	2.5	—	—	—	0.48

[a] M, males; F, females; A, age (years); W, weight (kg); H, height (cm); Na, sodium (mmol/24 h); K, potassium (mmol/24 h); Creat, creatinine (mg/24 h); R, multiple correlation coefficient; HR, heart rate (beats/min).
[b] The *t*-value obtained from the final multiple regression equation, containing factors significant at $P < 0.05$ level.

465

Table 18. BP vs A, A^2, A^3, W, W^2, W^3, H, H^2, H^3, Na, Na^2, Na^3, K, Creat (mean of ten days of measurement): men/Belgium (N = 133).

SBP = (mmHg)		t-value	DBP = (mmHg)		t-value
+56.08			+49.69		
+0.3166	A	+4.0	+0.1988	W	+3.4
+0.04281	A^2	+6.3	+0.3510	A	+6.1
+0.6127	W	+4.4			
+0.01496	W^2	+2.4			
−0.000819	W^3	−2.0			
+0.00000415	Na^3	+2.0			

R = 0.69, R^2 = 0.48, SEy = 9.3 mmHg   R = 0.54, R^2 = 0.29, SEy = 7.26 mmHg

Table 19. BP vs A, A^2, A^3, W, W^2, W^3, H, H^2, H^3, Na, Na^2, Na^3, K, Creat (mean of ten days of measurement): women/Belgium (N = 167).

SBP = (mmHg)		t-value	DBP = (mmHg)		t-value
+89.20			+51.03		
+0.5076	A	+7.1	+0.3590	A	+8.4
+0.02123	A^2	+4.5	+0.0008057	W^3	+3.2
+0.02832	W^2	+3.4	+0.04939	Na	+2.8
			−0.000004548	Na^3	−2.5

R = 0.62, R^2 = 0.38, SEy = 11.0 mmHg   R = 0.63, R^2 = 0.40, SEy = 0.59 mmHg

correlation coefficients obtained were higher than the values obtained in the previously mentioned more simple form of analysis. In Belgium, a significant correlation between Na and BP was demonstrated in certain subgroups. The results from the MRA for men and women in Belgium are presented in Tables 18 and 19, and the independent t-values for Na and K for all data are listed in Tables 20 and 21.

In MRA, the 24-h urinary calcium excretion was never correlated with BP. The independent significant correlation of Na and K with BP persisted when creatinine was omitted from the MRA.

Table 21. BP vs A, A^2, A^3, W, W^2, W^3, H, H^2, H^3, Na, Na^2, Na^3, K, Creat [a]: men and women/Belgium (N = 300).

t-value [b]		Na	Na^2	Na^3	K	R
M (N = 133)	SBP	—	—	2.0	—	0.69
	DBP	—	—	—	—	0.54
F (N = 167)	SBP	—	—	—	—	0.62
	DBP	2.8	—	− 2.5	—	0.63

[a], [b] For explanation, see footnotes to Table 20.

3. DISCUSSION

It is generally acknowledged that blood pressure in the population is one of the most difficult biological variables to be measured in a standardized way. In a large study in which blood pressure was measured in 42,804 men, less than 10% of its variation could be explained although, with the exception of heart rate, more factors were included in the MRA than in the present analysis [6]. At a symposium on the methodology of blood pressure measurement in epidemiological surveys, the procedure of home reading of ABP was recommended [7]. The major advantage of this method lies in the removal of one of the most important factors increasing the variability of blood pressure measurements, namely the presence of a doctor or medical technical personnel. The influence of hospital surroundings on BP is also automatically removed.

In the present study, highly significant correlations with both SBP and DBP were found for age, weight, height, heart rate, and some urinary electrolytes. Using a total group of only 758 participants, it was possible to explain 10%–45% of the total variation in ABP. The independent contribution of weight, age, and heart rate to ABP consists of a positive relationship, whereas ABP is negatively correlated with height. The statistical effect of the heart rate on ABP is of such an order of magnitude that its measurement merits inclusion in future epidemiological studies.

One of the most interesting findings in our study is the independent positive relationship between the 24-h sodium excretion and both SBP and DBP in several subgroups. Such a significant correlation does, however, not necessarily prove a causal role of dietary sodium in the genesis of arterial hypertension. MRA performed in a stepdown fashion does not select the variables in a logical way. Thus, the variables analyzed by MRA must be selected carefully and logic should prevail when interpreting the final results. We included age, height, weight, and heart rate in the MRA because these factors are known to influence BP and Na and K in order to investigate their possible independent correlation with BP. Our findings demonstrating a significant association of ABP with 24-h urinary sodium, both between Belgium and Korea, and within these populations, and in view of other existing evidence [8–10, 14], strongly support the concept of a causal association between BP and sodium intake.

Although many data demonstrate that ABP is low and does not increase with age in populations with low dietary sodium intake [8, 11, 12], conclusive evidence linking ABP to sodium intake within populations with a high dietary sodium intake remains scarce [8, 13, 14]. On the contrary, evidence was published showing a relative independence of ABP from daily dietary sodium intake in the range of 90–270 mmol/day, measured either by urinary excretion [15] or by questionnaire [16]. Comparing two Polynesian populations, a higher BP was found in the population with the highest salt intake, but no within-population association between BP and 24-h urinary sodium was demonstrated [17]. Salt intake diminished markedly in northern Japan, from 34.7 to 21.0 g daily, between 1959 and 1971, and was associated with a significant decrease in cerebral hemorrhage [18]. This can best be explained by a concomitant decrease in BP. In an epidemiological study in Newfoundland, the community with the highest BP also had the highest salt consumption [19]. A moderate decrease in sodium consumption was also found to influence blood pressure negatively [20].

In the present study, ABP increases only between 1 and 3 mmHg both for SBP and DBP for an increase of 100 mmol of urinary sodium excretion. Several explanations are possible for the relatively small influence of Na on BP in a within-population study. A prolonged period of high salt intake is probably necessary in order to increase BP markedly, in view of the existing mechanisms for the autoregulation of BP. The sodium/potassium ratio could also be important. Moreover, the issue of the relationship of Na consumption and BP within a population can be obscured by the fact that the level of Na consumption in a given population is relatively uniform. The difficulty of measuring BP and 24-h electrolyte excretion exactly also acts as a confounding factor. In this respect, the significant negative relationship between K and ABP established in this study is interesting, especially as its influence per mmol was about three times greater than that of sodium. This could point to dietary measures other than sodium restriction for lowering ABP. Potassium consumption is lower in Korea than in Belgium, and some populations with a low Na intake have a very high K intake [12]. More epidemiological data on the relationship between K and ABP are highly desirable.

Due to climatological influences, it is possible that in Korea some of the dietary sodium was eliminated through the sweat so that the value found here can be considered to be a minimum value of the daily sodium consumption. Our study confirms the very high sodium content in Korea compared with Belgium and the existent gradient between the city and the farming area. From the creatinine excretion, however, it appears that the urinary collection in the group of Seoul men could be underestimated by approximately 10%; as for a higher body weight, its value is lower than in the farming area.

Concomitantly, our study demonstrates that ABP is considerably higher in Korea than in Belgium, and this confirms the findings in another independent group of Korean subjects [4]. It also demonstrates that the differences in ABP are not due to differences in body build, as they have been included in the MRA. It should be noted that both SBP and DBP are considerably higher in Korea than in southern Japan, while both countries are situated within the same geographic region. In a group of men aged 45–49 years, a mean SBP of 125.7 mmHg and a mean DBP of 80.4 mmHg, measured in the conventional way, were found in southern Japan [21]. The real difference must still be higher, as the same group recorded a lower blood pressure of 9.8 mmHg for SBP and 7.1 mmHg for DBP during home reading [22]. It is known that the salt consumption is considerably lower in South Japan than in Korea, and this has been confirmed by published data on salt consumption in South Japan, which is in the range of 130–320 mmol/day [13, 23]. Comparative studies on ABP in Japanese subjects living in Japan, Hawaii, and California have not shown a higher blood pressure for Japanese living in Japan [22].

Differences in methodology and relative body weight could well explain these findings, as both the incidence of stroke and electrocardiographic signs of left-ventricular hypertrophy were more common in Japan [24]. The incidence of stroke in Korea is also very high and it is one of the major health problems in people aged 50 years and more. Comparison of ABP obtained in different populations has nearly been impossible until now due to differences in methodology, as already mentioned [25].

It would be very interesting to include the blood pressure, measured in a standardized way, and the daily urinary electrolyte excretion of more population groups in the covariance analysis performed in this study, in order to further extend the validity of the observations.

REFERENCES

1. Reid DD: International studies in epidemiology. Am J Epidemiol 102:469-476, 1975.
2. Joossens JV, Brems-Heyns E, Claessens J: The value of home blood pressure recordings: a tool for epidemiological studies. In: Kesteloot H (ed) Methodology and standardization of blood pressure measurement in epidemiological studies. Brussels: CRM/CREST, 1976, pp 85-91.
3. Kesteloot H: Epidemiology of arterial blood pressure. Arch Mal Cœur Vaiss [Suppl] 68:149-151, 1975.
4. Kesteloot H, Song CS, Song JS, Park BC, Brems-Heyns E, Joossens JV: An epidemiological survey of arterial blood pressure in Korea using home reading. In: Rorive E, Van Cauwenberge H (eds) The arterial hypertensive disease. New York: Masson, 1976, pp 141-148.
5. Kesteloot H, Van Houte O: An epidemiological survey of risk factors for ischemic heart disease in 42,804 men. Acta Cardiol [Fasc 5] 27:527-664, 1972.
6. Kesteloot H, Van Houte O: An epidemiological survey of arterial blood pressure in a large male population group. Am J Epidemiol 99:14-29, 1974.
7. Kesteloot H (ed): Methodology and standardization of non-invasive blood pressure measurement in epidemiological studies. Proceedings of a workshop organized in Leuven, 1974. Brussels: CRM/CREST, 1976 (EUR 5544e).
8. Joossens JV: Salt and hypertension, water hardness and cardiovascular death rate (Rev Articles). Triangle 12:9-16, 1973.
9. Joossens JV, Brems-Heyns E: Cerebrovaskulaire sterfte, maagkankersterfte en zoutverbruik. Tijdschr Soc Geneeskd 53:530-534, 1974.
10. Freis ED: Salt, volume and the prevention of hypertension (Rev Articles). Circulation 53:589-595, 1976.
11. Page LB, Damon A, Moellering LC: Antecedents of cardiovascular diseases in six Solomon Islands societies. Circulation 49:1132-1148, 1974.
12. Oliver WJ, Cohen EL, Neel JV: Blood pressure, sodium intake and sodium related hormones in the Yanomamo Indians, a 'no-salt' culture. Circulation 52:146-151, 1975.
13. Sasaki N: The relationship of salt intake to hypertension in the Japanese. Geriatrics 19:735-744, 1964.
14. Dahl LK: Salt and hypertension. Am J Clin Nutr 25:231-244, 1972.
15. Dawber TR, Kannel WE, Donabedian RK, McNamara PM, Pearson G: Environmental factors in hypertension. In: Stamler S, Stamler R, Pullman TN (eds) The epidemiology of hypertension. New York: Grune and Stratton, 1967, pp 225-587.
16. Miall WE: Follow-up study of arterial pressure in the population of a Welsh mining valley. Brux Med J 2:1204-1210, 1959.
17. Prior IAM, Grimley Evans J, Harvey EDB, Davidson F, Lindsey M: Sodium intake and blood pressure in two Polynesian populations. N Engl J Med 279:515-520.
18. Kimura T: An epidemiological study on hypertension. Clin Sci Mol Med 45:103-105, 1973.
19. Fodor JG, Abbott EC, Rusted JE: An epidemiological study of hypertension in Newfoundland. Can Med Assoc J 108:1365-1368, 1973.

20. Parijs J, Joossens JV, Van der Linden L, Verstreken G, Amery A: Moderate sodium restriction and diuretics in the treatment of hypertension. Am Heart J 85:22-34, 1973.
21. Kagan A, Harris BR, Winckelstein W, Johnson KG, Kato H, Syme SL, Rhoads GG, Gay ML, Nichaman MZ, Hamilton HB, Tillotson J: Epidemiologic studies of coronary heart disease and stroke in Japanese men living in Japan, Hawaii and California: demographic, physical and biochemical characteristics. J Chronic Dis 27:345-364, 1974.
22. Winckelstein W, Kagan A, Kato H, Sacks ST: Epidemiologic studies of coronary heart disease and stroke in Japanese men living in Japan, Hawaii and California: blood pressure measurements. Am J Epidemiol 102:502-513, 1975.
23. Komachi I, Iida M, Shimamoto T, Chikayama Y, Takahashi H, Konishi M, Tominaga S: Geographic and occupational comparisons of risk factors in cardio-vascular diseases in Japan. Jpn Circ J 35:189-207, 1971.
24. Marmot MG, Syme SL, Kagan A, Kato H, Cohen JB, Belsky J: Epidemiologic studies of coronary heart disease and stroke in Japanese men living in Japan, Hawaii and California: prevalence of coronary and hypertensive heart disease and associated risk factors. Am J Epidemiol 102:514-525, 1975.
25. Kesteloot H, Van Houte O: The epidemiology of arterial blood pressure. Symposium on hypertension and beta-receptor blockade. Brux Med [Suppl]:29-38, 1974.

29. PROBLEMS OF HYPERTENSION IN THE ASIAN-PACIFIC AREA

S. HATANO

Four years ago when I reviewed the state of art on hypertension in the Asian-Pacific area at the sixth Asian-Pacific Congress of Cardiology, Honolulu, the paucity of the information in many countries struck me, but small buds of research activities, observed here and there at that time [1], have been growing rapidly. The purpose of this paper is to introduce some of this research which, although still in a preliminary stage, has much research potential, and to indicate problems for future investigations.

1. BLOOD PRESSURES IN POPULATIONS

1.1. Limited comparability

Efforts have been made to standardize the procedures of blood pressure determination [2, 3]. The use of a zero-muddler machine [4] was recommended in order to diversify and evade apparent digit preference, but this does not eliminate other measurement errors. Human measurements are always subject to observer bias, and training of examiners is an obvious 'must' at the beginning of an epidemiological study. Not only technical failures but circadian variations of the blood pressure by the time of the day are well known [5], and seasonal variation has been reported [6]. It is also difficult to control the emotional tension of a subject in the encounter with a physician. The common finding of a spontaneous drop of blood pressures in the non-treated group in mild hypertension trials after repeated measurements [7] is partly due to regression toward the mean, but most likely is caused by gradual habituation to the measurement procedure and elimination of excitement of the subjects. Home measurement has been recommended to overcome this [8], but requires good cooperation from the subjects. These are warnings against a comparison of blood pressures when circumstances of the procedures are not thoroughly known and not rigorously controlled. In carefully performed blood pressure measurements, technical variations cannot be very large, though this is difficult to validate. Reported values from selected papers are thus compared as a first attempt.

H. Kesteloot, J.V. Joossens (eds.). Epidemiology of Arterial Blood Pressure, 471–487.

472

1.2. Indicators

Blood pressures in a population are distributed in a unimodal pattern with a slight skew to the right. In order to express the entire picture, medians and other percentiles or distributions provide precise information. Their use, however, is seldom reported in the available literature. In spite of skewness, the mean blood pressure and the standard deviation give a useful idea of blood pressure patterns of populations.

The prevalence of defined hypertension also provides a general idea on the magnitude of the problem and is helpful for planning control measures in a community or a country. In most publications, the WHO criteria have been used, and this facilitates understanding of the blood pressure situations in a given population. Though sensitive for discerning differences, the use of a cutoff point for blood pressures is more vulnerable to between-observer and between-center measurement bias.

Age/sex-specific or age-standardized data must be used for comparative purposes, because of the strong influence of age upon blood pressure. Just reporting prevalence rate of hypertension without referring to the age composition in a few publications does not promote our understanding.

In special cases, the distance of an individual blood pressure from the mean divided by the standard deviation (z-score) is used. This is suitable for the assessment of degrees of resemblance of blood pressures between family members[9] or between repeated measurements in the same subject.

1.3. Comparisons

The mean blood pressure or prevalence of hypertension in an age/sex-specific group varies between populations. These indicators increase with age in a similar manner, and their distributions are similar in American whites[10], Indians from Bombay[11], Japanese nationals[12], rural Koreans[13], Orang Asli from Malaysia[14], Micronesians[15, 16], Singaporeans[17], and Taiwanese[18]. Somewhat lower figures have been reported from rural India[19] and Iran[20], Pakistan[21] and the Philippines[22].

Persistence of low blood pressures and absence of hypertension until old age have been reported from several isolated areas that had little contact with modern civilization; to cite only a few reports from the Asian-Pacific area—Papua New Guinea[23], Pukapuka[24], and the Cook Islands and Solomon Islands[25]. At the other extreme, much higher figures for the blood pressure indicators were reported from some areas, e.g., Akita in northern Japan[26], Chamorros in Guam[15], Polynesians in Rarotonga[24], and workers in Seoul, Korea[27] (the reasons suggested for this are discussed in section 4). These populations are extremely interesting from an epidemiological viewpoint, but they are exceptions. We should not divert our sight from the mainstream: the worldwide 'epidemic of hypertension.'

2. HYPERTENSION IN THE YOUNG

Hypertension in the young has definite implications in Asia because of the predominantly young populations. A slight elevation of blood pressure plays a much worse role when it appears in the young [28] than in the elderly. This is probably because of cumulative effects in the long run, however minimal the cardiovascular strain may be at a younger age.

Rather stable blood pressure rankings of young people [29, 30] have been reported. Hyperreactivity of the sympathetic nervous system in some young subjects can cause hyperkinetic hypertension, but of a limited duration [31]. We therefore need much longer observations in order to confirm these. Distinction between stable and labile high blood pressure would give us more knowledge about the evolution of essential hypertension.

Frank hypertension found in the young [32] is very often secondary to renal, renovascular, or endocrine diseases; the frequency of these, however, is low. A large majority of secondary hypertension is chronic glomerulonephritis, which is difficult to cure. Prevention by treatment of skin and throat infections of infants would be the best way to control it. Some forms of secondary hypertension can be cured by surgery, and early and accurate diagnosis is important.

3. HYPERTENSION AS A COMMUNITY PROBLEM

3.1. Status of patients in the community

Significance of hypertension as a risk factor for a variety of cardiovascular diseases has been confirmed in Asia, too. Stroke is the commonest complication in the Western Pacific area [33–35], while heart failure is the commonest complication in Africa [36] and Pakistan [37, 38] as is renal failure followed by stroke in Indonesia [39].

Reports from Korea [40], the Philippines [22, 41], and Taiwan [34] showed unanimously insufficient identification of hypertensive patients and inadequate treatment of the known hypertensives, as had been reported elsewhere.

Improving the situation was possible when intensive education was given as in the case of Japan [42] and the USA [43].

3.2. Approaches

A well-controlled study by the VA Cooperative Study Group in the USA [44] produced strong evidence favoring the treatment of all hypertensive patients. Recent large-scale studies on mild hypertension [45, 46] showed less, but significant, benefit in treating borderline hypertension. To develop control of hypertension in the community is then a big problem.

In this paper, I refer mainly to the situation in Japan, since it is the only country that I know well, and the extent of hypertension control is probably the greatest in the world. In other countries in Asia, with the possible exception of China, control of hypertension is still at an infantile stage.

When pulmonary tuberculosis plagued Japan, a mass screening at schools and firms to detect pulmonary tuberculosis by using the tuberculin test and a miniature X-ray film had been supported by the government and widely carried out. Private agencies were established to undertake the mass screening. BCG vaccination or chemotherapy were administered when necessary.

A change of the target disease from the preceding leading cause of death, pulmonary tuberculosis, to the succeeding one, stroke, was accepted by people and screening agencies without much delay when tuberculosis had been suppressed. People want their health condition checked periodically and multiphasic screening, including blood pressure determination, became popular. Many municipal health centers assigned one day each week for cardiovascular screening at a modest cost. A free health check, at least blood pressure measurement and physical examination by a doctor, has been provided once a year for residents aged 40 to 64 years. The national government bears one-third of the cost, and the local government bears the remainder. An annual health check, including at least a blood pressure determination and urine sugar and protein examinations, for permanent employees aged 40 years and over became obligatory for all the firms in 1972 under the jurisdiction of the Ministry of Labor. These governmental supports have been promoting nationwide hypertension control. A battery of biochemical measurements of blood components and an electrocardiogram are often added.

In spite of these opportunities, participation rates varied. After-care services such as intensive education did not always follow. However, mass media, newspapers, journals, radio, and TV report advances of medical science every day, while the health check is repeated every year. Medical societies and private organizations, e.g., the Japan Heart Foundation, organize educational public lectures on medical topics from time to time. All these have played a significant role in decreasing high blood pressures among populations. Antihypertensive drugs are widely used without much financial constraints, thanks to a well-developed health insurance system in all the sectors of the Japanese population. Mortality rates from hypertensive disease, ischemic heart disease, and cerebrovascular disease have continuously declined in nearly all age/sex-specific population categories [47].

Because of the high costs involved, mass health screening has not been recommended by WHO. It may not be highly efficient, but seems at least partly to have contributed to a reduction in the number of deaths from cardiovascular disease.

Recent reports from Australia [45] and the United States [46] showed the favorable effects of vigorously treating mild hypertension, which is generally asymptomatic. Blood pressure measurements at various occasions thus should be encouraged when and where treatment is feasible. Education of physicians and the public should be strengthened. As the wait-and-measure blood pressure approach, however, does not appear to be promising [48], mass screening may be a more efficient way not only of identifying cases, but also of educating the public, and is particularly potent when repeated. Without actual measurement, people may not become interested in the problem of blood pressure.

Another experience to note is that participation in a hypertension detection project had never been successful by inviting individuals until a more aggressive door-to-door survey was undertaken in Bombay [49], involving the high as well as the low socioeconomical group. What is successful in one country, however, cannot be directly exported to another country. Available resources for hypertension control must be considered, and a flexible approach adapted to the attitudes and the behaviors of the local population must be sought and tried.

3.3. Compliance

Keeping hypertensive patients on an effective regimen is being gradually recognized as one of the most difficult problems of hypertension control at the community level in contrast to treating patients at the hypertension clinic of a large hospital where patients come with complaints, seeking medical care of their own accord. Most hypertensive patients detected in the community are symptom-free and are not ready to revisit a physician and pay for drugs that, at times, might have some adverse effects.

Rather poor outcomes have been reported in this respect. Unless intensified education was sustained, compliance with the advice on drug taking tended to wane [50].

In our survey of old population groups in urban and rural areas of Japan, 70%–80% of the hypertensive patients had been taking antihypertensive drugs regularly, and the average blood pressures of previously hypertensive subjects were normal in a rural area and near normal in an urban area [51]. The most popular antihypertensive drugs are thiazide diuretics and the

476

affirmative effects have been validated by the elevated mean serum concentrations of uric acid in a rural area, but not in an urban area. In a survey of another urban population [52], 35% of the hypertensive patients reported that they were taking antihypertensive tablets according to own judgment and feelings. Such self-controlled patients were less frequent in rural areas.

It would be useful to seek reasons for relatively high compliance in these populations. First, old people in Japan now enjoy free medical services and hence need not worry about financial constraints. Well-developed health insurance covers most, and often all, of the fees for medical services for the majority of people. Second, knowledge about the risk role that hypertension has in stroke is widely distributed to the population through the mass media. Over 90% of the households read newspapers and watch television. Third, Japanese people generally trust specialists' advice rather than make their own judgment on health, though this naive attitude may be exceptional in other cultures. Fourth, physicians welcome hypertensive patients because Japanese health insurance pays according to the amount of services (examinations and drug prescriptions) rendered to patients, with few restrictions. Fifth, a prescription is not valid for longer than two weeks. This legislation may have discouraged a few patients from continuing, but a patient or a family member is obliged to keep biweekly contact with a consulting physician so that the patient is continuously reminded of his latent illness. Physicians do not mind to see hypertensive patients so often because of the fourth reason. These reasons may not be applicable outside Japan, but some points may be applied when one plans hypertension control, for example, in selected occupational groups.

4. ETIOLOGICAL CONSIDERATIONS

So much for the community control of hypertension, where identification of hypertensive patients and maintenance of an effective drug regimen are practical goals for preventing multiple complications. This approach is less than ideal. We certainly prefer primary prevention of hypertension to a lifelong symptomatic treatment of high blood pressure drugs.

Hypertension is a symptom caused by various etiologies, encompassing essential hypertension and secondary hypertension of known causes. Studies on the pathogenesis of hypertension have identified some forms of secondary hypertension little by little but, so far, have been unsuccessful in determining the etiology of the larger core group, essential hypertension.

Animal models [53, 54] have greatly improved our understanding of the mechanisms of hypertension, but it is questionable to what extent a model represents human hypertension. Animal models help to produce useful hypotheses and to test them, but we eventually have to confirm them in men in a natural setting, i.e., in epidemiology. Few studies have followed up young cohorts long enough to observe the evolution of labile or fixed hypertension in normotensive subjects, and to elucidate risk factors of future hypertension at the entry. The large majority of studies have been case-control studies in which characteristics of hypertensive and normotensive populations were compared simultaneously. Since presuming causes and effects of hypertension is usually not difficult, this less time-consuming approach is useful. Topics on etiology referring to the report from Asia will be introduced.

4.1. Heredity

A classic work by Dahl on rats showed the presence of hypertension-prone and hypertension-resistant strains of rats [53]. The spontaneously hypertensive rat (SHR) of Okamoto and Aoki is another example of genetically predisposed hypertension [54].

Abundant reports on familial aggregation of high blood pressure in men have been published. Children of hypertensive parents start with higher blood pressure levels and show larger increments with age [9]. In studies in Korea [40] and the Philippines [55], family history of hypertension was associated with higher prevalence of hypertension; such observations support presence of family aggregation, but not necessarily its hereditary nature. Shared environment can also be a cause of aggregation. One of the most convincing supports for hereditary predisposition is the observation made by Biron et al., in which the blood pressure of real children showed a strong association with that of their natural parents ($r = 0.34$) whereas that of adopted children showed no association ($r = 0.03$) [56]. Feinleib et al. also demonstrated a stronger correlation of blood pressures between monozygot twins than between dizygot twins [57]. Therefore no doubt exists about the hereditary component in the blood pressure. What is necessary, then, is to investigate physiological responses through which genetic traits work and express themselves.

Predisposed persons may have higher sympathetic central nervous tone, more-sensitive vascular receptors, an inefficient kidney for salt excretion, or may have a metabolic tendency toward hypertrophy of the arteriolar media. Because of the polygenic nature of blood pressure expression and the complex networks of multiple physiological reactions, the mode of genetic influence may be difficult to elucidate fully. The statistical analysis of covariates could be the first step of disentanglement.

Despite these evidences, the genetic contribution to blood pressure is limited, and environmental factors take no less a part in determining the blood pressure. Japanese immigrants in California in the Ni-Hon-San study [58] and Tokelauan immigrants of New Zealand [59] became more obese, more hypertensive, and clearly indicated that the environment is a stronger influence than is ethnical identity. Environmental modification of the evolution of hypertension was possible even in genetically hypertension-prone rats.

4.2. Body build

Almost all epidemiological studies were in accordance in acknowledging the positive correlation between weight and various obesity indices, and blood pressure. In an Indian study in New Delhi, the differential weight appeared to be a more important cause of the higher blood pressure of a high socioeconomic group than of a lower socioeconomic group [19]. The appearance of high blood pressures in immigrants in urban areas [15, 16, 59] or in primitive tribes exposed to modern culture [25] was partly explained by an increase in weight caused by overeating and lack of physical exercise. In children, weight was a stronger predictor of the blood pressure than was age [60]. Not obesity with increased amount of fat deposit in the body, but overweight per se appeared to be related to high blood pressure. The exact mechanism is unknown. Reduction of weight was tested as a possible way of preventing or lowering high blood pressures with little success [61].

4.3. Diet and exercise

High calory intake, which leads to obesity, causes high blood pressure. Not only dietary intake but balance of energy input and output should be considered. A sedentary life accelerates obesity and rise of the blood pressure under a given diet. In a study of Micronesians, people on an isolated island, Ngerchelong, consumed higher calories and a larger amount of saturated fat from coconut, but showed lower serum cholesterol and lower blood pressures than people in the city of Koror [16]; the controversy possibly is explained by vigorous habitual physical activities. SHR that were fed with a protein and fat rich diet when allowed to do free exercise survived longer and manifested lower blood pressure than those without exercise [62]. This study suggests the need for another look at the famous observation made by McKay, who found that animals with limited calory intake and with a slow growth rate survived longer than those which were given calory- or protein-rich diet and had a rapid growth rate [63]. In the McKay experiments, physical activities, which are an important component of human life, were not considered, and prolongation of survival time in a confined condition was investigated. Applicability of these results to real human life may thus be limited.

On the contrary, the larger and more strenuous the physical workload, the higher the blood pressures and morbidity from stroke in the Japan National Railways (JNR) [64]. Fukuda postulated that they required greater calory intake for which Japanese workers tended to increase carbohydrate and salt, losing a good balance with other components. Such a diet is thought to accelerate hypertension.

Recent Japanese studies suggest that a shortage of fat (cholesterol inclusive) and protein in the diet may aggravate hypertension. The mean blood pressure of populations or morbidity from stroke in selected areas of Japan showed an inverse relation to the mean serum cholesterol concentrations[65]. In an animal experiment with SHR, feeding with fat or protein-enriched diets retarded development of hypertension[66]. Fish meat was most effective in preventing stroke, but soybean was less effective. Yamori observed a high amount of sulfur-containing amino acids in effective protein diets and demonstrated their blood-pressure-lowering effects in SHR[67]. Urinary inorganic sulfate excretion rate was inversely related to the prevalence rate of hypertension when Na excretion rate was identical in two contrasted populations[68].

Salt intake has been suggested as an accelerating agent. Among primitive tribes in Papua New Guinea[23], and the Solomon Islands[25], only those who washed foods with seawater customarily or those who learned the use of canned meat through contact with foreigners showed a slight trend of rising blood pressure with age. Without salt, there was no hypertension, even when plasma renin activity rises enormously[69]. A clear correlation between average blood pressures of populations and salt intake in various geographical locations has been demonstrated[70, 71]. However, many investigators have failed to show this association between individuals in one community[72, 73], and think that a drastic reduction of salt intake below 2–5 g is necessary to induce a definite reduction of blood pressure in an individual[74]. However, our experience with a modest reduction of daily Na intake from 250 meq to 200 meq resulted in the average of 10-mmHg reduction of systolic pressures in female patients[75]. Salt restriction was not successful in men, who did not follow our instructions rigorously. It is also possible that the response to salt varies between men and women, since we more often found that male patients were resistant after modest but successful salt restriction. A similar blood pressure reduction was induced by Parijs et al. by means of stronger reduction of Na intake from 191 meq to 92 meq in a Belgian population[76]. Salt reduction was more effective than weight control in one study[77]. Difficulty to demonstrate a clear relation would have come from the unrepresentative nature of 24-h urine[78], and noise effects by other blood-pressure-regulating factors[79]. Some hold the view that the role of Na should be considered in relation to potassium and calcium[78]. In animal models, an increased K intake decreased the hypertensive effect of Na intake[80].

4.4. Drinking and smoking habits

These habits are widely distributed in a modern life style as a means of distraction, relaxation, excitement or group enjoyment, and their association with blood pressure has been studied by many people. Drinking habits were reported to show a weak positive association [73, 81], which may be explained by additional calory intake from alcohol or overeating owing to the appetizing effect of alcoholic drinks. These correlations were weak, but still remained after removing the effect of weight. Smoking habit showed no association, and a tendency toward increasing weight but not blood pressure after subjects had quit smoking was reported in a seven year follow-up study [82].

4.5. Sociocultural factors

Numerous reports have dealt with the urban-rural difference, i.e., predominance of high blood pressure in urban areas. This has been observed in selected areas in China [83], Iran [20], and Pakistan [21]. Mental stress from noise [84], the rapid pace of life in urban environments, and weight gain due to diet and lack of physical exercise were counted as possible causes. The trend was reverse in Japan [12, 71, 85]. A plausible explanation is that salt intake is higher in rural areas, and that sociocultural gaps in Japan are not so large as to make urban life more stressful.

Immigrants from rural or less-industrialized areas provide a good opportunity to examine the influence of a change of environment. Weight gain from excess calory coupled with less physical activity in an urban environment was shown [58]. Salt intake also increased. High blood pressure in immigrants was not explained completely by changes in physical makeup. Studies on ethnic Japanese in California [86] and Tokelauans in New Zealand [87] showed that the more the sociocultural pattern of the native place was preserved, the less affected they were by cardiovascular problems such as high blood pressure. The prevalence rate of hypertension was higher in the population that immigrated to Manila, and particularly higher in those people with no previous experience of life in Manila before immigration. Difficulty in adjusting to an unfamiliar social system, or social instability and dissatisfaction, induce chronic sympathetic arousal, which supposedly accelerates high blood pressure [88].

Henry produced animal models of socially induced hypertension by breeding a mouse in isolation and then transferring the mouse to a different sociological environment so as to separate the mouse from its territory. Blood pressure elevation was accompanied by increased hormonal discharge stimulated by mental stress [89].

The problem of which component in urban life is the causative agent of higher blood pressure requires further investigation. Blacks in the United

States are more hypertensive than whites [10], but blacks in Africa have lower blood pressures [36]. Poor blacks in the Mississippi Delta have a particularly high prevalence of hypertension [90]. The struggle involved in living in an economically deprived area is harsh and stressful, and this may be a cause of hypertension. More-educated people generally had lower blood pressure than those with less education [91]. The poor and the less educated were more hypertensive in the Philippines, too [55].

Mental and physical stress cannot be entirely dissociated. Strenuous physical labor may be more stressful than desk work. Fukuda reported higher mean blood pressures, the highest incidence of stroke, and higher rates of heart attack among workers in the JNR whose job required hard physical labor [64]. Station masters and assistants who had more responsibility but did less physical work had moderately high blood pressures, a high incidence of heart attack, and a low incidence of stroke. This may represent a western model of hypertension. The workers who enjoyed the lowest incidence of cardiovascular complications and the lowest mean blood pressures were clerks, who were supposed to have the least mental and physical strain among the job categories. Likewise, SHR that were forced to run on a motor-driven wheel became more hypertensive, and those that were allowed to spin a wheel at leisure maintained lower blood pressures than control SHR without doing exercise [92]. Forced and unwilling exercise, and pleasureable and relaxing exercise, showed inverse effects on the blood pressure regulation, and should be distinguished.

Brunner, on the other hand, reported that workers in Kibbutzim who engaged in vigorous physical labour had lower morbidity and mortality of ischemic heart disease than sedentary workers [93]. This observation is in agreement with many western experiences, but differs from some Japanese experiences introduced in this paper. Careful separation of associated factors and further analysis of their mechanisms are needed for clarifying these controversies in Asia and extending our knowledge for more effective control of hypertension.

5. SUMMARY AND CONCLUSIONS

Based on available information mainly from the Asian-Pacific area, characteristics of community control of hypertension and etiological factors have been briefly reviewed.

1) Many hypotheses on etiology of hypertension have appeared from studies of varied population groups in this area. Some have been controversial and further in-depth investigations are warranted.

2) In the past, control of hypertension in the community has not been satisfactory in any community. Experiences in some countries show that the situation could be improved. Various approaches for better control should be sought. Mass screening approaches need not be rejected when appropriate conditions exist. It appears to have been effective in Japan.

3) Considering still younger population structures, secondary hypertension among young people should not be dismissed. The commonest type is chronic glomerulonephritis, and control of streptococcal skin infection should be intensified.

REFERENCES

1. Japan Heart Foundation (ed): Proceedings of the first Asian-Pacific symposium on hypertension. Jpn Circ J 41:1115-1178, 1977.
2. Rose G, Blackburn H: Cardiovascular survey methods. Geneva: WHO, 1968.
3. Kesteloot H (ed): Methodology and standardisation of noninvasive blood pressure measurement in epidemiological studies. Commission of the European Communities, 1976.
4. Rose GA, Holland WW, Crowley EA: A sphygmanometer for epidemiologists. Lancet 1:296-300, 1964.
5. Millar-Craig MW, Rafferty EB: Circadian variation of blood pressure. Lancet 1:795-797, 1978.
6. Takahashi E, Sasaki N, Takeda J, Ito H: Observations on the blood pressure in winter and summer of the same farmers in northeastern parts of Japan (in Japanese). Med Biol 36:64-67, 1955.
7. Perry Jr HM, Goldman AI, Schnaper HW, Fitz AE, Frohlich ED, Steele B, Richman HG, Tosch T, Lavin MA: Effects of chlorthalidone and reserpine in the treatment of blood pressure and chemistry. In: Gross F, Strasser T (eds) Mild hypertension: Natural history and management. Bath: Pitman Medical, 1979, pp 206-220.
8. Kesteloot H, Song CS, Song JS, Park BC, Brems-Heyns E, Joossens JV: An epidemiological study of arterial blood pressure in Korea using home reading. In: Rorive G, Cauwenberghe H van (eds) The arterial hypertensive disease. A symposium. New York: Masson, 1976, pp 141-148.
9. Zinner SH, Levy PS, Kass EH: Familial aggregation of blood pressure in childhood. N Engl J Med 284:401-404, 1971.
10. National Health Survey: Blood pressure of adults by race and area. United States 1960-1962. Washington DC: US Department of Health, Education and Welfare, 1964.
11. Dalal PM: Community survey of hypertension in 'Old' Bombay. In: Thurn, Phipps (eds) Essential hypertension symposium. Miami: Symposia Specialists, 1978.
12. Japan Ministry of Health and Welfare: Present status of national nutrition. (in Japanese). Tokyo: JMHW 1950-1971, Daiichi Shuppan 1972-1977.
13. Kim JS, Lee YW: Prevalence of diseases of circulatory system among rural Korean adults. Korean Circ J 5:87-94, 1975.
14. Burns-Cox MB, Maclean JD: Splenomegaly and blood pressure in an Orang Asli community in West Malaysia. Am Heart J 80:718-719, 1970.

483

15. Reed D, Labarthe D, Stallones R: Health effects of westernization and migration among Chamorros. Am J Epidemiol 92:94-112, 1970.
16. Labarthe D, Reed D, Brody J, Stallones R: Health effects of modernization in Palau. Am J Epidemiol 98:161-174, 1973.
17. Ree HP, Seah CS, Yik TY, Low LP, Leong SP, Wan SH, Ku G, Goh EH, Cheng WY: An epidemiological survey of blood pressure in Singapore. J Chronic Dis 30:793-802, 1977.
18. Lin TY, Hung TP, Chen CM: Studies on hypertension among urban Chinese in Taiwan. I. Mean blood pressure readings. J Formosa Med Assoc 55:131-138, 1956.
19. Padmavati S, Gupta S: Blood pressure studies in rural and urban groups in Delhi. Circulation 19:395-405, 1959.
20. Nadim A, Amini H, Malek-Afzali H: Blood pressure and rural-urban migration in Iran. Int J Epidemiol 7:131-138, 1978.
21. Rab SM, Shah MA: The epidemiology of hypertension in Karachi. Jpn Circ J 41:1142, 1977.
22. Icasas-Cabral EA, Paz AG de la, Yazon Jr JV, Morelos SI, Lammatao JC, Guzman SV: Hypertension (preliminary report). Philipp J Cardiol 5:24-35, 1977.
23. Maddocks I: Blood pressures in Melanesians. Med J Aust 54:1123-1126, 1967.
24. Prior IAM, Evans JG, Harvey HPB, Davidson F, Lindsey M: Sodium intake and blood pressure in two Polynesian populations. N Engl J Med 279:515-520, 1968.
25. Page LB, Damon A, Moellering Jr RC: Antecedents of cardiovascular diseases in six Solomon Islands societies. Circulation 49:1132-1146, 1974.
26. Komachi Y, Ozawa H, Iida M, Tominaga S, Chikayama Y, Shimamoto T: Epidemiological studies on Japanese hypertension and ischemic heart disease. Jpn Circ J 31:563-580, 1967.
27. Sohn ES: A study on hypertension and atherosclerosis in Koreans (in Korean with English abstract). Korean J Intern Med 18:251-325, 1975.
28. Lew EA: Blood pressure and mortality — life insurance experience. In: Stamler J, Stamler R, Pullman TN (eds) The epidemiology of hypertension. New York: Grune and Stratton, 1967, pp 302-397.
29. Kass EH, Zinner SH, Margolius HS, Lee Y-H, Rosner B, Donner A: Familial aggregation of blood pressure and urinary kallikrein in early childhood. In: Paul O (ed) Epidemiology and control of hypertension. Miami: Symposia Specialists, 1975, pp 359-374.
30. Frerichs RR, Webber LS, Voors AW, Srinivasan SR, Berenson GS: Cardiovascular disease risk factor variables in children at two successive years — the Bogalusa heart study. J Chronic Disc 32:251-262, 1979.
31. Julius S, Quadir H, Gajendragadkar S: Hyperkinetic state: a precursor of hypertension: a longitudinal study of borderline hypertension. In: Gross F, Strasser T (eds) Mild hypertension: natural history and management. Bath: Pitman Medical, 1979, pp 116-126.
32. Ooi BS, Chen BTM, Toh CCS, Khoo OT: Causes of hypertension in the young. Br Med J 3:744-746, 1970.
33. Omae T, Takeshita M: Causes of death of hypertensive subjects in a selected Japanese community. Jpn Circ J 41:1138, 1977.
34. Tseng W-P: Hypertension in Taiwan. Jpn Circ J 41:1133, 1977.

35. Icasas-Cabral E, Guzman SV: Mortality from hypertension at the Philippine General Hospital — 1971–1975. Philipp J Intern Med 16:102-112, 1978.
36. Akinkugbe OO: Epidemiology of hypertension and stroke in Africa. In: Hatano S, Shigematsu I, Strasser T (eds) Hypertension and stroke control in the community. Geneva: WHO, 1976, pp 28-42.
37. Rab SM, Shah MA: Incidence, mortality and morbidity of hypertension in large general hospital. Jpn Circ J 41:1126, 1977.
38. Ilyas M, Sherazi SH, Khan SM, Shan M: Hypertension in Peshawar: epidemiological profile, complications and management. Jpn Circ J 41:1143, 1977.
39. Darmadji T, Saleh M: Some clinical aspects of hypertension in Indonesia. Jpn Circ J 41:1165-1167, 1977.
40. Kim JY: A study on prevalence of hypertension at Iri City (in Korean with English abstract). Thesis, Seoul National University, 1979.
41. Guzman SV, Cabral E, Pas A de la, Morelos S, Lammatao JJ: Community survey of hypertension in the Phillippines. Jpn Circ J 41:1146-1149, 1977.
42. Kojima S: Practical aspects of hypertension and stroke control in a rural population. In: Hatano S, Shigematsu I, Strasser T (eds) Hypertension and stroke control in the community. Geneva: WHO, 1976, pp 149-162.
43. Hypertension Detection and Follow-up Program Cooperative Group: Blood pressure studies in 14 communities. A two stage screen for hypertension. JAMA 237:2385-2391, 1977.
44. Veterans Administration Cooperative Study Group on Antihypertensive Agents: Effects of treatment on morbidity in hypertension. II. Results in patients with diastolic blood pressure averaging 90 through 114 mmHg. JAMA 13:1143-1152, 1970.
45. Reader R: The Australian therapeutic trial in mild hypertension. Presented at 2nd Asian-Pacific symposium on hypertension, Manila, 1979.
46. Hypertension Detection and Follow-up Cooperative Group: Five-year findings of the hypertension detection and follow-up program. I. Reduction in mortality of persons with high blood pressure, including mild hypertension. JAMA 242:2562-2577, 1979.
47. WHO: World health statistics annual. Geneva: WHO.
48. Cypress BK: The role of ambulatory medical care in hypertension screening. Am J Public Health 69:19-24, 1979.
49. Dalal PM: The compliance of a community on screening program for the detection, diagnosis, treatment and prevention of cardiovascular diseases (personal communication, 1979).
50. Sackett DL, Taylor DW, Haynes RB, Johnson AL, Gibson ES, Roberts RS: Compliance with the therapeutic regimen. In: Gross F, Strasser T (eds) Mild hypertension: natural history and management. Bath: Pitman Medical, 1979, pp 309-327.
51. Ueno H, Hatano S: A survey of medical care usage in three communities (in Japanese). Jpn J Public Health [Suppl 10] 26:618, 1979.
52. Shibata H, Masuda T, Ueda A, Muto K, Matsuzaki T, Haga H, Hatano S: Perception and response of patients to antihypertensive drugs (in Japanese). Jpn J Public Health [Suppl 10] 23:353, 1976.
53. Dahl LK: Effects of chronic excess salt ingestion — experimental hypertension in the rat: correlation with human hypertension. In: Stamler J, Stamler R, Pullman TN (eds) The epidemiology of hypertension. New York: Grune and Stratton, 1967, pp 218-239.

54. Okamoto K, Aoki K: Development of a strain of spontaneously hypertensive rats. Jpn Circ J 27:283-293, 1963.
55. Icasas-Cabral E, Guzman SV, Hackenberg BY, Hackenberg R, Paz AG de la, Yason JV, Morelos SI: Survey of hypertension in two urban communities in the Philippines. Philipp J Cardiol 7:233-240, 1979.
56. Biron P, Mangean J-G, Bertrand D: Familial aggregation of blood pressure in adopted and natural children. In: Paul O (ed) Epidemiology and control of hypertension. Miami: Symposia Specialists, 1975, pp 397-406.
57. Feinleib M, Garrison R, Borhani N, Rosenman R, Christian L: Studies of hypertension in twins. In: Paul O (ed) Epidemiology and control of hypertension. Miami: Symposia Specialists, 1975, pp 3-17.
58. Winkelstein Jr W, Kagan A, Kato H, Sacks ST: Epidemiologic studies of coronary heart disease and stroke in Japanese men living in Japan, Hawaii and California: blood pressure distributions. Am J Epidemiol 102:502-513, 1975.
59. Prior IAM, Stanhope JM, Evans JG, Salmond CE: The Tokelau Island migrant study. Int J Epidemiol 3:225-232, 1974.
60. Voors AW, Webber LS, Frerichs RR, Berenson GS: Body height and body mass as determinants of blood pressure in children — the Bogalusa heart study. Am J Epidemiol 106:101-108, 1977.
61. Tyroler HA, Heyden S, Hames CG: Weight and hypertension: Evans County studies of blacks and whites. In: Paul O (ed) Epidemiology and control of hypertension. Miami: Symposia Specialists, 1975, pp 177-204.
62. Oshima S, Suzuki S: Influence of physical exercise on blood pressure using the spontaneously hypertensive rat (SHR) (in Japanese with English abstract). Jpn J Nutr 34:109-114, 1976.
63. McKay CM: Chemical aspects of ageing. In: Cowdry EV (ed) Problems of ageing. Baltimore: Williams and Wilkins, 1939.
64. Fukuda Y: Epidemiology of the occurrence of cerebral stroke and heart attack — with particular reference to influence of hypertension control and living conditions — Tokyo. Rodoigaku-Kenkyukai 1978.
65. Shigiya R, Komachi Y: Relationship between nutrition and cardiovascular diseases in Japanese. An epidemiological view. In: Shigiya R, Komachi Y, Watanabe T (eds) Nutrition and cardiovascular diseases in Japanese (in Japanese). Tokyo: Hokendojinsha, 1976, pp 1-42.
66. Okamoto K, Suzuki T, Ito H, Mitachi Y, Morita N: Further observations of stroke-prone SHR and dietary effects upon blood pressure and incidence of stroke. In: Spontaneous hypertension, 21-30. Washington DC: US Department of Health, Education and Welfare, 1977, pp 77-1179.
67. Yamori Y, Horie R, Nara Y, Ikeda K: Prophylactic trials for stroke in stroke-prone SHR (3) Amino acid analysis of various diets and their prophylactic effect. Jpn Heart J 19:624-626, 1978.
68. Yamori Y, Otaka M: Natural history and its modification of spontaneously hypertensive rat (SHR) as models for clinical and epidemiological studies (in Japanese). Sogo Rinsho 28:230-240, 1979.
69. Oliver WJ, Cohen EL, Neel JV: Blood pressure, sodium intake, and sodium related hormons in the Yanomamo Indians, a 'No-salt' culture. Circulation 52:146-151, 1975.
70. Dahl LK: Salt and hypertension. Am J Clin Nutr 25:231-244, 1972.
71. Sasaki N: The relationship of salt intake to hypertension in the Japanese. Geriatrics 19:735-744, 1964.

72. Miall WE: Follow-up study of arterial pressure in the population of a Welsh mining valley. Br Med J 2:1205-1210, 1959.
73. Dawber TR, Kannel WB, Kagan A, Donabedian RK, McNamara PM, Pearson G: Environmental factors in hypertension. In: Stamler J, Stamler R, Pullman TN (eds) The epidemiology of hypertension. New York: Grune and Stratton, 1967, pp 255-288.
74. Freis ED: Salt, volume and the prevention of hypertension. Circulation 53:589-595, 1976.
75. Shibata H, Hatano S: A salt restriction trial in Japan. In: Gross F, Strasser T (eds) Mild hypertension: natural history and management. Bath: Pitman Medical 1979, pp 147-160.
76. Parijs J, Joossens JV, Linden L van der, Verstreken G, Amery AKPC: Moderate sodium restriction and diuretics in the treatment of hypertension. Am Heart J 85:22-34, 1973.
77. Dole VP, Dahl LK, Cotzias GC, Eder HA, Krebs ME: Dietary treatment of hypertension. II. Clinical and sodium depletion as related to the therapeutic effect. J Clin Invest 30:584-595, 1951.
78. Langford HG, Watson RL: Electrolytes and hypertension. In: Paul O (ed) Epidemiology and control of hypertension. Miami: Symposia Specialists, 1975, pp 119-130.
79. Berglund G, Wikstrand J, Wallentin I, Wilhelmsen L: Sodium excretion and sympathetic activity in relation to severity of hypertensive disease. Lancet 1:324-327, 1976.
80. Dahl LK, Leitl G, Heine M: Influence of dietary potassium and sodium potassium molar ratios on development of salt hypertension. J Exp Med 136:318-330, 1972.
81. Kaltsky AL, Friedman GD, Siegelaub AB, Gerard MG: Alcohol consumption and blood pressure. N Engl J Med 296:1194-1200, 1977.
82. Greene SB, Aavedal MJ, Tyroler HA, Davis CE, Hames CG: Smoking habits and blood pressure change: a seven year follow-up. J Chronic Dis 30:401-413, 1977.
83. WHO Cardiovascular Disease Team: Report on the visit to the People's Republic of China. WHO internal document CHN/CVD/001-E, 1979.
84. Kavoussi N: The relationship between the length of exposure to noise and incidence of hypertension at a silo in Teheran. Pahlavi Med J 5:51-58, 1974.
85. Hatano S: Hypertension in Japan: a review. In: Paul O (ed) Epidemiology and control of hypertension. Miami: Symposia Specialists, 1975, pp 63-100.
86. Marmot MG, Syme SL: Acculturation and coronary heart disease in Japanese-Americans. Am J Epidemiol 104:225-247, 1976.
87. Beaglehole R, Salmond CE, Hooper A, Huntsman J, Stanhope JM, Cassel JC, Prior IAM: Blood pressure and social interaction in Tokelauan migrants in New Zealand. J Chronic Dis 30:803-812, 1977.
88. Henry JP, Cassel JC: Psychosocial factors in essential hypertension. Recent epidemiologic and animal experimental evidence. Am J Epidemiol 90:171-200, 1969.
89. Henry JP: Understanding the early pathophysiology of essential hypertension. Geriatrics 31:59-72, 1976.
90. Schoenberger JA, Carter M, Eckenfels EJ: Hypertension in Holmes county, Mississippi. In: Paul O (ed) Epidemiology and control of hypertension. Miami: Symposia Specialists, 1975, pp 485-501.

91. Hypertension Detection and Follow-up Program Cooperative Group: Race, education and prevalence of hypertension. Am J Epidemiol 106:351-361, 1977.
92. Suzuki S, Oshima S: Influences of physical exercise on blood pressure using spontaneously hypertensive rats. — Free and forced physical exercise (in Japanese). In: Bureau of Science and Technology of Japan (ed) Prevention of hypertension and stroke. Tokyo: Printing Office of Ministry of Finance, 1979.
93. Brunner D: Physical exercise in the primary prevention of ischemic heart disease. Presented at the 7th Asian-Pacific Congress of Cardiology, Bangkok, 1979.

30. STROKE, STOMACH CANCER AND SALT

A possible clue to the prevention of hypertension

J.V. JOOSSENS

A strong relationship exists between cerebrovascular (stroke, CVA) mortality and stomach cancer (SC) mortality, and this is true for both sexes [1]. This relation was unintentionally found in 1964, using mortality data from 1958 only. Since then, many more data have become available. This paper will deal with data covering the period from 1950 to 1974–1977.

1. METHODS

Data on mortality were provided by the World Health Organisation (WHO) on tape and through the annual WHO publications. This implies no responsibility whatsoever for WHO. The Registrar General in London, the 'Centraal Bureau voor de Statistiek,' Den Haag, and the 'Nationaal Instituut voor de Statistiek,' Brussels, made more recent data available. Cerebrovascular mortality was age adjusted for each sex between 45 and 75+ years of age, stomach cancer between ages 45 and 64. The weighting factors are proportional to the total population, in each age group, of England and Wales in 1951; namely 599 for the age group 45–54 years, 457 for 55–64, 324 for 65–74 and 156 for the 75+ age group.

As shown in Figures 1 and 2, the correlation for each sex ranges from good to excellent when taking CVA from all age groups above 45 years, and stomach cancer from the 45–54 and 55–64 year age groups. Since one of the aims of this study was to find an indicator for stroke, both between and within countries, the choice of these age groups was mandatory.

The average of both sexes, $(\male + \female)/2$, will be used from now on in order to save space, but the relations are true for each sex separately. Data were analyzed by classic linear regression; 5% confidence intervals for a point versus a given regression line were calculated [2], whenever necessary.

Supported by grants of NFWO, Brussels.

H. Kesteloot, J.V. Joossens (eds.), Epidemiology of Arterial Blood Pressure, 489–508.

490

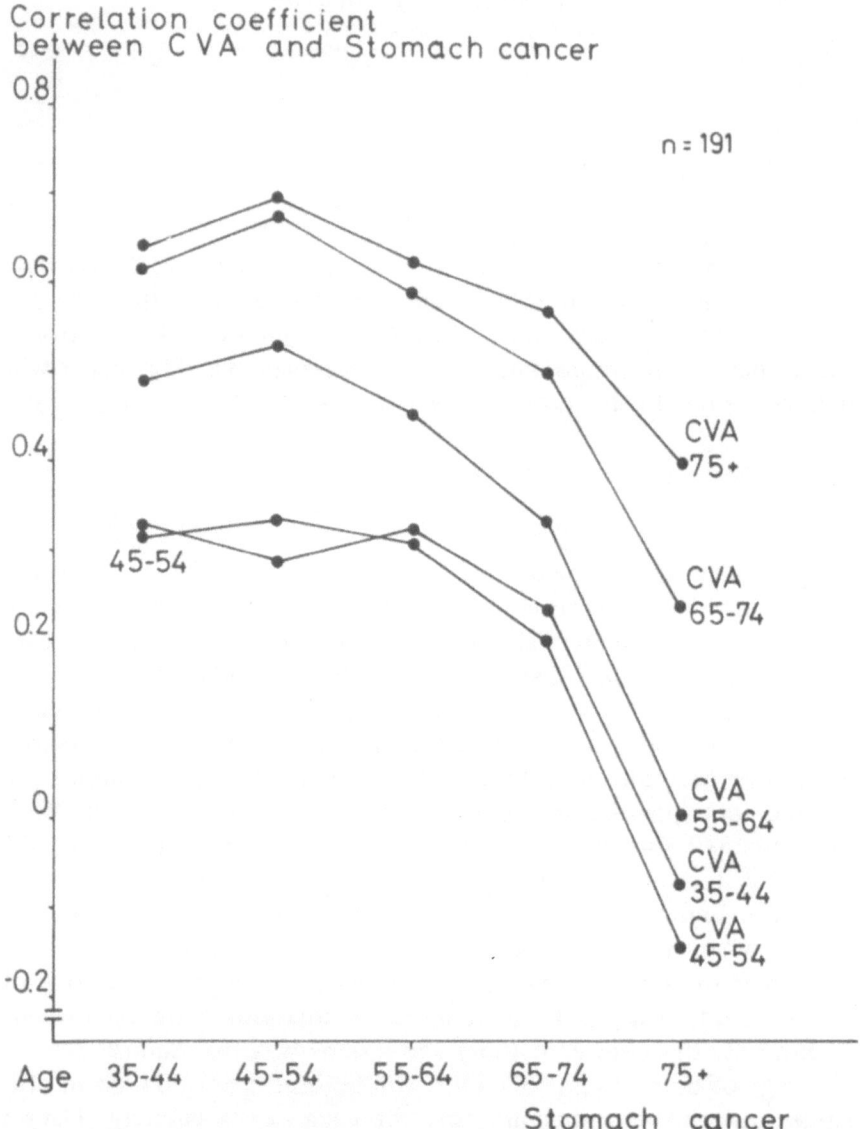

Figure 1. Correlation coefficient between CVA and stomach cancer, males (1955-1970) in 12 western countries.

The 12 western countries are defined in reference [38]. The $P < 0.05$ limit is for $r = \pm 0.14$, the < 0.01 for $r = \pm 0.19$ and the < 0.001 for $r = \pm 0.24$.

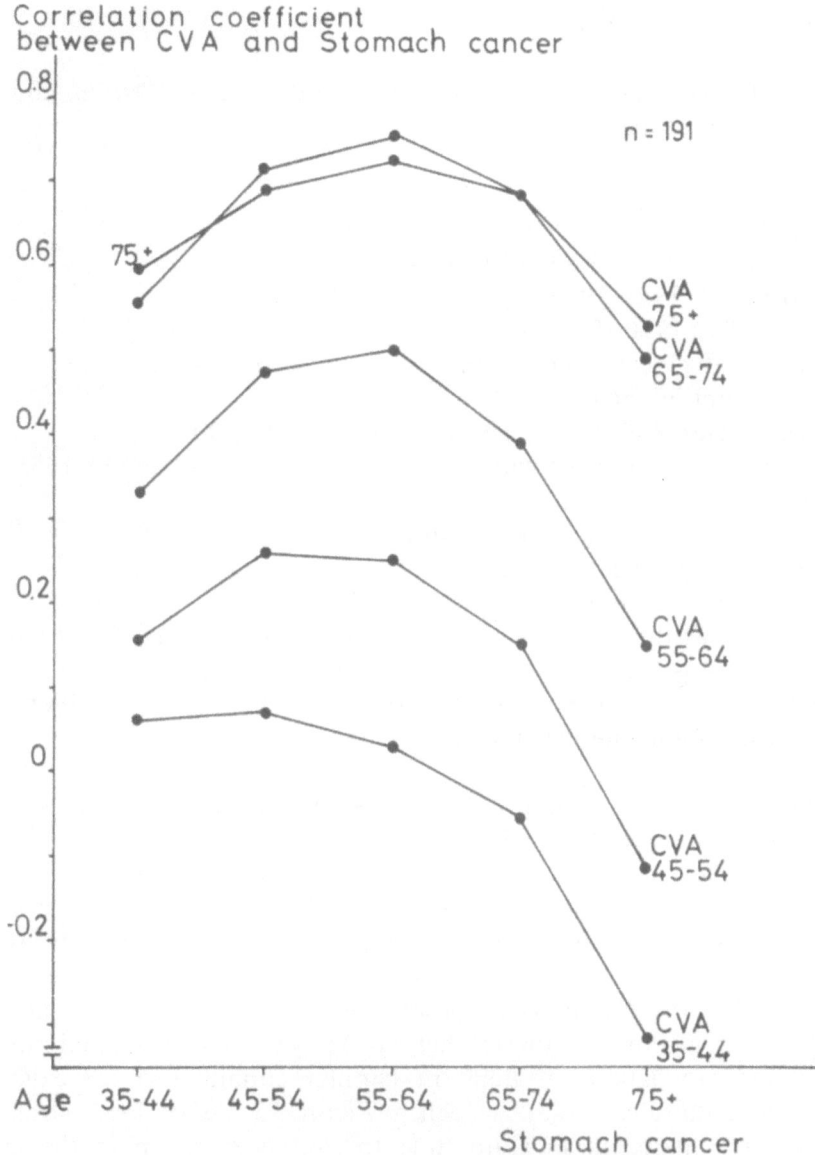

Figure 2. Correlation coefficient between CVA and stomach cancer, females (1955-1970) in 12 western countries.

The 12 western countries are defined in reference [38]. The $P < 0.05$ limit is for $r = \pm 0.14$, the < 0.01 for $r = \pm 0.19$ and the < 0.001 for $r = \pm 0.24$.

2. RESULTS AND DISCUSSION

The stroke-stomach cancer relationship is shown for the following countries and for certain time periods.

1) Between time periods
   a) England and Wales, 1950–1977 (Fig. 3)
   b) USA (all races), 1950–1975 (Fig. 4)
   c) Switzerland, 1951–1976 (Fig. 5)
   d) Japan, 1950-1976 (Fig. 6)
   e) Average of nine western countries as in 2b, 1955–1975 (Fig. 7)
2) Between countries or regions
   a) England and Wales, average of 1966–1974 (Fig. 8)
   b) Nine western countries with best vital statistics, average of 1955–1973 (Fig. 9)
   c) Western and east european countries, plus Japan in 1974 (Fig. 10)
3) Between time periods and countries
   a) Nine western countries, 1955–1973 (Fig. 11)
   b) The same as the previous one, with Japan for comparison. The regression line was calculated without Japan, which means an increase in range for stomach cancer from 0 to 0.6‰, to 1.2‰, i.e. a doubling of the observation interval (Fig. 12).

The figures for between time periods (series 1) show similar linear slopes at least between 1955 and 1968 in Figures 3–5 and 7, and between 1962 and 1974 in Figure 6.

Before 1955 (1962 in Japan), there is a lower stroke rate than predicted from stomach cancer. This is almost certainly due to underclassification of stroke and was already documented in 1948 in the USA when the change from the 5th to the 6th revision produced a drastic increase in stroke [3]. Another argument for the thesis that stroke was underclassified up to a certain period are data from Belgium (similar conditions have existed in Czechoslovakia up to ca. 1973), as seen in Figure 13. Before 1968, stroke was grossly underestimated in Belgium, due to overclassification in the arterial diseases group; upon correction, the observed stroke rate started decreasing versus increasing beforehand, and the observed rate fitted perfectly with the rate estimated from stomach cancer. A third reason is that in the 45–64 age group, where diagnosis is in general more easy, no deviation from linearity is seen from 1950 onwards, whereas this is obvious up to 1955 in the 65–75+ age group [4].

After the linear part (ca. 1955–1968), a new departure from linearity is observed (Figs. 3, 4, 7). This is in general not significant before 1973. From

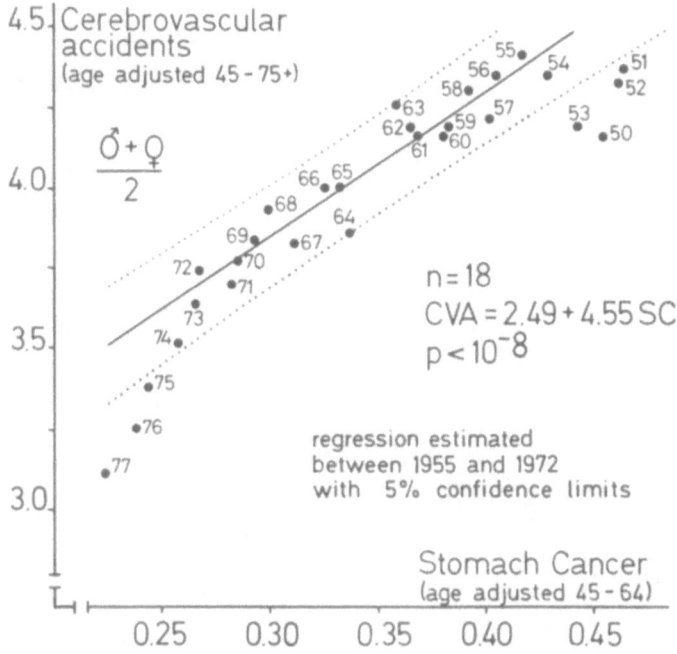

Figure 3. England and Wales, death rates ‰ (1950-1977). The three periods are clearly visible. The first from 1950 to 1954, the second from 1955 to 1972, the third after 1972 (see text). Each point gives a pair of mortality data. The year of the observation is indicated next to each point, e.g. 50 = 1950 a.s.o.

then on, stroke is decreasing much faster than stomach cancer, at least in countries like England and Wales, the USA, and Germany. This new deviation from linearity is most probably due to treatment of hypertension. Although antihypertensive drugs have been available since the end of the 1940s, they have not been used on a population-based level, but only in selected cases. From 1968 on, and gradually increasing over the years, there has been a progressive improvement in medical education, sponsored by drug companies, resulting in a much more effective treatment of hypertension. Recent surveys in the USA have shown that by treatment a modest reduction of 5 mmHg in diastolic blood pressure in the 90–104 mmHg range at entry produced a decline of 20% in total mortality [5]. If treatment had been effective on the population level before 1968, a curvilinear stroke-stomach cancer relationship, instead of a linear one, would have resulted. Treatment of hypertension is unlikely to improve stomach cancer and therefore, if effective, would only influence stroke. The kind of antihypertensive drug, in itself, is not important since similar results are seen in the USA and in England and

494

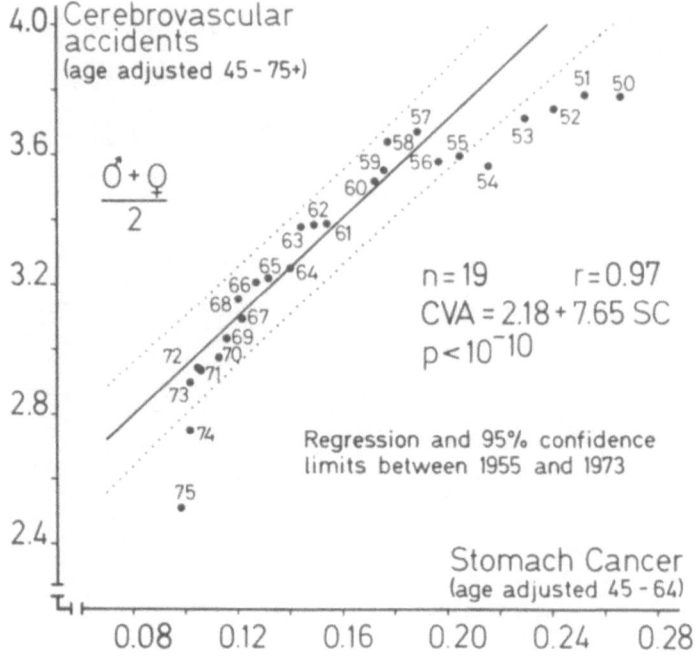

Figure 4. USA (all races), death rates ‰ (1950-1977). See legend of Figure 3.

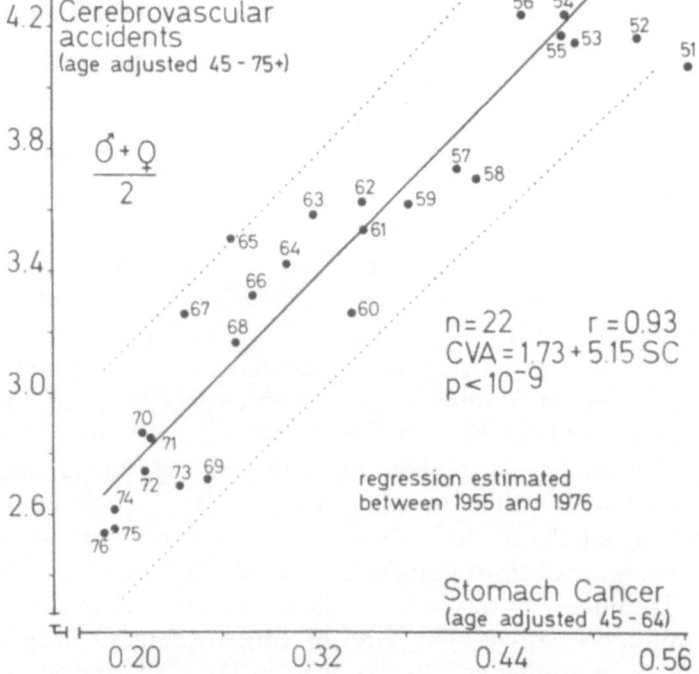

Figure 5. Switzerland, death rates ‰ (1951-1976). As in Figures 2 and 3, but the third period is not shown.

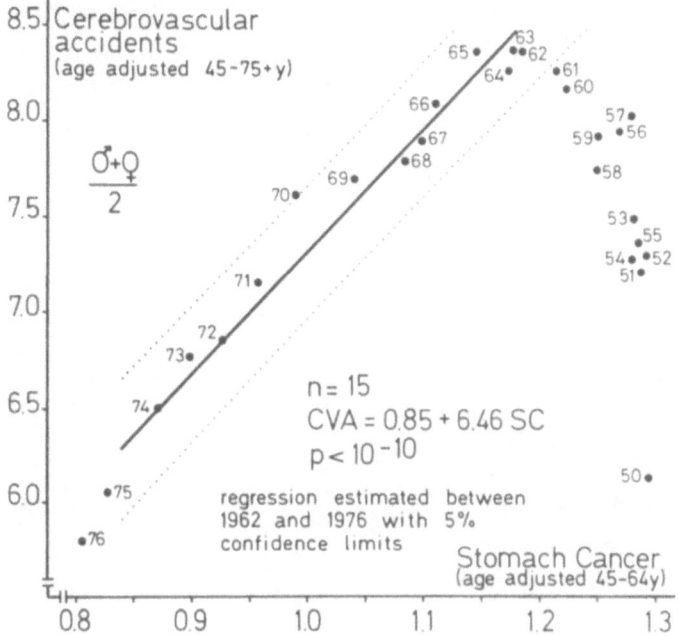

Figure 6. Japan, death rates ‰ (1950-1976). The first period lasts until 1961; there is an indication of a third period after 1974.

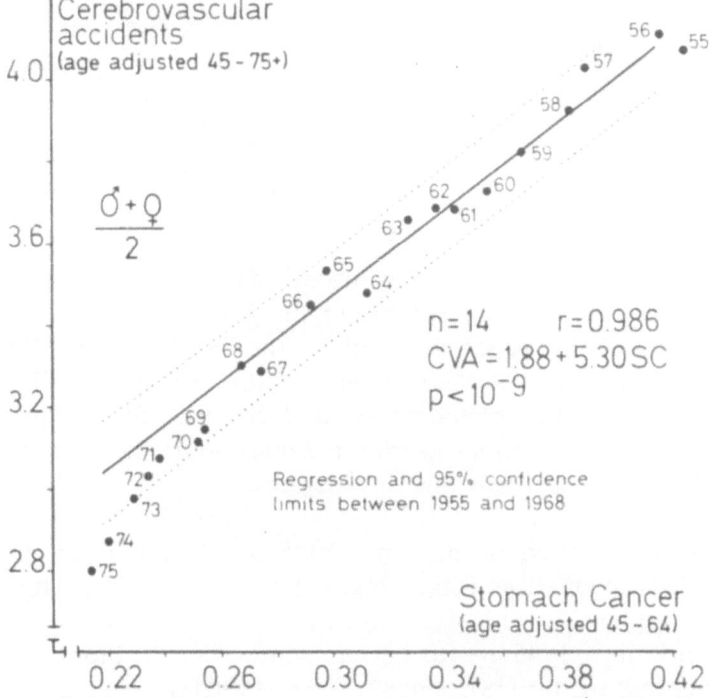

Figure 7. Mean of nine western countries, death rates ‰. The first period has been omitted from this figure. The third period starts after 1971.

496

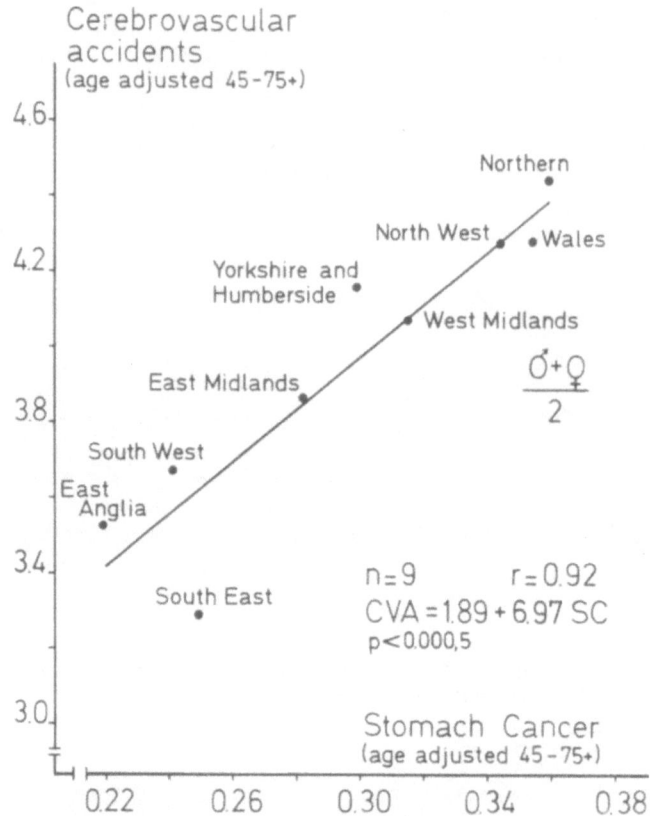

Figure 8. Standard regions of England and Wales, death rates ‰ (mean 1966-1974). The inter-regions regression line is not significantly different from the one obtained over time (Fig. 3).

Wales, although other drugs are used in both countries; e.g. more β-blockers in England and Wales, more reserpine in the USA.

The major aim of this paper is to explain the linear part (ca. 1955–1968 in western countries) of the stroke-stomach cancer relationship. This is (Figs. 3–7) a typical time-related phenomenon and can therefore be perfectly spurious (e.g. number of television sets and coronary mortality in males), but this can be ruled out by the following considerations:

1) The relationship existed already since 1925–30, at least in the USA. Stroke in the USA is reported as decreasing, since at least 1925, long before any available treatment [3]. This was confirmed since 1940 in Baltimore, Maryland [6], and since 1945 in Rochester, Minnesota [7]. Stomach cancer has been decreasing in the USA since at least 1930 [8].

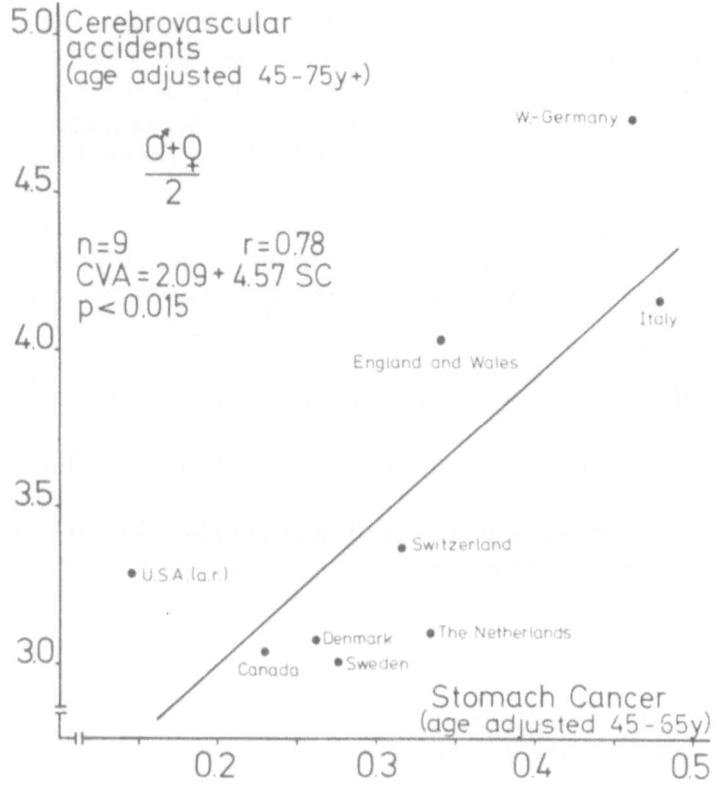

Figure 9. Mean of 19 years (1955-1973) in the nine western countries, death rates ‰. The between-countries slope is not different from the regression line obtained over the years (Fig. 7).

2) The time relation is not only very strong, but has a quantitative value, namely slope and intercept, which are very similar under extremely different environmental conditions (e.g. western countries versus Japan).

3) The most important argument against a spurious origin of the stroke-stomach cancer relation is the similarity of the regression lines between time periods (Figs. 3–7), between regions (Figs. 8 and 9), and combined (Figs. 10–12).

An almost identical relation that holds under conditions so varied must be a relatively simple one; i.e. each phenomenon separately (CVA or SC) can have a multifactorial causation, but the link between them must be either unique or at least predominant. A multifactorial link could not produce identical results under different conditions. The more factors involved in the link, the less chance there is to obtain identical relations between and within countries, the smaller the number of factors involved, and the more likely it is to get similar linking values. For a unique linking factor they must be identical. The relation between stroke mortality and lung cancer is a good example of a multifactorial link. Between countries there is a highly significant positive correlation between both types of mortality [4]. Within countries, however, with lung cancer increasing and stroke decreasing, a negative correlation is observed. It is therefore imperative to look out for the linking factor 'X.' Since it involves the stomach as well as the brain arteries, it may confidently be put as a nutritional factor. Factor X should have the following properties. It should:

1) raise blood pressure, since blood pressure is the most important risk factor in CVA [9, 10];
2) tend either to induce stomach cancer by itself or to facilitate the induction;
3) be present in western, east-european, and oriental diets; the concentration should be high in Japan and South Korea, medium in eastern Europe, and much lower in the West;

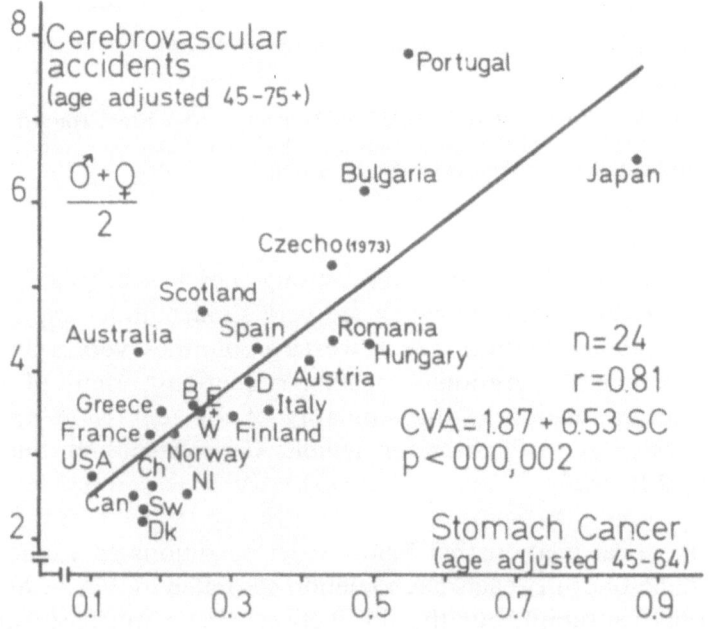

Figure 10. Death rates ‰, 1974. The high values obtained in east european countries, Portugal, and Japan should be noticed. For references on salt excretion in the two last countries, see references [25, 34].

4) it should be present in cereals, lard, sausages, miso sauce, smoked and pickled foods, nearly absent in milk, and absent in fresh fruits and vegetables [11–14];
5) decrease with time; in the USA the decline should start approximately around 1925.

Certain theories on the aetiology of stomach cancer do not fit into this pattern. For example, the soil trace element theory [15] could explain differences between regions or countries, but not what is happening with time. The

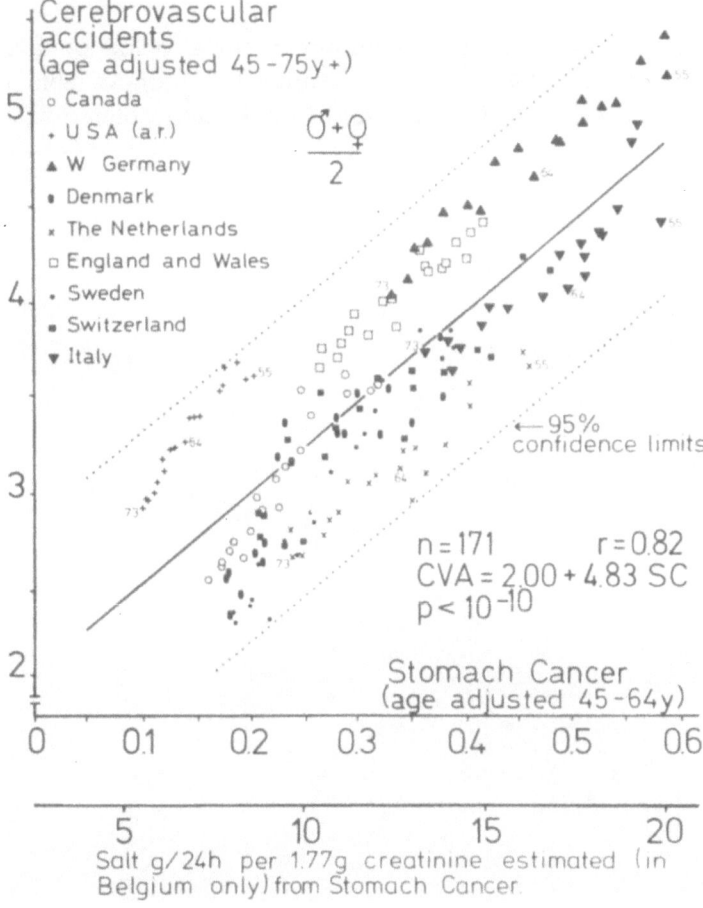

Figure 11. Death rates ‰, 1955-1973. The scale on salt excretion is only a preliminary estimate starting from the stomach cancer rates. The parallelism between the points obtained in each country over time is striking. The numbers 55, 64 and 73 are years of observation and have been indicated only for five countries.

500

soil theory cannot explain the decrease in stomach cancer. The same is true for blood groups and stomach cancer. The latter is more frequent in blood group A [16], but again, this cannot explain a decline quantitatively identical to the between region relationship.

In 1965 [17], the hypothesis was set forwart equating factor X to salt:

ad 1. Although not totally conclusive, salt is generally considered as an important factor in the genesis of essential hypertension [18–23].

The conclusion from the above-mentioned studies can be summarized as follows.

Evolutionary evidence. Mammals, including man, evolved on a diet low in sodium and high in potassium. This resulted in kidneys able to preserve sodium homeostasis on a very low sodium intake and potassium homeostasis

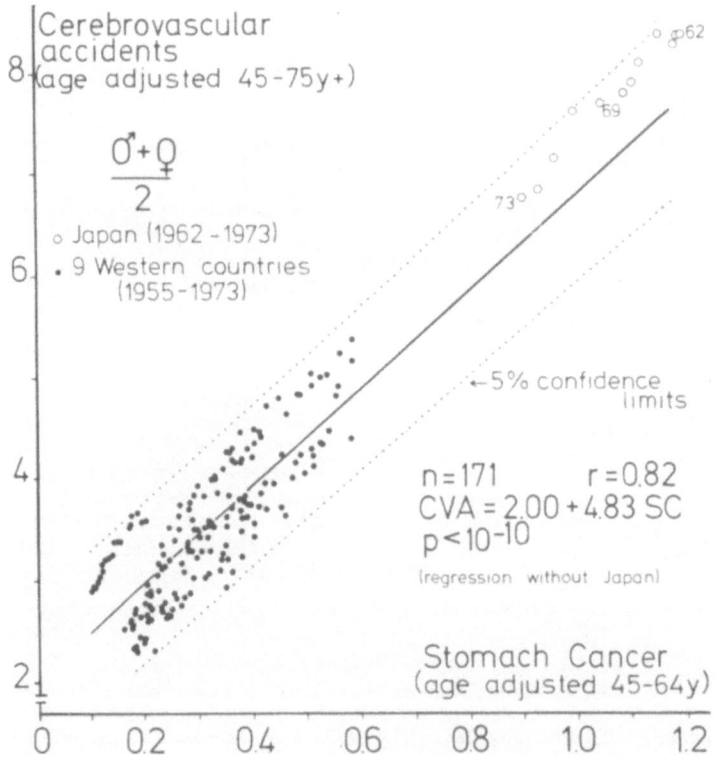

Figure 12. Death rates ‰. The same data as in Figure 11, but extrapolated so as to allow the comparison with Japan. Again the similarity of the slopes is striking.

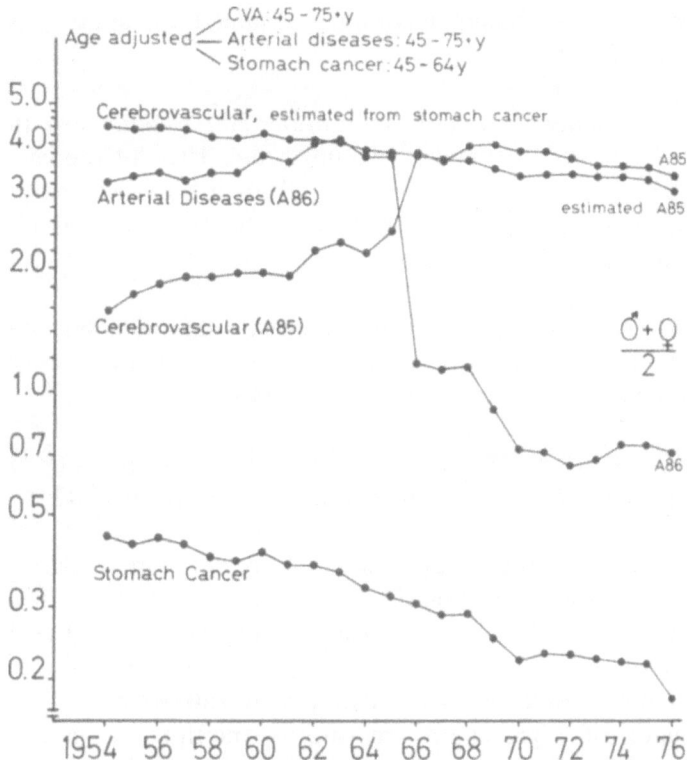

Figure 13. Belgium, death rates ‰ (1954-1967). An illustration of how classification errors may produce a spurious increase of cerebro-vascular mortality between 1954 and 1967. Stomach cancer mortality, being more accurate, is probably a better estimator of stroke than is stroke itself. The estimation was done with a regression equation from 12 other countries.

on a high potassium intake. The kidney has difficulties in handling a high sodium intake and a low potassium intake. The latter will result in serious troubles if persisting for some time. Heavy perspiration on a low sodium intake will not disturb the sodium homeostasis, but massive sweating on a high salt intake can result in severe sodium depletion. Maternal milk is very low in sodium, indicating that there is no need for a high intake in newborns.

The low-sodium, high-potassium diet, typical for the tropical setting in which man evolved, was drastically changed when man migrated to colder regions in the north. Absence of fresh food in winter was overcome by the salting technique. Hence the importance of salt for survival. Habitual salting of food damaged the taste-buds, creating the need for salting where no preservation was involved, e.g., bread and cereals. This situation was uncon-

502

sciously reserved when cooling techniques enabled the preservation of food without the use of salt.

Pharmacological evidence. All sodium diuretics are hypotensive from mercurials to amiloride, but the opposite is not true. The hypotensive action of diuretics can be blocked by an excessive sodium intake. All sodium-retaining drugs, such as mineralocorticoids, cortisone, licorice, and oestrogens, may increase the level of blood pressure.

Experimental evidence. Rats, dogs and baboons, but not rabbits, can be made hypertensive with salt. High doses of salt are in general necessary, but of course appearance time must be small in animals.

Clinical evidence. A lower Na intake lowers high blood pressure, not only as in the Kempner diet, but also with a moderate Na decrease [24].

Epidemiological evidence. The prevalence of hypertension is high in countries like Japan, South Korea, Portugal [25], and certain parts of the USSR [26], where salt intake is high. The age-adjusted prevalence of hypertension in Alexandrovka [26] with a salt intake of 350 mmol/24 h is three times higher than in neighbouring villages with an intake of 160 mmol.

The prevalence of high blood pressure is medium on a moderate salt intake, e.g. the USA, England and Wales, Belgium, New Zealand, and Australia.

There is no essential hypertension on a no added salt diet. Recently [27] it has been argued that the absence of hypertension is related to the absence of obesity in the same population. It should, however, be remembered that hypertension is very common in Japanese and South Koreans, who are at the same time very lean.

The most important objection against the salt hypothesis is the difficulty to prove a within-country relation from salt and high blood pressure. This situation has been discussed extensively in chapter 3 of this book [28].

ad 2. Chloride and sodium are, except for hydrogen, the smallest ions present in food and therefore osmotically the most active. Hunt and Pathak [29] provided evidence that stomach emptying is retarded by the presence of hypertonic solutions in the stomach. Hypertonic salt solutions can damage the stomach mucosa just as they damage the tastebuds, resulting, after many decades, in atrophic gastritis, an extremely common disease in Japan [30]. Recent observations have shown that the nitrite level of the stomach is inversely related to acidity [31]. Under those conditions, nitrosamides can be formed from guanidine bases present in the food. Such compounds are highly carcinogenic and produce glandular carcinoma from the stomach in animals. Vitamin C and other antioxydants may inhibit the formation of these nitroso-compounds [31].

ad 3. Salt is present in western, east european, and oriental diets. Salt intake is extremely high in Japan [33, 34] and in South Korea [35], medium high in eastern Europe [26] and much lower in the west [21], except in Portugal where high amounts have been found [25].

ad 4. All stated foods contain large amounts of salt except milk, fresh fruits and vegetables.

ad 5. The decrease of salt intake has been documented in Belgium [22], in Japan [34] and in Switzerland [36], but is probably present in all industrialized countries. A decrease from 15.2 g NaCl/24 h in 1966 to ±9 g in 1979 was observed in Belgium. In Japan, values from 30 g in 1937 to 18.5 (value not corrected for creatinine) in 1965 were noted, whereas in Switzerland a decrease per capita of about 9 g/day in iodized salt sales (about 90% of total salt sales) was observed over the period 1951–1976. Cooling techniques for the preservation of food together with a decreasing intake of cereals, salted fish, meat and vegetables are probably the origin of this decrease. Preservation by cold became first popular in the USA around 1925, in western Europe after world war II and in eastern Europe after 1970. This is consistent with the time sequence of changes in stroke and stomach cancer in those countries.

Although there are not many countries with documented decrease in salt intake, a simple calculation will show that the actual total intake of salt must be lower than the salt intake from bread and potatoes alone 40–60 years ago. In Belgium, for example the added salt to bread and potatoes must have amounted to more than 15 g NaCl in 1920 [21]. This is much higher than the actual total NaCl excretion/24 h. It should be remembered that in most west european countries, the total consumption of bread and potatoes was quite high in comparison with the present consumption.

The most important risk factors for stroke, namely hypertension and obesity, but not alcohol, are more or less related to salt. All the cited risk factors for stomach cancer (see under 4) contain salt, and the protecting factors do not. Talc in rice is an exception, but obviously this is of no importance in western food habits. Antioxydants are another exception, but it is difficult to see how this could influence stroke mortality. It is important to notice that the most frequent cardiac abnormality associated with stomach cancer, found at autopsy in Japan, was left-ventricle hypertrophy [37].

From the observed stomach cancer rates in the north of Belgium [38] and from the 24-h salt excretion (standardized to 1.77 g creatinine) [22] from 1966 to 1976, a preliminary regression line was fitted, namely ($n = 5$, $r = 0.97$): salt excretion g/day = 2.5 + 29.6 stomach cancer. The average of both sexes standardized per thousand between 45 and 64 years was used for stomach cancer. This regression line was used to give a rough estimate of the salt excretion in different countries (Fig. 11). The calculated salt excretion fits reasonably well into the still scarcely available data from other countries.

Table 1. Ten countries out of 29 with the highest decrease in cerebrovascular mortality since 1968 for the average of both sexes [a].

Country	Last year of observation	Cerebrovascular age-adj. 45–74+	Stomach cancer age-adj. 45–64	All causes age-adj. 45–74+
Finland	1974	61.7	53.5	24.3 [b]
Belgium	1978	38.0	46.8	13.6
Japan	1976	37.5	36.8	26.9
Denmark	1976	28.7	32.4	n.s.
Norway	1976	27.9	45.0	8.6
The Netherlands	1978	25.4	31.7	9.0
USA	1975	25.3	28.6	14.6
West Germany	1975	25.3	30.8	10.9
England and Wales	1977	24.1	31.0	8.2
Switzerland	1976	22.2	42.4	21.8

[a] Significant decrease in percent estimated as over 10 years (see text); ($P < 0.05$).
[b] Until 1976.

In Table 1, data from stroke, stomach cancer and all causes are provided for the ten countries out of 29 with the best results in both sexes since 1968. The percentual decrease was calculated as over a ten-year period with regression analysis:

$$10 \text{ year decrease } \% = \frac{1000 \times \text{slope of regression per year}}{\text{average mortality over the observed time interval}}$$

The observed decrease in mortality from stroke, stomach cancer and all causes in Belgium, Japan and Switzerland is consistent with the documented decline in salt intake in those countries.

From all data published here and elsewhere [1, 21–23] about the stroke-stomach cancer relationship, it can safely be concluded that stomach cancer can be used as an estimator of stroke levels in a given population. Stomach cancer was, in fact (e.g. before 1955), a better predictor of stroke mortality than stroke itself. This holds still true in certain countries like Poland and possibly also Chili [4].

If the salt hypothesis for the aetiology of stroke and stomach cancer is correct, a simple and inexpensive method is available to prevent these diseases and by the same token to decrease mortality from all causes. What should be done is to educate the population in order to accelerate the unconscious decrease in salt intake. The first limit can be set at 5 g/24 h in accordance with the dietary goals of the USA, but the final aim should be at less than 2–3 g [19]. When the decrease in salt intake is produced gradually, as it should and as it already is, there is no problem whatsoever with palatability, the contrary being true. Experience gained in Belgium in hundreds of families makes it clear that the lack of food palatability is not due to the absence of salt, but to the lack of taste resulting from damaged taste-buds. The latter comes from overindulgence in salty foods and is, except in some elderly, totally reversible.

In order to get more certainty, it is absolutely necessary to monitor salt intake (excretion) in different populations all over the world and at regular time intervals. This should be done with standardized methods [28] and, if possible, in a randomized sample of the population.

3. SUMMARY

The relation between stroke and stomach cancer mortality has been documented from 1950 to 1974–1977. In general, three periods can be described. In the first period, starting in 1950 and lasting in general up to 1955, stroke is lower than expected from stomach cancer. In Belgium, this period lasts until 1968. Evidence has been gathered to ascribe this to underclassification of stroke mortality. During the second period, an almost perfect linear relationship is observed from 1955 to 1968. This relation between time periods is quantitatively similar in all western countries and in Japan (1962–1970), and is not significantly different from the observed relation between regions. This already makes a spurious relation highly improbable. The third phase starts around 1969, with a gradual but still not significant departure from linearity. From 1973 onwards, a significant deviation from the expected stroke values is observed in the USA, England and Wales, and in a few other countries. This third phase is probably due to the effect of treatment of hypertension producing a faster decline in stroke than expected from stomach cancer.

For the second period, a linking factor X is postulated. Because of the similarity of the stroke-stomach cancer relation under totally different conditions—in western, east european and oriental countries, between regions as well as between time periods—it can be deduced that factor X must be unique or predominant. A multifactorial link should result in different relations between regions and between time periods. A unique factor must give an identical relation. From the known risk factors of stroke and stomach cancer, it appears that salt could be factor X. This is consistent, at least up to now, with all of what is known about measured salt excretion in certain countries, and about the decrease of salt intake over the years. The latter is documented in Belgium, Japan and Switzerland. The decrease of stroke and stomach cancer up to ±1973 can be ascribed to the unconscious decrease in salt intake, resulting from the use of refrigerators and deep-freezers, and from the decreasing intake of salted foods such as bread, potatoes, salted meat including lard, salted and smoked meat or fish and salted vegetables. The latter are nowadays more and more frequently replaced by fresh items, or at least by less salted varieties.

Because of the near to one correlations between stroke and stomach cancer, it is possible to use the second to estimate the first. This is important in countries or time periods where vital statistics are not optimal. It is easier to classify stomach cancer between ages 45 and 64 than stroke between age 45 and over. Stroke mortality reporting is especially deficient in the age group over 65 years. Stomach cancer rates have been used tentatively in order to get a rough estimate of the salt excretion in different populations and different years.

The observed decrease in stroke mortality, stomach cancer and even mortality from all causes in Belgium, Japan and Switzerland corresponds very well with the observed decrease in salt intake.

These observations make it very urgent to monitor salt excretion all over the world, if possible at regular time intervals and preferably under standardized conditions. This will make it possible to determine whether salt intake is truly a health risk factor. If so, a simple and inexpensive method will be available to lower not only stroke and stomach cancer mortality, but also total mortality in ages above 45 years.

If the salt hypothesis is confirmed by further research, it will lead to the rather unexpected conclusion that the most important contribution to public health in the field of non-infectious chronic diseases over the last 30–40 year has been the mass introduction of refrigerators and deep-freezers.

REFERENCES

1. Joossens JV, Willems J, Claessens J, Claes JH, Lissens W: Sodium and hypertension. In: Fidanza F, Keys A, Ricci G, Somogyi JC (eds) Nutrition and cardiovascular diseases. Rome: Morgagni Edizioni Scientifiche, 1971, pp 91-110.
2. Tables scientifiques Geigy, 6th edn. Basle: Geigy JR, 1963, p 179.
3. Acheson RM: Cerebrovascular disease epidemiology. Washington DC: DHEW Public Health Monogr 76, 1966, pp 23-40.
4. Joossens JV: unpublished data 1979.
5. Hypertension Detection and Follow-up Program Cooperative Group: Five year findings of the hypertension detection and follow-up program. I. Reduction in mortality of persons with high blood pressure, including mild hypertension. JAMA 242:2562-2571, 1979.
6. Miller GD, Kuller LH: Trends in mortality from stroke in Baltimore, Maryland: 1940–1941 through 1968–1969. Am J Epidemiol 98:233-242, 1973.
7. Garraway WM, Whisnant JP, Furlan AJ, Phillips II LH, Kurland LT, O'Fallon NM: The declining incidence of stroke. N Engl J Med 300:449-452, 1979.
8. Haenszel W: Incidence of and mortality from stomach cancer in the United States. Acta Unio Int Contra Cancrum 17:347-364, 1961.
9. McGee D, Gordon T: The results of the Framingham study applied to four other US-based epidemiologic studies of cardiovascular disease. In: The Framingham study: an epidemiological investigation of cardiovascular diseases. Washington DC: DHEW (NIH) 76-1083, 1976, sect 31.
10. Shurtleff D: Some characteristics related to the incidence of cardiovascular disease and death. In: The Framingham study: an epidemiological investigation of cardiovascular diseases. Washington DC: DHEW (NIH) 74-599, 1974, sect 30.
11. Sato T, Fukuyama T, Suzuki T, Takayanagi J, Murukami T, Shiotshuki N, Tanaka R, Tsuji R: Studies of the causation of gastric cancer. 2. The relation between gastric cancer mortality rate and salted food intake in several places in Japan. Bull Inst Public Health 8:187-198, 1959.
12. Hirayama T: The epidemiology of cancer of the stomach in Japan with special reference to the role of diet. In: Harris RJC (ed) Proceedings of the 9th international cancer congress, Tokyo, 1966. Berlin: Springer, 1967, pp 37-49.
13. Dungal N: The special problem of stomach cancer in Iceland, with particular reference to dietary factors. JAMA 178:789-798, 1961.
14. Higginson J: Etiological factors in gasto-intestinal cancer in man. J Natl Cancer Inst 37:527-545, 1966.
15. Stocks P, Davies RI: Zinc and copper content of soils associated with the incidence of cancer of the stomach and other organs. Br J Cancer 18:14-24, 1964.
16. Jones FA: The epidemiology of gastric cancer with special reference to causation. In: Proceedings of the 3rd world congress of gastroenterology, Tokyo, 1966. Tokyo: Nankodo, 1967, pp 93-98.
17. Joossens JV: Het probleem van de kankersterfte. Verh Vlaam Akad Geneesk Belg 27:489-545, 1965.
18. Dahl LK: Salt and hypertension. Am J Clin Nutr 25:231-244, 1963.
19. Freis ED: Salt, volume and the prevention of hypertension. Circulation 53:589-595, 1976.
20. Meneely GR, Battarbee HD: High sodium–low potassium environment and hypertension. Am J Cardiol 38:768-785, 1976.

508

21. Joossens JV, Brems-Heyns E: Cerebrovasculaire sterfte, maagkankersterfte en zoutverbruik. Tijdschr Soc Geneeskd 53:530-542, 1975.
22. Joossens JV: Dietary salt restriction. The case in favour. Proc R Soc Med (in press) 1980.
23. Joossens JV: Trends in cardiovascular mortality. In: Lequime J (ed) Prevention and treatment of coronary heart disease and its complications. Amsterdam: Excerpta Medica (in press) 1980.
24. Parijs J van, Joossens JV, Van der Linden L, Verstreken G, Amery KPC: Moderate sodium restriction and diuretics in the treatment of hypertension. Am Heart J 85:22-34, 1973.
25. Pereira Miguel JM, Padua F de: Epidemiology of arterial blood pressure in Portugal. In this book chapter 10.
26. Fatula MI: Effect of water with a high sodium chloride content on the incidence of arterial hypertension and temporary invalidity (in Russian). Gig Sanit 2:7-11, 1977.
27. Dustin HP: Research contributions toward prevention of cardiovascular disease. Research related to the underlying mechanism in hypertension. Circulation 60:1566-1568, 1979.
28. Joossens JV, Claessens J, Geboers J, Claes JH: Electrolytes and creatinine in multiple 24-hour urine collections. In this book, chapter 3.
29. Hunt JN, Pathak JD: The osmotic effect of some simple molecules and ions on gastric emptying. J Physiol 154:254-269, 1960.
30. Yoshitoshi Y: Incidence and pathogenesis of gastritis. In: Proceedings of the 3rd world congress of gastroenterology, Tokyo, 1966. Tokyo: Nankodo, 1967, pp 179-185.
31. Ruddel WSJ, Bone ES, Hill MJ, Blendis LM, Walters CI: Gastric-juice nitrite. A risk factor for cancer in the hypochlorhydric stomach? Lancet 2:1037-1039, 1976.
32. Weisburger JH: Current views on mechanisms concerned with the etiology of cancers in the digestive tract. In: Farber E, et al. (eds) Pathophysiology of carcinogenesis in digestive organs. Baltimore: University Park Press, 1977, pp 1-20.
33. Sasaki N: The relationship of salt intake to hypertension in the Japanese. Geriatrics 19:735-744, 1964.
34. Komachi Y, Shimamoto T: Salt intake and its relationship to blood pressure in Japan. Present and past. In this book, chapter 24.
35. Kesteloot H, Park BC, Lee CS, Brems-Heyns E, Joossens JV: A comparative study of blood pressure and sodium intake in Belgium and in Korea. In this book, chapter 28.
36. Société des salines suisses du Rhin réunis: La situation actuelle du sel iodé en Suisse. Schweizerhalle, Switzerland, 1980.
37. Miyaji Toru: Statistical analysis of myocardial infarction among 289,907 autopsies in Japan during 17 years from 1958 to 1974 (Abstr I). 8th World congress of cardiology, Tokyo, 1978, p 104.
38. Joossens JV: Food pattern and mortality in Belgium. Acta Cardiol [Suppl] 23:133-161, 1979.

INDEX

Page numbers followed by an asterisk refer to an entry in a figure or table.

512